Pharmacotherapy Casebook

NOTICE

Pharmacotherapy Casebook
A Patient-Focused Approach

Seventh Edition

Edited by

Terry L. Schwinghammer, PharmD, FCCP, FASHP, BCPS

Professor and Chair
Department of Clinical Pharmacy
West Virginia University
School of Pharmacy
Morgantown, West Virginia

Julia M. Koehler, PharmD

Associate Professor and Chair
Department of Pharmacy Practice
Butler University
College of Pharmacy and Health Sciences
and
Clinical Pharmacist in Family Medicine
Methodist Hospital and the Indiana University-Methodist Family Practice Center
Clarian Health Partners
Indianapolis, Indiana

A companion workbook for: *Pharmacotherapy: A Pathophysiologic Approach, 7th ed.*
DiPiro JT, Talbert RL, Yee GC, Matzke GR, Wells BG, Posey ML, eds. New York, NY: McGraw-Hill, 2008.

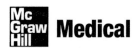

New York   Chicago   San Francisco   Lisbon   London   Madrid   Mexico City
Milan   New Delhi   San Juan   Seoul   Singapore   Sydney   Toronto

Pharmacotherapy Casebook: A Patient-Focused Approach, Seventh Edition

Copyright © 2009 by the McGraw-Hill Companies, Inc. All rights reserved. Printed in the United States of America. Except as permitted under the United States Copyright Act of 1976, no part of this publication may be reproduced or distributed in any form or by any means, or stored in a database or retrieval system, without the prior written permission of the publisher.

1 2 3 4 5 6 7 8 9 0 QPDQPD 12 11 10 9 8

ISBN 978-0-07-148835-8
MHID 0-07-148835-9

This book was set in Minion by Silverchair Science + Communications.
The editors were Michael Weitz and Peter J. Boyle.
The production supervisor was Catherine H. Saggese.
Project management was provided by Jennette L. Townsend, Silverchair Science + Communications.
The designer was Alan Barnett.
Quebecor Dubuque was printer and binder.

This book is printed on acid-free paper.

Cataloging-in-publication data is on file for this book at the Library of Congress.

CONTENTS

SECTION 1

Principles of Patient-Focused Therapy

SECTION 2

Cardiovascular Disorders

SECTION 3

Respiratory Disorders

SECTION 4

Gastrointestinal Disorders

SECTION 5

Renal Disorders

SECTION 6

Neurologic Disorders

SECTION 7

Psychiatric Disorders

SECTION 8

Endocrinologic Disorders

SECTION 9

Gynecologic Disorders

SECTION 10

Urologic Disorders

SECTION 11

Immunologic Disorders

CONTENTS

SECTION 17

Oncologic Disorders

SECTION 18

Nutrition and Nutritional Disorders

SECTION 19

Emergency Preparedness and Response

SECTION 20

Complementary and Alternative Therapies (Level III)

CONTRIBUTORS

Marie A. Abate, BS, PharmD

Professor and Director of the West Virginia Center for Drug and Health Information, Department of Clinical Pharmacy, West Virginia University School of Pharmacy, Morgantown, West Virginia

Cesar Alaniz, PharmD

Clinical Associate Professor of Pharmacy, Department of Clinical Sciences, University of Michigan College of Pharmacy; Clinical Pharmacist, Adult Medicine Intensive Care Unit, University of Michigan Health Systems, Ann Arbor, Michigan

Kwadwo Amankwa, PharmD

Clinical Assistant Professor, Department of Pharmacy Practice, School of Pharmacy, Purdue University; Clinical Pharmacy Specialist, The Indiana Heart Hospital, Indianapolis, Indiana

Jarrett R. Amsden, PharmD

Assistant Professor, Department of Pharmacy Practice, Butler University College of Pharmacy and Health Sciences, Indianapolis, Indiana

Peter L. Anderson, PharmD

Assistant Professor, School of Pharmacy, University of Colorado at Denver and Health Sciences Center, Denver, Colorado

Laurel Rodden Andrews, PharmD

Assistant Professor and Coordinator of Introductory Practice Experience, The University of Louisiana at Monroe College of Pharmacy, Monroe, Louisiana

Alexander J. Ansara, PharmD, BCPS

Assistant Professor of Pharmacy Practice, Butler University College of Pharmacy and Health Sciences, Indianapolis, Indiana

Edward P. Armstrong, PharmD, FASHP

Professor, Department of Pharmacy Practice and Science University of Arizona College of Pharmacy, Tucson, Arizona

Jacquelyn L. Bainbridge, BS Pharm, PharmD, FCCP

Associate Professor, School of Pharmacy Department of Clinical Pharmacy and School of Medicine Department of Neurology, University of Colorado at Denver and Health Sciences Center, Denver, Colorado

Chad Barnett, PharmD, BCOP

Clinical Pharmacy Specialist—Breast Medical Oncology, Division of Pharmacy, The University of Texas MD Anderson Cancer Center, Houston, Texas

Reina Bendayan, PharmD

Professor and Chair, Department of Pharmaceutical Sciences, Leslie Dan Faculty of Pharmacy, University of Toronto, Toronto, Ontario, Canada

Robert W. Bennett, MS, RPh

Professor, Department of Pharmacy Practice; Director, Pharmacy Continuing Education, Purdue University School of Pharmacy and Pharmaceutical Sciences, West Lafayette, Indiana

Scott J. Bergman, PharmD

Assistant Professor, Department of Pharmacy Practice, Southern Illinois University Edwardsville School of Pharmacy and Division of Infectious Diseases, Department of Medicine, Southern Illinois University School of Medicine, Springfield, Illinois

Scott Bolesta, PharmD

Assistant Professor, Department of Pharmacy Practice, Nesbitt College of Pharmacy and Nursing, Wilkes University, Wilkes-Barre, Pennsylvania

Tracy L. Bottorff, PharmD, BCPS

Assistant Professor of Pharmacy Practice, Butler University College of Pharmacy and Health Sciences, Indianapolis, Indiana

Gretchen M. Brophy, PharmD, BCPS, FCCP, FCCM

Associate Professor of Pharmacy and Neurosurgery, Virginia Commonwealth University, Medical College of Virginia Campus, Richmond, Virginia

Karim Anton Calis, PharmD, MPH, FASHP, FCCP

Director, Drug Information Service and Clinical Specialist, Endocrinology & Women's Health, Mark O. Hatfield Clinical Research Center, National Institutes of Health, Bethesda, Maryland; Professor, Department of Pharmacy, School of Pharmacy, Virginia Commonwealth University, Richmond, Virginia; Clinical Professor, Department of Pharmacy Practice and Science, School of Pharmacy, University of Maryland, Baltimore, Maryland; Clinical Professor, Department of Pharmacy Practice, School of Pharmacy, Shenandoah University, Winchester, Virginia

Bruce R. Canaday, PharmD, BCPS, FASHP, FAPhA

Clinical Professor and Vice Chair, Division of Pharmacy Practice and Experiential Education, School of Pharmacy, University of North Carolina, Chapel Hill, North Carolina; Director, Department of Pharmacotherapy, Coastal AHEC, Wilmington, North Carolina

Gina M. Carbonara, PharmD

Clinical Assistant Professor and Director of Introductory Pharmacy Practice Experiences, Department of Clinical Pharmacy, West Virginia University School of Pharmacy, Morgantown, West Virginia

Bruce C. Carlstedt, PhD, FASHP

Professor, Department of Pharmacy Practice, Purdue University School of Pharmacy and Pharmaceutical Sciences, West Lafayette, Indiana

Diana Hey Cauley, PharmD, BCOP

Clinical Pharmacy Specialist—Genitourinary Medicine, Division of Pharmacy, The University of Texas MD Anderson Cancer Center, Houston, Texas

Juliana Chan, PharmD

Clinical Assistant Professor, Department of Pharmacy Practice, College of Pharmacy and Department of Medicine; Sections of Digestive Diseases and Nutrition and Section of Hepatology, University of Illinois at Chicago, Chicago, Illinois

Kevin W. Cleveland, PharmD, ANP

Assistant Clinical Professor; Nontraditional Doctor of Pharmacy Curriculum Coordinator, Idaho State University College of Pharmacy, Pocatello, Idaho

Holly V. Coe, PharmD

Pharmacy Practice Resident, The University at Buffalo School of Pharmacy and Pharmaceutical Sciences and Buffalo Medical Group, Buffalo, New York

Lawrence J. Cohen, PharmD, BCPP, FASHP, FCCP

Professor of Pharmacotherapy, Washington State University College of Pharmacy; Assistant Director for Psychopharmacology Research and Training, Washington Institute for Mental Illness Research and Training (WIMIRT), Spokane, Washington

John R. Corboy, MD

Associate Professor, Department of Neurology, School of Medicine, University of Colorado Health Sciences Center, Denver, Colorado

James D. Coyle, PharmD

Assistant Professor, College of Pharmacy, and Director, Collaborative Antithrombotic, Management Program, Rardin Family Practice Center, The Ohio State University, Columbus, Ohio

Brian L. Crabtree, PharmD, BCPP

Associate Professor of Pharmacy Practice, School of Pharmacy, Associate Professor of Psychiatry, University of Mississippi Medical Center; Psychopharmacologist, Mississippi State Hospital, Jackson, Mississippi

Nicole S. Culhane, PharmD, BCPS

Associate Professor, Pharmacy Practice, Nesbitt College of Pharmacy and Nursing, Wilkes University, Wilkes-Barre, Pennsylvania

Lisa E. Davis, PharmD, FCCP, BCPS, BCOP

Associate Professor of Clinical Pharmacy, The University of the Sciences in Philadelphia, Philadelphia, Pennsylvania

Christopher M. Degenkolb, PharmD, BCPS

Assistant Professor of Pharmacy Practice, Butler University College of Pharmacy and Health Sciences; Clinical Pharmacy Specialist, Richard L. Roudebush Veterans Affairs Medical Center, Indianapolis, Indiana

John W. Devlin, PharmD, BCPS, FCCP, FCCM

Associate Professor, Department of Pharmacy Practice, Northeastern University School of Pharmacy; Adjunct Associate Professor, Tufts University School of Medicine; Clinical Pharmacist, Medical Intensive Care Unit, Tufts-New England Medical Center, Boston, Massachusetts

Mariela Díaz-Linares, PharmD

Clinical Assistant Professor, Department of Pharmacy Practice, College of Pharmacy, University of Illinois at Chicago, Chicago, Illinois

Margarita V. DiVall, PharmD, BCPS

Associate Clinical Specialist, School of Pharmacy, Bouvé College of Health Sciences, Northeastern University, Boston, Massachusetts

Holly S. Divine, PharmD, CGP, CDE

Associate Professor, Department of Pharmacy Practice and Science, University of Kentucky College of Pharmacy, Lexington, Kentucky

Jennifer A. Donaldson, PharmD

Clinical Pharmacist, Riley Hospital for Children; Adjunct Assistant Professor of Pharmacy Practice, Butler University College of Pharmacy and Health Sciences; Affiliate Assistant Professor of Clinical Pharmacy, Purdue University School of Pharmacy and Pharmaceutical Sciences, West Lafayette, Indiana

Victor G. Dostrow, MD

Assistant Professor of Neurology, University of Mississippi Medical Center; Associate Professor of Pharmacy Practice, School of Pharmacy, University of Mississippi; Neurology Service Chief, Mississippi State Hospital, Jackson, Mississippi

Scott R. Drab, PharmD, CDE, BC-ADM

Assistant Professor of Pharmacy and Therapeutics, University of Pittsburgh School of Pharmacy, Pittsburgh, Pennsylvania

Sharon M. Erdman, PharmD

Clinical Associate Professor, Purdue University School of Pharmacy and Pharmaceutical Sciences; Infectious Diseases Clinical Pharmacist, Wishard Health Services, Indianapolis, Indiana

Brian L. Erstad, PharmD, FCCP, FCCM, FASHP

Professor, University of Arizona College of Pharmacy, Department of Pharmacy Practice and Science, Tucson, Arizona

Jeffery Evans, PharmD

Assistant Professor, Department of Clinical and Administrative Sciences, University of Louisiana at Monroe College of Pharmacy, Shreveport, Louisiana

Patrick J. Fahey, MD

Professor, Department of Family Medicine, College of Medicine, The Ohio State University, Columbus, Ohio

Rochelle Farb, PharmD

Assistant Professor, Midwestern University, Chicago College of Pharmacy, Downers Grove, Illinois

Emily C. Farthing-Papineau, PharmD, BCPS

Assistant Professor of Pharmacy Practice, Butler University College of Pharmacy and Health Sciences; Clinical Pharmacist, Family Medicine Center of Community Health Network, Indianapolis, Indiana

Christopher A. Fausel, PharmD, BCPS, BCOP

Clinical Pharmacist, Hematology/Oncology/Bone Marrow Transplant, Indiana University Cancer Center, Indianapolis, Indiana

Charles W. Fetrow, PharmD

Clinical Pharmacy Specialist, Pharmacy Services, University of Pittsburgh Medical Center—Passavant Hospital, Pittsburgh, Pennsylvania

Courtney V. Fletcher, PharmD

Dean and Professor, University of Nebraska Medical Center College of Pharmacy, Omaha, Nebraska

Edward F. Foote, PharmD, FCCP, BCPS

Associate Professor and Chair, Department of Pharmacy Practice, Nesbitt College of Pharmacy and Nursing, Wilkes University, Wilkes-Barre, Pennsylvania

Pamela A. Foral, PharmD, BCPS

Associate Professor, Pharmacy Practice Department, School of Pharmacy and Health Professions, Creighton University; Clinical Pharmacist, Alegent Health Bergan Mercy Medical Center, Omaha, Nebraska

Allan D. Friedman, MD, MPH

Professor and Chair, Division of General Pediatrics, Virginia Commonwealth University, Richmond, Virginia

Michelle D. Furler, BSc Pharm, PhD

Pharmacist, Kingston, Ontario, Canada

William R. Garnett, PharmD, FCCP

Professor of Pharmacy, Virginia Commonwealth University School of Pharmacy, Richmond, Virginia

Sharon B. S. Gatewood, PharmD

Assistant Professor, Department of Pharmacy, Virginia Commonwealth University School of Pharmacy, Richmond, Virginia

Jane Gervasio, PharmD, BCNSP

Assistant Professor for Pharmacy Practice, Butler University College of Pharmacy and Health Sciences, Indianapolis, Indiana

Jasmine D. Gonzalvo, PharmD

Clinical Assistant Professor, Department of Pharmacy Practice, Purdue University School of Pharmacy and Pharmaceutical Sciences; Clinical Pharmacy Specialist, Primary Care, Wishard Health Services, Indianapolis, Indiana

Michael J. Gonyeau, BS, PharmD, BCPS

Associate Clinical Specialist, Northeastern University School of Pharmacy; Internal Medicine Clinical Pharmacist, Caritas St. Elizabeth's Medical Center, Boston, Massachusetts

Jean-Venable "Kelly" R. Goode, PharmD, BCPS, FAPhA, FCCP

Associate Professor; Director, Community Pharmacy Practice and Residency Programs, School of Pharmacy, Virginia Commonwealth University, Richmond, Virginia

A. Christie Graham, PharmD

Clinical Assistant Professor, University of Wyoming School of Pharmacy, Laramie, Wyoming

Wayne P. Gulliver, MD, FRCPC

Associate Professor of Medicine (Dermatology), Faculty of Medicine, Memorial University of Newfoundland, St. John's, Newfoundland, Canada

John G. Gums, PharmD

Professor of Pharmacy and Medicine, Departments of Pharmacy Practice and Family Medicine, University of Florida, Gainesville, Florida

Deanne L. Hall, PharmD, CDE

Assistant Professor of Pharmacy and Therapeutics, University of Pittsburgh School of Pharmacy; Clinical Specialist in Ambulatory Care, University of Pittsburgh Medical Center, Pittsburgh, Pennsylvania

Shawn R. Hansen, PharmD

Clinical Leader, Cardiology Services, St. Joseph's Hospital, Marshfield, Wisconsin; Clinical Instructor, University of Wisconsin School of Pharmacy, Madison, Wisconsin; Clinical Instructor, University of Minnesota College of Pharmacy, Minneapolis, Minnesota

Keith A. Hecht, PharmD, BCOP

Associate Professor of Pharmacy Practice, University of Southern Nevada, Nevada College of Pharmacy; Clinical Pharmacy Specialist, Hematology/Oncology, Henderson, Nevada

Brian A. Hemstreet, PharmD, BCPS

Associate Professor, University of Colorado at Denver and Health Sciences Center School of Pharmacy, Denver, Colorado

Richard N. Herrier, PharmD

Clinical Associate Professor, Department of Pharmacy Practice and Science, The University of Arizona College of Pharmacy, Tucson, Arizona

Catherine A. Heyneman, PharmD, MS, CGP, ANP, FASCP

Associate Professor of Pharmacy Practice, Director, Idaho Drug Information Service, Idaho State University College of Pharmacy, Pocatello, Idaho

Brian M. Hodges, PharmD, BCPS, BCNSP

Clinical Assistant Professor, West Virginia University School of Pharmacy; Clinical Pharmacy Specialist in Critical Care, Charleston Area Medical Center, Charleston, West Virginia

Mark T. Holdsworth, PharmD, BCOP

Associate Professor of Pharmacy and Pediatrics, College of Pharmacy, University of New Mexico, Albuquerque, New Mexico

Lisa M. Holle, PharmD, BCOP

Director, Medical Writing, Syntaxx Communications, Storrs, Connecticut

Jon D. Horton, PharmD

Clinical Manager, York Hospital Department of Pharmacy—A Division of WellSpan Health, York, Pennsylvania

Denise L. Howrie, PharmD

Associate Professor, Departments of Pharmacy and Therapeutics and of Pediatrics, Schools of Pharmacy and Medicine, University of Pittsburgh, Pittsburgh, Pennsylvania

Joseph R. Ineck, PharmD

Clinical Assistant Professor, Department of Pharmacy Practice and Administrative Sciences, College of Pharmacy, Idaho State University, Boise, Idaho

Timothy J. Ives, PharmD, MPH, BCPS, FCCP, FASHP, CPP

Associate Professor of Pharmacy and Medicine, Schools of Pharmacy and Medicine, University of North Carolina, Chapel Hill, North Carolina

Laura L. Jung, BS, PharmD

Medical Writer, Syntaxx Communications, Inc., Duluth, Georgia

Michael D. Katz, PharmD

Associate Professor, Department of Pharmacy Practice and Science, College of Pharmacy, University of Arizona, Tucson, Arizona

Michael B. Kays, PharmD, FCCP

Associate Professor of Pharmacy Practice, Purdue University School of Pharmacy and Pharmaceutical Sciences, Indianapolis, Indiana

Tien T. Kiat-Winarko, PharmD, BSc

Clinical Assistant Professor of Ophthalmology, Department of Ophthalmology, University of Southern California Keck School of Medicine, Los Angeles, California

Sandra L. Kim, PharmD

Clinical Assistant Professor and Clinical Pharmacist, University of Illinois at Chicago College of Pharmacy, Department of Ambulatory Care Pharmacy Services, Chicago, Illinois

Cynthia K. Kirkwood, PharmD, BCPP

Associate Professor, Virginia Commonwealth University School of Pharmacy; Clinical Specialist in Psychiatry, Virginia Commonwealth University Medical Center, Richmond, Virginia

Jennifer J. Kiser, PharmD

Research Assistant Professor, University of Colorado Health Sciences Center School of Pharmacy, Denver, Colorado

Joseph J. Kishel, PharmD, BCPS

Clinical Pharmacy Specialist in Infectious Diseases, Penn State Milton S. Hershey Medical Center, Hershey, Pennsylvania

Julie C. Kissack, PharmD, BCPP

Chair, Department of Pharmacy Practice, Harding University College of Pharmacy, Searcy, Arkansas

Julia M. Koehler, PharmD

Associate Professor and Chair, Department of Pharmacy Practice, Butler University College of Pharmacy and Health Sciences; Clinical Pharmacist in Family Medicine, Methodist Hospital and the Indiana University-Methodist Family Practice Center, Clarian Health Partners, Indianapolis, Indiana

Cynthia P. Koh-Knox, PharmD

Associate Director, Pharmacy Continuing Education, Clinical Assistant Professor, Pharmacy Practice, Purdue University School of Pharmacy and Pharmaceutical Sciences, West Lafayette, Indiana

Michael D. Kraft, PharmD

Clinical Assistant Professor, Department of Clinical Sciences, University of Michigan College of Pharmacy; Clinical Coordinator and Clinical Pharmacist, Surgery/Nutrition Support, University of Michigan Medical Center, Ann Arbor, Michigan

Poh Gin Kwa, MD, FRCPC

Clinical Associate Professor of Pediatrics, Faculty of Medicine, Memorial University of Newfoundland, St. John's, Newfoundland and Labrador, Canada

Elaine M. Ladd, PharmD

Primary Care Pharmacy Resident, Boise Veterans Affairs Medical Center, Boise, Idaho

Rebecca M. T. Law, BS Pharm, PharmD

Associate Professor, School of Pharmacy, Memorial University of Newfoundland, St. John's, Newfoundland and Labrador, Canada

W. Greg Leader, PharmD

Associate Dean, Academic Affairs; Professor, Clinical Pharmacy Practice, Department of Clinical and Administrative Sciences; College of Pharmacy, University of Louisiana Monroe, Monroe, Louisiana

Mary Lee, PharmD, BCPS, FCCP

Vice President and Chief Academic Officer, Pharmacy and Health Sciences Education, Midwestern University, Downers Grove, Illinois

Christina M. Lehane, MD, FAAP

Assistant Professor of Pediatrics, University of Pittsburgh School of Medicine, Pittsburgh, Pennsylvania

Cara Liday, PharmD, CDE

Associate Professor, Department of Pharmacy Practice and Administrative Sciences, Idaho State University College of Pharmacy, Pocatello, Idaho

John L. Lock, PharmD

Clinical Pharmacist, Infectious Diseases, St. Vincent Health, Indianapolis, Indiana

Kristen L. Longstreth, PharmD, BCPS

Clinical Pharmacy Specialist, Internal Medicine, St. Elizabeth Health Center, Youngstown, Ohio; Assistant Professor of Pharmacy Practice, Northeastern Ohio Universities College of Pharmacy, Rootstown, Ohio

Sherry A. Luedtke, PharmD

Associate Professor, Department of Pharmacy Practice and Associate Dean of Professional Affairs, Texas Tech University Health Sciences Center School of Pharmacy, Amarillo, Texas

Amy M. Lugo, PharmD, BCPS, CDM

Clinical Coordinator and Clinical Specialist, Internal Medicine, National Naval Medical Center, Bethesda, Maryland

Robert MacLaren, BSc, PharmD, FCCM, FCCP

Associate Professor, Department of Clinical Pharmacy, University of Colorado at Denver and Health Sciences Center School of Pharmacy, Denver, Colorado

Carrie Maffeo, PharmD, BCPS, CDE

Assistant Professor of Pharmacy Practice; Director, Health Education Center, Butler University College of Pharmacy and Health Sciences, Indianapolis, Indiana

Robert M. Malone, PharmD, CDE, CPP

Clinical Assistant Professor, School of Pharmacy; Assistant Medical Director, Division of General Internal Medicine, Department of Medicine, School of Medicine; University of North Carolina, Chapel Hill, North Carolina

Henry J. Mann, PharmD, FCCP, FCCM, FASHP

Professor and Associate Dean for Clinical Affairs, University of Minnesota College of Pharmacy; Director, Center for Excellence in Critical Care, Minneapolis, Minnesota

Margery H. Mark, MD

Associate Professor, Department of Neurology, UMDNJ—Robert Wood Johnson Medical School, New Brunswick, New Jersey

Joel C. Marrs, PharmD, BCPS
Clinical Assistant Professor, Department of Pharmacy Practice, College of Pharmacy, Oregon State University/Oregon Health and Science University, Portland, Oregon

Steven J. Martin, PharmD, BCPS, FCCP, FCCM
Professor and Chairman, Department of Pharmacy Practice, The University of Toledo College of Pharmacy, Toledo, Ohio

Barbara J. Mason, PharmD, FASHP
Professor and Interim Chair of Pharmacy Practice, Ambulatory Care Clinical Pharmacist, Idaho State University and Veterans Affairs Medical Center, Boise, Idaho

James W. McAuley, RPh, PhD
Associate Professor of Pharmacy Practice and Neurology, The Ohio State University College of Pharmacy, Columbus, Ohio

William McGhee, PharmD
Clinical Pharmacy Specialist, Children's Hospital of Pittsburgh; Adjunct Assistant Professor, Department of Pharmacy and Therapeutics, University of Pittsburgh School of Pharmacy, Pittsburgh, Pennsylvania

Sarah T. Melton, PharmD, BCPP, CGP
Associate Professor of Pharmacy Practice, University of Appalachia College of Pharmacy, Oakwood, Virginia

Renee-Claude Mercier, PharmD, BCPS, PhC
Associate Professor of Pharmacy and Medicine, University of New Mexico College of Pharmacy, Albuquerque, New Mexico

Pamela J. Murray, MD, MHP
Associate Professor of Pediatrics, University of Pittsburgh School of Medicine, Pittsburgh, Pennsylvania

James J. Nawarskas, PharmD, BCPS
Associate Professor of Pharmacy, University of New Mexico College of Pharmacy, Albuquerque, New Mexico

Amy S. Nicholas, PharmD, CDE
Associate Professor, Department of Pharmacy Practice and Science, PharmacistCARE Program, University of Kentucky College of Pharmacy, Lexington, Kentucky

Thomas D. Nolin, PharmD, PhD
Clinical Pharmacologist, Department of Pharmacy Services and Division of Nephrology and Transplantation, Department of Medicine, Maine Medical Center, Portland, Maine

Kimberly J. Novak, PharmD
Clinical Pharmacy Specialist, Pediatric Pulmonary Medicine, Children's Hospital; Adjunct Clinical Assistant Professor, Ohio State University College of Pharmacy, Columbus, Ohio

Kelly K. Nystrom, PharmD, BCOP
Assistant Professor, Department of Pharmacy Practice, Creighton University School of Pharmacy and Health Professions; Clinical Pharmacist, Alegent Health Bergan Mercy Medical Center, Omaha, Nebraska

Cindy L. O'Bryant, PharmD, BCOP
Assistant Professor, University of Colorado at Denver and Health Sciences Center School of Pharmacy, Denver, Colorado

Michelle O'Connor, PharmD
Ambulatory Care Pharmacy Resident, University of Iowa Hospitals and Clinics, Iowa City, Iowa

Dannielle C. O'Donnell, PharmD, BCPS, CDM
Clinical Assistant Professor, Department of Pharmacy Practice, College of Pharmacy, University of Texas, Austin, Texas

Christine K. O'Neil, PharmD, BCPS, FCCP, CGP
Professor, Department of Social, Clinical, and Administrative Sciences, Mylan School of Pharmacy, Duquesne University, Pittsburgh, Pennsylvania

Manjunath P. Pai, PharmD, BCPS
Associate Professor of Pharmacy, College of Pharmacy, University of New Mexico, Albuquerque, New Mexico

Nicole M. Paolini, PharmD
Clinical Assistant Professor, Department of Pharmacy Practice, The University at Buffalo School of Pharmacy and Pharmaceutical Sciences, Buffalo, New York

Dennis Parker, Jr., PharmD
Clinical Assistant Professor, Department of Pharmacy Practice, Eugene Applebaum College of Pharmacy and Health Sciences, Wayne State University; Neuroscience Clinical Specialist, Detroit Receiving Hospital, Detroit, Michigan

Robert B. Parker, PharmD, FCCP
Professor, Department of Clinical Pharmacy, University of Tennessee College of Pharmacy, Memphis, Tennessee

Beth Bryles Phillips, PharmD, FCCP, BCPS
Clinical Associate Professor, Department of Clinical and Administrative Pharmacy, University of Georgia College of Pharmacy, Athens, Georgia

Bradley G. Phillips, PharmD, BCPS, FCCP
Milliken-Reeve Professor and Head, Department of Clinical and Administrative Pharmacy, University of Georgia College of Pharmacy, Athens, Georgia

Charles D. Ponte, BS, PharmD, BC-ADM, BCPS, CDE, FAPhA, FASHP, FCCP
Professor, Departments of Clinical Pharmacy and Family Medicine, Robert C. Byrd Health Sciences Center, Schools of Pharmacy and Medicine, West Virginia University, Morgantown, West Virginia

Brian A. Potoski, PharmD
Assistant Professor, Department of Pharmacy and Therapeutics, University of Pittsburgh School of Pharmacy; Associate Director, Antibiotic Management Program, University of Pittsburgh Medical Center, Pittsburgh, Pennsylvania

Jane M. Pruemer, PharmD, BCOP, FASHP
Associate Professor of Clinical Pharmacy Practice, University of Cincinnati College of Pharmacy; Oncology Clinical Pharmacy Specialist, University Hospital, Health Alliance of Greater Cincinnati, Cincinnati, Ohio

Kelly R. Ragucci, PharmD, FCCP, BCPS, CDE
Associate Professor, Pharmacy and Clinical Sciences/Family Medicine, South Carolina College of Pharmacy, Medical University of South Carolina Campus, Charleston, South Carolina

Darin C. Ramsey, PharmD, BCPS

Assistant Professor of Pharmacy Practice, Butler University College of Pharmacy and Health Sciences; Clinical Pharmacy Specialist in Primary Care, Richard L. Roudebush VA Medical Center, Indianapolis, Indiana

Kristie C. Reeves-Cavaliero, PharmD, BCPS

Clinical Coordinator, Pharmacy Services, Seton Medical Center, Austin, Texas

Randolph E. Regal, BS, PharmD

Clinical Assistant Professor, University of Michigan College of Pharmacy; Clinical Pharmacist in Adult Internal Medicine/Infectious Diseases, University of Michigan Hospitals and Health Centers, Department of Pharmacy Services, Ann Arbor, Michigan

Denise H. Rhoney, PharmD, FCCP, FCCM

Associate Professor, Department of Pharmacy Practice, Eugene Applebaum College of Pharmacy and Health Sciences, Wayne State University; Neuroscience Clinical Specialist, Detroit Receiving Hospital, Detroit, Michigan

Michelle L. Rockey, PharmD, BCOP

Adjunct Assistant Professor of Clinical Pharmacy Practice, University of Cincinnati College of Pharmacy; Oncology Clinical Pharmacy Specialist, University Hospital, Cincinnati, Ohio

Keith A. Rodvold, PharmD, FCCP

Professor of Pharmacy Practice and Associate Professor of Medicine in Pharmacy, Colleges of Pharmacy and Medicine, University of Illinois at Chicago, Chicago, Illinois

Kelly C. Rogers, PharmD

Associate Professor of Clinical Pharmacy, University of Tennessee College of Pharmacy, Memphis, Tennessee

Carol J. Rollins, MS, RD, PharmD, BCNSP

Clinical Associate Professor, Department of Pharmacy Practice and Science, College of Pharmacy, University of Arizona; Coordinator, Nutrition Support Team and Clinical Pharmacist for Home Infusion Therapy, Arizona Health Sciences Center, Tucson, Arizona

Laurajo Ryan, PharmD, MSc, BCPS, CDE

Clinical Assistant Professor, University of Texas at Austin, College of Pharmacy, University of Texas Health Science Center San Antonio, Pharmacotherapy Education Research Center, San Antonio, Texas

Eric G. Sahloff, PharmD

Assistant Professor, Department of Pharmacy Practice, The University of Toledo College of Pharmacy, Toledo, Ohio

Elizabeth J. Scharman, PharmD, DABAT, BCPS, FAACT

Professor of Clinical Pharmacy and Director, West Virginia Poison Center, West Virginia University School of Pharmacy; Adjunct Associate Professor of Medicine, West Virginia University School of Medicine, Charleston, West Virginia

Marc H. Scheetz, PharmD, MSc

Assistant Professor of Pharmacy Practice, Midwestern University Chicago College of Pharmacy; Infectious Diseases Pharmacist, Northwestern Memorial Hospital, Chicago, Illinois

Kristine S. Schonder, PharmD

Assistant Professor, Department of Pharmacy and Therapeutics, University of Pittsburgh School of Pharmacy; Clinical Pharmacist in Transplantation, University of Pittsburgh Medical Center and Thomas E. Starzl Transplantation Institute, Pittsburgh, Pennsylvania

Terry L. Schwinghammer, PharmD, FCCP, FASHP, BCPS

Professor and Chair, Department of Clinical Pharmacy, West Virginia University School of Pharmacy, Morgantown, West Virginia

Christopher M. Scott, PharmD, BCPS

Clinical Associate Professor of Pharmacy Practice, Purdue University School of Pharmacy and Pharmaceutical Sciences, West Lafayette, Indiana; Pharmacy Manager of Clinical Services and Clinical Pharmacy Specialist, Trauma/Surgical Critical Care and Burn, Wishard Health Services, Indianapolis, Indiana

Mollie Ashe Scott, PharmD, BCPS, CPP

Director of Pharmacotherapy, Mountain Area Health Education Center, Asheville, North Carolina; Clinical Associate Professor of Pharmacy Practice and Assistant Professor of Family Medicine, University of North Carolina, Chapel Hill, North Carolina

Brian C. Sedam, PharmD

Clinical Pharmacist, Family Medicine, Jackson Memorial Hospital, Miami, Florida

Roohollah R. Sharifi, MD, FACS

Professor of Surgery and Urology, University of Illinois at Chicago College of Medicine; Section Chief of Urology, Jesse Brown VA Medical Center, Chicago, Illinois

Amy Heck Sheehan, PharmD

Associate Professor of Pharmacy Practice, Purdue University School of Pharmacy and Pharmaceutical Sciences, West Lafayette, Indiana; Drug Information Specialist, Clarian Health Partners, Indianapolis, Indiana

Justin J. Sherman, MCS, PharmD

Associate Professor of Pharmacy Practice, University of Louisiana at Monroe, College of Pharmacy, Monroe, Louisiana

Carrie A. Sincak, PharmD, BCPS

Associate Professor, Department of Pharmacy Practice, Midwestern University Chicago College of Pharmacy, Downers Grove, Illinois

Douglas Slain, PharmD, BCPS

Associate Professor, Department of Clinical Pharmacy, West Virginia University School of Pharmacy, Morgantown, West Virginia

Curtis L. Smith, PharmD, BCPS

Professor, Department of Pharmacy Practice, College of Pharmacy, Ferris State University, Lansing, Michigan

Denise R. Sokos, PharmD, BCPS

Assistant Professor, Department of Pharmacy and Therapeutics, University of Pittsburgh School of Pharmacy; Clinical Coordinator, Internal Medicine Pharmacy Services, UPMC Presbyterian Hospital, Pittsburgh, Pennsylvania

Suellyn J. Sorensen, PharmD, BCPS

Clinical Pharmacist, Infectious Diseases and Clinical Pharmacy Manager, Indiana University Hospital of Clarian Health Partners, Indianapolis, Indiana

Mikayla Spangler, PharmD

Assistant Professor, Creighton University School of Pharmacy and Health Professions; Clinical Pharmacist, Creighton Family Healthcare—John Galt, Omaha, Nebraska

William J. Spruill, PharmD, FASHP, FCCP

Professor, Department of Clinical and Administrative Sciences, University of Georgia College of Pharmacy, Athens, Georgia

Mary K. Stamatakis, PharmD

Associate Dean for Academic Affairs and Educational Innovation; Associate Professor of Clinical Pharmacy, West Virginia University School of Pharmacy, Morgantown, West Virginia

Lynne M. Sylvia, PharmD

Associate Professor, Department of Pharmacy Practice, Massachusetts College of Pharmacy and Health Sciences; Clinical Pharmacy Specialist, Department of Pharmacy, Tufts-New England Medical Center, Boston, Massachusetts

Christopher M. Terpening, PhD, PharmD

Assistant Professor, Departments of Clinical Pharmacy and Family Medicine, West Virginia University-Charleston Division, Charleston, West Virginia

Colleen Terriff, PharmD

Clinical Associate Professor, Washington State University College of Pharmacy; Deaconess Medical Center Pharmacy Department, Spokane, Washington

Matthew J. Thill, PharmD

Clinical/Staff Pharmacist, St. Joseph's Hospital, Marshfield, Wisconsin

James E. Tisdale, PharmD, BCPS, FCCP

Professor, School of Pharmacy and Pharmaceutical Sciences, Purdue University, West Lafayette, Indiana; Adjunct Associate Professor, School of Medicine, Indiana University, Indianapolis, Indiana

Margaret E. Tonda, PharmD

Director, Clinical Science, Exelixis, South San Francisco, California

Trent G. Towne, PharmD

PGY-2 Infectious Diseases Resident, South Texas Veterans Health Care System, The University of Texas Health Science Center at San Antonio, San Antonio, Texas

Sharon M. Tramonte, PharmD

Clinical Assistant Professor, Department of Pharmacotherapy, The University of Texas Health Sciences Center at San Antonio, San Antonio, Texas

Tate N. Trujillo, PharmD, BCPS, FCCM

Director of Pharmacy, Methodist Hospital, Clinical Pharmacist Trauma/Critical Care, Department of Pharmacy, Clarian Health, Indianapolis, Indiana

Maria Tsoras, PharmD

Pharmacy Fellow in Nutrition Support/Critical Care, Butler University College of Pharmacy and Health Sciences, Indianapolis, Indiana

Kevin M. Tuohy, PharmD, BCPS

Assistant Professor of Pharmacy Practice, Butler University College of Pharmacy and Health Sciences, Indianapolis, Indiana

Stephanie D. Vail, PharmD

Pharmacy Practice Resident, Maine Medical Center, Portland, Maine

J. Michael Vozniak, PharmD, BCOP

Hematology/Oncology Clinical Pharmacy Specialist, Hospital of the University of Pennsylvania, Department of Pharmacy Services, Philadelphia, Pennsylvania

William E. Wade, PharmD, FASHP, FCCP

Professor and Associate Head, Department of Clinical and Administrative Pharmacy, University of Georgia College of Pharmacy, Athens, Georgia

Mary Louise Wagner, PharmD, MS

Associate Professor, Department of Pharmacy Practice, Ernest Mario School of Pharmacy, Rutgers, The State University of New Jersey, Piscataway, New Jersey

Christine M. Walko, PharmD, BCOP

Assistant Professor, Division of Pharmacotherapy and Experimental Therapeutics, University of North Carolina School of Pharmacy, Chapel Hill, North Carolina

Geoffrey C. Wall, PharmD, BCPS, CGP

Internal Medicine Clinical Pharmacist, Iowa Methodist Medical Center; Associate Professor of Pharmacy Practice, Drake University College of Pharmacy and Health Sciences, Des Moines, Iowa

Amy L. Whitaker, PharmD

Assistant Professor, Virginia Commonwealth University, School of Pharmacy, Richmond, Virginia

Craig Williams, PharmD

Associate Professor, Department of Pharmacy Practice, Oregon State University School of Pharmacy, Portland, Oregon

Susan R. Winkler, PharmD, BCPS

Associate Dean and Professor, Department of Pharmacy Practice, Midwestern University Chicago College of Pharmacy, Downers Grove, Illinois

Peggy C. Yarborough, PharmD, MS, CPP, BC-ADM, CDE, FAPP, FASHP, NAPP

Professor Emeritus, Campbell University School of Pharmacy; Clinical Pharmacist Practitioner—pharmacotherapy and diabetes, Urban Ministries Open Door Clinic, Raleigh, North Carolina

Nancy S. Yunker, PharmD, BCPS

Assistant Professor, Department of Pharmacy, Virginia Commonwealth University School of Pharmacy—MCV Campus; Clinical Specialist in Internal Medicine, Virginia Commonwealth University Health System-Medical College of Virginia Hospitals, Richmond, Virginia

William C. Zamboni, PharmD, PhD

Assistant Member of the Program of Molecular Therapeutics and Drug Discovery, University of Pittsburgh Cancer Institute; Assistant Professor, Department of Pharmaceutical Sciences, School of Pharmacy; Assistant Professor, Department of Obstetrics, Gynecology, and Reproductive Sciences, School of Medicine, University of Pittsburgh, Pittsburgh, Pennsylvania

PREFACE

The purpose of the *Pharmacotherapy Casebook* is to help students in the health professions and practicing clinicians develop and refine the skills required to identify and resolve drug therapy problems by using case studies. Case studies can actively involve students in the learning process; engender self-confidence; and promote the development of skills in independent self-study, problem analysis, decision making, oral communication, and teamwork. Patient case studies can also be used as the focal point of discussions about pathophysiology, medicinal chemistry, pharmacology, and the pharmacotherapy of individual diseases. By integrating the biomedical and pharmaceutical sciences with pharmacotherapeutics, case studies can help students appreciate the relevance and importance of a sound scientific foundation in preparation for practice.

The patient cases in this book are intended to complement the scientific information presented in the seventh edition of *Pharmacotherapy: A Pathophysiologic Approach*. This edition of the casebook contains 150 unique patient cases, 35 more than the first edition. The case chapters are organized into organ system sections that correspond to those of the *Pharmacotherapy* textbook. Students should read the relevant textbook chapter to become thoroughly familiar with the pathophysiology and pharmacotherapy of each disease state before attempting to make "decisions" about the care of patients described in this casebook. The *Pharmacotherapy* textbook, *Casebook*, and other useful learning resources are also available on *AccessPharmacy.com* (subscription required). By using these realistic cases to practice creating, defending, and implementing pharmacotherapeutic care plans, students can begin to develop the skills and self-confidence that will be necessary to make the real decisions required in professional practice.

The knowledge and clinical experience required to answer the questions associated with each patient presentation vary from case to case. Some cases deal with a single disease state, whereas others have multiple diseases and drug therapy problems. As a guide for instructors, each case is identified as being one of three complexity levels; this classification system is described in more detail in Chapter 1.

The seventh edition has five introductory chapters:

Chapter 1 describes the format of case presentations and the means by which students and instructors can maximize the usefulness of the casebook. A systematic approach is consistently applied to each case. The steps involved in this approach include:

1. Identifying real or potential drug therapy problems
2. Determining the desired therapeutic outcome(s)
3. Evaluating therapeutic alternatives

4. Designing an optimal individualized pharmacotherapeutic plan
5. Developing methods to evaluate the therapeutic outcome
6. Providing patient education
7. Communicating and implementing the pharmacotherapeutic plan

In Chapter 2, the philosophy and implementation of active learning strategies are presented. This chapter sets the tone for the casebook by describing how these approaches can enhance student learning. The chapter offers a number of useful active learning strategies for instructors and provides advice to students on how to maximize their learning opportunities in active learning environments.

Chapter 3 presents an efficient method of patient counseling developed by the Indian Health Service. The information can be used as the basis for simulated counseling sessions related to the patient cases.

Chapter 4 describes the patient care process and delineates the steps necessary to create care plans that can help to ensure that the drug-related needs of patients are met. A blank care plan form is included at the end of the chapter. Students should be encouraged to practice using this form (or a similar one) when completing the case studies in this casebook.

Chapter 5 describes two methods for documenting clinical interventions and communicating recommendations to other health care providers. These include the traditional SOAP note and the more pharmacy-specific FARM note. Student preparation of SOAP or FARM notes for the patient cases in this book will be excellent practice for future documentation in actual patient records.

It should be emphasized that the focus of classroom discussions about these cases should be on the process of solving patient problems as much as it is on finding the actual answers to the questions themselves. Isolated scientific facts learned today may be obsolete or incorrect tomorrow. Health care providers who can identify patient problems and solve them using a reasoned approach will be able to adapt to the continual evolution in the body of scientific knowledge and contribute in a meaningful way to improving the quality of patients' lives.

We are grateful for the broad acceptance that previous editions of the casebook have received. In particular, it has been adopted by many schools of pharmacy and nurse practitioner programs. It has also been used in institutional staff development efforts and by individual pharmacists wishing to upgrade their pharmacotherapy skills. It is our hope that this new edition will be even more valuable in assisting health care practitioners to meet society's need for safe and effective drug therapy.

ACKNOWLEDGMENTS

It is my pleasure to introduce Julia M. Koehler, PharmD, as the co-editor for the *Pharmacotherapy Casebook*, Seventh Edition. Julia is Associate Professor and Chair of the Department of Pharmacy Practice at Butler University College of Pharmacy and Health Sciences and practices as a Clinical Pharmacist in Family Medicine at Methodist Hospital of Clarian Health Partners in Indianapolis, Indiana. She has served as a casebook author for the two previous editions and is a chapter author for the new textbook *Pharmacotherapy Principles & Practice*. She is always a joy to work with and produces only the best quality work. I look forward to working with her on many future editions.

Terry L. Schwinghammer, PharmD, FCCP, FASHP, BCPS

We would like to thank the 178 case and chapter authors from 94 schools of pharmacy, health care systems, and other institutions in the United States and Canada who contributed their scholarly efforts to this casebook. We especially appreciate their diligence in meeting deadlines, adhering to the unique format of the casebook, and providing the most current drug therapy information available. The next generation of pharmacists will benefit from the willingness of these authors to share their expertise.

We would also like to thank all of the individuals at McGraw-Hill Professional whose cooperation, advice, and commitment were instrumental in maintaining the high standards of this publication: James Shanahan, Michael Weitz, Peter Boyle, and Laura Libretti. We appreciate the meticulous attention to composition detail provided by Jennette Townsend of Silverchair Science + Communications. Finally, we are grateful to our spouses, Donna Schwinghammer and Brad Bowman, for their understanding, support, and encouragement during the preparation of this new edition.

Terry L. Schwinghammer, PharmD, FCCP, FASHP, BCPS
Julia M. Koehler, PharmD

CHAPTER 1

Introduction: How to Use This Casebook

TERRY L. SCHWINGHAMMER, PHARMD, FCCP, FASHP, BCPS

USING CASE STUDIES TO ENHANCE STUDENT LEARNING

The case method is used primarily to develop the skills of self-learning, critical thinking, problem identification, and decision making. When case studies from this casebook are used in the curricula of the health care professions or for independent study by practitioners, the focus of attention should be on learning the process of solving drug therapy problems, rather than simply on finding the scientific answers to the problems themselves. Students do learn scientific facts during the resolution of case study problems, but they usually learn more of them from their own independent study and from discussions with their peers than they do from the instructor. Working on subsequent cases with similar problems reinforces information recall. Traditional programs in the health care professions that rely heavily on the lecture format tend to concentrate on scientific content and the rote memorization of facts rather than the development of higher-order thinking skills.

Case studies in the health sciences provide the personal history of an individual patient and information about one or more health problems that must be solved. The learner's job is to work through the facts of the case, analyze the available data, gather more information, develop hypotheses, consider possible solutions, arrive at the optimal solution, and consider the consequences of the learner's decisions.[1] The role of the teacher is to serve as coach and facilitator rather than as the source of "the answer." In fact, in many cases there is more than one acceptable answer to a given question. Because instructors do not necessarily need to possess the correct answer, they need not be experts in the field being discussed. Rather, the students become teachers and learn from each other through thoughtful discussion of the case.

FORMAT OF THE CASEBOOK

BACKGROUND READING

The patient cases in this casebook should be used as the focal point for independent self-learning by individual students and for in-class problem-solving discussions by student groups and their instructors. If meaningful learning and discussion are to occur, students must come to discussion sessions prepared to discuss the case material rationally, to propose reasonable solutions, and to defend their pharmacotherapeutic plans. This requires a strong commitment to independent self-study prior to the session. The cases in this book were prepared to correspond with the scientific information contained in the seventh edition of *Pharmacotherapy: A Pathophysiologic Approach*.[2] For this reason, thorough understanding of the corresponding textbook chapter is recommended as the principal method of student preparation. The online learning center *AccessPharmacy.com* (subscription required) contains the *Pharmacotherapy* textbook and many other resources that will be beneficial in answering case questions. Primary literature should also be consulted as necessary to supplement textbook readings.

Most of the cases in the casebook represent common diseases likely to be encountered by generalist pharmacy practitioners. As a result, not all of the *Pharmacotherapy* textbook chapters have an associated patient case in the casebook. On the other hand, some of the textbook chapters that discuss multiple disease entities have several corresponding cases in the casebook.

LEVELS OF CASE COMPLEXITY

Each case is identified at the top of the first page as being one of three levels of complexity. Instructors may use this classification system to select cases for discussion that correspond to the experience level of the student learners. These levels are defined as follows:

Level I—An uncomplicated case; only the single textbook chapter is required to complete the case questions. Little prior knowledge of the disease state or clinical experience is needed.

Level II—An intermediate-level case; several textbook chapters or other reference sources may be required to complete the case. Prior clinical experience may be helpful in resolving all of the issues presented.

Level III—A complicated case; multiple textbook chapters and substantial clinical experience are required to solve all of the patient's drug therapy problems.

DEVELOPING ABILITY OUTCOMES

Several ability outcomes are included at the beginning of each case for student reflection. The focus of these outcomes is on achieving competency in the clinical arena, not simply on learning isolated scientific facts. These items indicate some of the functions that the student should strive to perform in the clinical setting after reading the textbook chapter, studying the case, preparing a pharmacotherapeutic plan, and defending his or her recommendations.

The ability outcome statements provided are meant to serve as a starting point to stimulate student thinking, but they are not intended to be all-inclusive. In fact, students should also generate their own personal ability outcomes and learning objectives for each case. By so doing, students take greater control of their own learning, which serves to improve personal motivation and the desire to learn.

PATIENT PRESENTATION

The format and organization of cases reflect those usually seen in actual clinical settings. The patient's medical history and physical examination findings are provided in the following standardized outline format.

CHIEF COMPLAINT

The chief complaint is a brief statement of the reason why the patient consulted the physician, stated in the patient's own words. In order to convey the patient's symptoms accurately, medical terms and diagnoses are generally not used. The appropriate medical terminology is used after an appropriate evaluation (i.e., medical history, physical examination, laboratory and other testing) leads to a medical diagnosis.

HPI

The history of present illness is a more complete description of the patient's symptom(s). Usually included in the HPI are:

- Date of onset
- Precise location
- Nature of onset, severity, and duration
- Presence of exacerbations and remissions
- Effect of any treatment given
- Relationship to other symptoms, bodily functions, or activities (e.g., activity, meals)
- Degree of interference with daily activities

PMH

The past medical history includes serious illnesses, surgical procedures, and injuries the patient has experienced previously. Minor complaints (e.g., influenza, colds) are usually omitted unless they might have a bearing on the current medical situation.

FH

The family history includes the age and health of parents, siblings, and children. For deceased relatives, the age and cause of death are recorded. In particular, heritable diseases and those with a hereditary tendency are noted (e.g., diabetes mellitus, cardiovascular disease, malignancy, rheumatoid arthritis, obesity).

SH

The social history includes the social characteristics of the patient as well as the environmental factors and behaviors that may contribute to the development of disease. Items that may be listed are the patient's marital status; number of children; educational background; occupation; physical activity; hobbies; dietary habits; and use of tobacco, alcohol, or other drugs.

MEDS

The medication history should include an accurate record of the patient's current use of prescription medications, nonprescription products, and dietary supplements. Because pharmacists possess extensive knowledge of the thousands of prescription and nonprescription products available, they can perform a valuable service to the health care team by obtaining a complete medication history that includes the names, doses, routes of administration, schedules, and duration of therapy for all medications, including dietary supplements and other alternative therapies.

ALL

Allergies to drugs, food, pets, and environmental factors (e.g., grass, dust, pollen) are recorded. An accurate description of the reaction that occurred should also be included. Care should be taken to distinguish adverse drug effects ("upset stomach") from true allergies ("hives").

ROS

In the review of systems, the examiner questions the patient about the presence of symptoms related to each body system. In many cases, only the pertinent positive and negative findings are recorded. In a complete ROS, body systems are generally listed by starting from the head and working toward the feet and may include the skin, head, eyes, ears, nose, mouth and throat, neck, cardiovascular, respiratory, gastrointestinal, genitourinary, endocrine, musculoskeletal, and neuropsychiatric systems. The purpose of the ROS is to evaluate the status of each body system and to prevent the omission of pertinent information. Information that was included in the HPI is generally not repeated in the ROS.

PHYSICAL EXAMINATION

The exact procedures performed during the physical examination vary depending upon the chief complaint and the patient's medical history. In some practice settings, only a limited and focused physical examination is performed. In psychiatric practice, greater emphasis is usually placed on the type and severity of the patient's symptoms than on physical findings. A suitable physical assessment textbook should be consulted for the specific procedures that may be conducted for each body system. The general sections for the PE are outlined as follows:

Gen (general appearance)

VS (vital signs)—blood pressure, pulse, respiratory rate, and temperature. In hospital settings, the presence and severity of pain is included as "the fifth vital sign." For ease of use and consistency in this casebook, weight and height are included in the vital signs section, but they are not technically considered to be vital signs.

Skin (integumentary)

HEENT (head, eyes, ears, nose, and throat)

Lungs/Thorax (pulmonary)

Cor or CV (cardiovascular)

Abd (abdomen)

Genit/Rect (genitalia/rectal)

MS/Ext (musculoskeletal and extremities)

Neuro (neurologic)

LABS

The results of laboratory tests are included with most cases in this casebook. **Appendix A** contains a number of commonly used conversion factors and anthropometric information that will be helpful in solving many case answers. Normal ranges for the laboratory tests used throughout the casebook are included in **Appendix B**. Values are provided in both traditional units and SI units (*le système International d'Unités*). The normal range for a given laboratory test is generally determined from a representative sample of the general population. The upper and lower limits of the range usually encompass two standard deviations from the population mean, which includes a range within which about 95% of healthy persons would fall. The term *normal range* may therefore be misleading, because a test result may be abnormal for a given individual even if it falls within the "normal" range. Furthermore, given the statistical methods used to calculate the range, about 1 in 20 normal, healthy individuals may have a value for a test that lies outside the range. For these reasons, the term *reference range* is preferred over normal range. Reference ranges differ among laboratories, so the values given in Appendix B should be considered only as a general guide. Institution-specific reference ranges should be used in actual clinical settings.

All of the cases include some physical examination and laboratory findings that are within normal limits. For example, a description of the cardiovascular examination may include a statement that the point of maximal impulse is at the fifth intercostal space; laboratory evaluation may include a serum sodium level of 140 mEq/L. The presentation of actual findings (rather than simple statements that the heart examination and the serum sodium were normal) reflects what will be seen in actual clinical practice. More importantly, listing both normal and abnormal findings requires students to carefully assess the complete database and identify the pertinent positive and negative findings for themselves. A valuable portion of the learning process is lost if students are only provided with findings that are abnormal and are known to be associated with the disease being discussed.

The patients described in this casebook have fictitious names in order to humanize the situations and to encourage students to remember that they will one day be caring for patients, not treating disease states. However, in the actual clinical setting, patient confidentiality is of utmost importance, and real patient names should not be used during group discussions in patient care areas unless absolutely necessary. To develop student sensitivity to this issue, instructors may wish to avoid using these fictitious patient names during class discussions. In this casebook, patient names are usually given only in the initial presentation; they are seldom used in subsequent questions or other portions of the case.

The issues of race, ethnicity, and gender also deserve thoughtful consideration. The traditional format for case presentations usually begins with a description of the patient's age, race, and gender, as in: "The patient is a 65-year-old white male. . . ." Single-word racial labels such as "black" or "white" are actually of limited value in many cases and may actually be misleading in some instances.[3] For this reason, racial descriptors are usually excluded from the opening line of each presentation. When ethnicity is pertinent to the case, this information is presented in the social history or physical examination. Patients in this casebook are referred to as men or women, rather than males or females, to promote sensitivity to human dignity.

The patient cases in this casebook include medical abbreviations and drug brand names, just as medical records do in actual practice.

Although these customs are sometimes the source of clinical problems, the intent of their inclusion is to make the cases as realistic as possible. **Appendix C** lists the medical abbreviations used in the casebook. This list is limited to commonly accepted abbreviations; thousands more exist, which makes it difficult for the novice practitioner to efficiently assess patient databases. Most health care institutions have an approved list of accepted abbreviations; these lists should be consulted in practice to facilitate one's understanding and to avoid using abbreviations in the medical record that are not on the official approved list. Appendix C also lists abbreviations and designations that should be avoided. Given the immense human toll resulting from medical errors, this section should be considered "must" reading for all students.

The casebook also contains some photographs of commercial drug products. These illustrations are provided as examples only and are not intended to imply endorsement of those particular products.

PHARMACEUTICAL CARE AND DRUG THERAPY PROBLEMS

Modern drug therapy plays a crucial role in improving the health of people by enhancing quality of life and extending life expectancy. The advent of biotechnology has led to the introduction of unique compounds for the prevention and treatment of disease that were unimagined just a decade ago. Each year the Food and Drug Administration approves approximately two dozen new drug products that contain active substances that have never before been marketed in the United States. Although the cost of new therapeutic agents has received intense scrutiny in recent years, drug therapy actually accounts for a relatively small proportion of overall health care expenditures. Appropriate drug therapy is cost-effective and may actually serve to reduce total expenditures by decreasing the need for surgery, preventing hospital admissions, and shortening hospital stays.

Several studies have indicated that improper use of prescription medications is a frequent and serious problem. Based on a decision analytic model, one study estimated that the cost of drug-related morbidity and mortality was more than $177 billion in 2000. Hospital admissions accounted for almost 70% ($121.5 billion) of total costs; long-term-care admissions were responsible for 18% of costs ($32.8 billion).[4] In 1999, the Institute of Medicine estimated that 7,000 patients die each year from medication errors that occur both within and outside hospitals. A societal need for better use of medications clearly exists. Widespread implementation of pharmaceutical care has the potential to positively impact this situation by the design, implementation, and monitoring of rational therapeutic plans to produce defined outcomes that improve the quality of patients' lives.[5]

The mission of the pharmacy profession is to render pharmaceutical care. Schools of pharmacy have implemented innovative instructional strategies and curricula that have an increased emphasis on patient-centered care, including more experiential training, especially in ambulatory settings. Many programs are structured to promote self-directed learning, develop problem-solving and communication skills, and instill the desire for lifelong learning.

In its broadest sense, pharmaceutical care involves the identification, resolution, and prevention of actual or potential drug therapy problems. A drug therapy problem has been defined as "any undesirable event experienced by a patient which involves, or is suspected to involve, drug therapy and that interferes with achieving the desired goals of therapy."[5] Seven distinct types of drug therapy problems have been identified that may potentially lead to an undesirable event that has physiologic, psychological, social, or economic ramifications.[6] These problems can be placed into four categories that include:

1. *Inappropriate indication* for drug use
   a. The patient requires additional drug therapy.
   b. The patient is taking unnecessary drug therapy.
2. *Ineffective* drug therapy
   a. The patient is taking a drug that is not effective for his/her situation.
   b. The medication dose is too low.
3. *Unsafe* drug therapy
   a. The patient is experiencing an adverse drug reaction.
   b. The medication dose is too high.
4. *Inappropriate adherence* or *compliance*
   a. The patient is unable or unwilling to take the medication as prescribed.

These drug therapy problems are discussed in more detail in **Chapter 4** of the casebook. Because this casebook is intended to be used in conjunction with the *Pharmacotherapy* textbook, one of its purposes is to serve as a tool for learning about the pharmacotherapy of disease states. For this reason, the primary problem to be identified and addressed for most of the patients in the casebook is the need for additional drug treatment for a specific medical indication (**problem 1.a.**, above). Other actual or potential drug therapy problems may coexist during the initial presentation or may develop during the clinical course of the disease.

PATIENT-FOCUSED APPROACH TO CASE PROBLEMS

In this casebook, each patient presentation is followed by a set of patient-centered questions that are similar for each case. These questions are applied consistently from case to case to demonstrate that a systematic patient care process can be successfully applied regardless of the underlying disease state(s). The questions are designed to enable students to identify and resolve problems related to pharmacotherapy. They help students recognize what they know and what they do not know, thereby guiding them in determining what information must be learned to satisfactorily resolve the patient's problems.[7] A description of each of the steps involved in solving drug therapy problems is included in the following paragraphs.

1. Identification of real or potential drug therapy problems

The first step in the patient-focused approach is to collect pertinent patient information, interpret it properly, and determine whether drug therapy problems exist. Some authors prefer to divide this process into two or more separate steps because of the difficulty that inexperienced students may have in performing these complex tasks simultaneously.[8] This step is analogous to documenting the subjective and objective patient findings in the *S*ubjective, *O*bjective, *A*ssessment, *P*lan (SOAP) format. It is important to differentiate the process of identifying the patient's drug therapy problems from making a disease-related medical diagnosis. In fact, the medical diagnosis is known for most patients seen by pharmacists. However, pharmacists must be capable of assessing the patient's database to determine whether drug therapy problems exist that warrant a change in drug therapy. In the case of preexisting chronic diseases, such as asthma or rheumatoid arthritis, one must be able to assess information that may indicate a change in severity of the disease. This process involves reviewing the patient's symptoms, the signs of disease present on physical examination, and the results of labora-

tory and other diagnostic tests. Some of the cases require the student to develop complete patient problem lists. Potential sources for this information in actual practice include the patient or his or her advocate, the patient's physician or other health care professionals, and the patient's medical chart or other records.

After the drug therapy problems are identified, the clinician should determine which ones are amenable to pharmacotherapy. Alternatively, one must also consider whether any of the problems could have been caused by drug therapy. In some cases (both in the casebook and in real life), not all of the information needed to make these decisions is available. In that situation, providing precise recommendations for obtaining additional information needed to satisfactorily assess the patient's problems can be a valuable contribution to the patient's care.

2. Determination of the desired therapeutic outcome

After pertinent patient-specific information has been gathered and the patient's drug therapy problems have been identified, the next step is to define the specific goals of pharmacotherapy. The primary therapeutic outcomes include:

- Cure of disease (e.g., bacterial infection).
- Reduction or elimination of symptoms (e.g., pain from cancer).
- Arresting or slowing of the progression of disease (e.g., rheumatoid arthritis, HIV infection).
- Preventing a disease or symptom (e.g., coronary heart disease).

Other important outcomes of pharmacotherapy include:

- Not complicating or aggravating other existing disease states.
- Avoiding or minimizing adverse effects of treatment.
- Providing cost-effective therapy.
- Maintaining the patient's quality of life.

Sources of information for this step may include the patient or his or her advocate, the patient's physician or other health care professionals, medical records, and the *Pharmacotherapy* textbook or other literature references.

3. Determination of therapeutic alternatives

After the intended outcome has been defined, attention can be directed toward identifying the types of treatments that might be beneficial in achieving that outcome. The clinician should ensure that all feasible pharmacotherapeutic alternatives available for achieving the predefined therapeutic outcome(s) are considered before choosing a particular therapeutic regimen. Nondrug therapies (e.g., diet, exercise, psychotherapy) that might be useful should be included in the list of therapeutic alternatives when appropriate. Useful sources of information on therapeutic alternatives include the *Pharmacotherapy* textbook and other references, as well as the clinical experience of the health care provider and other involved health care professionals.

There has been a resurgence of interest in dietary supplements and other alternative therapies in recent years. The public spends billions of dollars each year on supplements to treat diseases for which there is little scientific evidence of efficacy. Furthermore, some products are hazardous, and others may interact with a patient's prescription medications or aggravate concurrent disease states. On the other hand, scientific evidence of efficacy does exist for some dietary supplements (e.g., glucosamine for osteoarthritis). Health care providers must be knowledgeable about these products and prepared to answer patient questions regarding their efficacy and safety. The casebook contains a separate section devoted to this important topic (**Section 20**). This portion of the casebook contains 10 fictitious patient vignettes that are directly related to a patient case that was presented earlier in this casebook. Each scenario involves one or more questions asked by a patient about a specific remedy. Additional follow-up questions are then asked to help the reader provide a scientifically based answer to the patient's question(s). Eleven different dietary supplements are included in this section: garlic, omega-3 fatty acids, Ginkgo biloba, St. John's wort, valerian, black cohosh, saw palmetto, glucosamine, kava kava, Echinacea, and coenzyme Q10 (Co-Q10).

4. Design of an optimal individualized pharmacotherapeutic plan

The purpose of this step is to determine the drug, dosage form, dose, schedule, and duration of therapy that are best suited for a given patient. Individual patient characteristics should be taken into consideration when weighing the risks and benefits of each available therapeutic alternative. For example, an asthma patient who requires new drug therapy for hypertension might better tolerate treatment with a thiazide diuretic rather than a β-blocker. On the other hand, a hypertensive patient with gout may be better served by use of a β-blocker rather than by use of a thiazide diuretic.

Students should state the reasons for avoiding specific drugs in their therapeutic plans. Some potential reasons for drug avoidance include drug allergy, drug–drug or drug–disease interactions, patient age, renal or hepatic impairment, adverse effects, poor compliance, pregnancy, and high treatment cost.

The specific dose selected may depend upon the indication for the drug. For example, the dose of aspirin used to treat rheumatoid arthritis is much higher than that used to prevent myocardial infarction. The likelihood of adherence with the regimen and patient tolerance come into play in the selection of dosage forms. The economic, psychosocial, and ethical factors that are applicable to the patient should also be given due consideration in designing the pharmacotherapeutic regimen. An alternative plan should also be in place that would be appropriate if the initial therapy fails or cannot be used.

5. Identification of parameters to evaluate the outcome

Students must identify the clinical and laboratory parameters necessary to assess the therapy for achievement of the desired therapeutic outcome and for detection and prevention of adverse effects. The outcome parameters selected should be specific, measurable, achievable, directly related to the therapeutic goals, and have a defined endpoint. As a means of remembering these points, the acronym SMART has been used (*S*pecific, *M*easurable, *A*chievable, *R*elated, and *T*ime bound). If the goal is to cure a bacterial pneumonia, students should outline the subjective and objective clinical parameters (e.g., relief of chest discomfort, cough, and fever), laboratory tests (e.g., normalization of white blood cell count and differential), and other procedures (e.g., resolution of infiltrate on chest x-ray) that provide sufficient evidence of bacterial eradication and clinical cure of the disease. The intervals at which data should be collected are dependent on the outcome parameters selected and should be established prospectively. It should be noted that expensive or invasive procedures may not be repeated after the initial diagnosis is made.

Adverse effect parameters must also be well defined and measurable. For example, it is insufficient to state that one will monitor for potential drug-induced "blood dyscrasias." Rather, one should identify the likely specific hematologic abnormality (e.g., anemia, leukopenia, or thrombocytopenia) and outline a prospective sched-

ule for obtaining the appropriate parameters (e.g., obtain monthly hemoglobin/hematocrit, white blood cell count, or platelet count).

Monitoring for adverse events should be directed toward preventing or identifying serious adverse effects that have a reasonable likelihood of occurrence. For example, it is not cost-effective to obtain periodic liver function tests in all patients taking a drug that causes mild abnormalities in liver injury tests only rarely, such as omeprazole. On the other hand, serious patient harm may be averted by outlining a specific screening schedule for drugs associated more frequently with hepatic abnormalities, such as methotrexate for rheumatoid arthritis.

6. Provision of patient education

The concept of pharmaceutical care is based on the existence of a covenantal relationship between the patient and the provider of care. Patients are our partners in health care, and our efforts may be for naught without their informed participation in the process. For chronic diseases such as diabetes mellitus, hypertension, and asthma, patients may have a greater role in managing their diseases than do health care professionals. Self care is becoming widespread as increasing numbers of prescription medications receive over-the-counter status. For these reasons, patients must be provided with sufficient information to enhance compliance, ensure successful therapy, and minimize adverse effects. **Chapter 3** describes patient interview techniques that can be used efficiently to determine the patient's level of knowledge. Additional information can then be provided as necessary to fill in knowledge gaps. In the questions posed with individual cases, students are asked to provide the kind of information that should be given to the patient who has limited knowledge of his or her disease. Under the Omnibus Budget Reconciliation Act (OBRA) of 1990, for patients who accept the offer of counseling, pharmacists should consider including these items:

- Name and description of the medication (which may include the indication).
- Dosage, dosage form, route of administration, and duration of therapy.
- Special directions or procedures for preparation, administration, and use.
- Common and severe adverse effects, interactions, and contraindications (with the action required should they occur).
- Techniques for self-monitoring.
- Proper storage.
- Prescription refill information.
- Action to be taken in the event of missed doses.

Instructors may wish to have simulated patient-interviewing sessions for new and refill prescriptions during case discussions to practice medication education skills. Factual information should be provided as concisely as possible to enhance memory retention. An excellent source for information on individual drugs is the USP-DI Volume II, *Advice for the Patient: Drug Information in Lay Language.*[9]

7. Communication and implementation of the pharmacotherapeutic plan

The most well-conceived plan is worthless if it languishes without implementation because of inadequate communication with prescribers or other health care providers. Permanent, written documentation of significant recommendations in the medical record is important to ensure accurate communication among practitioners. Oral communication alone can be misinterpreted or transferred inaccurately to others. This is especially true because there are many drugs that sound alike when spoken but that have different thera-peutic uses.

The SOAP format has been used by clinicians for many years to assess patient problems and to communicate findings and plans in the medical record. However, writing SOAP notes may not be the optimal process for learning to solve drug therapy problems because several important steps taken by experienced clinicians are not always apparent and may be overlooked. For example, the precise therapeutic outcome desired is often unstated in SOAP notes, leaving others to presume what the desired treatment goals are. Health care professionals using the SOAP format also commonly move directly from an assessment of the patient (diagnosis) to outlining a diagnos-tic or therapeutic plan, without necessarily conveying whether care-ful consideration has been given to all available feasible diagnostic or therapeutic alternatives. The plan itself as outlined in SOAP notes may also give short shrift to the monitoring parameters that are required to ensure successful therapy and to detect and prevent adverse drug effects. Finally, there is often little suggestion provided as to the treatment information that should be conveyed to the most important individual involved: the patient. If SOAP notes are used for documenting drug therapy problems, consideration should be given to including each of these components.

In **Chapter 5** of this casebook, the FARM note (*Findings, Assess-ment, Recommendations, Monitoring*) is presented as a useful method of consistently documenting therapeutic recommendations and implementing plans.[10] This method can be used by students as an alternative to the SOAP note to practice communicating pharmaco-therapeutic plans to other members of the health care team. Although preparation of written communication notes is not included in writ-ten form with each set of case questions, instructors are encouraged to include the composition of a SOAP or FARM note as one of the requirements for successfully completing each case study assignment.

In addition to communicating with other health care profession-als, practitioners of pharmaceutical care must also develop a per-sonal record of each patient's drug therapy problems and the health care provider's plan for resolving them, interventions made, and actual therapeutic outcomes achieved. A pharmaceutical care plan is a well-conceived and scientifically sound method of documenting these activities. **Chapter 4** of this casebook discusses the philosophy of care planning and describes their creation and use. A sample care plan document is included in that chapter for use by students as they work through the cases in this book.

CLINICAL COURSE

The process of pharmaceutical care entails an assessment of the patient's progress in order to ensure achievement of the desired therapeutic outcomes. A description of the patient's clinical course is included with many of the cases in this book to reflect this process. Some cases follow the progression of the patient's disease over months to years and include both inpatient and outpatient treatment. Follow-up questions directed toward ongoing evaluation and prob-lem solving are included after presentation of the clinical course.

SELF-STUDY ASSIGNMENTS

Each case concludes with several study assignments related to the patient case or the disease state that may be used as independent study projects for students to complete outside class. These assign-ments generally require students to obtain additional information that is not contained in the corresponding *Pharmacotherapy* text-book chapter.

LITERATURE REFERENCES AND INTERNET SITES

Selected literature references that are specific to the case at hand are included at the end of the cases. These references may be useful to students for answering the questions posed. The *Pharmacotherapy* textbook contains a more comprehensive list of references pertinent to each disease state.

Some cases list Internet sites as sources of drug therapy information. The sites listed are recognized as authoritative sources of information, such as the Food and Drug Administration (*www.fda.gov*) and the Centers for Disease Control and Prevention (*www.cdc.gov*). Students should be advised to be wary of informa-tion posted on the Internet that is not from highly regarded health care organizations or publications. The uniform resource locators (URLs) for Internet sites sometimes change, and it is possible that not all sites listed in the casebook will remain available for viewing.

DEVELOPING ANSWERS TO CASE QUESTIONS

The use of case studies for independent learning and in-class discussion may be unfamiliar to many students. For this reason, students may find it difficult at first to devise complete answers to the case questions. **Appendix D** contains the answers to three cases in order to demonstrate how case responses might be prepared and presented. The authors of the cases contributed the recommended answers provided in the appendix, but they should not be consid-ered the sole "right" answer. Thoughtful students who have pre-pared well for the discussion sessions may arrive at additional or alternative answers that are also appropriate.

With diligent self-study, practice, and the guidance of instructors, students will gradually acquire the knowledge, skills, and self-confidence to develop and implement pharmaceutical care plans for their own future patients. The goal of the casebook is to help students progress along this path of lifelong learning.

REFERENCES

1. Herreid CF. Case studies in science: a novel method of science education. J College Sci Teaching 1994;23:221–229.
2. DiPiro JT, Talbert RL, Yee GC, et al., eds. Pharmacotherapy: A Pathophysiologic Approach, 7th ed. New York, McGraw-Hill, 2008.
3. Caldwell SH, Popenoe R. Perceptions and misperceptions of skin color. Ann Intern Med 1995;122:614–617.
4. Ernst FR, Grizzle AJ. Drug-related morbidity and mortality: updating the cost-of-illness model. J Am Pharm Assoc 2001;41:192–199.
5. Cipolle RJ, Strand LM, Morley PC. Pharmaceutical care practice: The clinician's guide, 2nd ed. New York, McGraw-Hill, 2004.
6. Strand LM, Morley PC, Cipolle RJ, et al. Drug-related problems: their structure and function. Drug Intell Clin Pharm 1990;24:1093–1097.
7. Delafuente JC, Munyer TO, Angaran DM, et al. A problem-solving active-learning course in pharmacotherapy. Am J Pharm Educ 1994;58:61–64.
8. Winslade N. Large-group problem-based learning: a revision from traditional to pharmaceutical care-based therapeutics. Am J Pharm Educ 1994;58:64–73.
9. Advice for the patient: Drug information in lay language (USP-DI volume II), 27th ed. Greenwood Village, CO; Thomson Healthcare, 2007.
10. Canaday BR, Yarborough PC. Documenting pharmaceutical care: creating a standard. Ann Pharmacother 1994;28:1292–1296.

CHAPTER 2

Active Learning Strategies

CYNTHIA K. KIRKWOOD, PHARMD, BCPP AND
GRETCHEN M. BROPHY, PHARMD, BCPS, FCCP, FCCM

Students in the health professions are faced with situations daily that require use of problem-solving skills—for example, trying to prioritize what courses they need to study for that day and developing a plan to use their time efficiently. Also, if they are involved in student professional organizations, they may need to do a service project that requires identifying an idea, developing a project plan, assigning tasks to different group members, and, finally, finishing the project and evaluating the results. On practice rotations, students often need to determine if a drug is causing an adverse event in a particular patient. To solve problems, we call upon our previous experiences with similar situations and we observe, investigate, ask appropriate questions, and finally come to a conclusion or resolution.

Students who finish their formal training in health care must recognize that learning is a lifelong process. Scores of new drugs are approved every year, and innovative research changes the way that many diseases are treated. Drug use practices change yearly, and students will have the opportunity to pursue many different career paths. They must be prepared to take direct responsibility for patient outcomes by practicing patient-centered care. Health care providers work in interprofessional environments that require active participation to provide optimal care. They will need to use their skills in communications, problem solving, independent learning, drug information retrieval, and knowledge of disease state management.[1-3] To prepare students to practice in this manner, many health care educators are using active learning strategies in the classroom.[4,5] In many therapeutics courses, students are given actual written patient cases as the basis for learning. Students may be asked to identify the significant subjective and objective findings; to develop a drug therapy problem list; to create an assessment statement; to consider all feasible therapeutic alternatives; to make therapeutic recommendations; to develop a monitoring plan; to formulate a written communication note for other health care providers; and to decide how they would educate the patient about his/her new drug therapies. This process actively engages students in problem solving because it requires them to integrate knowledge gained in other areas of the curriculum with specific patient information. As a result, students learn skills that they will use on a daily basis in their future practice sites.

TRADITIONAL TEACHING

Most students are taught using a teacher-centered approach before entering professional programs. At the beginning of the course, students are given a massive course syllabus packet that contains "everything they need to know" for the semester. In class, the teacher lectures on a predetermined subject that does not require student preparation. Students are passive recipients of information, and the testing method is usually a written examination that employs a multiple-choice or short-answer format. With this method, students are tested primarily on their ability to recall isolated facts that the teacher has identified as being important. They do not learn to apply

their knowledge to situations that they will ultimately encounter in practice. The reward is an external one (i.e., exam or course grade) that may or may not reflect a student's actual ability to use knowledge to improve patient care. To teach students to be lifelong learners, it is essential to stimulate them to be inquisitive and actively involved with the learning that takes place in the classroom. This requires that teachers move away from more comfortable teaching methods and learn new techniques that will help students "learn to learn."

ACTIVE LEARNING STRATEGIES

Active learning has numerous definitions, and various methods are described in the educational literature. Simply put, active learning is the process of having students engage in activities that require reflection on ideas and how students use them.[5] In classes with active learning formats, students are involved in much more than listening. The transmission of information is deemphasized and replaced with the development of skills. Most proponents agree that active learning allows students to become engaged in the learning process while developing cognitive skills. Learning is reinforced when students actually apply their knowledge to new situations.[5] Willing students, innovative teachers, and administrative support within the school are required for active learning to be successful.[6] Control of learning must be shifted from the teacher to the students; this provides an opportunity for students to become active participants in their own learning. Although it sounds frightening at first, students can take control of their own learning. Knowledge of career and life goals can help students make decisions about how to spend their educational time. Warren[7] identifies several traits that prepare students for future careers:

- Analytic thinking
- Polite assertiveness
- Tolerance
- Communication skills
- Understanding of one's own physical well-being
- The ability to continue to teach oneself after graduation

After going through the active learning process, most students realize that knowledge is easily acquired, but developing critical thinking skills aids in lifelong learning.[6]

Teachers implement active learning exercises into classes in a variety of ways. Some of the active learning strategies give students the opportunity to pause and recall information, cooperate and collaborate in groups, solve problems, and generate questions.[8] More advanced methods include use of simulation, role-playing, debates, peer teaching, problem-based learning (PBL), case studies, and team-based learning.[9,10] Tests and quizzes evaluate student comprehension of material. Each of these strategies allows students to demonstrate their skills.

Didactic lectures can be enhanced by several active learning strategies. The "pause procedure" is designed to enhance student retention and comprehension of material.[11] It involves 15- to 20-minute mini-lectures with 2- to 3-minute pauses for students to rework their notes, discuss the material with their peers for clarification, and develop questions.[12] Students are able to assess their understanding of the material and formulate opinions. The pause procedure is a useful method for classes that require retention of factual information.[9] With the "think-pair-share" exercise, students are asked to write down the answer to a question and turn to a classmate to compare answers. This method provides immediate feedback to students.[13] The "quick-thinks" technique allows students to quickly process the information they have learned.[14] Examples of "quick-thinks" include completing a sentence presented by the teacher on the treatment of a disease state, comparing and contrasting drug treatment strategies for a specific patient, drawing conclusions on the best treatment strategies for a disease state, and identifying and correcting errors in a case presentation.

Another active learning technique for classroom sessions is to involve the students in short writing assignments. Writing helps students identify knowledge deficits, clarify understanding of the material, and organize thoughts in a logical manner. Students can be asked to write questions related to the reading assignment and submit them for discussion at the next class session. The "shared paragraph" exercise requires students to write a paragraph at the end of class summarizing the major concepts that were presented. The paragraph is then shared with a partner to clarify the material and receive feedback.[9] Students can be asked to write a "minute paper" or "half-sheet response" to a question or issue raised in class to stimulate discussion.[15] Discussions of any misconceptions can be conducted in class or one-on-one with the teacher.

Students benefit by having access to pre- or post-class quizzes. Sample test questions can also be used to assess student comprehension of the presentation and facilitate class discussion. The Active Learning Centre (*http://www.med.jhu.edu/medcenter*) is an educational website designed to provide interactive exercises that engage students in active learning.[16]

Tests and quizzes are effective tools to help students review the class presentations or reading assignments. Quizzes can be administered several times during class (e.g., using electronic audience response systems) and may or may not be graded. Quizzes given at the beginning of class help stimulate students to review information they did not know and listen for clarification during class lecture. Quizzes at the end of the class session allow students to use their problem-solving skills by applying what they have just learned to a patient case or problem.

Problem-solving skills can be developed during a class period by applying knowledge of pharmacotherapy to a patient case. Application reinforces the previously learned material and helps students understand the importance of the topic in a real-life situation. PBL is a teaching and learning method in which a problem is used as the stimulus for developing critical thinking and problem-solving skills for acquiring new knowledge. The process of PBL starts with the student identifying the problem in a case. The student spends time either alone or in a group exploring and analyzing the problem and identifying learning resources needed to solve the problem. After acquiring the knowledge, the student applies it to solve the problem.[17] Small or large groups can be established for case discussions to help students develop communication skills, respect for other students' opinions, satisfaction for contributing to the discussion, and the ability to give and accept criticism.[17] Interactive PBL computer tools and the use of real patients also stimulate learning both outside and inside the classroom.[18,19] Computer technology can be used creatively in PBL cases as a tool for problem solving.[20]

Cooperative or collaborative learning strategies involve students in the generation of knowledge.[9] Students are randomly assigned to groups of four to six at the beginning of the school term. Several times during the term, each group is given a patient case and a group leader is selected. Each student in the group volunteers to work on a certain portion of the case. The case is discussed in class, and each member receives the same grade. After students have finished working in their small groups or during large group sessions, the teacher serves as a facilitator of the discussion rather than as a lecturer. The students actively participate in the identification and resolution of the problem. The integration of this technique helps with development of skills in decision making, conflict management, and communication.[8] Group discussions help students develop concepts from the material presented, clarify ideas, and develop new strategies for clinical problem solving. These skills are essential for lifelong learning and will be used by the students throughout their careers.

Team-based learning is an instructional strategy for use during the entire semester. The course is structured around the activity of teams of six to eight students that apply course content, assess student learning on both individual and team levels, and use peer assessment. Teams are formed in the classroom, students are held accountable for individual and team work, assignments are applications of course content performed during class time, and students receive frequent, prompt feedback.[9]

CASE STUDIES

Case studies are used by a number of professional schools to teach pharmacotherapy.[1,18,21,22] Case studies are a written description of a real-life problem or situation. Only the facts are provided, usually in chronologic sequence similar to what would be encountered in a patient care setting. Many times, as in real life, the information given is incomplete, or important details are not available. When working through a case, the student must distinguish between relevant and irrelevant facts and become accustomed to the fact that there is no single "correct" answer. The use of cases actively involves the student in the analysis of facts and details of the case, selection of a solution to the problem, and defense of his or her solution through discussion of the case.[23] In case-based learning, students use their recall of previously learned information to solve clinical cases.[24]

During class, active participation is essential for the maximum learning benefit to be achieved. Because of their various backgrounds, students learn different perspectives when dealing with patient problems. Some general steps proposed by McDade[23] for students when preparing cases for class discussion include:

- Skim the text quickly to establish the broad issues of the case and the types of information presented for analysis.
- Reread the case very carefully, underlining key facts as you go.
- Note on scratch paper the key issues and problems. Next, go through the case again and sort out the relevant considerations and decisions for each problem.
- Prioritize problems and alternatives.
- Develop a set of recommendations to address the problems.
- Evaluate your decisions.

EXPECTATIONS OF STUDENTS AND TEACHERS

Active learning provides students with an opportunity to take a dynamic role in the learning process. Students are expected to participate in class discussions and be creative in formulating their own opinions. This method also requires that students listen and be respectful of the thoughts and opinions of their classmates. Assigned readings and homework must be completed before class in order to use class time efficiently for questions that are not answered in other reference material. To prepare answers or appropriate therapeutic recommendations, students may have to look beyond the reference materials provided by the teacher; they may have to perform literature searches and use the library or Internet to retrieve additional information. It is important for students to justify their recommendations. The active learning strategies outlined previously allow students to comprehend the material presented, participate in peer discussions, and formulate opinions as in real-life situations.

To implement active learning strategies in the classroom, teachers must overcome the anxiety that change often creates. Experimenting with active learning methods such as the pause technique and slowly implementing a change in the classroom may work best. Using any of the active learning strategies requires teachers to encourage as much classroom discussion as possible instead of lecturing. Use of a wireless microphone is helpful in encouraging student participation in large classrooms. Teachers should make an effort to learn the names of all students so they can more easily interact with them. In addition, teachers should have a preconceived plan for how the class discussion will go and stick to it.

MAXIMIZING ACTIVE LEARNING OPPORTUNITIES: ADVICE TO STUDENTS

Taking initiative is the key to deriving the benefits of active learning. It is crucial to recognize the three largest squelchers of initiative: laziness, fear of change, and force of habit.[25] You will find that time management is important. Be sure to schedule adequate time for studying, prepare for class by reading ahead, use transition times wisely, identify the times of day that you are most productive, and focus on the results rather than the time to complete an activity.[7]

In active learning, you are expected to talk about what you are learning, write about it, relate it to previous patient cases, and apply it to the current case. In a sense, you repeatedly manipulate the information until it becomes a part of you. Some techniques to use when studying are to compare, contrast, and summarize similarities and differences among disease states, drug classes, and appropriate pharmacotherapy. In class, take advantage of every opportunity to present your own work. Attempt to relate personal experiences or outside events to topics discussed in class, and always be an active participant in class or group discussions; lively debates about pharmacotherapy issues allow more therapeutic options to be discussed.[26]

When reading assignments, summarize the information using tables or charts and take notes. These will be your personal set of notes to study for the course exams and to review for the pharmacy state board examination. While taking notes in class, leave a wide margin on the left to write down questions that you generate later when reviewing the notes.[13] Alternatively, make lists of questions from class or readings to discuss with your colleagues or faculty or try to answer them on your own. When time allows, seek out recent information on subjects that interest you. Use Web-based cases and other online resources to extend your knowledge on a particular disease state and drug therapy.[16] In class, always try to determine the "big picture."[26]

Some other methods for maximizing active learning are to review corrected assignments and exams for information that you do not understand and seek clarification from faculty. Complete assignments promptly and minimize short-term memorization. Give others a chance to contribute and try not to embarrass fellow classmates.[26]

In active learning, much of what you learn you will learn on your own. You will probably find that you read more, but you will gain understanding from reading. At the same time, you are developing a critical lifelong learning skill. Your reading will become more "depth processing" in which you focus on:

- The intent of the article.
- Actively integrating what you read with previous parts of the text.
- Using your own ability to make a logical construction.
- Thinking about the functional role of the different parts of an argument.

In writing, consider summarizing the major points of each class. Writing about a topic develops critical thinking, communication, and organization skills. In classes that involve active learning, you may write for "think-pair-share" exercises, quizzes, summary paragraphs, and other activities. Stopping to write allows you to reflect on the information you have just heard and reinforces learning. Discussions may occur in large or small groups. Discussing material helps you to apply your knowledge, verbalize the medical and pharmacologic terminology, engage in active listening, think critically, and develop interpersonal skills. When working in groups, all members should participate in problem solving. Teaching others is an excellent way to learn the subject matter.[7]

HOW TO USE THE CASEBOOK

The casebook was prepared to assist in the development of each student's understanding of a disease and its management as well as problem-solving skills. It is important for students to realize that learning and understanding the material is guided through problem solving. Students are encouraged to solve each of the cases individually or with others in a study group before discussion of the case and topic in class.

As cases are solved, the student begins to understand that each case may not have a single solution or answer; this may be frustrating initially but reflects real-world situations. The student will begin to appreciate the variety and complexity of diseases that are encountered in different patient populations. In some cases, more detailed information from the patient will play a pivotal role in drug therapy selection and monitoring. In others, some diagnoses can be resolved through use of laboratory analysis or specific medical tests. Some cases may require a much more in-depth assessment of the patient's disease state and treatment rendered so far. Other cases may involve initiation of both nonpharmacologic and pharmacologic therapy, ranging from single to multiple drug regimens.

Regardless of disease and/or treatment complexity, students must rely on knowledge previously learned in other courses (e.g., anatomy, biochemistry, microbiology, physiology, pathophysiology, medicinal chemistry, pharmacology, pharmacokinetics, pharmacoeconomics, drug literature evaluation, ethics, physical assessment). As a consequence, students may need to review previous notes, handouts, or textbooks. Students can use MEDLINE searches for primary literature, drug reference books, the Internet, and faculty experts as information sources. These resources and the textbook *Pharmacotherapy: A Pathophysiologic Approach* are essential in supporting each student's ability to solve the cases successfully. Understanding the usefulness and limitations of these resources will be beneficial in the future. Likewise, discussions in study groups and class should lead to a further understanding of disease states and treatment strategies.

SUMMARY

The use of case studies and other active learning strategies will enhance the development of essential skills necessary to practice in any setting, including community, ambulatory care, primary care, health-systems, long-term care, home health care, managed care, and the pharmaceutical industry. The role of the health care professional is constantly changing; thus, it is important for students to acquire knowledge and develop the lifetime skills required for continued learning. Teachers who incorporate active learning strategies into the classroom are facilitating the development of lifelong learners who will be able to adapt to change that occurs in their profession.

REFERENCES

1. Winslade N. Large-group problem-based learning: a revision from traditional to pharmaceutical care-based therapeutics. Am J Pharm Educ 1994;58:64–73.

2. Kane MD, Briceland LL, Hamilton RA. Solving problems. US Pharmacist 1995;20:55–74.

3. Kaufman DM, Laidlaw TA, Macleod H. Communication skills in medical school: exposure, confidence, and performance. Acad Med 2000;75(10, Suppl):S90–S92.

4. Brandt BF. Effective teaching and learning strategies. Pharmacotherapy 2000;20:307S–316S.

5. Michael J. Where's the evidence that active learning works? Adv Physiol Educ 2006;30:159–167.

6. Rangachari PK. Active learning: in context. Adv Physiol Educ 1995;13:S75–S80.

7. Warren G. Carpe diem: A student guide to active learning. Landover, MD; University Press of America, 1996.

8. Bonwell CC, Eison JA. Active learning: Creating excitement in the classroom. Washington, DC, George Washington University, School of Education and Human Development; 1991. ASHE-ERIC Higher Education Report no 1.

9. Shakarian DC. Beyond lecture: active learning strategies that work. JOPERD May-June 1995;21–24.

10. Michaelson LK, Knight AB, Fink LD. Team-based Learning: A Transformative Use of Small Groups in College Teaching. Sterling, VA; Stylus Publishing, 2002.

11. Ruhl KL, Hughs CA, Schloss PJ. Using the pause procedure to enhance lecture recall. Teacher Educ Spec Educ 1987;10:14–18.

12. Rowe MB. Pausing principles and their effects on reasoning in science. New Dir Com Coll 1980;8:27–34.

13. Elliot DD. Promoting critical thinking in the classroom. Nurs Educator 1996;21:49–52.

14. Johnson SP, Cooper J. Quick-thinks: active-thinking tasks in lecture classes and televised instruction. Coop Learn Coll Teach 1997;8:2–6.

15. McKeachie WJ. Teaching large classes (You can still get active learning!). In: McKeachie WJ, ed. Teaching Tips: Strategies, Research, Theory for College and University Teachers, 10th ed. Boston, Houghton Mifflin, 1999:209–215.

16. Turchin A, Lehmann CU. Active Learning Centre: Design and evaluation of an educational World Wide Web site. Med Inform 2000;25:195–206.

17. Walton HJ, Matthews MB. Essentials of problem-based learning. Med Educ 1989;23:542–558.

18. Raman-Wilms L. Innovative enabling strategies in self-directed, problem-based therapeutics: Enhancing student preparedness for pharmaceutical care. Am J Pharm Educ 2001;65:56–64.

19. Dammers J, Spencer J, Thomas M. Using real patients in problem-based learning: Students' comments on the value of using real, as opposed to paper cases, in a problem-based learning module in general practice. Med Educ 2001;35:27–34.

20. Lowther DL, Morrison GR. Integrating computers into the problem-solving protocol. New Dir Teach Learn 2003;95:33–38.

21. Hartzema AG. Teaching therapeutic reasoning through the case-study approach: Adding the probabilistic dimension. Am J Pharm Educ 1994;58:436–440.

22. Delafuente JC, Munyer TO, Angaran DM, et al. A problem-solving active-learning course in pharmacotherapy. Am J Pharm Educ 1994;58:61–64.

23. McDade SA. An Introduction to the Case Study Method: Preparation, Analysis, Participation. New York, Teachers College Press, 1988.

24. Williams B. Case-based learning—a review of the literature: Is there scope for this educational paradigm in prehospital education? Emerg Med J 2005;22:577–581.

25. Robbins A. Awaken the Giant Within. New York, Simon & Schuster, 1991.

26. Chickering AW, Gamson ZF, Barsi LM. Seven Principles for Good Practice in Undergraduate Education. Racine, WI, The Johnson Foundation, 1989.

RICHARD N. HERRIER, PHARMD

3 Case Studies in Patient Communication

CHAPTER

Delivering quality pharmaceutical care requires both strong technical and people skills. While all pharmacists are well versed in the technical aspects of the profession, many are not well prepared regarding interpersonal communication within the clinical context. In contemporary pharmacy practice, good communication skills are critical for achieving optimal patient outcomes and increasing pharmacists' satisfaction with their professional roles. The focus of this chapter is limited to the essential skills needed for symptom assessment, medication consultation, and strategies to improve compliance and monitor clinical progress. Readers are encouraged to review aspects of basic communication skills in other sources.[1–5]

THE IMPORTANCE OF ASKING OPEN-ENDED QUESTIONS IN HEALTH CARE SETTINGS

One of the most important techniques to effectively communicate with patients is the primary use of open-ended questions. Open-ended questions are ones that start with *who, what, where, when, why,* and *how.* Closed-ended can be answered with either a simple yes or no answer and start with *can, do, did, are, would,* or *could.* Open-ended questions have numerous advantages compared to closed-ended questions. They markedly increase the comprehensiveness and accuracy of patient responses compared to closed-ended questions. Open-ended questions help readily identify patients with special needs requiring interventions, including patients with cognitive impairment, hearing loss, or lack of fluency in English or other primary language. Closed-ended questions allow patients with special needs to go undetected by hiding behind their yes or no answers. Open-ended questions minimize the need for the professional to speak, maximizing opportunities for listening for patient understanding and symptom-defining answers. Finally, open-ended questions force the patient to answer with something other than yes or no, encouraging dialogue or further conversation with the patient. Closed-ended questions are perceived by patients as discouraging further response and are used to bring closure to conversations. Whether collecting information regarding a patient's symptoms or verifying that patients understand how to take their medication during medication counseling, the use of open-ended questions is the most effective communication technique and is therefore emphasized in this chapter.

BASIC MEDICATION CONSULTATION SKILLS

Consultation on prescription medication use is a fundamental and important activity of the pharmacist and is mandated by both state and federal law or regulation.[6] The primary goal of traditional methods of medication counseling is to provide information: the pharmacist "tells" and the patient "listens." Pharmacists may try and check for patient understanding by asking ineffective closed-ended questions

such as, "Do you understand?" or "Do you have any questions?" This traditional approach never verifies that the patient understands how to properly use his or her medication, which can lead to poor outcomes. Given the low level of patient health literacy in the United States, reliance on written patient handouts may also lead to a similar level of poor patient outcomes.[7] Using a modification of the effective educational approach, the "teachback" method, the Indian Health Service Pharmacy program developed a needs-based interactive medication counseling technique, *with the goal of verifying patient understanding.*

Using open-ended questions to initiate dialogue negates the disadvantages of the traditional lecture format. Retention of information is superior because patients forget 90% of *what you tell them* within 60 minutes, but they remember nearly 90% of *what they said* 24 hours later.[1] Using open-ended questions helps temporarily refocus the patient's attention, preventing the tendency to multi-task and lose focus after 45–60 seconds. Finally, the consultation is quicker, and you maintain the patient's attention span because you are not repeating boring facts the patient already knows.

Two sets of open-ended questions are used in the consultation. One is for new prescriptions (*Prime Questions*), and the other is for refill prescriptions (*Show-and-Tell Questions*), as shown in Table 3-1. These open-ended questions make the patient an active participant in the learning process. They provide an organized approach to ascertain what the patient already knows about the medication. Using a systematic approach has been associated with improved recall of prescription instructions.[8] The pharmacist can praise the patient for correct information recalled, clarify points misunderstood, and add new information as needed. It spares the pharmacist from repeating information already known by the patient, which is an inefficient use of time. The steps in the consultation process are described next.

Open the Consultation

When the patient is called for counseling, introduce yourself by name and state the purpose of the consultation. Next, verify the patient's identity, either by asking for identification or at least by asking, "And you are…?" If the patient is non-English speaking, hard of hearing, or otherwise unable to provide his or her name, or answers inappropriately to a question, you have identified a barrier in the consultation that must be overcome before discussing the medication.

Use of a private space is required for patients who have hearing problems or those needing extra privacy, such as patients receiving vaginal creams or those with AIDS. Sit facing the patient, and maintain the appropriate interpersonal distance (1.5–2 feet) during the consultation.

Conduct the Counseling Session for New Prescriptions

Begin by asking the *Prime Questions* if the prescription is a new one. The *Prime Questions* are a series of three structured questions that probe the patient's understanding of proper medication use. If the patient knows the answer to a question, the pharmacist moves on to the next question. If there are gaps in the patient's understanding, the pharmacist "fills in the gap" by providing the missing information before moving on to the next prime question. If the patient is able to tell you what the medication is for (the first question), move to the next question. If the patient does not know what the medication is for, or if the patient says, "Don't you know?" you should ask why the patient visited the physician. The patient may describe symptoms of a condition known to be treatable with the medication in question.

After verifying that the patient knows what the medication is for, ask the second prime question. Often, patients are unaware of the dosage instructions or indicate, "It's on the label, isn't it?" Be aware of the optimal dosing instructions, because the patient may correctly respond "twice a day," but you may need to ask about exact timing, or whether to take the drug with meals. Other questions to include under the second prime question are related to these areas of concern: a) how long to take the medication; b) exactly how much or how often to take it when the medication is prescribed as needed; c) what to do when a dose is missed; and d) how to store the medication. Rather than providing facts, consider asking the patient, "What did the doctor say about how long to take this medication?" or "What will you do if you miss a dose?" Asking a question of the patient prompts the patient's attention, whereas "telling" the information is less effective, and the patient may not listen as well. Keep the information you provide brief and to the point.

After verifying patient understanding about how to take the medication, proceed to the third prime question. This question verifies that the patient understands the beneficial effects that are expected and what to do if the medication doesn't work. In addition, the question verifies the patient's understanding of potential common and uncommon (but serious) adverse effects plus what to do if a bad effect occurs.

For example, for angiotensin-converting enzyme (ACE) inhibitors, the pharmacist should warn about mild cough (talk with your physician) and any sudden swelling in the face, mouth, or tongue (get to an emergency room), which may represent the uncommon but potentially serious adverse effect of angioedema. Research shows that patients want information about their medications, especially adverse effects, and that providing such information does not lead to the development of those reactions.[9–11] If the patient doesn't know a specific item of information, first probe with focused open-ended question such as "What side effects were you warned about?" or "What were you told to do if that happened?" before "filling in the gaps."

The manner in which the consultation is closed is extremely important. Most consultations are a combination of the patient knowing some information and the pharmacist "filling in the gaps" by providing additional information as the prime questions are reviewed. Because of this, it is important to close the consultation with the *final verification*. Think of the final verification as asking the patient to "play back" everything learned in order to check that the information is complete and accurate. Say to the patient, "Just to make sure I didn't leave anything out, please go over with me how you are going to use the medication." Avoid saying "Just to make sure you've got this . . ." because the patient may feel embarrassed if he or she does not recall important facts. At this point, the patient should describe correct use of the medication. Any errors can be corrected and any omissions clarified. Then ask the patient if there is anything else he or she needs and offer assistance as required.

Conduct the Counseling Session for Refill Prescriptions

A similar process is used for refill prescriptions. The *Show-and-Tell Questions* verify patient understanding of proper use of chronic medications or medications that the patient has used in the past.

TABLE 3-1	Indian Health Service Medication Counseling Technique

Prime questions

1. What did your doctor tell you the medication is for?
   or
   What were you told the medication is for?
   What problem or symptom is it supposed to help?
   What is it supposed to do?
2. How did your doctor tell you to take the medication?
   or
   How were you told to take the medication?
   How often did your doctor say to take it?
   How much are you supposed to take?
   What did your doctor say to do when you miss a dose?
   How did your doctor tell you to use it?
   What does three times a day mean to you?
3. What did your doctor tell you to expect?
   or
   What were you told to expect?
   What good effects are you supposed to expect?
   What bad effects did your doctor tell you to watch for?
   What should you do if a bad reaction occurs or if the medication doesn't work?

Show-and-tell questions

1. What do you take the medication for?
2. How do you take it?
3. What kind of problems are you having?

The pharmacist begins the process by showing the medication to the patient; that is, by opening the bottle and displaying the contents. Then, the patient tells the pharmacist how he uses the medication by answering the questions listed in Table 3-1. Note that the doctor is omitted as a reference, because the patient should have been counseled properly by the pharmacist before this and should have all information needed for proper medication usage. The show-and-tell technique enables the pharmacist to detect problems with compliance or unwanted drug effects. If the patient answers incorrectly to the second question, the patient may be noncompliant, or the physician may have changed the dosage. The pharmacist will need to further define the reason for the discrepancy. The second show-and-tell question also allows the pharmacist to ask the patient to demonstrate proper use of an inhaler, ophthalmic solution, or how to measure liquid doses to assure proper usage.

Some pharmacists have difficulty asking the third question, fearing that they may arouse suspicion in the patient. However, research discounts this notion, as previously discussed. If potential adverse effects were discussed when the patient was initially counseled, it seems natural, and certainly relevant and important, to query the patient about adverse effects at the refill visit. If new symptoms are present, explore this further using the *Chief Complaint history taking*. Because it is important to evaluate new symptoms critically, we will describe this in detail next.

EXPLORING SYMPTOMS

At the prescription counter, over the telephone, at a bedside visit, or in requesting assistance with self care via nonprescription products, the patient may mention symptoms that could be related to drug therapy or to an illness. Knowing how to explore the patient's symptoms and how to evaluate their relationship to either an acute disease or a chronic disease and its treatment or complications is a key assessment skill. The first step is to get the patient to reveal more information about the symptom. An introductory statement such as "Tell me more about it" encourages the patient to provide more specific details. After this, the *Basic 7 Questions* should be used. These seven focused, open-ended questions, based on *Chief Com-*

plaint history-taking techniques, seek specifics that will help to define whether the symptom is related to drug therapy or to a specific disease that may require referral or be suitable for self care with nonprescription products.[12] The *Basic 7 Questions* are:

1. *Location:* Where is it located? Where does it hurt the worst?

2. *Quality:* What do you bring up when you cough? How would you describe the pain? What does it feel like?

3. *Severity:* How bad is it?

4. *Context:* How did it happen? When do you notice it?

5. *Timing:* When did it start? *or* How long have you had it? How frequently does it happen?

6. *Modifying factors:* What makes it better? *or* What have you done about it? What makes it worse?

7. *Associated symptoms:* What other symptoms are you having?

Finally *summarize* what the patient has told you, allowing the patient to verify your understanding and correct any misinformation collected or add information omitted during initial questioning.

Without proper attention to detail, many pharmacists assume that the symptom expressed is caused by a disease state and do not adequately address it. Or they may jump to conclusions about the cause of the symptom and recommend a treatment without knowing the true cause. For example, a patient taking a nonsteroidal anti-inflammatory drug who complains of fatigue might be recommended a vitamin if the pharmacist thinks the patient is tired because of inadequate nutrition. Probing the symptom of fatigue with the questions listed above may reveal that the fatigue started after the medication was begun and is accompanied by gastric distress, suggesting anemia from GI blood loss as a possible cause for the fatigue.

The *Basic 7 Questions* are also important when there is a tendency to attribute every symptom to a medication, as patients are sometimes inclined to do. For instance, a pharmacy student reviewed the chart of a patient with bipolar illness, seizures, and parkinsonism. The patient was receiving several medications, including carbamazepine and carbidopa/levodopa. The patient complained of blurred vision and insomnia, which the student initially felt were caused by the medications. However, using all of the *Basic 7 Questions* disclosed that the patient had blurred vision only out of the left eye and that she had insomnia "since the day I was born." Her answers suggested that the symptoms were unlikely to be related to her drug therapy. The most important point in addressing symptoms is to obtain enough information to make an informed clinical judgment. This is accomplished by using the *Basic 7 Questions.*

BARRIERS DURING CLINICAL COMMUNICATION

The clinical skills described are easily applied in situations where there are few or no barriers in communication between patient and pharmacist. In reality, there are often obstacles to overcome in the environment or within the pharmacist or patient. Examples of problems within the pharmacy environment that deter optimal patient communication include lack of privacy, interruptions, high workload, and insufficient staff. Barriers present within the pharmacist include lack of desire or skills to adequately counsel patients, stereotyping patients and problems, and difficulty maintaining concentration, especially when stress is a factor. A detailed analysis of these barriers is beyond the scope of this discussion but can be found in the references.[3] The structured approach for patient consultation and exploring symptoms can be likened to knowing the road on which you are traveling. However, unforeseen events happen on every path and may arise at any time. Just as one must remove or negotiate around the obstacle on the highway, the pharmacist must recognize and manage barriers brought by the patient during the encounter for the consultation to reach the desired end.

Functional barriers include problems with hearing and vision that make it difficult for the patient to absorb information during the consultation. Language barriers and illiteracy are formidable obstacles to proper consultation. Language problems become apparent early in the counseling process when you use open-ended questions that require more than a yes/no answer. Strategies specific to each barrier are needed when these problems are identified. It is important to use translators, show picture diagrams, and involve English-speaking caregivers when language problems exist.

Emotional barriers are common in everyday pharmacist–patient interactions. When not handled properly, they give rise to further aggravation and break down communication, inhibiting effective consultation or history taking. Patients may express anger, hostility, sadness, depression, fear, anxiety, or embarrassment directly or indirectly during consultation with the pharmacist. They may also give the attitude of a "know-it-all," be suspicious of medications, or seem unmotivated or uninterested.

Unlike seeing the patient with a white cane and knowing that a vision problem exists, emotional barriers can be more difficult to discern. Because most patients will not say, "I'm angry and frustrated about feeling so ill," or "I'm upset that my doctor didn't spend much time with me," their feelings surface in statements such as, "I don't know why it takes all day to put a few pills in the bottle!" or "I don't know why I have to take this stupid medicine…nothing seems to help anyway." Unfortunately, we usually respond to the content of the message (e.g., "I'll have this ready for you as soon as I can") without recognizing that there may be other issues behind the statement, issues that will interfere with the effectiveness of counseling or interviewing and, more important, impact the patient's decision to comply with therapy.

OVERCOMING BARRIERS WITH REFLECTIVE RESPONSES

Reflective responding, also known as active listening or empathetic responding, is a skill that can be practiced to listen beyond just the words spoken. When we respond with a reflection of what the patient is saying, thinking, or feeling, we let the person know we are truly listening and give the person the opportunity to admit to feelings, clarify thoughts, and bring forth information. Making a reflective response is not natural for us because most of us have not been trained to use these skills. Reflective responding attempts to reflect in words what the patient is saying or feeling. The reflection may be based on the content or thought expressed by the patient, and/or the feelings associated with it that are often not outwardly expressed. Reflective responses are especially called for when the patient is demonstrating emotions. Angry looks, pounding fists, averted eye contact, and head drooping all convey certain emotional states. Hesitating gestures or remarks such as, "Well…I guess I could try it," call for reflective responses to bring concerns to light. Also, it calms the patient down and puts him or her in a better mental state for answering questions or receiving counseling.

The first step in effective reflective responding is to identify and label the emotional state. The four basic emotional states are mad, sad, glad, and scared. As you observe the patient during consultation, certain non-verbal or verbal signs (e.g., hesitating words) may suggest one of the four feeling states. The second step is to put the word describing the feeling state into a sentence to use as a response to the patient. Some basic structures for sentences include, "It sounds as if you are (frustrated, mad, happy)," or "I can see that you are (happy, confused, mad)." These remarks indicate to patients that you are truly attempting to understand their concerns; thus, the patient and his or her concerns remain the focus of the encounter.

To the patient who remarked, "I don't know why I have to take this...nothing helps anyway," the pharmacist might determine that the non-verbal tone of voice and choice of words indicate that the patient is disappointed with results of his or her therapy. Alternatively, the patient may be feeling hopeless about getting better. One reflective response is, "It sounds as if you have been frustrated with the things you have tried." This statement neither judges nor advises. It gives the patient an opportunity to open discussion of a difficult topic, if the patient so chooses. Contrast this with, "This is a good medicine, Joe, and I really think it will help." Although this may be true, maintaining the communication on a technical, information-providing level avoids dealing with the underlying issues of the patient's fears and markedly decreases the efficacy of the pharmacist's communication with the patient.

Emotional barriers can occur at any time throughout the consultation, and they must be dealt with first in order to put the patient in a receptive frame of mind. Embarrassment is a factor when vaginal preparations, condom use, and similar topics are the subject of the consultation. Observe for signs of embarrassment such as averted gaze or fidgeting, and respond with, "This can be hard to talk about, but it's important that we discuss ..." Also, be matter-of-fact, move to a private space, and speak in a normal tone of voice to help alleviate the embarrassment.

When faced with patients' emotional outbursts, acknowledge their expressed feelings before continuing with the consultation or the interview. The initial use of reflective responses will allow the consultation or interview to proceed with both parties devoting attention to the primary issues of drug therapy and usage, rather than to interpersonal difficulties. Remember, though, that reflective responses will not work in every situation nor with every type of patient.

COMPLIANCE AND DISEASE MONITORING

In no other situation is the pharmacist's role in monitoring and managing medication usage more vital than in the case of patients requiring chronic drug therapy, especially for diseases that are asymptomatic. Contemporary pharmacy practice continues to evolve into more direct patient care roles. The monitoring and management of common, chronic diseases such as hypertension, asthma, and diabetes are now being done in partnership between pharmacists and medical professionals. Models of community pharmacy practice now include private consultations and advanced practice techniques that were formerly limited to sites such as the Indian Health Service and the Department of Veterans Affairs. A majority of states now have regulations that allow pharmacists to assess and prescribe.[13]

WHOSE DISEASE IS IT ANYWAY?

A common misperception held by health care professionals regarding a patient with a chronic disease is that the professional manages the patient's disease. Nothing could be further from the truth, and this medical myth is probably a major contributor to compliance problems among patients with chronic diseases. In the traditional medical care model, health care professionals perceive their roles to be in the diagnosis, treatment, and management of disease. As drug therapy managers, pharmacists focus on blood levels, kinetic dosage calculations, and drug interactions. Guided by this focus on technical aspects of patient care, health care professionals often become frustrated and angry when patients do not follow instructions or, despite the provider's best efforts, achieve only partial results. In reality, the only time the professional manages the treatment is during an office

visit or while the patient is institutionalized in a hospital or long-term care facility. Almost all of the time, the patient controls the treatment of his or her disease, especially those that require continuous medication. Failure to recognize this basic truth has created: a) considerable tension in patient–provider relationships; b) provider frustration and anger; c) poor communication; d) negative provider attitudes toward individual patients; e) poor patient outcomes; f) patient distrust of providers; and g) legal consequences that have been a major contributor to rising health care costs.

One author strongly suggests that noncompliance in diabetes mellitus is due in large part to the failure of providers to recognize that their goal is not to treat the disease, but to *help the patient to treat the disease*.[14] That contention is supported by current medical literature on compliance that links good communication and a partnership style of provider–patient relationship to increased satisfaction, compliance, and better patient outcomes.[15,16]

To be successful in assisting patients to achieve good outcomes, the provider and pharmacist must adopt a partnership approach, with health professionals acting as facilitators to help patients manage their disease. That is, it is the patient's disease; the providers' job is *to help them manage it*.

GO SLOW/USE INTERACTIVE TECHNIQUES

Patients can absorb only a limited amount of new information at each encounter. In an attempt to do a thorough job, health care professionals often overwhelm the patient with information at or near the time of diagnosis or treatment initiation. Patients' active listening abilities last less than a minute during a monologue presentation, and they retain only a few pieces of information from a prolonged discussion and may miss key facts. In addition, a large volume of technical information may confuse or frighten patients, leading to the poor outcome that educational efforts are intended to prevent.[15] Also, newly diagnosed patients may not have accepted their diagnosis or the need for treatment.

Successful patient educators do three things: a) they give patients information in small manageable increments, b) they actively involve the patient in the educational process by creating an interactive dialogue and using other hands-on approaches that are consistent with adult learning principles,[16] and c) they understand patient readiness for information. For the pharmacist dispensing the initial prescription, this entails verifying that the patient understands how to take the medicine and its most common side effects. For example, with hydrochlorothiazide 25 mg daily for hypertension, the pharmacist should verify that the patient knows what it is for, knows to take it once daily in the morning to prevent nighttime voiding, knows that it takes a while before any changes in blood pressure occur, and knows that there will be a noticeable increase in urination the first week, which should lessen thereafter. Discussions about diet, exercise, and related issues can wait until later visits. Giving the patient a handout on hypertension and diuretics is appropriate and can lead to questions and subsequent education at later visits or during a follow-up phone call.

SET THE STAGE FOR FUTURE ENCOUNTERS

Many providers explain to patients what follow-up visits will entail so that patients view subsequent laboratory tests and examinations as a normal part of their care. However, few providers follow a similar process regarding medication compliance. Patients then perceive questions about compliance to be intrusive and, fearing parental-type sanctions from the provider, lie about being compliant. Using specific strategies during the *initial* patient visit when follow-up care is discussed can prevent this all-too-common problem. Explain that compliance is very important to successful outcomes, but that you know how hard it is to remember to take medication every day. Tell the patient that you expect that he or she will be like all patients and experience some difficulty remembering to take the medication. Ask the patient to keep track of those instances if possible, and further explain that you will be asking at each visit about the problems the patient has had with the medication so you can assist the patient to better remember to take the medication. It may be necessary to probe into his or her daily habits and to help him or her find a way to tie medication taking into a particular activity. For instance, if the patient always makes coffee in the morning, having the medication nearby may be a sufficient reminder to promote compliance. Be sure to use a partnership approach. Additional compliance-enhancing skills are discussed in the next section.

MONITORING PATIENT PROGRESS AT RETURN VISITS

Organizing an effective approach to evaluating and educating patients with chronic diseases at return visits may be problematic in a busy practice setting. One simple way to look at all patients returning for follow-up of chronic diseases is to use the "Three Cs": *Control, Complications,* and *Compliance* (Fig. 3-1). To evaluate the *control* of the chronic disease, couple objective findings (e.g., blood pressure or range of motion) with subjective findings from the consultation (e.g., reports of dizziness, nocturnal voiding, or degree of morning joint stiffness). *Complications* can occur both from disease progression and drug effects. As with the control parameters, a combination of subjective findings (e.g., symptoms) and objective findings from the health record or patient profile can disclose the presence of potential complications. For example, a patient with hypertension, diabetes mellitus, and osteoarthritis who takes lisinopril, glyburide, and ibuprofen can be queried about the presence of cough, difficulty sleeping, and exercise tolerance. These questions are primarily directed at detecting congestive heart failure or renal failure caused by hypertension and/or diabetes, but they also will help detect drug-related problems such as cough caused by the ACE inhibitor and renal effects from ibuprofen. Checking recent laboratory values for serum creatinine, electrolytes, and blood glucose will help assess diabetes and hypertension control and complications such as NSAID-induced renal impairment, excessive glyburide dosage, and ACE inhibitor–induced hyperkalemia. Collecting subjective information at each visit can be organized by integrating the "Three Cs" with broad open-ended questions similar to the *Basic 7 Questions.*

To identify potential compliance problems, review the health record or patient profile for objective evidence of potential non-compliance before talking with the patient. During profile review, three items should alert the pharmacist to potential compliance problems. The first and most common item is a discrepancy between the number of doses that should have been taken and the number of doses dispensed. Second, patients with incomplete refill requests (e.g., only one or two of multiple chronic medications due at the same time) raise suspicion for noncompliance. Third, the prescribing of a new medication for the same condition or one that may unknowingly be prescribed to offset adverse effects from another medication may indicate compliance problems. Patients often present to medical providers with new complaints. If the provider does not make the connection between the new symptom and the side effect, compliance or therapeutic problems may eventually occur. If patients taking ACE inhibitors present with new or repeat prescriptions for cough suppressants, the pharmacist should consider the potential for ACE inhibitor–induced cough.

Potential compliance problems found during profile or chart review call for further exploration before a definite compliance

Collecting Subjective Information as a Primary Care Provider

1. How have things been going with your _____ since your last visit? *(Control)*
2. What kind of problems have you had remembering to take your medication? *(Compliance)*
   - Tell me about the last time it happened.
   - How many times has it happened since your last visit?
3. What kind of changes have you noticed since your last visit? *(Complications)*
   - What problems are you having with your medication?
   - In order to make sure you aren't having any problems, are you experiencing:
   e.g., Drowsiness?   Yes ❏   No ❏
   Dizziness?   Yes ❏   No ❏
   Note: In this situation, using closed-ended questions covering major potential problems or complications is an efficient method.
4. If any problems are noted, shift gears to *Chief Complaint History Taking* and begin with:
   - Tell me more about it.
5. Follow with the *Basic 7 Questions* as needed.

FIGURE 3-1. Example form for collecting subjective information as a primary care provider. General approach to interviewing patients returning for chronic disease follow-up.

problem can be ascertained. There may be rational explanations for the objective findings. Gaps in refills may be a result of patients obtaining refills at another location, or the doctor may have told the patient to change the dosage schedule or to stop the drug altogether.

Begin the consultation using the *Show-and-Tell* technique for refill prescriptions when the profile indicates potential noncompliance. The patient may provide one or more clues during consultation to confirm your suspicions. Patients who tell the pharmacist during the *Show-and-Tell* questioning that they are taking their medication differently than prescribed are providing evidence of a potential compliance problem. Some clues are obvious, such as when a patient asks, "Why do I have to keep taking this medicine?" This is a "red flag" because it is clear that the patient wishes not to take the prescription. However, many statements are more subtle. Examples of these vague clues, called "pink flags," include: "My doctor says I *should* take it...," or "My doctor *wants* me to...," or "I'm *supposed* to be taking...." These are usually detected when the pharmacist asks the first two *Show-and-Tell* questions. "What kinds of problems are you having with the medication?" may prompt the following "pink flag" responses: "Well...none, really," or a hesitation before saying "No, none." Reflective responses discussed earlier in this chapter are appropriate in this situation. Responses include, "It seems as if you are not too sure about taking that," or "It sounds as if you think the medicine is causing a problem." These responses open the dialogue in a non-threatening manner and focus on the patient's perceptions or suggestion that a problem exists.

A *supportive compliance probe* is a more direct approach that must be initiated if the profile review reveals potential problems but the consultation does not confirm suspicions. This is a specific type of statement that uses "I" language to describe what the profile shows and to probe the discrepancy. For example, "I noticed when I reviewed your profile that you hadn't had your prednisone refilled in about 2 weeks. I was concerned that there might have been some changes that I'm not aware of." This combination of "I noticed...and

I'm concerned…" can be very effective in getting a dialogue started in a non-threatening manner. The *universal statement* is another useful approach, such as, "Most of my patients have problems remembering to take every dose of their medication. What kinds of problems are you having?" Open the discussion of compliance problems with non-threatening language, and there is a greater likelihood that the patient will disclose problems.

Patients may ask, "Does this medicine have any side effects?" or "What kind of side effects does this have?" or "Is this anything like (another specific drug)?" More often than not, pharmacists simply answer the question without really listening to the underlying concern. "Why do you ask?" is an appropriate response, especially if the patient looks hesitant or the intonation of the question suggests doubt about taking the medication. When the author uses this question, patients often disclose that a relative had it (or a similar medication) or the media has reported problems with the drug. These indirect experiences create enough doubt such that the patient wavers about taking the medication.

Compliance problems can be categorized into three groups. The first is a *knowledge* deficit. In these cases, patients have insufficient information or skills or misinformation that prevents compliance. An example is the patient who was never been shown or has forgotten how to use an inhaler. The second group involves *practical impediments* or barriers, such as complex drug regimens involving multiple drugs and/or different dosage schedules, difficulty in developing routines that facilitate medication compliance, difficulty in opening containers, or insufficient mental aptitude to comply. The final category is *attitudinal barriers.* Among the most difficult to identify and manage, these include patient beliefs about health, disease, and/or treatment that are inconsistent with the prescribed regimen. Once the specific cause is identified, a specific strategy to manage that problem can be attempted. Most knowledge and skill deficiencies can be successfully corrected with education and/or training. Practical impediments respond well to specific measures such as simplifying regimens, use of easy-open containers, and enlisting the aid of a spouse or caregiver. Attitudinal issues tend to be the most complex and difficult to solve.

CONCLUSIONS

Contemporary pharmacy practice is changing at a very rapid pace. Pharmaceutical care, which focuses on the outcomes of drug therapy, is the founding principle for today's practitioners. The delivery of quality pharmaceutical care involves the skills and techniques discussed in this chapter and many others that support the pharmacist–patient interaction and medication use process. As direct patient contact and responsibility for drug therapy outcomes become the main task for pharmacists, the skills of interpersonal communication, medication history taking, patient consultation, plus compliance monitoring and enhancement become the "tools of the trade." The consistent application of a high level of interpersonal and applied clinical skills by pharmacists will lead to optimal outcomes for patients.

REFERENCES

1. Bolton R. People Skills. New York, Simon & Schuster, 1979.
2. Gardner M, Boyce RW, Herrier RN. Pharmacist–Patient Consultation Program, Unit 1: An Interactive Approach to Verify Patient Understanding. New York, Pfizer, 1991.
3. Pharmacist–Patient Consultation Program, Unit 2: Counseling Patients in Challenging Situations. New York, Pfizer, 1993.
4. Meldrum H. Interpersonal Communication in Pharmaceutical Care. New York, Haworth Press, 1994.
5. Muldary TW. Interpersonal Relations for Health Professionals: A Social Skills Approach. New York, Macmillan, 1983.
6. Meade V. OBRA '90: How has pharmacy reacted? Am Pharm 1995; NS35:12–16.
7. Parker RM, Williams MV, Weiss BD, et al. Health literacy: Report of the council on scientific affairs. JAMA 1999;281:552–557.
8. Gardner M, Hurd PD, Slack M. Effect of information organization on recall of medication instructions. J Clin Pharm Ther 1989;14:1–7.
9. Lamb GC, Green SS, Heron J. Can physicians warn patients of potential side effects without fear of causing those side effects? Arch Intern Med 1994;154:2753–2756.
10. Howland JS, Baker MG, Poe T. Does patient education cause side effects? A controlled trial. J Fam Pract 1990;31:62–64.
11. Meldrum H, Hardy M. Challenges in communicating about risk. In: Communicating Risk to Patients: Proceedings of the Conference. Rockville, MD; United States Pharmacopeial Convention, 1995:36–49.
12. Boyce RW, Herrier RN. Obtaining and using patient data. Am Pharm 1991;NS31:65–71.
13. Hammond RW, Schwartz AH, Campbell MJ, et. al. Collaborative drug therapy management. Pharmacotherapy 2003;23:1210-1225.
14. Anderson RM. Is the problem of noncompliance all in our heads? Diabetes Educ 1985;11:31–34.
15. Herrier RN, Boyce RW. Compliance with prescribed drug regimens. In: Bressler R, Katz M, eds. Geriatric Pharmacology. New York, McGraw-Hill, 1993:63–77.
16. Eraker SA, Kirscht JP, Becker MH. Understanding and improving patient compliance. Ann Intern Med 1984;100:258–268.

PATIENT CASES

This section includes three scenarios with patient profiles and prescriptions that require education. First, review the profile and prescription and think about issues that may arise during the consultation. Then provide written answers to the questions asked. Use concepts from the preceding material on education strategies, as well as any other techniques you think are useful or have found useful through your own experience or by observing others in practice.

CASE NO. 1: SALLY M. JOHNSON

NAME	**Johnson, Sally M.**	DATE 2/20/08
ADDRESS	1862 Briar Court Lansdale, PA 18018	AGE IF CHILD
R$_x$	FULL DIRECTIONS FOR USE	Rx No. 148647
		Date filled
	Tamoxifen 10 mg	Cost
	#60	Fee
	Sig: 1 po BID	Total Price
		❏ Do not refill
		No. of refills authorized: 6

❏ IDENTIFY CONTENTS ON LABEL UNLESS CHECKED
❏ NONPROPRIETARY EQUIVALENT UNLESS CHECKED

S. Mayer M.D.

Sally comes to the pharmacy alone to pick up a tamoxifen prescription. You have reviewed the profile and are ready to educate her on the medication.

1. Before talking with the patient, what functional and emotional barriers would you expect during the consultation? What else would you like to know about your patient?

2. How are you going to begin the consultation?

Patient Medication Profile

Name:	Sally M. Johnson	**Known Diseases**	**Allergies and Sensitivities**	**Additional Information**
Address:	1862 Briar Court	S/P hysterectomy 9/00 with estrogen replacement	Sulfa: rash	
	Lansdale, PA 18018	S/P surgery, CA breast 2/08		
Telephone:	832-7358			
Date of Birth:	4/15/48			

Date	Rx No.	Medication	Strength	Quantity	Dosage Regimen	R.Ph.	Physician
07/18/07	83104	Premarin	0.625 mg	#100	1 QD	JD	Hepler
10/25/07	89436	Premarin	0.625 mg	#100	1 QD	HV	Hepler
12/04/07	145922	Tylox		#12	1–2 Q 4 h PRN	JD	Cavanaugh
12/04/07	145923	Dicloxacillin	250 mg	#40	2 QID	JD	Cavanaugh

CA, cancer; S/P, status post.

3. Listed below are three different responses by the patient to the first *Prime Question*. For each statement, consider what each statement reveals about what the patient knows or feels, and state what should happen next in the consultation.

   Patient Response A[1]: *"He gave it to me after my surgery."*

   Patient Response B: *"I just had surgery for breast cancer."*

   Patient Response C: *"I know what it's for."*

4. Listed below are three different responses to the second *Prime Question*. Consider what each tells you, and state what you would do next in the consultation.

   Patient Response A: *"I'm going to take it twice a day."*

   Patient Response B: *"It's on the label, isn't it?"*

   Patient Response C: *"I don't remember. He didn't tell me."*

5. Listed below are three different responses to the third *Prime Question*. Consider what each tells you, and state what you would do next in the consultation.

   Patient Response A: *"I hope it will keep my cancer in check."*

   Patient Response B: *"The doctor says things look good, but I thought I heard something about uterine cancer?"*

   Patient Response C: *"Nothing. I'm not sure anything is going to help me now."*

CASE NO. 2: THOMAS GORDON

NAME	**Gordon, Thomas**	DATE 2/15/08
ADDRESS	38 Main Street Muncie, IL 82695	AGE IF CHILD
R$_x$	FULL DIRECTIONS FOR USE	Rx No. 148647
		Date filled
	Cephalexin 500 mg	Cost
	#40	Fee
	Sig: 1 po QID	Total Price
		❏ Do not refill
		No. of refills authorized: 0
❏ IDENTIFY CONTENTS ON LABEL UNLESS CHECKED		
❏ NONPROPRIETARY EQUIVALENT UNLESS CHECKED		
		B. Higley M.D.

Tom is a 53-year-old man with type 2 diabetes mellitus who is picking up an antibiotic for an infected cut on his arm. He owns his own construction company and is always "on the go." You are ready to educate him about his antibiotic prescription.

1. What concerns do you have based on review of the patient's medication profile? What else would you like to know about your patient? Before talking with the patient, what functional

and emotional barriers would you expect during education? What are the goals of the education?

2. How are you going to begin the education?

3. Listed below are Tom's responses to the *Prime Questions*. Consider what each response reveals about what the patient knows or feels, and state how you would address any concerns you detect.

   Pharmacist: "What did the doctor tell you the medication was for?"

   Tom: "He said he was giving me an antibiotic for this infection on my arm. It started as just a scratch, but it's gotten really bad."

   Pharmacist: "How did the doctor tell you to take the medicine?"

   Tom: "I don't know. He said it was on the label. I know I'm supposed to take it all."

   Pharmacist: "What did the doctor tell you to expect?"

   Tom: "I guess it will kill the infection and make the cut heal."

4. You have decided to ask about glipizide. Listed next is Tom's answer to your inquiry about the glipizide. Consider what the statement reveals, and state how you would address his concerns.

   Tom: "Yeah, well, I'm really busy with my business and it's hard to remember to take it."

CASE NO. 3: WILLIAM HODGES

NAME	**Hodges, William**	DATE 7/12/08
ADDRESS	4212 W. Mission Lane Albuquerque, NM 87546	AGE IF CHILD
R$_x$	FULL DIRECTIONS FOR USE	Rx No. 148647
	1. Digoxin 0.125 mg #45	Date filled
	Sig: 1 tab po Q AM on Sat M W F	Cost
	2 tabs po Q AM on Tues Thurs Sun	Fee
		Total Price
	2. Captopril 25 mg #180	❏ Do not refill
	Sig: 2 po TID	No. of refills authorized: 6
❏ IDENTIFY CONTENTS ON LABEL UNLESS CHECKED		
❏ NONPROPRIETARY EQUIVALENT UNLESS CHECKED		
		Ames M.D.

Bill is a 65-year-old man with an 8-year history of congestive heart failure secondary to an anterior wall myocardial infarction. Shortly after his recovery, he had a four-vessel coronary artery bypass graft performed. In addition to his prescription medications, he takes aspirin 81 mg daily to prevent re-infarction.

Bill has seen his physician today and brings in renewal prescriptions for digoxin and captopril (captopril replaced nifedipine due to lack of efficacy). His condition worsened enough that he had to cancel his June trip to Disneyland with his grandchildren.

[1]Patient statements A, B, and C do not necessarily correspond throughout the consultation.

Patient Medication Profile

		Known Diseases		Allergies and Sensitivities		Additional Information	
Name:	Thomas Gordon	Diabetes since 1997		NKA			
Address:	38 Main Street						
	Muncie, IL 82695						
Telephone:	542-5016						
Date of Birth:	01/10/52						

Date	Rx No.	Medication	Strength	Quantity	Dosage Regimen	R.Ph.	Physician
01/10/07	75243	Glipizide	10 mg	100	1 Q AM	EM	B. Higley
06/20/07	75243R	Glipizide	10 mg	100	1 Q AM	EM	B. Higley
10/28/07	75243R	Glipizide	10 mg	100	1 Q AM	JR	B. Higley

NKA, no known allergies.

1. Review the patient's profile. What concerns do you have based on your review of the patient profile? What are the goals of the education?

2. How are you going to begin the education?

3. Listed below are Bill's responses to Show-and-Tell questions. What do you notice?

    a. Digoxin

    Pharmacist: "What is this for?" (as he shows the patient the tablets)

    Bill: "That's digoxin, my heart pill."

    Pharmacist: "How do you take it?"

    Bill: "I take it once a day in the morning."

    Pharmacist: "What kind of problems are you having?"

    Bill: "None. I'm doing great!"

    b. Captopril

    Pharmacist: "What is this for?" (while showing the patient the tablets)

    Bill: "Also for my heart."

    Pharmacist: "How do you take it?"

    Bill: "Uh … two, three times a day."

    Pharmacist: "What kind of problems are you having?"

    Bill: "None…What kind of problems could this medicine cause?"

4. How should you respond to Bill's last question?

5. Bill tells you that captopril made him feel funny when he first started taking it. What should be your next response, and what technique should you now use?

6. The patient's response to your questions was:

    a. "I felt real dizzy."

    b. "It started about 24 hours after I started taking it."

    c. "It was bad enough that I saw spots and almost fell."

    d. "It happened primarily when I got up out of bed or from a chair."

    e. "I tried getting up slowly and it only helped some, so I stopped it for a day and it went away. Then I started back at one pill twice a day for a couple of weeks. I'm back up to one pill three times a day and I'm not having any problems. I'm going to try to slowly increase it to what the doctor wants me to take. I meant to ask him about it, but I forgot."

    f. "I haven't noticed anything else except this new medicine seems to be working better than the other. I've got lots more energy and I can make that six-block walk to the store without getting winded."

    What clinical assessment do you make from these responses?

7. Before taking action to correct the problem, what should you do now in the education?

8. What about the problem with his digoxin?

9. You need to call Dr. Ames. How would you phrase your comments to Dr. Ames regarding the two problems you detected?

10. What would you recommend to Dr. Ames?

Patient Medication Profile

Name:	William Hodges	**Known Diseases**	**Allergies and Sensitivities**	**Additional Information**
Address:	4212 W. Mission Ln.	S/P CABG 1999	Penicillin	
	Albuquerque, NM	Angina		
	87546			
Telephone:	505/425-7219	CHF		
Date of Birth:	3/22/39			

Date	Rx No.	Medication	Strength	Quantity	Dosage Regimen	R.Ph.	Physician
04/20/08	18591	Digoxin	0.125 mg	45	1 Sat M W F 2 Sun T Th	BR	Ames
04/20/08	18592	K Tabs	10 mEq	60	2 QD	BR	Ames
04/20/08	18593	Furosemide	40 mg	15	½ tab QD	BR	Ames
04/20/08	18594	Nifedipine XL	30 mg	60	1 BID	BR	Ames
05/15/08	21052	Digoxin	0.125 mg	45	1 Sat M W F 2 Sun T Th	JC	Ames
05/15/08	21053	K Tabs	10 mEq	120[a]	2 QD	JC	Ames
05/15/08	21054	Furosemide	40 mg	30[a]	½ tab QD	JC	Ames
05/15/08	21055	Nifedipine XL	30 mg	60	1 BID	JC	Ames
6/16/08	24273	Digoxin	0.125 mg	45	1 Sat M W F 2 Sun T Th	DT	Ames
6/16/08	24274	K Tabs	10 mEq	60	2 QD	DT	Ames
6/16/08	24275	Furosemide	40 mg	15	½ tab QD	DT	Ames
6/16/08	24276	Captopril	25 mg	180	2 TID	DT	Ames

BID, twice daily; CABG, coronary artery bypass graft; CHF, congestive heart failure; QD, every day; S/P, status post; TID, three times daily.
[a]Vacation supply.

TERRY L. SCHWINGHAMMER, PHARMD, FCCP, FASHP, BCPS

CHAPTER 4

Care Planning: A Component of the Patient Care Process

THE PATIENT CARE PROCESS

The *patient care process* for pharmacists is a systematic and comprehensive method that is employed to identify, solve, and prevent drug therapy problems.[1] A drug therapy problem is "any undesirable event experienced by a patient which involves, or is suspected to involve, drug therapy and that interferes with achieving the desired goals of therapy."[1] The patient care process includes three essential elements: 1) assessment of the patient's drug-related needs; 2) creation of a care plan to meet those needs; and 3) follow-up evaluation to determine whether positive outcomes were achieved. Consequently, development of a patient care plan is only one component of the overall patient care process. Before developing a patient-specific care plan, it is important for the clinician to have an understanding of the comprehensive nature of the patient care process. This process offers a logical and consistent framework that can be most useful in care planning and serves as the framework for this chapter.

ASSESSMENT OF DRUG-RELATED NEEDS

The first step in assessment is to identify the patient's drug-related needs by collecting, organizing, and integrating pertinent patient, drug, and disease information. In the patient care process, as with all direct patient care services, the patient is the primary source of information. This involves asking patients what they *want* (expectations) and what they *don't want* (concerns) and determining how well they understand their drug therapies. For example, the clinician may ask, "How may I help you today?" or "What concerns do you have that I may address for you today?" In addition to speaking with the patient, data can also be obtained from: 1) family members or caretakers when appropriate; 2) the patient's current and past medical records; and 3) discussions with other health care providers. The types of information that may be relevant are described below.[1,2]

Patient Information

- Demographics and background information: age, gender, race, height, weight.
- Social history: living arrangements, occupation, special needs (e.g., physical abilities, cultural traits, drug administration devices).
- Family history: relevant health histories of parents and siblings.
- Insurance/administrative information: name of health plan, primary care physician.

Disease Information

- Past medical history.
- Current medical problems.
- History of present illness.

- Pertinent information from the review of systems, physical examination, laboratory results, x-ray/imaging results.
- Medical diagnoses.

Drug Information

- Allergies, side effects (include the name of the medication and the reaction that occurred).
- Current prescription medications:
  ✓ How the medication was prescribed.
  ✓ How the patient is actually taking the medication.
  ✓ Effectiveness and side effects of current medications.
  ✓ Questions or concerns about current medications.
- Current nonprescription medications, vitamins, dietary supplements, and other alternative/complementary therapies.
- Past prescription and nonprescription medications (i.e., those discontinued within the past 6 months).

The information obtained is then organized, analyzed, and integrated to: 1) determine whether the patient's drug therapy is appropriate, effective, safe, and convenient for the patient; 2) identify drug therapy problems that may interfere with goals of therapy; and 3) identify potential drug therapy problems that require prevention. One method of organizing and integrating this information with appropriate pharmacotherapeutic knowledge has been described as the Pharmacotherapy Workup© (copyright 2003, the Peters Institute of Pharmaceutical Care).[1]

Drug therapy problems are uncovered through careful assessment of the patient, drug, and disease information to determine the appropriateness of each medication regimen. This process involves a logical sequence of steps. It begins with evaluating each medication regimen for appropriateness of indication; then optimizing the drug and dosage regimen to ensure maximum effectiveness; and finally, individualizing drug therapy to make it as safe as possible for the patient. After completing these three steps, the practitioner considers other issues such as cost, compliance, and convenience.

Drug therapy problems can be placed into distinct categories, as summarized below. See Table 4-1 for a useful checklist that can be used in actual practice situations.[1]

1. *Inappropriate indication* for drug use
   a. The patient requires additional drug therapy.
   b. The patient is taking unnecessary drug therapy.
2. *Ineffective* drug therapy
   a. The patient is taking a drug that is not effective for his/her situation.
   b. The medication dose is too low.

TABLE 4-1	Drug Therapy Problems to Be Resolved or Prevented
Assessment	**Drug Therapy Problem**
Indication	**Unnecessary drug therapy**
	No medical indication
	Duplicate therapy
	Nondrug therapy indicated
	Treating avoidable adverse drug reaction
	Addictive/recreational use
	Needs additional drug therapy
	Untreated condition
	Preventive/prophylactic
	Synergistic/potentiating
Effectiveness	**Needs different drug product**
	More effective drug available
	Condition refractory to drug
	Dosage form inappropriate
	Not effective for condition
	Dosage too low
	Wrong dose
	Frequency too long
	Duration too short
	Drug interaction
	Incorrect administration
Safety	**Adverse drug reaction**
	Undesirable effect
	Unsafe drug for patient
	Drug interaction
	Dose administered or changed too rapidly
	Allergic reaction
	Contraindications present
	Dosage too high
	Wrong dose
	Frequency too short
	Duration too long
	Drug interaction
	Incorrect administration
Compliance	**Nonadherence**
	Directions not understood
	Patient prefers not to take
	Patient forgets to take
	Drug product too expensive
	Cannot swallow or administer
	Drug product not available

Adapted with permission from Cipolle RJ, Strand LM, Morley PC. Pharmaceutical Care Practice: A Clinician's Guide, 2nd ed. New York, McGraw-Hill, 2004:168.

3. *Unsafe* drug therapy

　a. The patient is experiencing an adverse drug reaction.

　b. The medication dose is too high.

4. Inappropriate *adherence* or *compliance*

　a. The patient is unable or unwilling to take the medication as prescribed.

A drug therapy problem can be resolved or prevented only when the cause of the problem is clearly understood. Therefore, it is necessary to identify and categorize both the drug therapy problem and its cause (Table 4-2).[1]

CREATION OF A PATIENT CARE PLAN

Care plan development is a cooperative effort that should involve the patient as an active participant. It may also involve an interdisciplinary team of care providers and the patient's family. Care planning involves establishing therapeutic goals and determining appropriate interventions to:

1. Resolve all existing drug therapy problems.

TABLE 4-2	Causes of Drug Therapy Problems
Drug Therapy Problem	**Possible Causes of Drug Therapy Problems**
Unnecessary drug therapy	No valid medication indication for the drug at this time.
	Multiple drug products are used when only single-drug therapy is required.
	The condition is better treated with nondrug therapy.
	Drug therapy is used to treat an avoidable adverse drug reaction associated with another medication.
	The medical problem is caused by drug abuse, alcohol use, or smoking.
Need for additional drug therapy	A medical condition exists that requires initiation of new drug therapy.
	Preventive therapy is needed to reduce the risk of developing a new condition.
	A medical condition requires combination therapy to achieve synergism or additive effects.
Ineffective drug	The drug is not the most effective one for the medical problem.
	The drug product is not effective for the medical condition.
	The condition is refractory to the drug product being used.
	The dosage form is inappropriate.
Dosage too low	The dose is too low to produce the desired outcome.
	The dosage interval is too infrequent.
	A drug interaction reduces the amount of active drug available.
	The duration of therapy is too short.
Adverse drug reaction	The drug product causes an undesirable reaction that is not dose-related.
	A safer drug is needed because of patient risk factors.
	A drug interaction causes an undesirable reaction that is not dose-related.
	The regimen was administered or changed too rapidly.
	The product causes an allergic reaction.
	The drug is contraindicated because of patient risk factors.
Dosage too high	The dose is too high for the patient.
	The dosing frequency is too short. The duration of therapy is too long.
	A drug interaction causes a toxic reaction to the drug product.
	The dose was administered too rapidly.
Noncompliance	The patient does not understand the instructions.
	The patient prefers not to take the medication.
	The patient forgets to take the medication.
	Drug product is too expensive.
	The patient cannot swallow or self-administer the medication properly.
	The drug product is not available for the patient.

Adapted with permission from Cipolle RJ, Strand LM, Morley PC. Pharmaceutical Care Practice: A Clinician's Guide, 2nd ed. New York, McGraw-Hill, 2004:178–179.

2. Achieve the goals of therapy intended for each active medical problem.

3. Prevent future drug therapy problems that have a potential to develop.

Although care plans have been a standard component of the practice of other health professionals (e.g., nurses, physical therapists, respiratory therapists) for many years, there is still no standard, widely accepted method of care planning in pharmacy. In 1995, the Joint Commission on Accreditation of Healthcare Organizations (JCAHO) made pharmaceutical care planning a requirement for accreditation in all settings that it accredits. This requirement mandates that pharmaceutical care planning be included in the overall plan of care for the patient.[3] Implementation of a systematic care planning process serves to organize the pharmacist's practice, to communicate activities to other health care professionals, and to provide a record of drug therapy interventions in the event that questions arise regarding the standard of care provided to a patient.

It cannot be overemphasized that a plan of care is not merely a document; rather, it is a systematic, ongoing process of planning, action, and documentation. It is a dynamic instrument that reflects the continuing care that is modified according to the patient's changing needs.[4] The most essential element to remember is that the needs of the patient drive the plan, regardless of the care-planning format used. In short, the plan must be tailored to the needs of each unique patient. All care providers and the patient should agree on the care plan because each participant has a responsibility for implementing a portion of the plan. In the ambulatory care setting, the patient often assumes much of the responsibility for plan implementation.

Organization of a care plan is important, and each medical problem should be addressed separately and in its entirety so that the drug therapy problems associated with each condition and the plans for intervention are logically organized and implemented. The elements of a care plan include:

- *Medical condition:* List the disease state for which the patient has drug-related needs.
- *Drug therapy problems:* State the drug therapy problems by including the patient's problem or condition, the drug therapy involved, and the association between the drug(s) and the patient's condition(s).
- *Goals of therapy:* State the goals in the future tense. Goals should be realistic, measurable and/or observable, specific, and associated with a definite time frame.
- *Interventions:* In collaboration with the patient, the practitioner develops and prioritizes a list of activities to address the patient's drug-related needs. The patient's input is important because the plan should adequately address the patient's unique concerns, needs, and preferences. The list of activities may be stated in the past, present, or future tense. Include the recommendations made to the patient, the caregiver on the patient's behalf, or to the prescriber to resolve (or prevent) the patient's drug therapy problems.
- *Follow-up plan:* Determine when the patient should return for follow-up and what will occur at that subsequent visit.

An example of how each of these components might be incorporated into a care plan is given in the following case vignette:

Patrick Murphy is a 73-year-old man who underwent coronary artery bypass grafting 2 months ago and was started on simvastatin 10 mg by mouth (po) once daily 6 weeks ago for dyslipidemia. The results of this week's fasting lipid profile revealed total cholesterol 230 milligrams/deciliter (mg/dL), low density lipoprotein (LDL) cholesterol 141 mg/dL, high density lipoprotein cholesterol 45 mg/dL, and triglycerides 220 mg/dL. He continues to smoke 1.5 packs of cigarettes per day.

- *Medical condition:* Dyslipidemia.
- *Drug therapy problems:* Dyslipidemia treated with an inadequate dose of a lipid-lowering agent.
- *Goals of therapy:* The patient's LDL cholesterol will be lowered to <100 mg/dL within 6 weeks. (Note: Because the patient has known coronary artery disease, his goal LDL cholesterol is <100 mg/dL.[5])
- *Interventions:* The maximum dose of simvastatin is 80 mg, so the dose should be increased in an attempt to achieve the target LDL level. Increase simvastatin to 20 mg po once daily; #30 dispensed. Reviewed possible side effects of simvastatin with patient (constipation, rare muscle weakness) and monitored for liver injury (serum alanine aminotransferase measurements). Recommended that the patient consider stopping smoking—advised to keep a log of smoking habits, including number of cigarettes, time of day, and trigger events.

- *Follow-up plan:* Patient will return to clinic in 6 weeks for a repeat fasting lipid profile, questioning about potential adverse effects, and discussion of a plan for smoking cessation.

FOLLOW-UP EVALUATION

The purpose of a follow-up evaluation is to evaluate the positive and negative impact of the care plan on the patient, to uncover new drug therapy problems, and to take appropriate action to address new problems or adjust previous therapies as needed. Follow-up evaluation requires direct contact with the patient to obtain feedback about the benefits of therapy achieved, the occurrence of problems such as side effects, and patient concerns about the treatment. Additionally, relevant data are gathered from current clinical assessments, laboratory tests, radiographs, and other procedures. The practitioner evaluates and documents the patient's progress in achieving the goals of therapy.

The evaluation involves comparing goals of therapy with the patient's current status. Cipolle, Strand, and Morley developed terminology to describe the patient's status, the medical conditions, and the comparative evaluation of that status with the previously determined therapeutic goals.[1] These terms also describe the actions taken as a result of the follow-up evaluation:

Status	Definition
Resolved	Therapeutic goals achieved for the acute condition, discontinue therapy
Stable	Therapeutic goals achieved, continue the same therapy for chronic disease management
Improved	Progress is being made in achieving goals, continue the same therapy because more time is required to assess the full benefit of therapy
Partial improvement	Progress is being made, but minor adjustments in therapy are required to fully achieve the therapeutic goals before the next assessment
Unimproved	Little or no progress has been made, but continue the same therapy to allow additional time for benefit to be observed
Worsened	A decline in health is observed despite an adequate duration using the optimal drug; modify drug therapy (e.g., increase the dose of the current medication, add a second agent with additive or synergistic effects)
Failure	Therapeutic goals have not been achieved despite an adequate dose and duration of therapy; discontinue current medication(s) and start new therapy
Expired	The patient died while receiving drug therapy; document possible contributing factors, especially if they may be drug related

Example: If the patient Mr. Murphy described above returns in 6 weeks with a repeat fasting LDL cholesterol of 120 mg/dL without complaints of side effects, the outcome status of this patient would be partial improvement. Another adjustment in therapy is indicated to further reduce his LDL cholesterol (e.g., increase the simvastatin dose to 40 mg po once daily).

EXAMPLE OF CARE PLAN DOCUMENTATION

Each step in the patient care process must be documented. Documentation should take place on an ongoing basis to provide an updated record of the patient's current and changing needs, care activities in response to those needs, the patient's progress, and plans for future care and follow-up evaluation. This document provides a means for communication among health care providers and is now required for accreditation by JCAHO. What JCAHO requires is not merely a list of the patient's current medications but a document that reflects the systematic and dynamic process of patient care. The example provided in Fig. 4-1 is intended to demonstrate to students how a care plan might be created.

A blank care plan form is also included at the end of this chapter for use by students who are completing the cases for this casebook (see Appendix A). Students may practice using this form when completing the case studies in this casebook. The vast amount of medical information available and the widespread computerization of patient records make the use of electronic pharmaceutical care records virtually mandatory. Consequently, use of this relatively simple hard-copy form should be considered only the first step in developing the student's ability to electronically organize and manage large volumes of complex medical information.

On the electronic resource *AccessPharmacy.com* (subscription required), care plans from the casebook can be completed electronically and e-mailed to course instructors for grading. The patient cases from this casebook are also available on *AccessPharmacy.com*, providing a seamless resource for creating and evaluating the patient care plans written by students.

Example Case Vignette: Donald Benferardo is a 64-year-old man with osteoarthritis currently treated with nabumetone. He has been diagnosed with hypertension based on the average of two blood pressure (BP) readings taken at three previous clinic visits.[6] The hypertension is presently untreated. What information must be included in the patient's care plan?

Patient Information

- *The patient's name* is essential to identify the patient to whom the record belongs. The name, Donald Benferardo, should be the first information placed on the chart. Although this guideline seems logical, it sometimes does not happen. When in a hurry, a care provider may grab a blank form and begin to make notes with the intention of placing the patient's personal information on it later, and in the midst of distractions, the name is not recorded.

- *Current address and phone number* are necessary for future contact and follow-up evaluation. The information should be complete (621 E. Greene Street, Washington, PA 15301), and the telephone number should include the area code (412-555-1950).

- *Insurance* information should include the name of the insurance plan and policy number (Metro United Health Plan #1234789) to ensure accurate billing of services.

- *Demographic* information including *age (birth date), gender, race, height, and weight* should be recorded for the purpose of individualizing drug therapy. Mr. Benferardo is a 64-year-old Caucasian man who is 5'11" tall and weighs 177 lbs. Include weight information in both pounds (lbs) and kilograms (kg). The equation for converting lbs to kg is as follows: weight in lbs/2.2 = weight in kg. Mr. Benferardo weighs 177 lbs or 80.4 kg (177/2.2 = 80.4). This information is used to determine the appropriate drug and dosage regimens for treatment. *Ideal body weight (IBW)* is necessary for calculating appropriate dosage for medications that do not distribute into fatty tissues. IBW is calculated as follows: For men, IBW = 50 kg + [2.3 × (height in inches above 5 feet)]. For women, IBW = 45.5 kg + [2.3 × (height in inches above 5 feet)]. For Mr. Benferardo, 50 kg + (2.3 × 11) = 75.3 kg.

- *Allergies and adverse drug reactions* should be documented with specific descriptions of the reactions that occurred. Reactions should be clearly identified as allergies or side effects. Mr. Benferardo has an allergic reaction to penicillin that resulted in hives. He also has experienced dyspepsia, a well-documented side effect of ibuprofen. This information is critical to avoiding

patient harm. Allergies are distinct from side effects. An allergy is an immune-mediated reaction that often precludes future use of the medication except in rare cases in which the benefit of using the drug outweighs the risk of the reaction. However, a side effect may sometimes be self-limiting with continued use, or it may be successfully managed with adjustments in the dosage regimen or administration. For example, a drug that is taken once daily and causes drowsiness may be administered at bedtime. A drug that causes GI upset may be successfully managed by taking it with meals.

- *Tobacco/alcohol/substance use* information is important for appropriate drug selection, dosing calculation, and patient education. Include the name of the substance, the amount, and frequency, when possible. Mr. Benferardo occasionally smokes approximately 3 cigars each week and drinks 1 ounce of whiskey with each cigar. It is important to record pertinent negatives for substance use. For example, caffeine may increase BP acutely, although tolerance to this effect develops quickly. Nevertheless, caffeine use may be relevant to this patient and should be recorded. Alcohol and tobacco may affect the metabolism of certain drugs and potentiate or counteract the benefits of other drugs. For example, tobacco enhances the metabolism of theophylline. Therefore, smokers generally require higher doses of theophylline to achieve therapeutic benefits. Substances such as cocaine, caffeine, or tobacco may enhance the sympathomimetic effect of some drugs while counteracting the sympatholytic effects of others, such as some antihypertensive medications.

- *Medical conditions* should be listed to offer a general overview of the patient's medical problems. The care plan is also organized according to the medical condition whereby all drug therapy problems associated with each medical condition are addressed separately and in their entirety.

Medication Record

- The list of medications should include the date each was started; the indication for use; and the drug name, strength, and regimen that the patient is actually taking. The *actual* regimen may differ from the *prescribed* regimen because patients don't always take medications as directed. Assessment of therapy must be made based upon the actual therapy the patient is receiving. Mr. Benferardo is currently taking nabumetone two 750-mg tablets po daily. A stop date should be recorded for medications that have been discontinued.

- Relevant clinical impressions or comments can also be recorded, for example: "Discontinued ibuprofen secondary to dyspepsia that occurred even when taken with food." Also note the antihypertensive regimen, which was initiated with hydrochlorothiazide 25 mg po once daily and subsequently changed to triamterene/hydrochlorothiazide 37.5/25 mg po once daily. Atenolol 50 mg po once daily was added later because only partial improvement in hypertension was achieved with diuretic therapy.

Assessment, Plan, and Follow-Up Evaluation

This section of the patient's chart provides a record of therapeutic interventions and the patient's responses to them. Information is documented as events occur, providing a "flow chart" of the patient's progress to date. The historical information contained in this chart is important to incorporate in therapeutic decision making.

- *The Date* should be recorded in the far-left column to document when each encounter occurred. Mr. Benferardo's chart shows that he has been seen three times: on May 3, May 17, and May 31, 2008.

PHARMACEUTICAL CARE PATIENT RECORD

Patient Name: Donald Benferardo		**Gender:** M	
Address: 621 E. Greene St., Washington PA 15301		**Race:** W	
Telephone: 412-555-1950	**Age:** 64	**Actual Weight:** 177 lb (80 kg)	
Insurance: Metro United Health Plan #1234789		**Ideal Weight:** 166 lb (75.3 kg)	
Medical Conditions: Osteoarthritis left knee (stable)		**Allergies:** Penicillin ⟶ hives	
Tobacco/Alcohol/Substance Use: Occasional cigar 3×/wk; EtOH 3×/wk; no caffeine		**Adverse Reactions:** Ibuprofen ⟶ dyspepsia	

Medication Record

Start Date	Stop Date	Indication	Drug Name	Actual Strength	Regimen	Clinical Impressions
12/14/05		Osteoarthritis	Nabumetone	750 mg	2 tablet po once daily	Tolerating well minor knee pain
5/03/08	5/17/08	HTN	Hydrochlorothiazide	25 mg	1 tablet po once daily	5/17/08: D/C due to hypokalemia
5/17/08		HTN	Triamterene/ Hydrochlorothiazide	37.25/25 mg	1 tablet po once daily	5/31/08: K^+ WNL; HTN partially improved
5/31/08		HTN	Atenolol	50 mg	1 tablet po once daily	

Assessment, Plan, and Follow-Up Evaluation

Date	Medical Condition	Drug-Therapy Problem	Goal	Current Status	Interventions	Follow-Up Plan
5/3/08	HTN	Untreated HTN	Lower BP to 110–138/70–88 within 4 wks	Untreated (BP 160/104)	Start hydrochlorothiazide 25 mg po once daily × 4 wks	Return for BP check & serum K+ in 2 wks
5/17/08	HTN	Hypokalemia secondary to hydrochlorothiazide	K+ 3.5–5.0 mEq/L	Untreated (K+ 3.2 mEq/L)	Discontinue HCT Start triamterene/HCT 3.75/25 mg po once daily	Recheck K^+ in 2 wks
5/17/08	HTN	HTN inadequately treated with hydrochlorothiazide	BP 110–138/70–88	Partial improvement (BP 150/92)	Change to triamterene/HCT as above	Return in 2 wks for BP & K+ check
5/31/08	HTN	Hypokalemia requiring drug therapy	K+ 3.5–5.0 mEq/L	Stable (K+ 3.6 mEq/L)	Continue current therapy	Check symptoms of ↓K+ in 1 mo
5/31/08	HTN	HTN inadequately treated with hydrochlorothiazide	Same as above	Partial improvement (BP 146/92)	Add atenolol 50 mg po once daily × 4 wks	Return for BP check in 1 mo

FIGURE 4-1. Sample pharmaceutical care patient record. (BP, blood pressure; HTN, hypertension; WNL, within normal limits.)

- In the next column, *Medical Condition* specifies the medical diagnosis for which the medications are indicated. On May 3, Mr. Benferardo was diagnosed with hypertension; his subsequent visits also were for evaluation of hypertension.

- The *Drug Therapy Problem* is recorded in the next column to indicate the drug therapy problem(s) associated with each medical diagnosis. Each medical diagnosis may have one or more drug therapy problems associated with it. On May 3, Mr. Benferardo had one drug therapy problem—untreated hypertension. That is, he had an indication for drug therapy but was not receiving treatment. On May 17 and May 31, the dates were recorded twice because on these days he had two drug therapy problems that were being addressed. Each drug therapy problem should be recorded in a separate row. Although he had only one active diagnosis (hypertension), he had two drug therapy problems associated with that diagnosis as shown on May 17 and May 31. He had hypokalemia possibly secondary to hydrochlorothiazide and hypertension inadequately treated with hydrochlorothiazide.

- The *Goal* of therapy is recorded in the next column. Using the SMART acronym, therapy goals should be *Specific, Measurable* (or observable), and *Achievable*. The goal should also be directly *Related* to the drug therapy problem. In this case, the systolic BP goal should be less than 140 mm Hg with a diastolic pressure of less than 90 mm Hg. Treatment to lower levels may be useful if tolerated by the patient. For example, the clinician may establish an acceptable range of BP control, such as systolic BP between 110 and 138 mm Hg and diastolic BP between 70 and 88 mm Hg. The *Timeline* to achieve the goal should also be specified. For example, his BP should be reduced to within the indicated range within 4 weeks of therapy.

- The *Current Status* includes the patient's actual BP at each encounter. In this case, Mr. Benferardo's BP was 160/104 mm Hg on May 3 prior to starting drug therapy. Notice that his BP continues to decline with treatment. On May 17 and 31, his BPs were 150/92 and 146/92 mm Hg, respectively. The status on May 31 (4 weeks after treatment) is considered partially improved because the BP did decrease with treatment, but an adjustment in treatment is still required to achieve the BP goal.

- *Interventions* that were implemented must be recorded. The drug name, dose, route, frequency, and duration of therapy should be documented. On May 3, hydrochlorothiazide was started at a dose of 25 mg orally once a day. As you look down this column, you can see that the therapy was adjusted on May 17 and May 31. These interventions were made in response to the patient's BP as recorded in the previous column. By looking across the row, you can see the supportive evidence for the intervention: a clearly documented problem (hypertension) and the patient's status measured objectively (BP). Looking down the columns, one can see what interventions have been made and also how the patient has responded over time.

- The *Follow-Up Plan* specifies details of how the outcome of therapy will be assessed. This column should contain information about who will do what and when they will do it. The plan made on May 3 indicated that Mr. Benferardo was to return to the clinic in 2 weeks to have his BP and serum potassium level measured. This flow chart provides an easy way to see whether the patient is appearing for the follow-up visits. Mr. Benferardo did return for follow-up in 2 weeks (May 17) according to the plan. There should continue to be a follow-up plan as long as a person is receiving drug therapy. After the patient's condition is stabilized, the follow-up intervals may be much longer, such as every 6 months or once a year. However, the assessment, plan, and follow-up must continue for the duration of drug therapy. In this case, after Mr. Benferardo's BP is stabilized, he may be responsible for monitoring his own BP and assessing the side effects by self-monitoring while keeping a twice-yearly appointments for a more formal evaluation at the clinic. The patient's care plan remains active and represents the ongoing and dynamic process of providing pharmaceutical care.

Patient Summary

Based on the information documented in the care plan, the practitioner providing care to this patient and other health care professionals who have access to this information should be able to extract the following summary of this patient's past and present status regarding hypertension treatment and response.

Mr. Benferardo is a 64-year-old man diagnosed with osteoarthritis and hypertension. He was seen on May 3, 2008, at which time his BP was 160/104 mm Hg. His goal BP range was set as systolic BP of 110–138 mm Hg and diastolic BP of 70–88 mm Hg. This was the standard against which future BP measurements would be compared. He was started on hydrochlorothiazide 25 mg orally once daily for 2 weeks and was to return to clinic for a follow-up BP check and serum potassium level 2 weeks later. He returned according to the plan, but the BP reading of 152/98 indicated only a partial improvement. The BP reduction had not yet reached the goal level; it may take 4 weeks for the full effect of diuretic therapy to be manifested. Consequently, no adjustment in therapy was made pending an adequate trial of single-agent diuretic therapy. However, the low serum potassium value of 3.2 mEq/L (reference range 3.5–5.0 mEq/L) indicated hypokalemia that required treatment. Because the hypokalemia may have resulted from the thiazide diuretic, hydrochlorothiazide 25 mg was discontinued and a combination product containing triamterene 37.5 mg + hydrochlorothiazide 25 mg, 1 tablet orally once daily, was begun. He returned 2 weeks later as planned and his BP continued to show improvement (148/96 mm Hg), but it was not at the therapeutic goal that had been established 4 weeks earlier. This indicated partial improvement requiring further adjustment of his antihypertensive therapy. However, his potassium level had risen to within the normal range. Therefore, atenolol 50 mg orally once daily was added to the regimen. The patient was scheduled to return for a follow-up visit in 1 month.

CONCLUSIONS

Implementation of a care planning process is necessary for providing consistent pharmaceutical care and for documenting the outcomes of that care. It is also essential for obtaining compensation for care provided. Care planning captures past and current events occurring in a dynamic patient care process that is provided in response to changing patient needs. This process should be incorporated into the practice of each provider of pharmaceutical care, regardless of the practice setting.

REFERENCES

1. Cipolle RJ, Strand LM, Morley PC. Pharmaceutical Care Practice: The Clinician's Guide, 2nd ed. New York, McGraw-Hill, 2004.
2. ASHP Council on Professional Affairs. ASHP Guidelines on a standard method for pharmaceutical care. Am J Hosp Pharm 1996;53:1713–1716.
3. Rich DS. JCAHO's pharmaceutical care plan requirements. Hosp Pharm 1995;30(4):315–319.
4. McCallian DJ, Carlstedt BC, Rupp MT. Elements of a pharmaceutical care plan. Am J Pharm Assoc 1999;39(1):82–83.
5. Expert Panel on Detection, Evaluation, and Treatment of High Blood Cholesterol in Adults. Executive summary of the third report of the National Cholesterol Education Program (NCEP) Expert Panel on

detection, evaluation, and treatment of high blood cholesterol in adults (Adult Treatment Panel III). JAMA 2001;285:2486–2497.

6. The Seventh Report of the Joint National Committee on Prevention, Detection, Evaluation, and Treatment of High Blood Pressure: the JNC 7 report. JAMA 2003;289(19):2560–2572.

ACKNOWLEDGMENTS

This chapter is based on the chapter written for the Sixth Edition with co-author Grace D. Lamsam, PharmD, PhD.

Appendix A

Sample Pharmaceutical Care Patient Record for Creating a Care Plan

PHARMACEUTICAL CARE PATIENT RECORD

Patient Name:	**Gender:**
Address:	**Race:**
Telephone: **Age:**	**Actual Weight:**
Insurance:	**Ideal Weight:**
Medical Conditions:	**Allergies:**
Tobacco/Alcohol/Substance Use:	**Adverse Reactions:**

Medication Record

Start Date	Stop Date	Indication	Drug Name	Actual Strength	Regimen	Clinical Impressions

Assessment, Plan, and Follow-Up Evaluation

Date	Medical Condition	Drug-Therapy Problem	Goal	Current Status	Interventions	Follow-Up Plan

CHAPTER 5

Documentation of Pharmacotherapy Interventions

BRUCE R. CANADAY, PHARMD, BCPS, FASHP, FAPHA
PEGGY C. YARBOROUGH, PHARMD, MS, CPP, BC-ADM, CDE, FAPP, FASHP, NAPP
ROBERT M. MALONE, PHARMD, CDE, CPP
TIMOTHY J. IVES, PHARMD, MPH, BCPS, FCCP, FASHP, CPP

If there is no documentation, then it didn't happen! This philosophy is the standard in all health care settings as physicians, nurses, respiratory therapists, physical therapists, social workers, and other health care providers generate and maintain detailed notes regarding the patient's situation and their efforts to achieve the best possible outcomes for the patient. Documentation chronologically outlines the care the patient received and serves as a form of communication among health care practitioners, an important element that contributes to the quality of care provided. Each practitioner involved knows what evaluation has occurred, what the plan for the patient's treatment is, and who will provide it. Furthermore, third-party payers require reasonable documentation from practitioners that assures that the services provided are consistent with the insurance coverage.[1] General components of documentation include:

- A complete and legible record;
- Documentation for each encounter with a rationale for the encounter, physical findings, prior test results, assessment, clinical impression (or diagnosis), and plan for care;
- Identified health risk factors, and an easily inferred rationale for ordering diagnostic tests or ancillary services; and
- The patient's progress, response to and changes in treatment, and revision of the original diagnosis/assessment.

Traditionally, this documentation was paper based. These records are often inaccessible at the point of patient care, not easily transferable or transportable, illegible, poorly organized, and often may be missing key information. Due to these limitations, many academic centers and health care systems have developed and implemented electronic medical records (EMRs). Further, *Crossing the Quality Chasm* was published in 2001 by the Institute of Medicine. This report identified the EMR as a key component to improve access to medical information, facilitate decision support and collection of data, and reduce medical errors.[2] The EMR may also assist in proper documentation, reduce clinical variation, and improve the provision of quality preventative and chronic care.[3–6]

PRINCIPLES OF DOCUMENTATION

Documentation in the record is required to record pertinent facts, findings, and observations about a patient's health history, including past and present illnesses, examinations, tests, treatments, and outcomes. Particularly in an era of evolution of electronic databases,[7] it also facilitates:

- The ability of providers to evaluate and plan the patient's immediate treatment and monitor his/her health care over time;
- Communication and continuity of care among providers involved in the patient's care;

- Accurate and timely claims review and payment;
- Appropriate utilization review and quality of care evaluations;
- Collection of data that may be useful for research and education; and
- Appropriate coding (i.e., CPT [Current Procedural Terminology] and ICD-10-CM [International Statistical Classification of Diseases and Related Health Problems, Tenth Revision, Clinical Modification], from the World Health Organization) for use on health insurance claim forms should be supported by documentation in the patient record.

Much of this documentation is derived from a systematic patient care process of evaluation that is standardized within each discipline. For example, physicians are taught to perform a history and physical examination based upon a standardized review of body systems and to document their results using a universally accepted, standardized, systematic process.

Several evaluation/documentation systems have been suggested for health care professionals. More than 30 years ago, the use of a Problem-Oriented Medical Record was proposed[8] and most, if not all, physicians, nurse practitioners, physician associates, and other health care practitioners have been taught to write progress notes using the Subjective, Objective, Assessment, Plan (SOAP) format. The example elements of SOAP are as follows:

S = Subjective: Chief complaint; history of present illness; why the patient is being seen;
O = Objective: Evaluation of the patient, which may include appearance, mood, affect, mental status;
A = Assessment: Analysis or conclusion about the patient's current status/behavior, evidence of progress, response to intervention or medication, and change in functional status;
P = Plan: Interventions or actions taken in response to assessment, collaboration with others, plan for the next session, change in diagnosis, and documentation that the patient was informed of changes in interventions or medications.

Institutional consultant notes often use an abbreviated version of the SOAP format. This abbreviated version usually includes Findings (i.e., subjective and objective information), Assessment (or Impression), and Diagnosis (or Recommendations). In most cases, the EMR has embraced many of the key components of the above formats. EMR documentation is tailored to documenting medical encounters and history and also to maximize billing by meeting requirements established by the federal Centers for Medicare & Medicaid Services. Traditionally this documentation has been performed by dictation and transcription. Most EMRs use templates to accept automated insertion of clinical data and fields with "copy and paste" capabilities, both of which facilitate documentation.

Historically, pharmacy has not had a corresponding standard approach to the evaluation and documentation of the patient's pharmacotherapy that is applicable to all types of pharmacy practice settings. Thus, pharmacy has not been as active as other disciplines in documenting its contributions to patient care.

EVOLUTION OF PHARMACIST-PROVIDED CARE AND THE IMPORTANCE OF DOCUMENTATION

Pharmacist-provided care has gone through a long evolutionary process that, like all evolutionary processes, continues to bring change. Early descriptors such as *clinical pharmacy* continue to hold meaning[9] but have also spawned terms such as *pharmaceutical care* and, most recently, *medication therapy management* (MTM).

PHARMACEUTICAL CARE

Pharmaceutical care uses a process through which a pharmacist cooperates with a patient and other health care professionals in designing, implementing, and monitoring a therapeutic plan that will produce specific therapeutic outcomes for the patient.[10] This process involves three major functions:

1. Identifying potential and actual drug-related problems.
2. Resolving actual drug-related problems.
3. Preventing potential drug-related problems.

These functions aid in the provision of patient care through the identification of medication-related problems, development of a pharmacotherapeutic plan to address the problems, and the ultimate resolution or prevention of those problems.

As described in **Chapter 1**, a systematic approach is used in this casebook to identify and resolve the medication-related problems of patients. The steps can be summarized as follows:

1. Identification of real or potential medication therapy problems.
2. Determination of desired therapeutic outcomes and therapeutic endpoints.
3. Determination of therapeutic alternatives.
4. Design of an optimal pharmacotherapeutic plan for the patient.
5. Identification of parameters to evaluate the outcome.
6. Provision of patient education.
7. Communication and implementation of the pharmacotherapeutic plan.

Step 7 is crucial; the tenets of pharmaceutical care suggest that pharmacists should document, at the very least, the actual or potential drug therapy problems identified, as well as the associated interventions that they desire to implement or have implemented. Pharmacists must adequately communicate their recommendations and actions to non-pharmacy health care practitioners (e.g., physicians, nurses), the patient or caregiver (e.g., parents), or other pharmacists. The goal is to provide a clear, concise record of the actual/potential problem,[11,12] the thought process that led the pharmacist to select an intervention, and the intervention itself. Additionally, the ability to receive remuneration for services provided also necessitates an acceptable documentation strategy.

MEDICATION THERAPY MANAGEMENT

Eleven national pharmacy organizations achieved consensus on a definition of MTM in July 2004.[13] MTM was defined as a distinct service or group of services that optimize therapeutic outcomes for individual patients. MTM services are independent of, but can occur in conjunction with, the provision of a medication product. MTM encompasses a broad range of professional activities and responsibilities within the scope of practice of the licensed pharmacist or other qualified health care providers. These services include but are not limited to the following, according to the individual needs of the patient:

1. Performing or obtaining necessary assessments of the patient's health status;
2. Formulating a medication treatment plan;
3. Selecting, initiating, modifying, or administering medication therapy;
4. Monitoring and evaluating the patient's response to therapy, including safety and effectiveness;
5. Performing a comprehensive medication review to identify, resolve, and prevent medication-related problems, including adverse drug events;
6. Documenting the care delivered and communicating essential information to the patient's other primary care providers;
7. Providing verbal education and training designed to enhance patient understanding and appropriate use of his/her medications;
8. Providing information, support services, and resources designed to enhance patient adherence with his/her therapeutic regimens;
9. Coordinating and integrating MTM services within the broader health care–management services being provided to the patient.

In concert with this definition, patients, providers, payers, and health information technology system vendors have been encouraged to develop a documentation format that meets individual and customer needs.[14] This documentation format, while not a standard, can be useful in achieving the goals of the process. The white paper notes that the pharmacist is responsible for documenting services in a manner appropriate for evaluating patient progress and sufficient for billing purposes, and that the use of core documentation elements will help to create consistency in professional documentation and information sharing among members of the health care team, while facilitating practitioner, organization, or regional variations.[13] Documentation of MTM services includes the following information categories:

- Patient demographics.
- Known allergies, diseases, or conditions.
- A record of all medications, including prescription, nonprescription, herbal, and other dietary supplement products.
- Assessment of medication therapy problems and plans for resolution.
- Therapeutic monitoring performed.
- Interventions or referrals made.
- Education provided to the patient.
- Schedule and plan for follow-up appointment.
- Amount of time spent with the patient.
- Feedback provided to providers or patients.

While the precise format may not be critical at this point, standardization of documentation must and will evolve to provide for clarity in the history and plan, timely feedback, consistent follow-up, and enhanced continuity of care.

TRADITIONAL DOCUMENTATION FORMAT: SOAP NOTES

As noted above, in the SOAP note format subjective (S) and objective (O) data are recorded and then assessed (A) to formulate a plan (P). Subjective data include patient symptoms, things that may be observed about the patient, or information obtained about the patient. By its nature, subjective information is descriptive and generally cannot be confirmed by diagnostic tests or procedures. Much of the subjective information is obtained by speaking with the patient while obtaining the medical history, as described in **Chapter 1** (i.e., chief complaint, history of present illness, past medical history, family history, social history, medications, allergies, and review of systems). Important subjective information may also be obtained by direct interview with the patient after the initial medical history has been performed (e.g., a description of an adverse drug effect, rating of pain severity using standard scales).

A primary source of objective information (O) is the physical examination. Other relevant objective information includes laboratory values, serum drug concentrations (along with the target therapeutic range for each level), and the results of other diagnostic tests (e.g., electrocardiogram [ECG], x-rays, culture and sensitivity tests). Risk factors that may predispose the patient to a particular problem should also be considered for inclusion. The communication note should include only the pertinent positive and negative findings. Pertinent negative findings are signs and symptoms of the disease or problem that are not present in the particular patient being evaluated.

The assessment (A) section outlines what the practitioner thinks the patient's problem is, based upon the subjective and objective information acquired. This assessment often takes the form of a diagnosis or differential diagnosis. This portion of the SOAP note should include all of the reasons for the clinician's assessment. This helps other health care providers reading the note to understand how the clinician arrived at his or her particular assessment of the problem.

The plan (P) may include ordering additional diagnostic tests or initiating, revising, or discontinuing treatment. If the plan includes changes in pharmacotherapy, the rationale for the specific changes recommended should be described. The drug, dose, dosage form, schedule, route of administration, and duration of therapy should be included. The plan should be directed toward achieving a specific, measurable goal or endpoint, which should be clearly stated in the note. The plan should also outline the efficacy and toxicity parameters that will be used to determine whether the desired therapeutic outcome is being achieved and to detect or prevent drug-related adverse events. Ideally, information about the therapy that should be communicated to the patient should also be included in the plan. The plan should be reviewed and referred to in the note as often as necessary.

AN ALTERNATIVE APPROACH TO DOCUMENTING DRUG THERAPY PROBLEMS AND PLANS

There is a pharmacist equivalent of a physician's progress note in a systematized approach for the construction and maintenance of a record reflecting the pharmacist's contributions to care.[15] This process includes provisions for the identification and assessment of actual or potential medication-related problems, description of a therapeutic plan, and appropriate follow-up monitoring of the problems. Although there is no current uniform documentation system for the profession of pharmacy, students are encouraged to try this system as they learn to document patient interventions and compare its effectiveness with the SOAP format. In this system, problems that have been identified are addressed systematically in a pharmacist's note under the headings Findings, Assessment, Resolution, and Monitoring. The sections of the pharmacist's note can be easily recalled with the mnemonic F-A-R-M.

IDENTIFICATION OF DRUG THERAPY PROBLEMS

The first step in the construction of a FARM note is to clearly state the nature of the drug-related problem(s). Each problem in the FARM note should be addressed separately and assigned a sequential number. Understanding the types of problems that may occur facilitates identification of pharmacotherapy problems. Seven types of medication-related problems have been identified (see **Chapter 1**)[16]:

1. Unnecessary drug therapy
2. Needs additional drug therapy
3. Ineffective drug
4. Dosage too low
5. Adverse drug reaction
6. Dosage too high
7. Noncompliance

Use of a classification system such as this for the various types of medication-related problems offers at least two advantages. First, it presents a framework, applicable in any practice setting, to assure that the pharmacist has considered each possible type of problem. Second, categorization allows optimal data analysis and retrieval capabilities. Thus, problems as well as the interventions to resolve them can be stored in a standardized format in a computer. When an analysis of this information is needed at a later date, such as determining how much money was saved through an intervention, how outcomes were improved by the pharmacist, or how many problems of a certain type have occurred, the problems and interventions can be reviewed by groups rather than individually.

DOCUMENTATION OF FINDINGS

Each statement of a drug-related problem should be followed by documentation of the pertinent findings (F) indicating that the problem may (potential) or does (actual) exist. Information included in this section should include a summary of the pertinent information obtained after collection and thorough assessment of the available patient information. Demographic data that may be reported include a patient identifier (e.g., name, initials, or medical record number), age, race (if pertinent), and gender. As noted earlier under the section on SOAP notes, medical information included in the note should include both subjective and objective findings that indicate a drug-related problem.

ASSESSMENT OF PROBLEMS

The assessment (A) section of the FARM note includes the pharmacist's evaluation of the current situation (i.e., the nature, extent, type, and clinical significance of the problem). This part of the note should delineate the thought process that led to the conclusion that a problem did or did not exist and that an active intervention either was or was not necessary. If additional information is required to satisfactorily assess the problem and make recommendations, this data should be stated along with its source (e.g., the patient, pharmacist, physician). The severity or urgency of the problem should be indicated by stating whether the interventions that follow should be made immediately or within 1 day, 1 week, 1 month, or longer. The desired therapeutic endpoint or outcome should be stated. This may include both short-term goals (e.g., lower blood pressure to <140/90 mm Hg in a patient with primary hypertension [therapeutic endpoint]) and long-term goals (e.g., prevent cardiovascular complications in that patient [therapeutic outcome]).

PROBLEM RESOLUTION

The resolution (R) section should reflect the actions proposed (or already performed) to resolve the drug-related problem based upon the preceding analysis. The note should convey that, after consideration of all appropriate therapeutic options, the option(s) considered to be the most beneficial was either carried out or suggested to someone else (e.g., the physician, patient, or caregiver). Recommendations may include nonpharmacologic therapy, such as dietary modification or assisting devices (e.g., canes, walkers); the rationale for this method of treatment should be described. If pharmacotherapy is recommended, a specific drug, dose, route, schedule, and duration of therapy should be specified. It is not sufficient to simply provide a list of choices for the prescriber. Importantly, the rationale for selecting the particular regimen(s) should be stated. It is reasonable to include alternative regimens that would be satisfactory if the patient is unable to complete treatment with the initial regimen because of adverse effects, allergy, cost, or other reasons. If patient education is recommended, the information that will be included in the session should be described. Conversely, if certain types of information will be withheld from the patient, the reasons for doing so should be stated. If no action is recommended or was taken, that should be documented as well. In this situation, the note serves as a record of the pharmacist's involvement in the patient's care. The pharmacist then has documentation that patient care activities were performed.

MONITORING FOR ENDPOINTS AND OUTCOMES

It is not enough, however, to only provide a clear, concise record of the nature of a problem, the assessment that led to the conclusion that a problem exists, and the selection of a plan for resolution of the problem. In the spirit of pharmaceutical care, the patient must not be abandoned after an intervention has been made. A plan for follow-up monitoring of the patient must be documented and adequately implemented. This process is likely to include questioning the patient, gathering laboratory data, and performing the ongoing physical assessments necessary to determine the effect of the plan that was implemented to assure that it results in an optimal outcome for the patient.

Monitoring parameters to assess efficacy generally include improvement in or resolution of the signs, symptoms, and laboratory abnormalities that were initially assessed. The monitoring parameters used to detect or prevent adverse reactions are determined by the most common and most serious events known to be associated with the therapeutic intervention. Potential adverse reactions should be precisely described along with the method of monitoring. For example, rather than stating "monitor for GI complaints," the recommendation may be to "question the patient about the presence of dyspepsia, diarrhea, or constipation." The frequency, duration, and target endpoint for each monitoring parameter should be identified. The points at which changes in the plan may be warranted should be included. For example, in the case of a patient with dyslipidemia, one may recommend to "obtain fasting high density lipoprotein, low density lipoprotein (LDL), total cholesterol, and triglycerides after 3 months of treatment. If the goal LDL of <100 mg/dL is not achieved with good compliance at 3 months, increase simvastatin to 40 mg by mouth (po) once daily. If goal LDL is achieved, maintain simvastatin 20 mg po once daily and repeat fasting lipoprotein profile annually."

SUMMARY

A SOAP or FARM progress note constructed in the manner described identifies each drug-related problem and states the pharmacist's Findings observed, an Assessment of the findings, the actual or proposed Resolution of the problem based upon the analysis, and the parameters and timing of follow-up Monitoring. Either form of note should provide a clear, concise record of process, activity, and projected follow-up. When written for each medication-related problem, these notes should provide data in a standardized, logical system.

Based upon recommendations from organizations such as the Institute of Medicine, Centers for Medicare & Medicaid Services, and those who focus on the provision of quality of care, EMRs will proliferate and may change the way pharmacists and other health care providers document encounters. Documentation may occur by transcription, voice recognition, or direct provider entry. Although the format of the documentation may not strictly follow the SOAP or FARM format, the common principles of documentation will remain.

SAMPLE CASE PRESENTATION

The following case presentation illustrates how such a system can be used in practice.

HISTORY OF PRESENT ILLNESS

Geraldine Johns is a 70-year-old woman seen Monday morning in clinic for her first visit. She has just moved to town to be near her son following the death of her husband. She has a history of atrial fibrillation, type 2 diabetes, COPD, mild heart failure, and is S/P MI 4 years ago. She lives alone and maintains a good level of activity and self care. Denies pain in legs upon walking. She is maintained on metformin 500 mg po BID, glyburide 10 mg po Q AM, famotidine 20 mg po daily, digoxin 0.125 mg po Q AM, warfarin 5 mg po Q AM, aspirin 81 mg po Q AM, furosemide 80 mg po BID, and metoprolol XL 100 mg po Q AM.

PHYSICAL EXAMINATION

VS

B/P 169/88, P 68 and regular, RR 13, T 99°F; Wt 100 lbs, Ht 5'2"

Skin

No rashes

Cardiac

No murmurs or rubs. (+) S_3 gallop; PMI in the 6th intercostal space 3 cm distal to the midclavicular line

Chest

Slight crackles at the right and left bases; no rales, e-to-a changes or tactile fremitus

Ext

1–2+ pedal edema bilaterally. ABI (ankle brachial index) = 1.02 (negative)

HEENT

Slight AV nicking, otherwise unremarkable

GI, GU, & Neuro

Unremarkable

Laboratory Values Are Unremarkable with the Following Exceptions

INR 3.5
Glucose 198 mg/dL
A_{1c} 11.3%
Serum creatinine 1.3 mg/dL
Digoxin level 1.0 ng/mL

Chest X-Ray

Some diffuse patchiness at the bases. Enlarged cardiac silhouette. Decreased density of the vertebrae consistent with mild osteoporosis.

ECG

Normal sinus rhythm

Medical Assessment

1. Mild to moderate heart failure with pedal edema and slight pulmonary edema on digoxin and metoprolol

2. Type 2 DM, not optimally controlled on metformin and glyburide

3. Hypertension not optimally managed on metoprolol and furosemide

4. Atrial fibrillation, currently controlled on digoxin and metoprolol

5. Possible moderate renal insufficiency; SCr 1.3, estimated CLcr = 28 mL/min (Cockcroft & Gault)

6. Possible dyslipidemia, as suggested by history of MI

7. Osteoporosis suggested by chest radiographs

8. COPD requiring no additional intervention at this time

9. S/P MI, on aspirin; lipid status unknown

CONSTRUCTION OF A SOAP OR FARM NOTE

Note: The Subjective and Objective findings of the SOAP note are combined into Findings for a FARM note. The Plan of the SOAP note is split into Recommendations/Resolution and Monitoring/Follow-Up in the FARM note.

Findings

Subjective 70-year-old woman recently moved here after the death of her husband. Patient complains of slight shortness of breath when walking up stairs and long distances. She voices no other complaints. She has a history of atrial fibrillation, type 2 diabetes, COPD, mild heart failure, and is S/P MI 4 years ago. She lives alone and maintains a good level of activity and self care. She is maintained on metformin 500 mg po BID, glyburide 10 mg po Q AM, famotidine 20 mg po daily, digoxin 0.125 mg po Q AM, warfarin 5 mg po Q AM, aspirin 81 mg po Q AM, furosemide 80 mg po BID, and metoprolol XL 100 mg po Q AM. She states that she takes her medications as prescribed, but she has some difficulty describing precisely how she takes them and is not quite certain what each medication does for her.

Objective

VS: BP 169/88, P 68 and regular, RR 13, T 99°F; Wt 100 lb, Ht 5'2"
Cardiac: S_3 gallop, PMI in the 6th intercostal space 3 cm distal to the midclavicular line
Chest: Slight crackles at the right and left bases
Extremities: 1–2+ pedal edema bilaterally, ABI negative
HEENT: Slight AV nicking, otherwise unremarkable
Medications:
    Metformin 500 mg po BID
    Glyburide 10 mg po Q AM
    Famotidine 20 mg po daily
    Digoxin 0.125 mg po Q AM
    Warfarin 5 mg po Q AM
    Aspirin 81 mg po Q AM
    Furosemide 80 mg po BID
    Metoprolol XL 100 mg po Q AM
Labs:
    INR 3.5
    Glucose 198 mg/dL
    A_{1c} 11.3%
    Serum creatinine 1.3 mg/dL
    Serum digoxin level 1.0 ng/mL
Chest X-Ray: Some diffuse patchiness at the bases. Enlarged cardiac silhouette. Decreased density of the vertebrae consistent with mild osteoporosis.
ECG: NSR

Assessment

1. Possible nonadherence/concordance and lack of knowledge about medications.

2. Mild to moderate heart failure as suggested by pedal edema, DOE, and cardiomegaly on chest x-ray. Maintained on a β-blocker and is not currently prescribed an ACE inhibitor.

3. Type 2 diabetes mellitus, not optimally controlled on metformin and glyburide; A_{1c} above goal of <7%. Not prescribed either an ACE inhibitor or an ARB for renal protective effects.

4. Hypertension, not optimally controlled on metoprolol, as suggested by increased BP, elevated serum creatinine, and AV nicking. The renal and ophthalmic findings are suggestive of significant, sustained hypertension. Repeated measurements will be necessary to confirm this assessment.

5. Atrial fibrillation

   a. Rate control: Rate currently under control with metoprolol and digoxin. No adjustment indicated.

   b. Anticoagulation: INR above target range of 2.0–3.0, without clinical complications at this time. No cause could be identified, although a change in diet associated with recent life events is suspected.

6. Possible moderate renal insufficiency as indicated by increased SCr. Renal dose adjustments may be necessary.

7. S/P MI on aspirin.

8. Possible dyslipidemia as suggested by history of MI.

9. R/O osteoporosis: Chest radiography suggestive of osteoporosis. Her petite frame and age are consistent with postmenopausal osteoporosis.

10. COPD: Mild DOE may suggest that the COPD is contributing to the heart failure symptoms. COPD appears to be an untreated indication.

11. Adverse medication effects: Although metoprolol may be considered appropriate for both the post-MI and CHF indications and is a β_1-selective β-blocker, its β_2-blocking properties (usually at higher doses) may contribute to worsening COPD and/or CHF due to bronchoconstriction, negative inotropic effects, or both.

12. Medication without indication (famotidine): On further questioning, the patient recalls being started on it while hospitalized for MI 4 years ago. She was given a prescription for it when she left the hospital. She has no complaints related to GERD or PUD. No need for famotidine can be identified.

Plan (Recommendations/Resolution)

1. Assess and reinforce adherence/concordance with recommended therapy. Educate on purpose of each medication.

2. Mild to moderate heart failure: Continue both the β-blocker metoprolol and digoxin, pending evaluation by the Cardiology Service to determine appropriateness. Suggest initiation of an ACE inhibitor at low doses and increasing furosemide to 100 mg po BID until her return next week because of persistent pedal and pulmonary edema. No added dietary salt. May consider adding spironolactone at next visit.

3. Type 2 diabetes mellitus:

   a. Medication: Suggest initiation of an ACEI (as above) per current ADA guidelines. Suggest changing glyburide 10 mg to glipizide XL 10 mg po daily to improve control and enhance compliance/concordance. Continue to follow blood glucose readings and, if indicated, may supplement glyburide with insulin lispro for elevated pre-meal BG, based upon an estimated insulin sensitivity of 1 unit per 30 to 40 mg/dL:

If blood glucose:	Give insulin lispro:
180 mg/dL	2 units
220	3 units
260	4 units
300	5 units
340	6 units, and test for urinary ketones. Call PCP if ketones are moderate or large.

   b. Diet: Suggest 3 meals and bedtime snack, with no concentrated carbohydrate (CHO) choices. Limit CHO intake per meal to 60 g; snacks 15–20 g CHO. No added salt. Check blood glucose AC and HS.

4. Hypertension: Suggest initiation of an ACEI (as above), started at low doses. If repeated measurements confirm the diagnosis of hypertension, they may be titrated to maintain blood pressure control. Blood pressure goal is <130/80 mm Hg in patients with diabetes. Currently, the patient is stage 2, ≥160/100 mm Hg.

5. Atrial fibrillation:

   a. Rate control: Suggest continuing metoprolol and digoxin unless Cardiology suggests otherwise. No adjustment indicated at this time.

   b. Anticoagulation: INR is above target range of 2.0–3.0. Recommend warfarin 2.5 mg today and then resume 5 mg po daily; dose to be adjusted as needed to maintain INR between 2.0 and 3.0.

6. Renal insufficiency: Suggest hydration regimen and repeat serum creatinine. No medication dosage adjustments are indicated currently.

7. S/P MI: Recommend continuation of aspirin 81 mg po Q AM. Suggest initiation of ACEI/ARB as noted above, and a statin (e.g., pravastatin 10 mg po at bedtime). Continue metoprolol, if acceptable to Cardiology.

8. Possible dyslipidemia: Treat based upon lipid panel; goal LDL is <100 mg/dL in patient with existing CAD or diabetes; this patient has both.

9. Possible osteoporosis: If DXA scan indicates osteoporosis, begin a bisphosphonate (e.g., alendronate 70 mg po weekly) and calcium 1,500 mg daily.

10. COPD: COPD appears to be an untreated indication. Suggest initiation of ipratropium 2 puffs QID.

11. Adverse medication effects: As noted above, will await Cardiology opinion on need for/appropriateness of β-blocker and digoxin to manage CHF.

12. Medication without indication: Suggest discontinuation of famotidine.

Monitoring/Follow-Up

1. RTC in 1 week.

2. Prior to RTC:

   a. Laboratory (slips given)

      i. Baseline electrolytes (K, Na, Ca, and Mg levels in light of unopposed furosemide therapy of unknown duration and use of digoxin) today

      ii. Serum creatinine today

      iii. Fasting lipid panel next week prior to RTC

      iv. INR next week prior to RTC

   b. DXA scan. Patient referred to Jones Pharmacy.

   c. Cardiology education. Appointment made with Dr. Welford's office.

3. Patient instructed to monitor blood glucose AC and HS and bring information on RTC.

4. Prescribed medication after this visit:

   a. Enalapril 5 mg po daily for CHF, hypertension, and type 2 DM

   b. Metformin 500 mg po BID for type 2 DM

   c. Glipizide XL 10 mg po daily for type 2 DM substituted for glyburide 10 mg po Q AM

   d. Lispro, as indicated

   e. Digoxin 0.125 mg po Q AM for CHF and rate control

   f. Furosemide 100 mg po BID for CHF

   g. Warfarin 5 mg po Q AM for S/P MI and CVA prevention

   h. Aspirin 81 mg po daily for S/P MI

   i. Metoprolol XL 100 mg po Q AM for S/P MI and rate control

   j. Pravastatin 10 mg po at bedtime for hyperlipidemia

   k. Ipratropium 2 puffs QID for COPD, and

   l. D/C Famotidine 20 mg po BID.

REFERENCES

1. Evaluation & Management Services Guide. Washington, DC, Centers for Medicare & Medicaid Services, July 2006. *www.cms.hhs.gov/MLNEdWebGuide/25_EMDOC.asp*. Accessed January 1, 2007.

2. Institute of Medicine. Crossing the Quality Chasm: A New Health System for the 21st Century. Washington DC, National Academy Press, 2001.

3. Embi PJ, Yackel TR, Logan JR, et al. Impacts of computerized physician documentation in a teaching hospital: perceptions of faculty and resident physicians. J Am Med Inform Assoc 2004;11:300–309.

4. Adams WG, Mann AM, Bauchner H. Use of an electronic medical record improves the quality of urban pediatric primary care. Pediatrics 2003;111:626–632.

5. O'Conner PJ, Crain AL, Rush WA, et al. Impact of an electronic medical record on diabetes quality of care. Ann Fam Med 2005;3:300–306.

6. Asch SM, McGlynn EA, Hogan MM, et al. Comparison of quality of care for patients in the Veterans Health Administration and patients in a national sample. Ann Intern Med 2004;141:938–945.

7. Shortliffe EH. The evolution of electronic medical records. Acad Med 1999;74:414–419.

8. Weed LL. Medical records that guide and teach. N Engl J Med 1968;278:593–600, 652–657.

9. Hepler CD. Clinical pharmacy, pharmaceutical care, and the quality of drug therapy. Pharmacotherapy 2004;24:1491–1498.

10. Hepler CD, Strand LM. Opportunities and responsibilities in pharmaceutical care. Am J Hosp Pharm 1990;47:533–543.

11. Donnelly WJ. The language of medical case histories. Ann Intern Med 1997;127:1045–1048.

12. Voytovich AE. Reduction of medical verbiage. Ann Intern Med 1999;131:146–147.

13. Bluml BM. Definition of medication therapy management: Development of professionwide consensus. J Am Pharm Assoc 2005;45:566–572.

14. American Pharmacists Association and the National Association of Chain Drug Stores Foundation. Medication therapy management in community pharmacy practice. Core elements of an MTM service. Version September 19, 2007. Available online at *www.pharmacist.com*. Accessed March 16, 2008.

15. Canaday BR, Yarborough PC. Documenting pharmaceutical care: creating a standard. Ann Pharmacother 1994;28:1292–1296.

16. Cipolle RJ, Strand LM, Morley PC. Pharmaceutical Care Practice: The Clinician's Guide, 2nd ed. New York, McGraw-Hill, 2004.

6

CARDIAC ARREST

A Near-Death Experience . . . . Level II

Tate N. Trujillo, PharmD, BCPS, FCCM

Christopher M. Scott, PharmD, BCPS

LEARNING OBJECTIVES

After completing this case study, the reader should be able to:

- Discuss possible causes for cardiac arrest.

- Outline medications used to treat cardiac arrest.

- List the pharmacologic actions of medications used in cardioversion.

- Outline the Advanced Cardiac Life Support (ACLS) guidelines.

- Identify appropriate parameters to monitor a patient who has just been cardioverted.

PATIENT PRESENTATION

Chief Complaint

"I don't know what happened. I don't remember a thing."

HPI

Jaclyn Lee is a 68-year-old female driver of a motor vehicle brought from an outside hospital by air ambulance who was involved in a crash. She was T-boned at high speed by a semitruck on the driver's side. There was no alcohol involved. The extrication time was 15 minutes. There was a loss of consciousness, and she does not remember the event.

PMH

Cervical dystonia
Endometriosis
Thyroid disease
HTN
Hyperlipidemia
Type 2 DM—diet controlled

PSH

Hysterectomy in 1985

FH

Mother had HTN and died of an AMI at age 69; no information available for father; one brother is alive with HTN and DM at age 73

SH

Smoker; quit 8 years ago; previously 1.5 ppd

Meds PTA

Atorvastatin 20 mg po daily
Metoprolol 50 mg po twice daily

Meds

Metoclopramide 10 mg IV Q 6 h
Famotidine 20 mg IV Q 12 h
Labetalol 10 mg IV Q 10 min PRN for SBP >160 (3 uses)
Enalaprilat 1.25 mg IV Q 6 h PRN SBP >120 (2 uses—late evening)
Lorazepam 2 mg IV Q 4 h PRN (9 uses)
Morphine 2–4 mg IV Q 2 h PRN (2 uses)
Fentanyl 150 mcg/h
Midazolam 3 mg/h
Nitroprusside 1.5 mcg/kg/min

All

Sulfa

ROS

Frequent chest pain and back pain with difficulty breathing

Physical Examination

Gen

Obese white woman

VS

BP 98/60, P 112, RR 24, T 37.9°C; dry Wt 120 kg

Skin

Warm, dry

HEENT

PERRLA; EOMI; arteriolar narrowing on funduscopic exam; no hemorrhages, exudates, or papilledema; oral mucosa clear

Neck

Supple with no JVD or bruits; no lymphadenopathy or thyromegaly

Chest

Mild bibasilar rales with decreased breath sounds on the left

CV

Tachycardic; S_1, S_2 normal; no S_3 or S_4; no murmurs or rubs

Abd

Obese, soft, nontender; (+) BS; no HSM

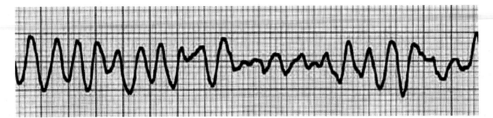

FIGURE 6-1. Electrocardiogram showing ventricular fibrillation.

Genit/Rect

Stool heme (−)

MS/Ext

Capillary refill <2 sec; age-appropriate strength and ROM

Neuro

A & O × 3, GCS 15, CN II–XII intact

▉ Labs

Na 140 mEq/L	Mg 2.5 mg/dL	Hgb 9.3 g/dL
K 3.9 mEq/L	Phos 2.5 mg/dL	Hct 28%
Cl 106 mEq/L	Alb 2.5 g/dL	Plt 229 × 10³/mm³
CO_2 20 mEq/L		WBC 9.9 × 10³/mm³
BUN 25 mg/dL		79% PMNs
SCr 0.9 mg/dL		1% Bands
Glu 245 mg/dL		17% Lymphs
Ca 6.7 mg/dL		3% Monos

▉ ECG

Sinus tachycardia at a rate of 112 bpm

▉ Clinical Course

The patient's clinical condition deteriorated and she was subsequently intubated for respiratory failure and taken to CT scan for further work-up. The CT showed a normal head, bilateral acetabular fractures, bilateral inferior and superior pubic ramus fractures, a 50% left pneumothorax, and an aortic tear. She was emergently taken to the operating room for repair of the aortic tear by cardiovascular surgery. Postoperatively, she was taken to the intensive care unit. Approximately 36 hours S/P aortic repair, the patient developed multifocal PVCs that quickly changed to ventricular fibrillation (Fig. 6-1). A code was called.

▉ Assessment

68-year-old multiple trauma patient S/P aortic repair currently in cardiac arrest 36 hours postoperatively

QUESTIONS

Problem Identification

1.a. What actual and potential drug related problems does this patient have just prior to the development of ventricular fibrillation?

1.b. Discuss the possible causes for the development of ventricular fibrillation.

Desired Outcome

2. What are the short-term goals of pharmacotherapy for this patient?

Therapeutic Alternatives

3.a. What nonpharmacologic maneuvers should be taken immediately in a patient with ventricular fibrillation?

3.b. What pharmacotherapeutic agents are available for the acute therapy of this patient's condition?

Optimal Plan

4.a. A pharmacist was not available to participate in this resuscitation effort. Assess the appropriateness of the treatment used to obtain a cardiac conversion in this patient (see Clinical Course: Cardiopulmonary Resuscitation Record of Events and Orders).

4.b. Upon conversion to normal sinus rhythm, what is your pharmacotherapeutic plan to maintain the patient's stability?

▉ CLINICAL COURSE

Cardiopulmonary Resuscitation Record of Events and Orders (see table below)

Time	BP	Cardiac Rhythm	HR	Defib. (joules)	Rhythm after Defib.	Drugs Given
0220	56/?	VF (see Fig. 6-1)	98	100	Torsades (Fig. 6-2)	
0221	46/?	Torsades		200	Torsades	
0222	116/?	Torsades		300	Agonal	
0225	88/?	Torsades		360	Agonal to Torsades	Epi 1 mg IVP
						Atropine 1 mg IVP
						Amio 150 mg IVP
0232	302/133	SVT	160	360	SVT	
0238	160/84	SVT	180	360	NSR	Amio 150 mg IVP
0247	133/50	NSR	96		Torsades to NSR with PVC	
0252					NSR with PVC	

Key: ?, not recorded; Amio, amiodarone; BP, blood pressure; HR, heart rate; Defib., defibrillation; Epi, epinephrine; IVP, intravenous push; NSR, normal sinus rhythm; PVC, premature ventricular contraction; SVT, supraventricular tachycardia; VF, ventricular fibrillation.

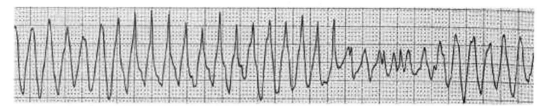

FIGURE 6-2. Electrocardiogram showing torsades de pointes.

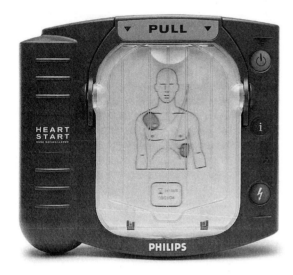

FIGURE 6-3. The Heartstart Home Defibrillator, an automated external defibrillator (AED) device approved by the FDA for home use. *(Photograph courtesy of Philips Medical Systems, Bothell, Washington.)*

Outcome Evaluation

5. How should the patient be monitored to assess drug efficacy and to prevent or detect adverse effects? Describe how the therapy should be adjusted if adverse events occur.

■ SELF-STUDY ASSIGNMENTS

1. Search the Internet for commercially available automated external defibrillator (AED) devices (see Fig. 6-3 for one example). Explain how such a device would be used by a layperson during a cardiac arrest that occurred in the home or workplace.

2. Perform a literature search to determine the odds of surviving a cardiac arrest while hospitalized.

3. List medications that can be administered through an endotracheal tube in an emergent situation.

CLINICAL PEARL

During a cardiac arrest, a patient's serum potassium will increase dramatically due to the presence of metabolic acidosis; this can worsen or complicate arrhythmia conversion.

REFERENCES

1. Hazinski MF, Chameides L, Elling B, et al. (eds). 2005 American Heart Association Guidelines for Cardiopulmonary Resuscitation and Emergency Cardiovascular Care. Circulation 2005;112(24):Suppl IV.

2. Zipes DP, Camm AJ, Borggrefe M, et al. ACC/AHA/ESC 2006 guidelines for management of patients with ventricular arrhythmias and the prevention of sudden cardiac death: a report of the American College of Cardiology/American Heart Association Task Force and the European Society of Cardiology Committee for Practice Guidelines (Writing Committee to Develop Guidelines for Management of Patients With Ventricular Arrhythmias and the Prevention of Sudden Cardiac Death). Circulation 2006;114:e385–e484.

3. Wenzel V, Krismer AC, Arntz HR, et al. A comparison of vasopressin and epinephrine for out-of-hospital cardiopulmonary resuscitation. N Engl J Med 2004;350:105–113.

7

HYPERTENSION

Salty Sam . . . . Level II

Julie M. Koehler, PharmD

James E. Tisdale, PharmD, BCPS, FCCP

LEARNING OBJECTIVES

After completing this case study, the reader should be able to:

• Classify blood pressure according to JNC 7 Guidelines, and discuss the correlation between blood pressure and risk for cardiovascular morbidity and mortality.

• Identify medications that may cause or worsen hypertension.

• Discuss complications (e.g., target organ damage, clinical cardiovascular disease) that may occur as a result of uncontrolled and/or long-standing hypertension and identify cardiovascular risk factors.

• Establish goals for the treatment of hypertension, and choose appropriate lifestyle modifications and antihypertensive regimens based on patient-specific characteristics and co-morbid disease states.

• Provide appropriate patient counseling for antihypertensive drug regimens.

PATIENT PRESENTATION

■ Chief Complaint

"I just moved to town, and I'm here to see my new doctor for a checkup. I'm just getting over a cold. Overall, I'm feeling fine, except for occasional headaches and some dizziness in the morning. My other doctor prescribed a low-salt diet for me, but I don't like it!"

HPI

Sam Street is a 62-year-old African-American male who presents to his new family medicine physician for evaluation and follow-up of his medical problems. He generally has no complaints, except for occasional mild headaches and some dizziness after he takes his morning medications. He states that he is dissatisfied with being placed on a low sodium diet by his former primary care physician. He reports a "usual" chronic cough and shortness of breath, particularly when walking moderate distances (states, "I'm just out of shape").

PMH

Hypertension × 15 years
Type 1 diabetes mellitus
Chronic obstructive pulmonary disease, Stage 2 (Moderate)
Benign prostatic hyperplasia
Chronic kidney disease

FH

Father died of acute MI at age 71. Mother died of lung cancer at age 64. Mother had both HTN and DM.

SH

Former smoker (quit 3 years ago; smoked 1 ppd × 28 years); reports moderate amount of alcohol intake. He admits he has been nonadherent to his low sodium diet (states, "I eat whatever I want.") He does not exercise regularly and is limited somewhat functionally by his COPD. He is retired and lives alone.

Meds

Triamterene/hydrochlorothiazide 37.5 mg/25 mg po Q AM
Insulin 70/30, 24 units Q AM, 12 units Q PM
Doxazosin 2 mg po Q AM
Albuterol INH 2 puffs Q 4–6 h PRN shortness of breath
Tiotropium DPI 18 mcg 1 capsule INH daily
Salmeterol DPI 1 INH BID
Entex PSE 1 capsule Q 12 h PRN cough and cold symptoms
Acetaminophen 325 mg po Q 6 h PRN headache

All

PCN—Rash

ROS

Patient states that overall he is doing well and just getting over a cold. He has noticed no major weight changes over the past few years. He complains of occasional headaches, which are usually relieved by acetaminophen, and he denies blurred vision and chest pain. He states that his shortness of breath is "usual" for him, and that his albuterol helps. He denies experiencing any hemoptysis or epistaxis; he also denies nausea, vomiting, abdominal pain, cramping, diarrhea, constipation, or blood in stool. He denies urinary frequency, but states that he used to have difficulty urinating until his physician started him on doxazosin a few months ago.

Physical Examination

Gen

WDWN, African-American male; moderately overweight; in no acute distress

VS

BP 168/92 mm Hg (sitting; repeat 170/90), HR 76 bpm (regular), RR 16 per min, T 37°C; Wt 95 kg, Ht 6'2"

HEENT

TMs clear; mild sinus drainage; AV nicking noted; no hemorrhages, exudates, or papilledema

Neck

Supple without masses or bruits, no thyroid enlargement or lymphadenopathy

Lungs

Lung fields CTA bilaterally. Few basilar crackles, mild expiratory wheezing

Heart

RRR; normal S_1 and S_2. No S_3 or S_4

Abd

Soft, NTND; no masses, bruits, or organomegaly. Normal BS.

Genit/Rect

Enlarged prostate; benign

Ext

No CCE

Neuro

No gross motor-sensory deficits present. CN II–XII intact. A & O × 3.

Labs

		Fasting Lipid Panel	Spirometry (6 months ago)
Na 142 mEq/L	Ca 9.7 mg/dL		
K 4.8 mEq/L	Mg 2.3 mEq/L	Total Chol 169 mg/dL	FVC 2.38 L (54% pred)
Cl 101 mEq/L	HbA$_{1C}$ 6.2%		
CO_2 27 mEq/L	Alb 3.5 g/dL	LDL 99 mg/dL	FEV$_1$ 1.21 L (38% pred)
BUN 22 mg/dL	Hgb 13 g/dL	HDL 40 mg/dL	
SCr 1.6 mg/dL	Hct 40%	TG 151 mg/dL	FEV$_1$/FVC 51%
Glucose 136 mg/dL	WBC 9.0×10^3/mm^3		
	Plts 189×10^3/mm^3		

UA

Yellow, clear, SG 1.007, pH 5.5, (+) protein, (−) glucose, (−) ketones, (−) bilirubin, (−) blood, (−) nitrite, RBC 0/hpf, WBC 1–2/hpf, neg bacteria, 1–5 epithelial cells

ECG

Normal sinus rhythm

ECHO (6 months ago)

Mild LVH, estimated EF 45%

Assessment

1. Hypertension, uncontrolled
2. Type 1 diabetes mellitus, controlled on current insulin regimen
3. Moderate COPD, stable on current regimen
4. BPH, symptoms improved on doxazosin

QUESTIONS

Problem Identification

1.a. Create a list of this patient's drug-related problems, including any medications which may be contributing to the patient's uncontrolled hypertension.

1.b. How would you classify this patient's HTN (e.g., Prehypertension, Stage 1, or Stage 2), according to JNC 7 Guidelines?

1.c. What are the patient's known cardiovascular risk factors, and what is the patient's Framingham risk score?

1.d. What evidence of target organ damage or clinical cardiovascular disease does this patient have?

Desired Outcome

2. List the goals of treatment for this patient (including the patient's goal blood pressure, according to JNC 7 Guidelines).

Therapeutic Alternatives

3.a. What lifestyle modifications should be encouraged for this patient to achieve and maintain adequate blood pressure reduction?

3.b. What reasonable pharmacotherapeutic options are available for controlling this patient's blood pressure, and what co-morbidities and individual patient considerations should be taken into account when selecting pharmacologic therapy for his HTN? How might Mr. Street's HTN medications potentially affect his other medical problems?

Optimal Plan

4.a. Outline specific lifestyle modifications for this patient.

4.b. Outline a specific and appropriate pharmacotherapeutic regimen for this patient's uncontrolled hypertension, including drug(s), dose(s), dosage form(s), and schedule(s).

Outcome Evaluation

5. Based on your recommendations, what parameters should be monitored after initiating this regimen and throughout the treatment course? At what time intervals should these parameters be monitored?

Patient Education

6. Based on your recommendations, provide appropriate education to this patient.

■ SELF-STUDY ASSIGNMENTS

1. Review the American Heart Association Scientific Statement on the treatment of hypertension in the prevention of and management of ischemic heart disease, and highlight the key differences in recommendations for managing a hypertensive patient with known CHD.

2. Outline the changes, if any, that you would make to the pharmacotherapeutic regimen for this patient if he had a history of each of the following co-morbidities or characteristics:

   • Severe-persistent asthma
   • Major depression
   • Gout
   • Cerebrovascular disease
   • Peripheral arterial disease
   • Isolated systolic hypertension
   • Migraine headache disorder
   • Liver disease

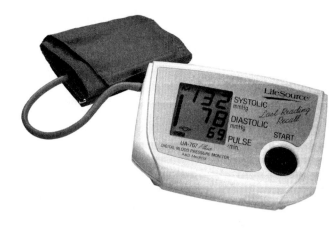

FIGURE 7-1. The LifeSource UA-767 Plus—One-Step Plus Memory digital home blood pressure monitor. *(Photo courtesy of A&D Medical, Milpitas, California.)*

• Renovascular disease (bilateral or unilateral renal artery stenosis)
• Heart failure due to left ventricular systolic dysfunction

3. Describe how you would explain to a patient how to use a digital home blood pressure monitor such as the one shown in Fig. 7-1.

CLINICAL PEARL

The risk of hemorrhagic stroke may be increased by the use of aspirin therapy in patients with uncontrolled hypertension.

REFERENCES

1. Salerno SM, Jackson JL, Berbano EP. Effect of oral pseudoephedrine on blood pressure and heart rate: a meta-analysis. Arch Intern Med 2005;165:1686–1694.

2. Chobanian AV, Bakris GL, Black HR, et al. and the National High Blood Pressure Education Program Coordinating Committee. Seventh report of the Joint National Committee on Prevention, Detection, Evaluation, and Treatment of High Blood Pressure. Hypertension 2003;42:1206–1252.

3. Rosendorff C, Black HR, Cannon CP, et al. Treatment of hypertension in the prevention and management of ischemic heart disease: a scientific statement from the American Heart Association Council for High Blood Pressure Research and the Councils on Clinical Cardiology and Epidemiology and Prevention. Circulation 2007;115:2761–2788.

4. Sacks FM, Svetkey LP, Vollmer WM, et al. Effects on blood pressure of reduced dietary sodium and the Dietary Approaches to Stop Hypertension (DASH) diet. DASH-Sodium Collaborative Research Group. N Engl J Med 2001;344:3–10.

5. Douglas JG, Bakris GL, Epstein M, et al. Management of high blood pressure in African Americans: Consensus Statement of the Hypertension in African Americans Working Group of the International Society on Hypertension in Blacks. Arch Intern Med 2003;163:525–541.

6. ALLHAT Officers and Coordinators for the ALLHAT Collaborative Research Group. Major outcomes in high-risk hypertensive patients randomized to angiotensin-converting enzyme inhibitor or calcium channel blocker vs diuretic: The Antihypertensive and Lipid-Lowering Treatment to Prevent Heart Attack Trial (ALLHAT). JAMA 2002;288:2981–2997.

7. UKPDS 39. Efficacy of atenolol and captopril in reducing risk of macrovascular and microvascular complications in type 2 diabetes: UKPDS 39. UK Prospective Diabetes Study Group. BMJ 1998;317:713–720.

8. Heart Outcomes Prevention Evaluation Study Investigators. Effects of an angiotensin-converting enzyme inhibitor, ramipril, on cardiovascular events in high-risk patients. N Engl J Med 2000;342:145–153.

9. Heart Outcomes Prevention Evaluation Study Investigators. Effects of ramipril on cardiovascular and microvascular outcomes in people with diabetes mellitus: results of the HOPE study and the MICRO-HOPE substudy. Lancet 2000;355:253–259.

10. American Diabetes Association. Treatment of hypertension in adults with diabetes. Diabetes Care 2002;25:S71–S73.

11. The ALLHAT Officers and Coordinators for the ALLHAT Collaborative Research Group. Major cardiovascular events in hypertensive patients randomized to doxazosin vs chlorthalidone: The Antihypertensive and Lipid-Lowering Treatment to Prevent Heart Attack Trial (ALLHAT). JAMA 2000;283:1967–1975.

12. Hou FF, Zhang X, Xie D, et al. Efficacy and safety of benazepril for advanced chronic renal insufficiency. N Engl J Med 2006;354:131–140.

13. Hansson L, Zanchetti A, Carruthers SG, et al. Effects of intensive blood-pressure lowering and low-dose aspirin in patients with hypertension: principal results of the Hypertension Optimal Treatment (HOT) randomized trial. HOT Study Group. Lancet 1998;351:1755–1762.

8

HYPERTENSIVE URGENCY/EMERGENCY

I Thought I Was Cured . . . . Level I

James J. Nawarskas, PharmD, BCPS

LEARNING OBJECTIVES

After completing this case study, the reader should be able to:

- Distinguish a hypertensive urgency from a hypertensive emergency.

- Identify treatment goals for a patient with a hypertensive crisis.

- Develop an appropriate treatment plan for a patient with a hypertensive crisis.

- Describe how a pharmacist can educate a patient about hypertension and the importance of providing this education.

PATIENT PRESENTATION

▥ Chief Complaint

"I need my prescriptions refilled."

▥ HPI

Reynaldo Santos is a 55-year-old man with a history of HTN (well-controlled on medication), hypercholesterolemia, and gastroesophageal reflux who presents to your community pharmacy stating he needs his blood pressure medications refilled. Upon entering his information into your computer, you discover that Mr. Santos last picked up his antihypertensive medications about 9 weeks ago. When you ask Mr. Santos about this he comments, "I was feeling fine and my doctor said my blood pressure was good, so I thought I was cured and didn't need the medications any more. Besides, I think I feel better without the medicines." When you ask Mr. Santos what prompted him to come to the pharmacy to pick up these medications, his response was "I haven't been feeling well lately and figured maybe my blood pressure was high." Mr. Santos admits to not having a home blood pressure monitoring device and has never routinely monitored his blood pressure.

▥ PMH

HTN × 15 years
Hypercholesterolemia × 10 years
GERD × 25 years

▥ FH

Both parents had HTN. Father had a heart attack in his early 50's and died in his 70's of a second heart attack; mother died a few years later from a stroke. Two brothers, 57 and 60 years old, are both alive and have hypercholesterolemia; the oldest also has HTN and underwent coronary artery bypass graft surgery 3 years ago. Two sisters, one is 53 years old and in good health with no known chronic diseases and the other is 50 years old with HTN and hypercholesterolemia.

▥ SH

Married for 35 years with 4 children (2 boys, 2 girls all over 25 years of age with no notable medical problems); works as a groundskeeper at a cemetery. States he started smoking cigarettes when he was 17 years old and smoked about one pack per day until he was diagnosed with HTN 15 years ago. Drinks about one can of beer daily, up to 3 cans on weekends, but rarely drinks hard liquor. He denies ever using recreational drugs. He does not exercise, but his job keeps him active. Against his wife's wishes, he usually eats fast food for breakfast and lunch, although his wife does make him eat a healthy dinner.

▥ Meds

Atenolol 100 mg once daily (has not taken for over a month)
Amlodipine 10 mg once daily (has not taken for over a month)
Lovastatin 20 mg once daily
OTC famotidine PRN gastric reflux (takes about every other day)

▥ All

NKDA

▥ ROS

No visual disturbances or hearing problems; denies headaches. Denies palpitations and chest pain, but states that he did almost pass out while trimming trees a couple of weeks ago. He had an episode of dizziness and had to sit down; he felt like he was going to pass out but never did. He also gets short of breath more easily in the past few weeks and has felt a loss of energy over this same time period. He feels nauseated when he exerts himself at work, but has never vomited. He denies any muscle weakness or mental status changes.

▥ Physical Examination

Gen

The patient is a middle-aged Hispanic man appearing to be in no acute distress.

VS

BP 200/120 mm Hg right arm, 198/122 mm Hg left arm (manual readings performed by yourself). A repeat measurement in the right arm after several minutes yields a BP of 192/124 mm Hg.
P 58, RR 24, T 36.8°C; Wt 72 kg, Ht 5'7"

Skin

Cool to touch, good turgor

HEENT

PERRLA; EOMI; funduscopic exam revealed arterial tortuosity, but no nicking, hemorrhages or exudates; oropharynx clear

Neck/Lymph Nodes

Neck supple, no JVD, no bruits, no thyromegaly

Chest

CTA

CV

PMI shifted laterally, RRR, no murmurs or rubs appreciated; $+S_4$ heard at apex

Abd

Soft, NT/ND, no guarding, (+) BS, no abdominal bruits appreciated, liver span about 12 cm

Genit/Rect

Normal male genitalia, heme-negative stool

MS/Ext

Normal ROM, no CCE, pulses 2+ throughout

Neuro

A & O × 3, CN II–XII intact, motor/sensory normal, DTRs 2+

▓ Labs

Na 140 mEq/L	Hgb 13.8 g/dL	AST 27 IU/L
K 4.0 mEq/L	Hct 44.0%	ALT 45 IU/L
Cl 100 mEq/L	WBC $6.6 \times 10^3/mm^3$	Cholesterol 196 mg/dL
CO_2 28 mEq/L	Plt $222 \times 10^3/mm^3$	HDL 36 mg/dL
BUN 14 mg/dL		Triglycerides 142 mg/dL
SCr 1.1 mg/dL		LDL 132 mg/dL
Glu 100 mg/dL		

▓ UA

Specific gravity 1.020; pH 5.8; negative for protein or blood; negative for recreational drugs

▓ Chest X-Ray

Enlarged heart, no infiltrates

▓ ECG

Normal sinus rhythm; LVH by voltage criteria. There are no ST-segment changes, although there does appear to be some T-wave flattening in the anterior leads.

▓ Assessment

55-year-old man with a history of HTN, hypercholesterolemia, and GERD presents with an extremely elevated blood pressure and nonspecific symptoms. He admits to not taking any antihypertensive drug therapy for over a month due to lack of understanding about his disease state.

QUESTIONS

Problem Identification

1.a. Did this patient's situation result from a drug-related problem? Why or why not?

1.b. What signs and symptoms are present that may be related to the severity of this patient's hypertension?

1.c. Is this a hypertensive urgency or an emergency? Explain your answer.

Desired Outcome

2.a. What are the goals of pharmacotherapy for this patient's hypertension?

2.b. How would the treatment goals differ if this patient presented with the same blood pressure, but had symptoms of blurred vision and chest pressure and retinal hemorrhages on funduscopic exam?

Therapeutic Alternatives

3.a. As a community pharmacist presented with this patient and his blood pressure, what is your most immediate course of action?

3.b. What nondrug therapies might be useful for this patient?

3.c. What feasible pharmacotherapeutic alternatives are available for the treatment of this patient's acute hypertension?

Optimal Plan

4.a. What drug and dosage form are best for treating this patient's acute hypertension?

4.b. How would your treatment recommendations differ if this patient presented with the same blood pressure, but had symptoms of blurred vision and chest pressure and retinal hemorrhages on funduscopic exam?

Outcome Evaluation

5. Which clinical and laboratory parameters are necessary to evaluate your therapy for reducing this patient's blood pressure and monitoring for adverse events?

Patient Education

6. What information can you provide to Mr. Santos to enhance adherence, ensure successful therapy, and minimize adverse effects?

Clinical Course

Once Mr. Santos' blood pressure is lowered to an acceptable level, his provider consults with you regarding chronic therapy for Mr. Santos.

7.a. Do you recommend Mr. Santos resume his atenolol and amlodipine as prescribed or would you recommend alternative drug therapy? Rationalize your answer. If you would recommend alternative drug therapy, which drug(s) would you recommend and why?

7.b. What economic considerations are applicable to this patient regarding drug selection?

■ SELF-STUDY ASSIGNMENTS

1. Compare and contrast the various types of home blood pressure monitoring devices with regard to finger, wrist, and arm cuff devices in terms of accuracy, cost, and ease of use.

2. Describe all aspects of proper manual blood pressure measurement.

3. List examples of target organ damage that can occur with extremely elevated blood pressure.

4. State the LDL-cholesterol goal for Mr. Santos and provide the reference to one large clinical trial to justify your answer.

CLINICAL PEARL

Hypertension is largely an asymptomatic disease. The presence of symptoms usually indicates blood pressure that is extremely elevated or chronically elevated. Educating patients regarding the expected benefits and risks of treating hypertension can go a long way toward improving outcomes.

REFERENCES

1. Joint National Committee on Prevention, Detection, Evaluation, and Treatment of High Blood Pressure. The JNC 7 Report. JAMA 2003;289:2560–2572.
2. Varon J, Marik PE. The diagnosis and management of hypertensive crises. Chest 2000;118:214–227.
3. Mansoor GA, Frishman WH. Comprehensive management of hypertensive emergencies and urgencies. Heart Dis 2002;4:358–371.
4. Handler J. Hypertensive urgency. J Clin Hypertens 2006;8:61–64.
5. Joint National Committee on Prevention, Detection, Evaluation, and Treatment of High Blood Pressure, 6th report. Arch Intern Med 1997;157:2413–2446.
6. Aggarwal M, Khan I. Hypertensive crisis: hypertensive emergencies and urgencies. Cardiol Clin 2006;24:135–146.
7. Thach AM, Schultz PJ. Nonemergent hypertension. New perspectives for the emergency medicine physician. Emerg Med Clin North Am 1995;13:1009–1035.
8. Abdelwahab W, Frishman W, Landau A. Management of hypertensive urgencies and emergencies. J Clin Pharmacol 1995;35:747–762.
9. Gales MA. Oral antihypertensives for hypertensive urgencies. Ann Pharmacother 1994;28:274–284.
10. Ross S, Walker A, MacLeod MJ. Patient compliance in hypertension: role of illness perceptions and treatment beliefs. J Hum Hypertens 2004;18:607–613.

9

HEART FAILURE: SYSTOLIC DYSFUNCTION

The Pump Organist. . . . . Level III

Jon D. Horton, PharmD

LEARNING OBJECTIVES

After completing this case study, the reader should be able to:

- Recognize the signs and symptoms of heart failure.
- Develop a pharmacotherapeutic plan for treatment of heart failure due to systolic dysfunction.
- Outline a monitoring plan for heart failure that includes both clinical and laboratory parameters.
- Initiate, titrate, and monitor β-adrenergic blocker therapy in heart failure when indicated.

PATIENT PRESENTATION

■ Chief Complaint

"I think I might have the flu. I have been feeling run down, and I haven't been able to get up the stairs to my bedroom because I get winded."

■ HPI

Richard Anderson is a 65-year-old African American man who was brought to the ED by ambulance upon request of his endocrinologist. The patient had called the physician's office this morning to cancel his routine visit for diabetes follow-up because he became short of breath and diaphoretic after attempting to climb a flight of stairs. When evaluated by the paramedics in his home, the diaphoresis had resolved, and his heart rate was in the range of 100–120 bpm. The patient states that he has been gaining weight and having progressively worsening dyspnea on exertion over the last 5 days. His shortness of breath is often worse at night, forcing him to "sit bolt upright." He began sleeping in his recliner about 3 days ago. He is unable to complete physical activities that he could do 2 weeks ago without difficulty.

■ PMH

Type 2 DM × 15 years, untreated until 3 years ago; neuropathy × 2 years and retinopathy × 1 year
HTN × 20 years
Hypercholesterolemia (documented 6 months ago)
CVA × 2 (2 and 3 years ago)
Recurrent TIAs × 1 year

■ FH

Father died at age 65 of a heart attack. Mother died in her 70's in an MVA. One brother age 70 alive with DM.

■ SH

Retired musician living alone. Prior to his CVAs, his hobby was repairing and playing antique pump organs. He has a 30 pack-year history of smoking but reports quitting 22 years ago. He has a positive history for alcohol use but states he "hasn't had a drop in 12 years."

■ Meds

Rosiglitazone 4 mg po once daily
Metformin XR 1,000 mg po once daily
Glyburide 5 mg po BID
Atorvastatin 20 mg po once daily (LDL 90 mg/dL 1 month ago)
Lisinopril 10 mg po once daily
Aspirin/extended-release dipyridamole 25 mg/200 mg po twice daily

■ All

NKDA

■ ROS

Reports having headaches recently, but nothing that he would consider unusual or out of the ordinary. Denies any recent chest pain. No chronic cough, but has had recent episodes of coughing spells without productivity. Complains of recent abdominal bloating and of being awakened the past four evenings to relieve his bladder. He reports some weakness in his right lower extremity but states that it is unchanged from his most recent stroke. He denies chronic joint pain.

Physical Examination

Gen

The patient is sitting up on the gurney in the ED in moderate distress.

VS

BP 150/95, P 100–120, RR 22, T 35°C; Wt 103 kg (usual weight 93 kg), Ht 5'11"

Skin

Color pale and diaphoretic; no unusual lesions noted

HEENT

PERRLA, EOMI, fundi were not examined. He has a complete upper denture and about two-thirds of the teeth in the lower jaw are remaining and are in fair repair.

Neck

(+) JVD at 30° (8 cm). Carotid bruit is not appreciated. No lymphadenopathy or thyromegaly.

Lungs/Thorax

Respirations are even. There are fine crackles in both lung fields posteriorly noted two-thirds of the way up the lung fields. No CVAT.

Heart

Regular rhythm, no rubs, variation in intensity of S_1 as expected. S_3 is appreciated at apex in lateral position. PMI displaced laterally and difficult to discern.

Abd

Soft, NT/ND, (+) HJR, liver and spleen slightly enlarged, no masses, hypoactive bowel sounds

Genit/Rect

Guaiac (−), genital examination not performed

MS/Ext

3+ pitting pedal edema bilaterally; radial and pedal pulses are of poor intensity bilaterally; grip strength greater on left than on right

Neuro

A & O × 3, CNs intact. Some sensory loss in both LE below the knee. DTR 1+

Labs

Na 139 mEq/L	Hgb 12.6 g/dL	Mg 1.2 mEq/L	CK 20 IU/L
K 3.4 mEq/L	Hct 39.5%	Ca 8.8 mg/dL	CK-MB 0.8 IU/L
Cl 99 mEq/L	Plt 339 × 10³/mm³	AST 36 IU/L	PT 20.6 sec
CO₂ 27 mEq/L	WBC 8.6 × 10³/mm³	ALT 43 IU/L	INR 2.8
BUN 20 mg/dL	70% PMNs	Alk phos 150 IU/L	TSH 1.42 mIU/L
SCr 1.8 mg/dL	23% Lymphs	GGT 37 IU/L	A1C 6.9%
Glucose 139 mg/dL	7% Monos	T. bili 0.2 mg/dL	
BNP 1,200 pg/mL	Troponin I 1.8 ng/mL		

ECG

Sinus tachycardia rate of 112, QRS 0.08. Diffuse non specific ST-T wave changes. Low voltage.

Chest X-Ray

PA and lateral views (Fig 9-1) show evidence of congestive failure with cardiomegaly, interstitial edema, and some early alveolar edema. There is a small right pleural effusion.

Assessment

Diabetic patient with new-onset congestive heart failure

Clinical Course

The patient was admitted to a step-down unit and placed on telemetry. A 2D echocardiogram was obtained to evaluate LV and

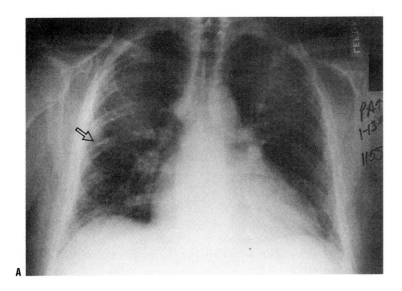
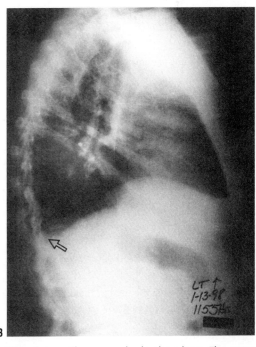

FIGURE 9-1. *A.* PA CXR demonstrates increased vascular markings representative of interstitial edema, with some early alveolar edema. The *arrow* points out fluid lying in the fissure of the right lung. Note the presence of cardiomegaly. *B.* Lateral view of CXR. *Arrow* points out the presence of pulmonary effusion.

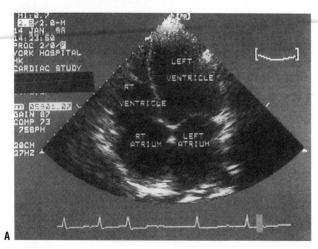
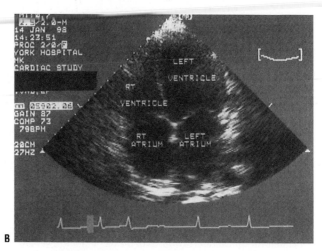

FIGURE 9-2. 2D echocardiogram. *A.* End systole. *B.* End diastole. Note the presence of severe left ventricular dilation and increased left atrial dimension in end diastole *(B)* that appear to be unchanged from the photographs of end systole *(A)*. The ventricular septum appears to be in nearly the identical position in both films, thus representing akinesia.

valvular function (see Fig. 9-2). The results showed severe LV dilation and increased left atrial dimension, akinesia of the septum, and severe LV dysfunction. EF was estimated at 15–20%, with no visible clots.

QUESTIONS

Problem Identification

1.a. Create a list of this patient's drug-related problems.

1.b. What signs, symptoms, and other information indicate the presence and severity of the patient's heart failure?

1.c. What is the classification and staging of heart failure for this patient upon presentation?

1.d. Could any of this patient's problems have been caused by drug therapy?

Desired Outcome

2.a. What are the goals for the pharmacologic management of heart failure in this patient?

2.b. Considering his other medical problems, what other treatment goals should be established?

Therapeutic Alternatives

3. What medications are indicated in the long-term management of this patient's heart failure based upon his stage of heart failure?

Optimal Plan

4. What drugs, doses, schedules, and duration are best suited for the management of this patient?

Outcome Evaluation

5. What clinical and laboratory parameters are needed to evaluate the therapy for achievement of the desired therapeutic outcome and to detect and prevent adverse events?

■ CLINICAL COURSE

Over the next 3 days, the patient received maximal drug therapy, and his condition improved. He underwent a cardiac catheteriza-

tion and bare metal stent placement for a 90% LAD lesion. He was discharged on lisinopril 20 mg po daily, carvedilol 6.25 mg po BID, furosemide 40 mg po daily, potassium chloride 40 mEq po daily, magnesium oxide 400 mg po daily, insulin glargine 20 units SC hs, aspart insulin 5 units SC AC, clopidogrel 75 mg po daily, aspirin 325 mg po daily, and atorvastatin 40 mg po daily.

Patient Education

6. What information should be provided to the patient about the medications used to treat his heart failure?

■ CLINICAL COURSE

Upon follow-up at the clinic the patient is noted to have sustained a 5-pound weight gain from baseline dry weight at discharge. His ability to climb stairs and symptoms of shortness of breath have all improved from prior to his admission.

■ FOLLOW-UP QUESTIONS

1. What is the role of routine monitoring of BNP levels in the management of this patient's heart failure?

2. The patient's development of worsening symptoms may be a result of initiation of carvedilol therapy. Outline information that should be provided to the patient about common adverse effects when initiating or titrating carvedilol therapy. Describe how they should be managed if they occur.

3. Outline a therapeutic plan for transitioning this patient from carvedilol immediate release to the controlled release product.

■ CLINICAL COURSE

The patient returns to your clinic site 3 weeks later stating that his weight is improved. He notes that in general he feels much better than he did just 1 week ago and is happily back to playing his pump organ.

■ SELF-STUDY ASSIGNMENTS

1. Develop a list of vitamins and/or minerals that should be considered secondary to the patient's chronic diuretic use.

2. This patient may develop diuretic resistance. Write a one-page essay describing what this phenomenon is, and how it might be overcome.

3. Describe how you would evaluate and monitor this patient's quality of life.

CLINICAL PEARL

The presence of pitting edema is associated with a substantial increase in body weight; it typically takes a weight gain of 10 pounds to result in the development of pitting edema.

REFERENCES

1. Grundy SM, Cleeman JI, Noel Bairey Merz N, et al. Implications of recent clinical trials for the National Cholesterol Education Program Adult Treatment Panel III Guidelines. Circulation 2004;110:227–239.
2. Smith SC, Allen J, Blair SN, et al. AHA/ACC guidelines for secondary prevention for patients with coronary and other atherosclerotic vascular disease: 2006 Update. Circulation 2006;113:2363–2372.
3. Nesto RW, Bell D, Bonow RO, et al. AHA/ADA consensus statement for thiazolidinedione use, fluid retention, and congestive heart failure. Circulation 2003;108:2941–2948.
4. Tang WH, Francis GS, Morrow DA, et al. National Academy of Clinical Biochemistry Laboratory Medicine practice guidelines: clinical utilization of cardiac biomarker testing in heart failure. Circulation 2007;116:99–109.
5. Hunt SA, Abraham WT, Chin MH, et al. ACC/AHA 2005 guideline update for the diagnosis and management of chronic heart failure in the adult: A report of the American College of Cardiology/American Heart Association Task Force on Practice Guidelines (Writing Committee to Update the 2001 Guidelines for the Evaluation and Management of Heart Failure). J Am Coll Cardiol 2005;46:1–82.
6. Adams KF, Lindenfeld J, Arnold JMO, et al. Executive Summary: HFSA 2006 Comprehensive Heart Failure Practice Guideline. J Card Fail 2006;12:10–38.
7. Rosendorff C, Black HR, Cannon CP, et al. Treatment of hypertension in the prevention and management of ischemic heart disease. Circulation 2007;115:2761–2788.
8. Pitt B, Poole-Wilson PA, Segal R, et al. Effect of losartan compared with captopril on mortality in patients with symptomatic heart failure: randomised trial—the Losartan Heart Failure Survival Study ELITE II. Lancet 2000;355:1582–1587.
9. Cohn JN, Tognoni, G; Valsartan Heart Failure Trial Investigators. A randomized trial of the angiotensin-receptor blocker valsartan in chronic heart failure. N Engl J Med 2001;345:1667–1675.
10. McMurray JJ, Ostergren J, Swedberg K, et al. Effects of candesartan in patients with chronic heart failure and reduced left ventricular systolic function taking angiotensin-converting-enzyme inhibitors: the CHARM-added trial. Lancet 2003;362:759–771.
11. Pitt B, Zannad F, Remme WJ, et al. The effect of spironolactone on morbidity and mortality in patients with severe heart failure. Randomized Aldactone Evaluation Study Investigators. N Engl J Med 1999;341:709–717.
12. Pitt B, Remme W, Zannad F, et al. Eplerenone, a selective aldosterone blocker, in patients with left ventricular dysfunction after myocardial infarction. N Engl J Med 2003;348:1309–1321.
13. Taylor AL, Ziesche S, Yancy C, et al; for the African-American Heart Failure Trial Investigators. Combination of isosorbide dinitrate and hydralazine in blacks with heart failure. N Engl J Med 2004;351:2049–2057.
14. Colucci WS, Elkayam U, Horton DP, et al. Intravenous nesiritide, a natriuretic peptide, in the treatment of decompensated congestive heart failure. Nesiritide Study Group. N Engl J Med 2000;343:246–253.
15. Packer M, Poole-Wilson PA, Armstrong PW, et al. Comparative effects of low and high doses of the angiotensin-converting enzyme inhibitor, lisinopril, on morbidity and mortality in chronic heart failure. ATLAS Study Group. Circulation 1999;100:2312–2318.
16. Svensson M, Gustafsson F, Galatius S, et al. Hyperkalaemia and impaired renal function in patients taking spironolactone for congestive heart failure: retrospective study. BMJ 2003;327:1141–1142.
17. Tang WH, Girod JP, Lee MJ, et al. Plasma B-type natriuretic peptide levels in ambulatory patients with established chronic symptomatic systolic heart failure. Circulation 2003;108:2964–2966.

10

HEART FAILURE: DIASTOLIC DYSFUNCTION

Be Still My Racing Heart. . . . . Level III

Jon D. Horton, PharmD

LEARNING OBJECTIVES

After completing this case study, the reader should be able to:

- Recognize the signs and symptoms of diastolic heart failure.
- Develop a pharmacotherapeutic plan for treatment of diastolic heart failure.
- Outline a monitoring plan for heart failure that includes both clinical and laboratory parameters.
- Initiate, titrate, and monitor β-adrenergic blocker therapy in heart failure when indicated.

PATIENT PRESENTATION

Chief Complaint

"I can't catch my breath."

HPI

Nina Orendorff is an 83-year-old woman who presented to the ED with generalized complaints, feeling run down and unable to breathe. When evaluated by the ED nursing staff, her heart rate was in the range of 110–120 beats per minute. The patient states that she has had progressively worsening dyspnea on exertion over the last 2 weeks. Her shortness of breath has severely limited her activities and has increased to persist even at rest.

PMH

Type 2 DM × 5 years, diet controlled
HTN × 40 years

FH

Father died at age 85 of "old age"; mother died at 88 after a hip fracture; one brother (age 80) alive with no significant history

SH

Retired schoolteacher who lives at home alone; reports enjoying a cocktail while playing cards with friends

Meds

Minoxidil 10 mg po bid

All

NKDA

■ ROS

Gen

Patient reports a recent weight gain along with a general reduction in her state of health primarily related to an inability to get around as she usually has in the past.

CV

She has no complaints of any chest pain but does report dyspnea on exertion, as well as orthopnea and paroxysmal nocturnal dyspnea. She has noted peripheral edema.

Resp

She reports shortness of breath and a new cough that is not productive. She has not had any recent respiratory infections.

GI

She reports no recent changes in bowel habits.

GU

No complaints

MS

No complaints of MS pain or weakness, just a general inability to exercise secondary to becoming "winded"

Neuro

No abnormalities noted

■ Physical Examination

Gen

The patient is sitting up on the gurney in the ED in moderate distress.

VS

BP 150/100, P 100–130 (regular), RR 28, T 35°C; Wt 73 kg (usual weight 65 kg), Ht 5'3"

Skin

Color pale; no unusual lesions noted

HEENT

PERRLA, EOMI, fundi were not examined. She has complete dentition, and her teeth are in fair repair.

Neck

(+) JVD at 30° (6 cm). Carotid bruit is not appreciated. No lymphadenopathy or thyromegaly

Lungs/Thorax

Respirations are even. There are crackles in both lung fields posteriorly noted one-third of the way up the lung fields. There is no CVAT.

Heart

Regular rhythm, no rubs, variation in intensity of S_1 as expected; S_3 appreciated at the apex in the lateral position; PMI displaced laterally and difficult to discern

Abd

Soft, NT/ND; (+) HJR; liver and spleen slightly enlarged; no masses; hypoactive bowel sounds

Genit/Rect

Guaiac (−), genital examination not performed

MS/Ext

2+ pitting pedal edema bilaterally; radial and pedal pulses are of poor intensity bilaterally; grip strength even

Neuro

A & O × 3; CNs intact; DTR intact

■ Labs

Na 144 mEq/L	Hgb 11.6 g/dL	Mg 1.8 mEq/L	CK 20 IU/L
K 4.4 mEq/L	Hct 38.5%	Ca 9.1 mg/dL	CK-MB 0.8 IU/L
Cl 101 mEq/L	Plt 239 × 10³/mm³	AST 41 IU/L	PT 12.6 sec
CO_2 27 mEq/L	WBC 6.6 × 10³/mm³	ALT 27 IU/L	INR 1.1
BUN 12 mg/dL	40% PMNs	Alk phos 80 IU/L	TSH 1.12 mIU/L
SCr 1.4 mg/dL	13% Lymphs	GGT 24 IU/L	A1C 6.7%
Glucose 148 mg/dL	7% Monos	T. bili 0.3 mg/dL	
BNP 1,100 pg/mL	Troponin I 1.1 ng/mL		

■ ECG

Sinus tachycardia rate of 112; QRS 0.08; diffuse nonspecific ST-T wave changes; low voltage

■ CXR

PA and lateral views (see Fig. 9-1) show evidence of interstitial edema and some early alveolar edema

■ Assessment

Diet-controlled patient with Type 2 DM and new-onset congestive heart failure

■ Clinical Course

The patient was admitted to a telemetry unit. A 2D echocardiogram was obtained to evaluate LV and valvular function. Results revealed evidence of impaired ventricular relaxation and elevated left atrial filling pressures consistent with grade II diastolic dysfunction. EF was estimated at 45–50%; there was no evidence of mitral stenosis or pericardial disease.

QUESTIONS

Problem Identification

1.a. Create a list of this patient's drug-related problems.

1.b. What signs, symptoms, and other information indicate the presence and severity of the patient's heart failure?

1.c. What are the classification and staging of this patient's heart failure upon presentation?

1.d. Could any of this patient's problems have been caused by drug therapy?

Desired Outcome

2.a. What are the goals for the pharmacologic management of heart failure in this patient?

2.b. Considering her other medical problems, what other treatment goals should be established?

Therapeutic Alternatives

3. What medications are indicated in the long-term management of this patient's heart failure based on her stage of heart failure?

Optimal Plan

4. What drugs, doses, schedules, and duration are best suited for the management of this patient?

Outcome Evaluation

5. What clinical and laboratory parameters are needed to evaluate the therapy for achievement of the desired therapeutic outcome and to detect and prevent adverse events?

■ CLINICAL COURSE

Over the next 3 days, the patient received maximal drug therapy, and her condition improved. She was discharged on lisinopril 20 mg po daily, metoprolol 25 mg po bid, furosemide 40 mg po daily, and aspirin 325 mg po daily.

Patient Education

6. What information should be provided to the patient about the medications used to treat her heart failure?

■ CLINICAL COURSE

On follow-up with her geriatrician, the patient is noted to have sustained a 2-kg weight gain from baseline dry weight at discharge. Her exercise tolerance and ability to conduct activities of daily living have improved.

■ FOLLOW-UP QUESTIONS

1. Outline a plan for maximizing the patient's current medication regimen for heart failure.

2. Outline a therapeutic plan for titration of metoprolol for this patient.

3. What common adverse effects should be anticipated with metoprolol, and how should they be managed if they occur?

■ CLINICAL COURSE

The patient returns to your geriatric clinic 2 weeks later, stating that her weight is improved. Despite this improvement, her blood pressure is now 100/50 mm Hg, her heart rate is 100–110 beats per minute, and she still has symptoms.

4. You suspect the patient may have been overdiuresed. What impact might this have on the patient?

■ SELF-STUDY ASSIGNMENTS

1. Describe the common causes of heart failure in patients with a preserved LVEF.

2. Develop a list of pharmacologic agents that can be used to reduce ventricular filling pressures in patients with diastolic dysfunction. Compare and contrast the evidence for, advantages of, and any potential disadvantages of the use of each agent.

3. Describe how you would evaluate and monitor this patient's quality of life.

CLINICAL PEARL

Patients with heart failure and a preserved LVEF are typically particularly sensitive to the loss of atrial kick. This supports the need for restoration of sinus rhythm in patients with atrial fibrillation and diastolic dysfunction.

REFERENCES

1. Tang WHW, Francis GS, Morrow DA, et al. National Academy of Clinical Biochemistry Laboratory Medicine Practice Guidelines: clinical utilization of cardiac biomarker testing in heart failure. Circulation 2007;116:99–109.
2. Hunt SA, Abraham WT, Chin MH, et al. ACC/AHA 2005 guideline update for the diagnosis and management of chronic heart failure in the adult—summary article: a report of the American College of Cardiology/American Heart Association Task Force on Practice Guidelines (Writing Committee to Update the 2001 Guidelines for the Evaluation and Management of Heart Failure). Available at http://content.onlinejacc.org/cgi/content/full/46/6/1116. Accessed February 3, 2008.
3. Rosendorff C, Black HR, Cannon CP, et al. Treatment of hypertension in the prevention and management of ischemic heart disease: a scientific statement from the American Heart Association Council for High Blood Pressure Research and the Councils on Clinical Cardiology and Epidemiology and Prevention. Circulation 2007;115:2761–2788.
4. The Digitalis Investigation Group. The effect of digoxin on mortality and morbidity in patients with heart failure. N Engl J Med 1997;336:525–533.
5. Aronow WS, Kronzon I. Effect of enalapril on congestive heart failure treated with diuretics in elderly patients with prior myocardial infarction and normal left ventricular ejection fraction. Am J Cardiol 1993;71:602–604.
6. Philbin EF, Rocco TA Jr, Lindenmuth NW, et al. Systolic versus diastolic heart failure in community practice: clinical features, outcomes, and the use of angiotensin-converting enzyme inhibitors. Am J Med 2000;109:605–613.
7. Warner JG Jr, Metzger DC, Kitzman DW, et al. Losartan improves exercise tolerance in patients with diastolic dysfunction and a hypertensive response to exercise. J Am Coll Cardiol 1999;33:1567–1572.
8. Yusuf S, Pfeffer MA, Swedberg K, et al. Effects of candesartan in patients with chronic heart failure and preserved left-ventricular ejection fraction: the CHARM-Preserved Trial. Lancet 2003;362:777–781.
9. Aronow WS, Ahn C, Kronzon I. Effect of propranolol versus no propranolol on total mortality plus nonfatal myocardial infarction in older patients with prior myocardial infarction, congestive heart failure, and left ventricular ejection fraction > or = 40% treated with diuretics plus angiotensin-converting enzyme inhibitors. Am J Cardiol 1997;80:207–209.
10. Chen HH, Lainchbury JB, Redfield MM, et al. Factors influencing survival of patients with diastolic heart failure in Olmsted County, MN in 1996–1997. Circulation 2000;102:II412–13.
11. Setaro JF, Zaret BL, Schulman DS, et al. Usefulness of verapamil for congestive heart failure associated with abnormal left ventricular diastolic filling and normal left ventricular systolic performance. Am J Cardiol 1990;66:981–986.

11

ISCHEMIC HEART DISEASE AND ACUTE CORONARY SYNDROME

Drip and Ship . . . . Level III

Shawn R. Hansen, PharmD

Matthew J. Thill, PharmD

LEARNING OBJECTIVES

After completing this case study, the reader should be able to:

• Identify modifiable risk factors for IHD and discuss the potential benefit to be gained by their modification in an individual patient.

- Optimize medical therapy in a patient with persistent angina, considering response to current therapy and the presence of comorbidities.

- Assess clinical response to antianginal therapy by identifying relevant monitoring parameters for efficacy and adverse effects.

- Outline contemporary antithrombotic therapy in catheter-based intervention for acute coronary syndromes, with an emphasis on appropriate long-term therapy.

PATIENT PRESENTATION

■ Chief Complaint
"I don't think the drugs are working for my chest pain."

■ HPI
David Lassee is a 67-year-old man with coronary artery disease. He has had two coronary artery bypass operations. He has been seen on several occasions recently because of frequent angina. A coronary angiogram performed 1 month ago revealed significant disease in the RCA proximal to his graft, but this was considered high risk for angioplasty. His dose of isosorbide mononitrate was increased at that time from 60 mg to 120 mg once daily. This had no effect on his angina. He is still using approximately 30 nitroglycerin tablets a week, and these do relieve his chest pain. He reports that most often the chest discomfort comes on with activity, such as walking. The discomfort is located in the center of his chest and rated as a 3–4 out of 10 on average. He reports that the chest discomfort slowly fades as he slows his activity. He also complains of occasional lightheadedness, with a pulse of around 50 beats per minute and SBP near 100 mm Hg.

■ PMH
Acute anterior wall MI with CABG in 1976
Posterior lateral MI in 1990 and PTCA to the circumflex at that time
Redo CABG in 1998
Ischemic cardiomyopathy
Heart failure with an ejection fraction of 40%
Dyslipidemia
COPD (mild)
Chronic low back pain
Depression

■ FH
Noncontributory for premature coronary artery disease

■ SH
Retired dairy farmer; lives with wife; drinks occasionally; previous smoker; quit in 1998

■ Meds
Carvedilol 6.25 mg twice daily
Lisinopril 5 mg once daily
Furosemide 40 mg once daily
Aspirin 325 mg once daily
Isosorbide mononitrate 120 mg once daily
Diltiazem extended-release 240 mg once daily
Escitalopram 20 mg once daily
Celecoxib 200 mg once daily
Atorvastatin 20 mg once daily
Nitroglycerin 0.4 mg SL PRN

■ All
NKDA

■ ROS
No fever, chills, or night sweats. No recent viral illnesses. No shortness of breath; occasional cough with cold weather. No nausea, vomiting, diarrhea, constipation, melena, or hematochezia. No dysuria or hematuria. No myalgias or arthralgias.

■ Physical Examination
Gen

Pleasant, cooperative man in no acute distress

VS

BP 105/68, P 50, RR 22, T 36.4°C; Wt 90 kg, waist circumference 43 inches, Ht 5'11"

Skin

Intact, no rashes or ulcers

HEENT

PERRL; EOMI; oropharynx is clear

Neck

Supple, no masses; no JVD, lymphadenopathy, or thyromegaly

Lungs

Bilateral air entry is clear. No wheezes.

CV

RRR, S_1, S_2 normal; no murmurs or gallops; PMI palpated at left fifth ICS, MCL

Abd

Soft, NT/ND; bowel sounds normoactive

Genit/Rect

Heme (–) stool

Ext

No CCE; pulses 2+ throughout

Neuro

A & O × 3, CNs II–XII intact; speech is fluent; no motor or sensory deficit; no facial asymmetry; tongue midline

■ Labs

Na 137 mEq/L	Hgb 11.8 g/dL	*Fasting Lipid Profile*
K 4.8 mEq/L	Hct 35.1%	Chol 202 mg/dL
Cl 103 mEq/L	Plt 187 × 10³/mm³	LDL 125 mg/dL
CO_2 21 mEq/L	WBC 7.9 × 10³/mm³	HDL 38 mg/dL
BUN 24 mg/dL	MCV 77 μm³	Trig 215 mg/dL
SCr 1.2 mg/dL	MCHC 29 g/dL	
Glu 98 mg/dL		

■ ECG
Sinus rhythm; first-degree AVB; 50 beats per minute; old AWMI; no ST-T wave changes noted; QT/QTc 406/431

■ Assessment
A 67 yo man with poorly controlled angina on multiple medications who is a poor candidate for angioplasty

QUESTIONS

Problem Identification
1.a. What drug-related problems appear to be present in this patient?

1.b. Could any of these problems potentially be caused or exacerbated by his current therapy?

Desired Outcome

2. What are the goals of pharmacotherapy for IHD in this case?

Therapeutic Alternatives

3.a. Does this patient possess any modifiable risk factors for IHD?

3.b. What pharmacotherapeutic options are available for treating this patient's IHD? Discuss the agents in each class with respect to their relative usefulness in his care.

Optimal Plan

4. Given the patient information provided, construct a complete pharmacotherapeutic plan for optimizing management of his IHD.

Outcome Evaluation

5. When the patient returns to the clinic in 2 weeks for a follow-up visit, how will you evaluate the response to his new antianginal regimen for efficacy and adverse effects?

■ CLINICAL COURSE

Mr. Lassee improved hemodynamically after a switch from diltiazem to amlodipine. However, because of continued frequent episodes of angina, his amlodipine was titrated to 10 mg once daily. He returns to cardiology clinic today, stating that his angina frequency has improved somewhat on the maximum dose of amlodipine but is still bothersome to him. His cardiologist decided to add ranolazine 500 mg twice daily to his regimen in an attempt to further decrease his angina frequency.

Patient Education

6. What information will you communicate to the patient about his antianginal regimen to help him experience the greatest benefit and fewest adverse effects?

■ CLINICAL COURSE

Two months later, the patient's cardiologist is notified of his arrival at the ED of a regional hospital. The patient is complaining of severe substernal chest pain that came on at rest. He rated the pain as 10 out of 10 on presentation and said that it radiated to his left arm. He has received only partial relief with IV NTG and morphine. An ECG revealed 1-mm ST-segment depression in the inferior leads consistent with inferior wall ischemia. A troponin level was drawn but is not yet available for interpretation. He is diagnosed with acute coronary syndrome, and his cardiologist has requested that he be given clopidogrel 600 mg orally × 1, enoxaparin 90 mg subcutaneously × 1, and eptifibatide 180 mcg/kg bolus followed by 2 mcg/kg/min and transferred for cardiac catheterization. On arrival, angiography revealed a high-grade lesion with thrombus in the RCA proximal to his graft. Despite the high risk of the procedure, the decision was made to perform percutaneous coronary intervention (PCI), with deployment of a 3.5-mm CYPHER sirolimus-eluting coronary stent.

■ FOLLOW-UP QUESTIONS

1. What is the recommended duration of dual-antiplatelet therapy with aspirin plus clopidogrel in the setting of percutaneous coronary intervention with drug-eluting stents?

2. What data support antithrombotic therapy with bivalirudin alone as an alternative to the combination of enoxaparin plus eptifibatide in this patient?

■ SELF-STUDY ASSIGNMENTS

1. Review and describe the role of low-molecular-weight heparins and fondaparinux in the management of acute coronary syndromes.

2. Describe the epidemiology and potential mechanisms of aspirin and clopidogrel resistance and their relationship to clinical outcomes in primary and secondary prevention scenarios.

3. Discuss precautions related to the use of sildenafil, vardenafil, and tadalafil in the setting of IHD and assess the relative risk to patient subgroups based on disease and therapy considerations.

CLINICAL PEARL

In patients receiving drug-eluting stents, compliance with dual-antiplatelet therapy (aspirin plus clopidogrel) is critical to prevent late stent thrombosis, which may lead to heart attack or death. Patients must not discontinue antiplatelet therapy for any reason, including surgery or procedures, without first discussing with their cardiologist.

REFERENCES

1. Hunt SA, Abraham WT, Chin MH, et al. ACC/AHA 2005 guideline update for the diagnosis and management of chronic heart failure in the adult—summary article: a report of the American College of Cardiology/American Heart Association Task Force on Practice Guidelines (Writing Committee to Update the 2001 Guidelines for the Evaluation and Management of Heart Failure). Circulation 2005;112:1825–1852.

2. Adams KF, Lindenfeld J, Arnold JMO, et al. Executive Summary: HFSA 2006 Comprehensive Heart Failure Practice Guideline. J Cardiac Failure 2006;12:10–38.

3. Antman EM, Bennett JS, Daugherty A, et al. Use of nonsteroidal antiinflammatory drugs: an update for clinicians. A scientific statement from the American Heart Association. Circulation 2007;115: 1634–1642.

4. Executive summary of the third report of the National Cholesterol Education Program (NCEP) Expert Panel on Detection, Evaluation, Treatment of High Blood Cholesterol in Adults (Adult Treatment Panel III). JAMA 2001;285:2486–2497.

5. Grundy SM, Cleeman JI, Merz CNB, et al. Implications of recent clinical trials for the National Cholesterol Education Program Adult Treatment Panel III Guidelines. Circulation 2004;110:227–239.

6. Grundy SM, Cleeman JI, Daniels SR, et al. Diagnosis and management of the metabolic syndrome: an American Heart Association/National Heart, Lung, and Blood Institute scientific statement. Circulation 2005;112:2735–2752.

7. Gibbons RJ, Abrams J, Chatterjee K, et al. ACC/AHA 2002 guideline update for the management of patients with chronic stable angina—summary article: a report of the American College of Cardiology/American Heart Association Task Force on Practice Guidelines (Committee on the Management of Patients with Chronic Stable Angina). J Am Coll Cardiol 2003;41:159–168.

8. The CAPRICORN Investigators. Effect of carvedilol on outcome after myocardial infarction in patients with left-ventricular dysfunction: The CAPRICORN randomized trial. Lancet 2001;357:1385–1390.

9. Chaitman BR. Ranolazine for the treatment of chronic angina and potential use in other cardiovascular conditions. Circulation 2006; 113:2462–2472.

10. Antithrombotic Trialists' Collaboration. Collaborative meta-analysis of randomised trials of antiplatelet therapy for prevention of death, myocardial infarction, and stroke in high risk patients. BMJ 2002; 324:71–86.

11. Smith SC, Allen J, Blair SN, et al. AHA/ACC guidelines for secondary prevention for patients with coronary and other atherosclerotic vascular disease: 2006 update. J Am Coll Cardiol 2006;47:2130–2139.

12. CAPRIE Steering Committee. A randomised, blinded, trial of clopidogrel versus aspirin in patients at risk of ischaemic events (CAPRIE). Lancet 1996;348:1329–1339.

13. Smith SC Jr, Feldman TE, Hirshfeld JW Jr, et al. ACC/AHA/SCAI 2005 guideline update for percutaneous coronary intervention: a report of the American College of Cardiology/American Heart Association Task Force on Practice Guidelines (ACC/AHA/SCAI Writing Committee to Update the 2001 Guidelines for Percutaneous Coronary Intervention). Circulation 2006;113:e166–e286.

14. Grines CL, Bonow RO, Casey DE Jr, et al. Prevention of premature discontinuation of dual antiplatelet therapy in patients with coronary artery stents: a science advisory from the American Heart Association, American College of Cardiology, Society for Cardiovascular Angiography and Interventions, American College of Surgeons, and American Dental Association, with representation from the American College of Physicians. Circulation 2007;115:813–818.

15. Lincoff AM, Bittle JA, Harrington RA, et al. Bivalirudin and provisional glycoprotein IIb/IIIa blockade compared with heparin and planned glycoprotein IIb/IIIa blockade during percutaneous coronary intervention: REPLACE-2 randomized trial. JAMA 2003;289:853–863.

16. Stone GW, McLaurin BT, Cox DA, et al. Bivalirudin for patients with acute coronary syndromes. N Engl J Med 2006;355:2203–2216.

12

ACUTE CORONARY SYNDROME: ST-ELEVATION MYOCARDIAL INFARCTION

I'm Too Young to Die . . . . Level II

Kelly C. Rogers, PharmD

Robert B. Parker, PharmD, FCCP

LEARNING OBJECTIVES

After completing this case study, the reader should be able to:

- Determine the goals of pharmacotherapy for patients with STEMI.

- Discuss interventional strategies for patients with STEMI and understand the pharmacotherapeutic agents used with interventions.

- Design an optimal therapeutic plan for management of STEMI and describe how the selected drug therapy achieves the therapeutic goals.

- Identify appropriate parameters to assess the recommended drug therapy for both efficacy and adverse effects.

- Provide appropriate education to a patient who has suffered a STEMI.

PATIENT PRESENTATION

▓ Chief Complaint

"It feels like an elephant is sitting on my chest! I'm too young to die!"

▓ HPI

Larry Stanton is a 46-year-old man transported by paramedics to the ED of a large community hospital. He presents with severe, substernal chest pain for the last 6 hours. He states he was fine until about an hour after he ate breakfast. The pain radiates to his jaw and neck and is accompanied by N/V and diaphoresis. In the ambulance, his chest pain is unrelieved by three SL NTG tablets.

▓ PMH

No significant past medical history

▓ FH

Father with heart failure and Type 2 DM and questionable history of "mild heart attack" at age 42; mother alive with HTN. He has one sister who is 48, alive and well, and one brother who died suddenly at age 46.

▓ SH

(+) tobacco × 20 years; drinks beer usually on weekends; states he hasn't been to a physician since his appendectomy 10 years ago

▓ Meds

Acetaminophen PRN
Pepcid AC PRN

▓ All

NKDA

▓ ROS

Positive for some baseline CP for "some time"

▓ Physical Examination

Gen

WDWN man A & O × 3, still with chest pain, somewhat anxious

VS

BP 145/92, P 89, RR 18, T 37.1°C; Wt 102 kg, Ht 5'10"

HEENT

PERRLA, EOMI, fundi benign; TMs intact

Neck

No bruits; mild JVD; no thyromegaly

Lungs

Few dependent inspiratory crackles; bibasilar rales; no wheezes

CV

PMI displaced laterally, normal S_1 and S_2, no S_3 or S_4, I/VI SEM @ LUSB

Abd

Soft, nontender; liver span 10–12 cm; no bruits

Genit/Rect

Deferred

MS/Ext

Normal ROM; muscle strength on right 5/5 UE/LE; on left 4/5 UE/LE; pulses 2+; no femoral bruits or peripheral edema

Neuro

CNs II–XII intact; DTRs decreased on left; negative Babinski's sign

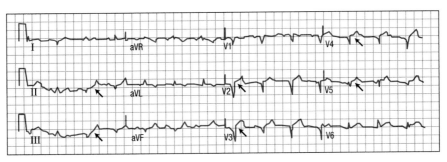

FIGURE 12-1. ECG taken on arrival in the emergency department showing ST-segment elevation (*arrows*) in leads V_2–V_6, consistent with acute anterior myocardial infarction.

■ Labs

Na 134 mEq/L	Ca 9.8 mg/dL	Hgb 14.0 g/dL	*Fasting Lipid Profile*
K 4.4 mEq/L	Mg 2.0 mg/dL	Hct 44%	T. chol 230 mg/dL
Cl 102 mEq/L	PO_4 2.4 mg/dL	WBC 5.0×10^3/mm^3	Trig 105 mg/dL
CO_2 23 mEq/L	AST 22 U/L	Plt 268×10^3/mm^3	LDL 182 mg/dL
BUN 15 mg/dL	ALT 30 U/L	PT 12.5 sec	HDL 30 mg/dL
SCr 1.0 mg/dL	Alk Phos 75 U/L	aPTT 32.4 sec	
Glu 76 mg/dL	Troponin I 4.2 ng/mL	INR 1.0	

■ ECG

Two- to five-mm ST-segment elevation in leads V_2–V_6 (Fig. 12-1)

■ Assessment

Acute anterolateral STEMI

QUESTIONS

Problem Identification

1.a. Which findings in this patient's case history are consistent with acute STEMI?

1.b. What risk factors for the development of coronary artery disease are present in this patient?

Desired Outcome

2.a. What is the immediate goal of therapy in this patient?

2.b. How can this goal be achieved using pharmacotherapy?

Therapeutic Alternatives

3.a. What nonpharmacologic therapeutic alternative can also achieve the immediate goal in this patient?

3.b. What is the role of glycoprotein IIb/IIIa inhibitors (GPIs) in the setting of PCI with coronary artery stenting, and how should these agents be used?

3.c. How should therapy with GPIs be monitored?

Optimal Plan

4.a. What are other important goals of therapy in this patient?

4.b. Based on the history and presentation, what initial drug therapy is indicated in this patient?

Outcome Evaluation

5. How should the recommended therapy be monitored for efficacy and adverse effects?

■ CLINICAL COURSE

The patient received aspirin, morphine, oxygen, IV unfractionated heparin, IV nitroglycerin, and IV metoprolol. An interventional cardiologist was consulted and discussed with the patient the need for primary PCI to restore blood flow to the heart. Within 1 hour of his arrival to the ED, the patient was transported to the cardiac catheterization lab. The catheterization revealed a 60% proximal stenosis in the LAD coronary artery, with thrombus present. The other major coronary arteries had only minor luminal irregularities. The patient then underwent PCI, which consisted of PTCA of the LAD lesion followed by successful placement of a sirolimus drug-eluting coronary artery stent. After the stent was placed, the patient received an eptifibatide infusion, and therapy with clopidogrel and aspirin was initiated. The left ventricular ejection fraction by echocardiogram 3 days postinfarct was 45%. The remainder of the patient's hospital stay was uncomplicated, and he was discharged 5 days post-MI.

Patient Education

6.a. Based on his hospital course, which discharge medications would be most appropriate for this patient?

6.b. What education should you provide to this patient?

■ CLINICAL COURSE

Eight months after he received his sirolimus DES, the patient developed a cough with hemoptysis. His primary care physician did a chest X-ray and discovered a new lung mass and referred him to pulmonary medicine. The pulmonologist scheduled the patient for a CT-guided biopsy and told him to discontinue his aspirin and clopidogrel 1 week before this test. Six days after stopping clopidogrel and aspirin, the patient presented to the ED with a large anterior STEMI, with troponins peaking at 500 ng/mL. He was taken emergently to the catheterization lab, and it was found that the DES in his LAD was totally occluded with thrombus.

■ FOLLOW-UP QUESTION

1. Why did this patient develop late stent thrombosis, and how can this potential life-threatening catastrophe be prevented in the future?

■ SELF-STUDY ASSIGNMENTS

1. A patient comes into your pharmacy and asks you whether he really needs to take two "blood-thinner drugs" (aspirin and clopidogrel). He is concerned about having bleeding complications and the cost of all of his medications. Review the indications for combination therapy with aspirin and clopidogrel, and review the cost of this treatment. How should you respond to him?

2. A 54 yo man is admitted to the hospital for an acute MI. He states that he heard on the news that taking fish oil supplements or eating fish might help his heart. Review the available literature on the cardiovascular impact of fish oil supplements and dietary fish intake. How would you respond to him?

3. Perform a literature search and evaluate recent clinical trials discussing the use of thienopyridines in patients receiving drug-eluting stents.

CLINICAL PEARL

Signs of successful thrombolysis include disappearance of chest pain, presence of reperfusion arrhythmias, resolution of ST-segment changes, and early peak of cardiac isoenzymes.

REFERENCES

1. Antman EM, Anbe DT, Armstrong PW, et al. ACC/AHA guidelines for the management of patients with ST-elevation myocardial infarction: a report of the American College of Cardiology/American Heart Association Task Force on Practice Guidelines (Committee to Revise the 1999 Guidelines for the Management of Patients with Acute Myocardial Infarction). Circulation 2004;110:588–636.

2. Braunwald E, Antman EM, Beasley JW, et al. ACC/AHA 2002 guideline update for the management of patients with unstable angina and non-ST-segment elevation myocardial infarction: a report of the American College of Cardiology/American Heart Association Task Force on Practice Guidelines (Committee on the Management of Patients with Unstable Angina). 2002. Available at: http://circ.ahajournals.org/cgi/content/full/107/1/149. Accessed September 25, 2007.

3. Smith SC, Feldman TE, Hirshfeld JW, et al. ACC/AHA/SCAI 2005 guideline update for percutaneous coronary intervention: a report of the American College of Cardiology/American Heart Association Task Force on Practice Guidelines (ACC/AHA/SCAI Writing Committee to Update the 2001 Guidelines for Percutaneous Coronary Intervention). American Heart Association Web Site. Available at: http://www.americanheart.org. Accessed September 25, 2007.

4. Levine GN, Berger PB, Cohen DJ, et al. Newer pharmacotherapy in patients undergoing percutaneous coronary interventions: a guide for pharmacists and other health care professionals. Pharmacotherapy 2006;26:1537–1556.

5. Smith SC, Allen J, Blair SN, et al. AHA/ACC guidelines for secondary prevention for patients with coronary and other atherosclerotic vascular disease: 2006 update. J Am Coll Cardiol 2006;47:2130–2139.

6. Grines CL, Bonow RO, Casey DE, et al. Prevention of premature discontinuation of dual antiplatelet therapy in patients with coronary artery stents. A science advisory from the American Heart Association, American College of Cardiology, Society for Cardiovascular Angiography and Interventions, American College of Surgeons, and American Dental Association, with representation from the American College of Physicians. Circulation 2007;115:813–818.

7. Ong AT, McFadden EP, Regar E, et al. Late angiographic stent thrombosis (LAST) events with drug-eluting stents. J Am Coll Cardiol 2005;45:2088–2092.

8. Pfisterer M, Brunner-LaRocca HP, Buser PT, et al. for the BASKET-LATE Investigators. Late clinical events after clopidogrel discontinuation may limit the benefit of drug-eluting stents. J Am Coll Cardiol 2006;48:2584–2591.

9. Cannon CP, Braunwald E, McCabe CH, et al. for the Pravastatin or Atorvastatin Evaluation and Infection Therapy-Thrombolysis in Myocardial Infarction 22 Investigators. Intensive versus moderate lipid lowering with statins after acute coronary syndromes. N Engl J Med 2004;350:1495–1504.

10. Grundy SM, Cleeman JI, Merz NB, et al. Implications of recent clinical trials for the national cholesterol education program adult treatment panel III guidelines. Circulation 2004;110:227–239.

13

DRUG-INDUCED ARRHYTHMIA

Syncopal Julia! . . . . Level III

Kwadwo Amankwa, PharmD

LEARNING OBJECTIVES

After completing this case study, the reader should be able to:

- Understand the risk factors for development of drug-induced torsades de pointes (TdP).

- Differentiate TdP from other cardiac arrhythmias.

- Select appropriate first-line therapy for acute treatment of TdP.

- Identify appropriate dosing, common adverse effects, and monitoring parameters for pharmacologic agents used to treat TdP.

- Discuss long-term approaches to prevention of drug-induced TdP.

PATIENT PRESENTATION

▓ Chief Complaint

"I was not feeling well, and I think I passed out."

▓ HPI

Julia Doellefeld is a 60-year-old woman who experiences a syncopal episode while being evaluated in the emergency department. She reports being in her usual state of relatively good health until she developed a "cold" approximately 4 days before admission. She called her primary care physician complaining of her upper respiratory tract symptoms, and the physician called in a prescription for erythromycin 500 mg QID (for 10 days) to her pharmacy. She took the first dose on the morning of admission. She started feeling worse approximately 1 hour after taking the second dose of erythromycin. She reports feeling lightheaded and short of breath. She experienced palpitations as well and eventually passed out for a few minutes. She awoke on the floor of her living room and called for an ambulance. On medic arrival, she was awake and alert but looked shaken. She was transported to the ED without further events.

While being evaluated in the ED, she had another syncopal episode. ACLS protocol was initiated, and a rhythm strip showed TdP.

▓ PMH

CAD S/P PTCA
Heart failure (EF 30%)
Dyslipidemia
Paroxysmal atrial fibrillation

▓ SH

She lives with her husband and does not smoke or drink alcohol.

▓ Meds

Carvedilol (Coreg) 3.125 mg po bid
Pravastatin (Pravachol) 40 mg po daily
Furosemide (Lasix) 40 mg bid (increased from 40 mg po once a day due to increased edema)

Warfarin (Coumadin) 4 mg po daily as directed
Amiodarone 200 mg po bid
Centrum Silver po daily
Ranitidine (Zantac) 150 mg po daily
Candesartan (Atacand) 8 mg po daily
Aspirin 325 mg po daily
Erythromycin 500 mg po QID, started day of admission

▨ All

NKDA

▨ ROS

The patient has no complaints other than those mentioned in the HPI.

▨ Physical Examination
Gen

The patient is awake on an ED bed in moderate distress.

VS

BP 104/50, P 98 (200 during syncope), RR 30, T 36.3°C; Ht 5'7", Wt 90 kg

Skin

Warm and dry; no rashes seen

HEENT

Normocephalic, atraumatic. PERRLA. EOMI. Oropharynx is clear.

Neck/Lymph Nodes

Supple; no JVD or bruits; no lymph nodes palpated

Lungs/Thorax

CTA bilaterally

Breasts

Nontender

CV

RRR with no murmurs or gallops

Genit/Rect

Deferred

Abd

NTND; no rebound or guarding; (+) bowel sounds

MS/Ext

Trace edema in the lower extremities; pulses intact

Neuro

A & O × 3

▨ Labs

Na 140 mEq/L	Hgb 12.1 g/dL	WBC 12 × 10³/mm³
K 2.8 mEq/L	Hct 35%	
Cl 100 mEq/L	RBC 3.88 × 10⁶/mm³	
CO₂ 29 mEq/L	Plt 200 × 10³/mm³	
BUN 36 mg/dL	MCV 90.5 μm³	
SCr 1.4 mg/dL	MCHC 34.4 g/dL	
Glu 110 mg/dL	INR 2.3	
Mg 1.2 mg/dL		

▨ ECG

NSR, QTc 605 ms; rhythm strip from oscilloscope during syncope: TdP (Fig. 13-1)

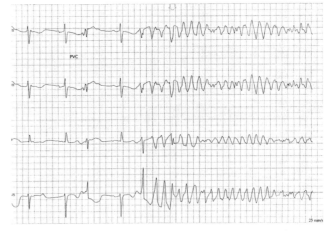

FIGURE 13-1. Electrocardiogram showing torsades de pointes.

▨ Assessment

60-year-old woman S/P syncopal episodes from drug-induced TdP
Upper respiratory tract symptoms
Drug-induced electrolyte imbalance

QUESTIONS

Problem Identification

1.a. What risk factors predisposed the patient to drug-induced arrhythmia?

1.b. What features of the patient's ECG are characteristic of TdP?

1.c. Discuss pharmacologic and nonpharmacologic factors that may have contributed to drug-induced TdP in this patient.

Desired Outcome

2. What are the short-term goals of pharmacotherapy for this patient?

Therapeutic Alternatives

3.a. What nonpharmacologic therapies may be useful for this patient?

3.b. What pharmacotherapy options are available for acute treatment of TdP?

Optimal Plan

4. Design a pharmacotherapeutic plan for the treatment of acute drug-induced TdP for this patient.

Outcome Evaluation

5. What monitoring parameters should be used to assess efficacy and toxicity of treatment?

Patient Education

6. What medication counseling should be provided for the patient to prevent recurrence?

■ CLINICAL COURSE

The patient was treated with magnesium infusion, and she converted to normal sinus rhythm. The erythromycin was stopped. Potassium and magnesium were replaced, and the patient was admitted for further electrophysiology workup.

■ SELF-STUDY ASSIGNMENTS

1. List the most common drug classes associated with TdP.
2. List 10 commonly used medications that have a potential to cause TdP.

CLINICAL PEARL

There is a need for increased pharmacovigilance regarding drug-induced arrhythmias in the outpatient setting because a large number of pharmacologic agents and/or conditions that cause QT prolongation and TdP are present in the outpatient population.

REFERENCES

1. Gowda RM, Khan IA, Wilbur SL, et al. Torsades de pointes: the clinical considerations. Int J Cardiol 2004;95:219–222.
2. Arizona CERT—Center for Education and Research on Therapeutics. Available at: QTdrugs.org. Accessed January 24, 2007.
3. Yee GY, Camm AJ. Drug induced QT prolongation and torsades de pointes. Heart 2003:89;1363–1372.
4. Owens RC, Nolin TD. Antimicrobial-associated QT interval prolongation: pointes of interest. CID 2006;43:1603–1611.
5. Tisdale JT. Torsades de pointes. In: Tisdale JE, Miller DA, eds. Drug-Induced Diseases: Prevention, Detection and Management. Bethesda, MD, American Society of Health-Systems Pharmacists, 2005:310–317.
6. ACC/AHA/ESC 2006 Guidelines for management of patients with ventricular arrhythmias and the prevention of sudden cardiac death: a report of the American College of Cardiology/American Heart Association Task Force and the European Society of Cardiology Committee for Practice Guidelines (Writing Committee to Develop Guidelines for Management of Patients With Ventricular Arrhythmias and the Prevention of Sudden Cardiac Death): Developed in Collaboration With the European Heart Rhythm Association and the Heart Rhythm Society. J Am Coll Cardiol 2006;48:247–346.
7. Berul CI, Seslar SP, Zimetbaum PJ, et al. Acquired QT syndrome. In: Rose BD, ed. UpToDate, Waltham, MA. http://www.uptodateonline.com. Accessed January 4, 2007.

14

ATRIAL FIBRILLATION

Not Sleeping with Atrial Fibrillation . . . . Level III

Bradley G. Phillips, PharmD, BCPS, FCCP

LEARNING OBJECTIVES

After completing this case study, the reader should be able to:

• Determine therapeutic goals for attaining ventricular rate control or normal sinus rhythm in patients with heart disease presenting with recurrent paroxysmal atrial fibrillation.

• Describe the difference between recurrent paroxysmal and persistent atrial fibrillation.

• Understand the influence of obstructive sleep apnea on the recurrence and risk of incident atrial fibrillation.

• Recognize the importance of identifying and alleviating sleep-disordered breathing in patients with atrial fibrillation, hypertension and obstructive sleep apnea.

PATIENT PRESENTATION

■ Chief Complaint

"I feel tired and dizzy during the day, and my heart feels like it is pumping too fast."

■ HPI

Mark Finley is a 53-year-old man who presents to the Emergent Care Clinic with heart palpitations and dizziness. He has a 2-year history of recurrent paroxysmal atrial fibrillation. He now has morning headaches and feels tired throughout the day despite sleeping 7–8 hours each night. At his last visit 6 months ago he was in normal sinus rhythm. He has gained 6 kg since his last visit. The severity of his dizziness fluctuates; the dizziness is worst in the morning and during exercise. He has been seen by his primary care provider in the Internal Medicine Clinic for many years for HTN and recurrent paroxysmal atrial fibrillation.

■ PMH

HTN (previously well controlled on current antihypertensive regimen)
Recurrent paroxysmal atrial fibrillation (rate controlled)

■ FH

Both parents had HTN; father had obstructive sleep apnea and died of an early morning stroke at age 52, mother died in MVA at age 63. He has one brother who has hypertension.

■ SH

Mr. Finley manages a local grocery store and lives at home with his wife. He smoked 1 ppd for 10 years and quit 2 years ago. He drinks 1–2 glasses of wine each week.

■ Meds

Lisinopril 20 mg po daily
Metoprolol 50 mg po twice daily
Amlodipine 10 mg po daily
Hydrochlorothiazide 25 mg po daily
Warfarin 5 mg po daily

■ All

NKDA

■ ROS

Headache but no blurred vision, chest pain, or fainting spells; complains of being tired during the day; mild SOB; 2+ pitting edema

■ Physical Examination

Gen

Cooperative overweight man in moderate distress

VS

BP 149/84 (supine), P 118 (irregular), RR 20, T 36.3°C; Wt 108.3 kg, Ht 5'11"

Skin

Cool to touch, normal turgor and color

HEENT

PERRLA, EOMI; funduscopic exam reveals mild arteriolar narrowing but no hemorrhages, exudates, or papilledema

Neck

Large and supple, no carotid bruits; no lymphadenopathy or thyromegaly, (–) JVD

Lungs/Thorax

Inspiratory and expiratory wheezes and rales bilaterally no rhonchi

CV

Tachycardia with irregular rate; normal S_1, S_2; (+) S_3; no S_4

Abd

NT/ND, (+) BS; no organomegaly, (–) HJR

Genit/Rect

Stool heme (–)

MS/Ext

Pulses 1+ weak, full ROM, no clubbing or cyanosis

Neuro

A & O × 3; CN II–XII intact; DTR 2+, negative Babinski

■ Labs (non-fasting)

Na 140 mEq/L	Hgb 15.2 g/dL	Ca 9.1 mg/dL
K 4.2 mEq/L	Hct 48%	Mg 2.1 mEq/L
Cl 99 mEq/L	Plt 293 × 10³/mm³	CRP 14.3 mg/L
CO_2 24 mEq/L	WBC 9.1 × 10³/mm³	
BUN 23 mg/dL	Polys 71%	
SCr 1.3 mg/dL	Bands 2%	
Glu 101 mg/dL	Lymphs 24%	
INR 2.7	Monos 3%	

■ ECG

Atrial fibrillation, ventricular rate 97 bpm, mild LVH

■ Echo

Evidence of diastolic dysfunction (LVEF 59%, LVEDP 15 mm Hg) and moderate left atrial enlargement (5.3 cm). No thrombus seen.

■ Chest X-Ray

Bilateral basilar infiltrates

■ Assessment

Recurrent paroxysmal atrial fibrillation: moderately symptomatic.
Diastolic heart failure: preserved ejection fraction with increased LVEDP, pulmonary and peripheral edema; start furosemide.
Possible sleep apnea: schedule sleep study during hospitalization.
HTN: maintain meds for blood pressure control.

QUESTIONS

Problem Identification

1.a. List and prioritize the patient's drug therapy problems.

1.b. Can OSA increase risk for and recurrences of AF in this patient? Please elaborate in your answer.

1.c. What are the common signs and symptoms of OSA? Which signs and symptoms are suggestive that this patient may have sleep apnea?

1.d. This patient has recurrent paroxysmal AF. How is this different from recurrent persistent AF?

1.e. What is the optimal therapy for prevention of cardioembolic stroke?

Desired Outcome

2. What are the goals for pharmacotherapy in this case?

Therapeutic Alternatives

3.a. Mr. Finley is now symptomatic, likely due to his diastolic heart failure, with this episode of AF despite chronic β-blocker and anticoagulation therapies. If Mr. Finley continues or becomes more symptomatic, what antiarrhythmic drug therapy would you recommend to chemically cardiovert him to normal sinus rhythm? Provide your rationale including the risks and benefits of antiarrhythmic therapy.

3.b. What nondrug therapies might be useful for this patient?

Optimal Plan

4. What therapy and dosage regimen would you recommend acutely to manage his AF?

■ CLINICAL COURSE

The patient is diuresed successfully. The drug regimen that you recommended to moderate ventricular rate control was initiated. Blood pressure is now 127/84 mm Hg, and he has spontaneously converted to normal sinus rhythm with a resting pulse of 73 bpm. He states that he feels better and no longer feels dizzy. His sleep study was diagnostic for severe obstructive sleep apnea. His Apnea Hypopnea Index was 52 events per hour with an average oxygen saturation of 92% and an oxygen saturation low of 71%. He had episodes of atrial fibrillation during apneic events (Fig. 14-1). He was started on nasal continuous positive airway pressure (CPAP), which was titrated to 8 cm H_2O to alleviate sleep disordered breathing. He is scheduled to return to the Heart Failure Clinic in 1 week for his diastolic heart failure.

Outcome Evaluation

5. How would you monitor and adjust his drug therapies for rate control and prophylaxis for thromboembolic events?

Patient Education

6. What patient education would you provide Mr. Finley about his AF and newly diagnosed OSA to enhance adherence and ensure successful therapy and to minimize side effects?

■ FOLLOW-UP QUESTIONS

1. Which mechanism might explain why untreated OSA may increase the recurrence of and risk for incident AF?

2. Which antiarrhythmic agent would you recommend if this patient requires chronic antiarrhythmic therapy to maintain normal sinus rhythm?

3. The patient has an elevated CRP level. Explain the association between systemic inflammation and AF. Do patients with obstructive sleep apnea have evidence of systemic inflammation?

■ SELF-STUDY ASSIGNMENTS

1. Obstructive sleep apnea may impact the management of atrial fibrillation. Outline therapies for the treatment of obstructive sleep apnea. How would you evaluate each of these therapies for effectiveness? Mr. Finley was started on nasal CPAP therapy to al-

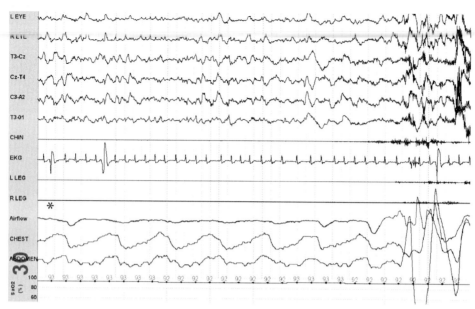

FIGURE 14-1. Polysomnogram obtained from this patient on second night of hospitalization. Electrocardiogram *(EKG lead, middle)* shows atrial fibrillation during apneic episode. Obstructive apnea is observed at the beginning of the recording *(left, *)* for over 30 seconds with no airflow from mouth or nose *(Airflow lead)* despite rhythmic chest *(Chest lead)* and abdominal *(Abdomen lead)* efforts to breath. Subject experiences micro-arousals from sleep on electroencephalogram leads *(top leads, right)* following apneic episode. The remaining leads are chin electromyogram *(Chin)*, left *(L Leg)* and right *(R Leg)* leg electromyograms, and blood oxygen saturation *(SaO$_2$)*. Nasal CPAP therapy is initiated and increased to alleviate sleep disordered breathing *(not shown)*.

leviate sleep disordered breathing. How frequently should you reevaluate this therapy?

2. This patient had self-terminating episodes of atrial fibrillation during untreated obstructive sleep apnea. How would you classify these episodes of atrial fibrillation?

3. This patient has diastolic heart failure and recurrent paroxysmal atrial fibrillation. Is there clinical evidence that inhibiting the RAAS is beneficial for treating diastolic heart failure and reducing the risk of developing recurrent AF? Would you recommend ARB therapy in this patient?

CLINICAL PEARL

Obstructive sleep apnea may be associated with risk for incident atrial fibrillation and recurrence. Complete a sleep history and sleep study in those patients that may be at risk for obstructive sleep apnea. Optimizing therapy to alleviate sleep-disordered breathing is prudent in sleep apneic patients with concomitant cardiovascular disease and atrial fibrillation.

REFERENCES

1. Fuster V, Ryden LE, Cannom DS, et al. ACC/AHA/ESC 2006 Guidelines for the Management of Patients With Atrial Fibrillation: A Report of the American College of Cardiology/American Heart Association Task Force on Practice Guidelines and the European Society of Cardiology Committee for Practice Guidelines (Writing Committee to Revise the 2001 Guidelines for the Management of Patients With Atrial Fibrillation). Developed in Collaboration with the European Heart Rhythm Association and the Heart Rhythm Society. Circulation 2006;114:e257–e354.

2. Gami AS, Hodge DO, Herges RM, et al. Obstructive sleep apnea, obesity, and the risk of incident atrial fibrillation. J Am Coll Cardiol 2007;49:565–571.

3. Gami AS, Pressman G, Caples SM, et al. Association of atrial fibrillation and obstructive sleep apnea. Circulation 2004;110:364–367.

4. Mehra R, Benjamin EJ, Shahar E, et al. Association of nocturnal arrhythmias with sleep-disordered breathing: The Sleep Heart Health Study. Am J Respir Crit Care Med 2006;173:910–916.

5. Kanagala R, Murali NS, Friedman PA, et al. Obstructive sleep apnea and the recurrence of atrial fibrillation. Circulation 2003;107:2589–2594.

6. Caples SM, Gami AS, Somers VK. Obstructive sleep apnea. Ann Intern Med 2005;142:187–197.

7. Singer DE, Albers GW, Dalen JE, et al. Antithrombotic Therapy in Atrial Fibrillation: The Seventh ACCP Conference on Antithrombotic and Thrombolytic Therapy. Chest 2004;126:429S–456S. (NOTE: See pages 449–450 regarding atrial fibrillation and anticoagulation.)

15

DEEP VEIN THROMBOSIS

Trouble from Deep Within. . . . . .Level II

James D. Coyle, PharmD

Patrick J. Fahey, MD

LEARNING OBJECTIVES

After completing this case study, the reader should be able to:

• Define acute deep vein thrombosis (DVT) and discuss its pathophysiology.

• Discuss the clinical presentation of patients with a DVT.

• Develop a pharmacotherapeutic care plan for the management of a patient with a DVT.

- Educate a patient receiving anticoagulation therapy for the treatment of a DVT.

PATIENT PRESENTATION

■ Chief Complaint

"I'm having pain in my leg."

■ HPI

Robert Roberts is a 54-year-old man who presented to his primary care physician because of pain in his right leg. He states that he awoke with the pain 3 days ago and that it has been continuous, although it hurts more when he walks. The patient denies chest pain, shortness of breath, fever, headache, and leg trauma. The patient started ezetimibe 10 mg daily for treatment of hyperlipidemia approximately 3 weeks prior to this visit. He stopped the ezetimibe 3 days ago because he thought it might be causing his leg pain, but the pain has continued. Physical examination reveals a tight, warm, right calf with mild tenderness. Lower extremity pulses and sensation are normal bilaterally. The physician's differential diagnosis includes deep vein thrombosis and rhabdomyolysis, and the patient is referred to the emergency department for further evaluation.

The emergency department history includes persistent pain in the right calf that is exacerbated by walking, with no remitting factors. The patient rates the pain intensity as 3/10 at this time.

■ PMH

Graves' disease with thyroid ablation
Gout
Hyperlipidemia
Left ankle fracture 9 years ago that required a cast but no surgery
Remote history of depression

■ PSH

Left herniorrhaphy about 10 years ago
Pilonidal cyst excision in remote past

■ FH

Father died at age 81 of liver failure. Mother, one brother, and son all alive and well. No family history of venous thromboembolism or clotting disorders.

■ SH

Married, one adult child. Drinks one to two alcoholic beverages daily. Smokes one cigar per month, no cigarettes. Denies illicit drug use.

■ Meds

Allopurinol 300 mg po daily
Levothyroxine 150 mcg po daily
Ezetimibe 10 mg po daily (discontinued 3 days ago)

■ All

NKDA

■ ROS

Constitutional: No chills, no fatigue
Eyes: No eye pain or changes in vision
ENT: No sore throat
Skin: No pigmentation changes, no nail changes
Cardiovascular: No chest pain, palpitations, or syncope
Respiratory: No cough, SOB, wheezing, or stridor

GI: No abdominal pain, nausea, diarrhea, or vomiting
Musculoskeletal: No neck pain, back pain, or injury
Neurologic: No dizziness, headache, or focal weakness
Psychiatric/Behavioral: No depression

■ Physical Examination

Gen

Somewhat obese, Caucasian man who appears comfortable. Cooperative, A & O × 3, normal affect.

VS

BP 106/78, P 75 regular, R 16, T 98.3°F, O_2 sat 97/ra; Wt 245 lb, Ht 6'0"

Skin

Warm, dry, normal color. No rash or induration.

HEENT

Pupils equal and reactive to light. EOM intact. Mucous membranes moist and pink.

Neck

Normal range of motion with no meningeal signs

Lungs/Thorax

Breath sounds normal, no respiratory distress

CV

RRR, no rubs, murmurs, or gallops

Abd

Non tender, no masses, no distension, no peritoneal signs

MS/Ext

Upper extremities: normal by inspection, no CCE, normal ROM.
Lower extremities: no CCE, normal ROM. Right calf tender with mild swelling. No obvious compartment syndrome.

Neuro

Glasgow coma scale of 15, no focal motor deficits, no focal sensory deficits

■ Labs

Na 140 mEq/L	WBC $5.9 \times 10^3/\mu$L
K 3.9 mEq/L	RBC $4.28 \times 10^6/\mu$L
Cl 103 mEq/L	Hgb 13.5 g/dL
CO_2 27 mEq/L	Hct 39.3%
BUN 10 mg/dL	MCV 92.0 fL
SCr 0.84 mg/dL	MCHC 34.4 g/dL
Glucose 88 mg/dL	RBC dist 14.3
Uric acid 5.0 mg/dL	Platelets $118 \times 10^3/\mu$L
CK 117 U/L	Mean platelet volume 7.2 fL
	Granulocytes, electronic 51.0%
	Lymphocytes, electronic 38.2%
	Monocytes, electronic 8.4%
	Eosinophils, electronic 1.9%
	Basophils, electronic 0.5%
	ESR, Westergren 9 mm/h

Lower extremity venous duplex ultrasonography: acute DVT of right distal superficial femoral, popliteal, and peroneal veins. No compression or flow in these vessels.

■ Assessment

Acute DVT in right superficial femoral, popliteal, and peroneal veins

QUESTIONS

Problem Identification

1.a. Create a list of this patient's medication-related problems.

1.b. What subjective and objective findings support the diagnosis of a lower extremity DVT?

Desired Outcome

2. What are the short- and long-term goals of pharmacotherapy for this patient's DVT?

Therapeutic Alternatives

3. What therapeutic alternatives are available for the pharmacologic management of this patient's DVT?

Optimal Plan

4. Design a treatment plan for the initial management of this patient's DVT. Be sure to include dosage form, dose, schedule, and duration of therapy for each drug that is part of the plan.

Outcome Evaluation

5. Design a monitoring plan for this patient's DVT therapy. Be sure to include monitoring for both safety and efficacy.

Patient Education

6. What education should be provided for this patient to optimize the probability of therapeutic success while minimizing the risk of adverse events?

■ CLINICAL COURSE

Mr. Roberts presents to his primary care physician 2 days after his emergency department visit, and again 6 days after that visit. He reports no missed warfarin doses, no changes in his other medications, a diet with consistent vitamin K intake, no exacerbation or recurrence of acute DVT symptoms, and no acute health problems. His INR at the first post-ED visit (after two doses of warfarin 5 mg) is 1.1 and his INR at the second post-ED visit (after six doses of warfarin 5 mg) is 1.2.

Follow-Up Question

1. Identify the patient's anticoagulation therapy-related drug therapy problem(s) and design treatment and monitoring plans for managing each problem you identify.

■ CLINICAL COURSE

Mr. Roberts presents to his primary care physician's office approximately 3 months after his acute DVT episode. He reports that he experienced an episode of very dark brown, "cola"-colored urine 2 days before this visit. He has had no recurrences. The patient denies dysuria, back or groin pain, and blood in his bowel movements. His current dose of warfarin is 5 mg on Monday, Wednesday, Friday, and Saturday and 7.5 mg on Tuesday, Thursday, and Sunday. Physical examination reveals no CVA tenderness. His INR is 2.4.

Follow-Up Question

1. Identify the patient's anticoagulation therapy-related drug therapy problem(s) and design treatment and monitoring plans for managing each problem you identify.

■ CLINICAL COURSE

Five months after his initial presentation, you see Mr. Roberts in the new anticoagulation clinic at his primary care physician's office. He is currently taking warfarin 5 mg on Monday, Wednesday, Friday, and Saturday and 7.5 mg on Tuesday, Thursday, and Sunday. His INR is 3.3. The patient's INR 2 weeks ago was 2.1 on the same dose. Mr. Roberts has not experienced any symptoms suggesting DVT recurrence or PE occurrence. He states that he has not had any problem with bleeding, has not missed doses or taken extra doses of warfarin in the past month, and has not changed his diet. His medications have been unchanged, except for the addition of rosuvastatin 5 mg every other day for the treatment of his hyperlipidemia approximately 2–3 weeks ago. You note that the following thrombophilia tests were completed prior to the initiation of anticoagulation therapy:

Test	Result	Reference Interval
Antithrombin III (% activity)	101%	85–118%
Protein C (% activity)	122%	72–220%
Protein S (% activity)	111%	50–168%
Factor V Leiden mutation	Negative	Normal: negative
Prothrombin G-20210-A mutation	Negative	Normal: negative
Anticardiolipin antibodies IgG	5.0 GPL units	0.0–15.0 GPL units
Anticardiolipin antibodies IgM	<4.7 MPL units	0.0–12.5 MPL units
Thrombin time	15.5 sec	13.0–20.0 sec
DRVVT	63.2 sec	35.0–47.0 sec
DRVVT confirm	36.3 sec	–
DRVVT ratio	1.74	1.10–1.41
StaClot LA	Positive	Normal: negative
ANA	Positive, 1:640, speckled pattern	Normal: negative, <1:20
Smith antibody	Negative	Normal: negative
RNP antibody	Positive	Normal: negative
SS-A antibody	Negative	Normal: negative
SS-B antibody	Negative	Normal: negative
Homocysteine, plasma	10.0 μmol/L	3.7–13.9 μmol/L

The laboratory summarizes the above results as consistent with the presence of lupus anticoagulants. Even though "anticoagulants" are present, many patients with this condition experience thrombotic events.

Follow-Up Question

1. Identify this patient's anticoagulation therapy-related drug problem(s) and design a treatment and monitoring plan for each problem that you identify. Be sure to specify the anticipated duration of his anticoagulation therapy.

■ SELF-STUDY ASSIGNMENTS

1. Create a summary of antiphospholipid syndrome, including its definition, clinical presentation, and management.

2. Summarize the existing literature regarding possible interactions between statins and warfarin. Is it likely that the initiation of rosuvastatin therapy increased this patient's INR? Does warfarin alter the effects of statins?

CLINICAL PEARL

Current evidence does not clearly establish the appropriate duration of anticoagulation therapy for many patients with DVTs. A decision must therefore be based on a careful comparison of the benefits of continuing anticoagulation (primarily a decreased risk of DVT recurrence and potential sequelae) versus the risk of adverse events (primarily bleeding) in each patient.

61

CHAPTER 16

Pulmonary Embolism

REFERENCES

1. Buller HR, Agnelli G, Hull RD, et al. Antithrombotic therapy for venous thromboembolic disease: the Seventh ACCP Conference on Antithrombotic and Thrombolytic Therapy. Chest 2004;126(Suppl):401S–428S.
2. Snow V, Qaseem A, Barry P, et al. Management of venous thromboembolism: a clinical practice guideline from the American College of Physicians and the American Academy of Family Physicians. Ann Intern Med 2007;146:204–210.
3. Segal JB, Streiff MB, Hoffman LV, et al. Management of venous thromboembolism: a systematic review for a practice guideline. Ann Intern Med 2007;146:211–222.
4. Kearon C, Ginsberg JS, Julian JA, et al. Comparison of fixed-dose weight-adjusted unfractionated heparin and low-molecular-weight heparin for acute treatment of venous thromboembolism. JAMA 2006;296:935–942.
5. Nutescu EA, Wittkowsky AK, Dobesh PP, et al. Choosing the appropriate antithrombotic agent for the prevention and treatment of VTE: a case-based approach. Ann Pharmacother 2006;40:1558–1571.
6. Jindal D, Tandon M, Sharma S, et al. Pharmacodynamic evaluation of warfarin and rosuvastatin co-administration in healthy subjects. Eur J Clin Pharmacol 2005;61:621–625.
7. Simonson SG, Martin PD, Mitchell PD, et al. Effect of rosuvastatin on warfarin pharmacodynamics and pharmacokinetics. J Clin Pharmacol 2005;45:927–934.
8. Miyakis S, Lockshin MD, Atsumi T, et al. International consensus statement on an update of the classification criteria for definite antiphospholipid syndrome (APA). J Thromb Haemost 2006;4:295–306.
9. Lim W, Crowther MA, Eikelboom JW. Management of antiphospholipid antibody syndrome: a systematic review. JAMA 2006;295:1050–1057.

16

PULMONARY EMBOLISM

One HIT Wonder. . . . . Level II

Kristen L. Longstreth, PharmD, BCPS

LEARNING OBJECTIVES

After completing this case study, the reader should be able to:

- Identify the signs, symptoms and risk factors associated with pulmonary embolism.
- Evaluate a patient for heparin-induced thrombocytopenia (HIT).
- Select an appropriate anticoagulant for a patient with HIT.
- Recommend a pharmacotherapeutic plan to initiate and monitor anticoagulation for the treatment of pulmonary embolism in a patient with HIT.
- Provide patient education on anticoagulation therapy.

PATIENT PRESENTATION

Chief Complaint

"My chest hurts and I feel like I can't get enough air."

HPI

Michael Veder is a 52-year-old man who was transferred to the hospital's skilled nursing unit to complete IV antibiotic therapy for a gangrenous chronic wound infection on his left ankle secondary to poorly controlled diabetes. The patient is S/P BKA left leg (post-op day #11) and has completed 11/14 days of the IV antibiotic regimen. He has tolerated the antibiotics well and his pain is improving daily, although he often refuses physical therapy in the skilled nursing unit. Early this morning, the patient complained of sharp chest pain and shortness of breath. The pain does not radiate. He denies nausea, vomiting, and dizziness. The patient is anxious. He has a non-productive cough and he claims that he has been having trouble with deep inspiration since yesterday.

PMH

HTN × 12 years
Type 2 DM × 10 years; uncontrolled due to noncompliance with diet and medications at home
Diabetic nephropathy (baseline creatinine 1.4 mg/dL)
Obesity
Chronic wound infection left ankle (previously failed 2 courses of IV antibiotics)
S/P BKA left leg (post-op day #11)

FH

Father has Type 2 DM

SH

The patient performs with a local rock band and leads an unhealthy lifestyle (poor diet, no exercise). Significant for tobacco abuse (20 pack-year history). Denies illicit drug use. Drinks alcohol socially on the weekends.

Meds

Home medications:
    Novolin 70/30 40 units Q AM and 30 units Q PM
    Lisinopril 10 mg po once daily
Additional medications started in the skilled nursing unit:
    Unfractionated heparin 5,000 units subcutaneously every 8 hours
    Nicotine transdermal patch 21 mg/day
    Cefepime 2 g IV every 24 hours
    Vancomycin 2 g IV every 24 hours
    Meperidine 50 mg po every 4–6 hours PRN pain
    Metformin 500 mg po twice daily
Regular insulin sliding scale subcutaneous coverage AC and HS:
    Glucose 150 to 199 mg/dL—2 units
    Glucose 200 to 249 mg/dL—4 units
    Glucose 250 to 299 mg/dL—6 units
    Glucose 300 to 349 mg/dL—8 units
    Glucose greater than or equal to 350 mg/dL—call physician for orders

All

NKDA

ROS

The patient denies headache, fever, chills. Positive for shortness of breath, non-productive cough. Positive for chest pain. No palpitations. No abdominal pain. No nausea, vomiting, or diarrhea.

Physical Examination

Gen

The patient is alert and oriented × 3; moderate respiratory distress

VS

BP 132/66, P 88, RR 21, T 36.5°C; Wt 102 kg, Ht 5'10'', O₂ sat 96% on room air

Skin

Warm and dry

HEENT

Head: Atraumatic; PERRLA; EOMI

Neck/Lymph Nodes

No carotid bruits; no lymphadenopathy

Lungs/Thorax

Clear to auscultation bilaterally; no wheezing or crackles

CV

RRR; normal heart sounds; no murmurs, rubs, or gallops

Abd

Soft; NT/ND; good bowel sounds

Genit/Rect

Patient refused at this time

MS/Ext

S/P BKA left leg; range of motion within normal limits; no swelling or redness; no cyanosis

Neuro

No focal deficits noted; cranial nerves intact

■ Labs

Na 140 mEq/L	Hgb 14 g/dL	Albumin 4.3 g/dL	D-Dimer 885 ng/mL
K 4.3 mEq/L	Hct 40%	AST 19 IU/L	CK 32 IU/L
Cl 102 mEq/L	Plt 61 × 10³/mm³	ALT 11 IU/L	(Time:0305)
CO₂ 28 mEq/L	WBC 8 × 10³/mm³	Alk Phos 76 IU/L	CK-MB 0.4 IU/L
BUN 18 mg/dL			(Time:0305)
SCr 1.6 mg/dL			Troponin I 0.01 ng/mL
Glu 125 mg/dL			(Time:0305)

■ ECG

Normal sinus rhythm at 88 bpm. No Q waves or ST changes present. No ectopy. Normal QRS axis, normal QRS morphology.

■ Assessment

1. Chest pain, SOB—most likely non-cardiac, R/O PE, R/O pneumonia

2. Thrombocytopenia—R/O heparin-induced thrombocytopenia (HIT)

3. Chronic wound infection, S/P BKA—continue current antibiotic regimen to complete 14 days, continue wound care and pain management

4. Diabetes mellitus—blood glucose well controlled on current medications and hospital no-added sugar diet

5. HTN—stable on current regimen

■ Clinical Course

The patient was transferred to a monitored unit within the hospital for further work-up. A chest x-ray and spiral CT of the chest were ordered. The spiral CT was later canceled due to the patient's elevated creatinine and the risk of contrast nephropathy. A V/Q scan was ordered. A platelet count history was obtained from the skilled nursing unit.

Chest x-ray report: no evidence of acute cardiopulmonary disease. Cardiac enzymes (second set):

CK 30 IU/L (Time:0915)	
CK-MB 0.4 IU/L (Time:0915)	
Troponin I 0.01 ng/mL (Time:0915)	

V/Q scan report: multiple segmental perfusion defects, indicating a ventilation perfusion mismatch and high probability of pulmonary embolism (Fig. 16-1).

Platelet count history from skilled nursing unit:

Post-op day #2	Plt 229 × 10³/mm³	Admission to skilled nursing unit
Post-op day #4	Plt 231 × 10³/mm³	Unfractionated heparin
Post-op day #6	Plt 227 × 10³/mm³	started for DVT prophylaxis
Post-op day #7	Plt 142 × 10³/mm³	
Post-op day #8	Plt 120 × 10³/mm³	
Post-op day #9	Plt 92 × 10³/mm³	
Post-op day #10	Plt 76 × 10³/mm³	
Post-op day #11	Plt 61 × 10³/mm³	Transferred to monitored unit

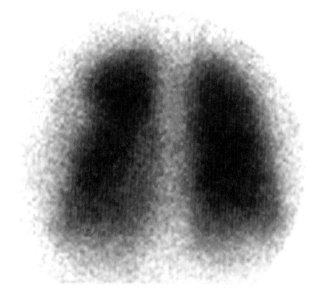

A   1ST Breath

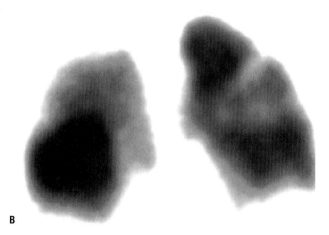

B

FIGURE 16-1. Ventilation-perfusion lung scan. *(A)* normal ventilation; *(B)* multiple segmental perfusion defects, indicating a ventilation perfusion mismatch and high probablilty of pulmonary embolism. *(Reproduced with permission from Goldhaber SZ. Pulmonary embolic disease. In Crawford MH ed. Current Diagnosis and Treatment in Cardiology, 2nd ed. New York, McGraw-Hill, 2003.)*

TABLE 16-1 Estimating the Pre-Test Probability of HIT: The "Four T's"

	Points (0, 1, or 2 for Each of 4 Categories: Maximum Possible Score = 8)		
	2	**1**	**0**
Thrombocytopenia	>50% Platelet fall to nadir ≥20	30–50% Platelet fall, or nadir 10–19	<30% Platelet fall, or nadir <10
Timing[a] of onset of platelet fall (or other sequelae of HIT)	Days 5–10, or ≤day 1 with recent heparin (past 30 days)	>Day 10 or timing unclear; or <day 1 with recent heparin (past 31–100 days)	<Day 4 (no recent heparin)
Thrombosis or other sequelae	Proven new thrombosis; skin necrosis; or acute systemic reaction after intravenous UFH bolus	Progressive or recurrent thrombosis; erythematous skin lesions; suspected thrombosis (not proven)	None
Other cause(s) of platelet fall	None evident	Possible	Definite

[a]First day of immunizing heparin exposure considered day 0.
Pretest probability score: 6–8 indicates high; 4–5, intermediate; and 0–3, low.
Reproduced with permission from Warkentin TE. Heparin-induced thrombocytopenia: diagnosis and management. Circulation 2004;110:e454–e458.

QUESTIONS

Problem Identification

1.a. What subjective and objective information is consistent with a diagnosis of PE in this patient?

1.b. What risk factors for PE are present for this patient?

1.c. Calculate this patient's pre-test probability score for HIT (Table 16-1).

1.d. Develop a list of the potential drug therapy problems related to this patient's increased serum creatinine.

Desired Outcome

2.a. What are the goals of therapy for the treatment of PE?

2.b. What additional goals of therapy exist for this patient with HIT?

Therapeutic Alternatives

3.a. Which agents are available to initiate anticoagulation for the treatment of PE in this patient?

3.b. What non-anticoagulant alternatives (pharmacologic and non-pharmacologic) are available? Is this patient an appropriate candidate for any of these alternatives?

Optimal Plan

4.a. Choose an appropriate anticoagulant to initiate therapy and calculate the dose for this patient.

4.b. When can warfarin be started for long-term management of PE in this patient? Design a pharmacotherapeutic plan for the transition to warfarin.

■ CLINICAL COURSE

The patient was started on an IV infusion of lepirudin at 10:00 AM. A heparin-induced platelet antibody ELISA (enzyme-linked immu-nosorbent assay) was drawn and sent to an outside laboratory for confirmation of HIT. An order was written to avoid all heparin (including catheter flushes). Prior to initiating lepirudin, a baseline aPTT (27.3 sec; reference: 23.8–34.6 sec), PT (11.1 sec; reference: 9.8–12.3 sec), and INR (1.0) were obtained to assist with anticoagulation dosing. Table 16-2 provides a summary of anticoagulation dosing and monitoring in this patient.

Outcome Evaluation

5.a. Determine the therapeutic aPTT range for the direct thrombin inhibitor administered to this patient.

5.b. After reviewing the dosing information in Table 16-2, determine what lepirudin dosage adjustment is necessary on day 4 to maintain this patient within the therapeutic aPTT range.

5.c. What clinical and laboratory parameters will you use to monitor the efficacy and safety of anticoagulation in this patient?

Patient Education

6.a. Prior to discharge, what information should be provided to this patient about warfarin therapy to enhance compliance and ensure efficacy and safety?

6.b. Discuss the information that you will provide to this patient concerning the future use of heparin and low molecular weight heparin therapy.

■ SELF-STUDY ASSIGNMENTS

1. Compare the risk of the development of HIT with unfractionated heparin and low molecular weight heparin. List other risk factors that influence the development of HIT.

2. Investigate the sensitivity and specificity of the various activation and antigen assays available to confirm the diagnosis of HIT.

3. Considering the potential for combined effects on the INR, list the steps necessary to transition a patient receiving argatroban to warfarin therapy.

TABLE 16-2 Anticoagulation Dosing and Monitoring

Anticoagulation Day and Time		Lepirudin Dose	Warfarin Dose	aPTT (sec)	PT (sec)/INR	Platelet Count (×10³/mm³)
1	10:00 AM	Infusion started at initial calculated rate (see question 4.a.)	Not given	27.3	11.1/1.0	61
	2:00 PM			61.0		
	6:00 PM			60.4		
2	6:15 AM	Initial calculated rate	Not given	59.5	12.9/1.1	89
3	6:05 AM	Initial calculated rate	Not given	64.4	13.3/1.1	96
4	5:57 AM	Initial calculated rate	Not given	79.2	14.1/1.2	117

Reference ranges: aPTT 23.8–34.6 sec; PT 9.8–12.3 sec.

4. Review the literature for available options to reverse the effects of the direct thrombin inhibitors if excessive anticoagulation occurs.

CLINICAL PEARL

Heparin-associated thrombocytopenia (HIT Type 1), which is more common than heparin-induced thrombocytopenia (HIT Type 2), is a nonimmunogenic mild decrease in platelet count (nadir greater than $100 \times 10^3/mm^3$) that occurs within 1 to 3 days after the initiation of heparin and does not increase the patient's risk of thrombosis or require heparin discontinuation.

REFERENCES

1. Fedullo PF, Tapson VF. The evaluation of suspected pulmonary embolism. N Engl J Med 2003;349:1247–1256.
2. Warkentin TE. Heparin-induced thrombocytopenia: diagnosis and management. Circulation 2004;110:e454–e458.
3. Warkentin TE, Greinacher A. Heparin-induced thrombocytopenia: recognition, treatment, and prevention: the Seventh ACCP Conference on Antithrombotic and Thrombolytic Therapy. Chest 2004;126:311–337.
4. Lo GK, Juhl D, Warkentin TE, et al. Evaluation of pretest clinical score (4 T's) for the diagnosis of heparin-induced thrombocytopenia in two clinical settings. J Thromb Haemost 2006;4:759–765.
5. Eichler P, Friesen HJ, Lubenow N, et al. Antihirudin antibodies in patients with heparin-induced thrombocytopenia treated with lepirudin: incidence, effects on aPTT, and clinical relevance. Blood 2000;96:2373–2378.
6. Greinacher A, Lubenow N, Eichler P. Anaphylactic and anaphylactoid reactions associated with lepirudin in patients with heparin-induced thrombocytopenia. Circulation 2003;108:2062–2065.
7. Tardy B, Lecompte T, Boelhen F, et al. Predictive factors for thrombosis and major bleeding in an observational study in 181 patients with heparin-induced thrombocytopenia treated with lepirudin. Blood 2006;108:1492–1496.
8. Bartholomew JR. Transition to an oral anticoagulant in patients with heparin-induced thrombocytopenia. Chest 2005;127:27–34.
9. Buller HR, Agnelli G, Hull RD, et al. Antithrombotic therapy for venous thromboembolic disease: the Seventh ACCP Conference on Antithrombotic and Thrombolytic Therapy. Chest 2004;126:401–428.
10. Baroletti SA, Goldhaber SZ. Heparin-induced thrombocytopenia. Circulation 2006;114:355–356.

17

CHRONIC ANTICOAGULATION

Anticoagulate and Anticipate . . . . Level II

Mikayla Spangler, PharmD

Beth Bryles Phillips, PharmD, FCCP, BCPS

LEARNING OBJECTIVES

After completing this case study, the reader should be able to:

- List the goals of oral anticoagulant therapy in preventing recurrent thromboembolism.

- Appropriately assess a patient's response to chronic warfarin therapy.

- Recognize common drug–drug interactions associated with warfarin therapy.

- Develop patient-specific pharmacotherapeutic plans for patients receiving chronic anticoagulation.

- Educate patients appropriately about chronic warfarin therapy.

PATIENT PRESENTATION

■ Chief Complaint

"I'm here to get my blood drawn."

■ HPI

Willow Bradley is a 47-year-old woman with a past medical history of a deep venous thrombosis (DVT), pulmonary embolus (PE), and Factor V Leiden gene mutation who presents to the clinic for anticoagulation follow-up. In the interval since the last anticoagulation appointment, Ms. Bradley reports she had an outpatient surgical procedure 13 days ago to remove a superficial malignant melanoma on her right thigh. Ms. Bradley states she has not missed any of her warfarin doses during the last month. She uses a medication box and states no warfarin tablets were left over in her medication box at the end of each week. She denies any bleeding, excessive bruising, severe headaches, abdominal pain, chest pain, shortness of breath, or pain or swelling in the lower extremities. She does not drink alcoholic beverages. She states that she has cut out her daily intake of spinach salads lately because of some diarrhea. When asked about recent medication changes, she reports she was started on a 10-day course of dicloxacillin 500 mg QID for a post-operative cellulitis 6 days ago and attributes her diarrhea to the antibiotic. She was also seen in the acute care clinic today with the complaint of dysphagia, which has worsened over the last 2 weeks. She describes the symptoms as a "pulling/contracting" sensation and tightness over her lower chest every time she swallows food or liquid. She denies regurgitating food back into her throat. She feels that she has more problems with swallowing cold liquids than warm liquids or food. The symptoms only occur when swallowing and are not related to activity. She has no associated lightheadedness or diaphoresis and has no pleuritic chest pains. Her weight has been stable over the last year.

■ PMH

DVT $1^1/_2$ years ago
PE $1^1/_2$ years ago
Homozygous Factor V Leiden gene mutation
Dysthymia
Malignant melanoma of the right thigh

■ FH

Ms. Bradley has two sisters and two brothers—one with basal cell carcinoma. Her father had colon polyps removed when he was in his 50's but is currently alive and well in his 80's. Her mother has high blood pressure and is 79 years of age. She has three children who are alive and well.

■ SH

(–) ETOH; (–) smoking

■ Meds

Acetaminophen 500 mg po daily PRN minor pain
Multivitamin one tablet po daily
Celexa 30 mg po once daily
Dicloxacillin 500 mg po QID × 10 days
Vitamin E 400 units po once daily
Warfarin 7.5 mg po M, W, F; 5 mg 4 days/wk

All

Tetracycline—bumps, rash/hives
Polysporin—swelling

ROS

(–) For CP, SOB, severe headaches, abdominal pain, leg pain, bruises, or change in color of stool or urine; (+) for difficulty swallowing

Physical Examination

Gen

Pleasant obese woman in NAD

VS

BP 104/71, HR 65, RR 14, T 36.5°C; Wt 85.9 kg, Ht 5'6"

Skin

Normal turgor and color; warm; healing melanoma excision site on right thigh

HEENT

PERRLA, EOMI; disks flat; fundi with no hemorrhages or exudates

Neck/Lymph Nodes

No lymphadenopathy, thyromegaly, or carotid bruits

Lungs

CTA bilaterally

CV

RRR; normal S_1 and S_2; no S_3 or S_4; no MRG

Abd

Obese, soft, non-distended, moderate tenderness on palpitation of the epigastric as well as right lower quadrant with no rebound or guarding, (+) BS

Genit/Rect

Deferred

Ext

Warm with no clubbing, cyanosis, or edema

Neuro

A & O × 3; CN II–XII intact; DTR 2+; Babinski negative

Labs

Date	INR	Warfarin Dose
Today	1.7	7.5 mg Mon, Wed, Fri; 5 mg 4 days/wk
1 Mo. ago	2.4	7.5 mg Mon, Wed, Fri; 5 mg 4 days/wk
2 Mo. ago	2.1	7.5 mg Mon, Wed, Fri; 5 mg 4 days/wk
3 Mo. ago	2.6	7.5 mg Mon, Wed, Fri; 5 mg 4 days/wk
4 Mo. ago	2.5	7.5 mg Mon, Wed, Fri; 5 mg 4 days/wk
5 Mo. ago	2.5	7.5 mg Mon, Wed, Fri; 5 mg 4 days/wk
6 Mo. ago	2.0	7.5 mg Mon, Wed, Fri; 5 mg 4 days/wk

Assessment

History of venous thromboembolism (VTE) and homozygous Factor V Leiden gene mutation requiring chronic anticoagulation with a target INR 2.5 (range, 2.0–3.0)
Subtherapeutic INR
Esophageal dysphagia

QUESTIONS

Problem Identification

1.a. Create a list of this patient's drug-related problems.

1.b. What signs or symptoms might patients experience if they are under-anticoagulated?

1.c. What questions would you ask this patient to assess her current warfarin therapy?

1.d. What are possible causes for the subtherapeutic INR?

Desired Outcome

2. What are the goals of oral anticoagulation in this patient?

Therapeutic Alternatives

3. What are the options for anticoagulation in this patient?

Optimal Plan

4.a. Based on today's laboratory result, what is your recommendation for this patient's warfarin therapy?

4.b. What can she do to help prevent subtherapeutic INRs in the future?

Outcome Evaluation

5. How will you monitor this patient's warfarin therapy?

Patient Education

6. What information should this patient know about her warfarin therapy, especially to minimize sub- or supratherapeutic INRs and potential hemorrhagic and thromboembolic complications?

■ CLINICAL COURSE

Upon return to clinic 3 days later, the patient reports she missed a couple of doses of her dicloxacillin. As a result, she will need to continue dicloxacillin for 4 more days in order to complete the full course of therapy. Her INR is 2.7. She continues to eat less dietary vitamin K due to antibiotic-associated diarrhea.

Follow-Up Question

1. Based on this information, what are your recommendations for her warfarin therapy?

■ ADDITIONAL CASE QUESTION

1. Ms. Bradley is being referred to Gastroenterology for further work-up of her dysphagia. In the meantime, the physician would like to prescribe a medication to relieve her symptom. He would like to give her either a proton pump inhibitor or an H_2-receptor antagonist. What pharmacotherapeutic recommendation would be least likely to interact with her warfarin therapy?

■ SELF-STUDY ASSIGNMENTS

1. There are several mechanisms by which drugs may interact with warfarin. What are the major mechanisms of these interactions? Give examples of drugs that interact by each mechanism.

2. Develop a list of antibiotics that may interact with warfarin, and indicate appropriate alternatives to the antibiotics.

CLINICAL PEARL

Because the effects of the interaction may persist for up to 3 weeks after discontinuation of dicloxacillin in patients receiving warfarin therapy, frequent monitoring and potential dose adjustment are needed during this period.

REFERENCES

1. Hirsh J, Dalen J, Anderson DR, et al. Oral anticoagulants: mechanism of action, clinical effectiveness, and optimal therapeutic range. Chest 2001;119(1 suppl):8S–21S.
2. Taylor AT, Pritchard DC, Goldstein AO, et al. Continuation of warfarin-nafcillin interaction during dicloxacillin therapy. J Fam Pract 1994;39:182–185.
3. Krstenansky PM, Jones WN, Garewal HS. Effect of dicloxacillin sodium on the hypothrombinemic response to warfarin sodium. Clin Pharm 1987;6:804–806.
4. Mailloux AT, Gidal BE, Sorkness CA. Potential interaction between warfarin and dicloxacillin. Ann Pharmacother 1996;30:1402–1407.
5. Halvorsen S, Husebye T, Arnesen H. Prosthetic heart valve thrombosis during dicloxacillin therapy. Scand Cardiovasc J 1999;33:366–368.
6. Ridker PM, Goldhaber SZ, Danielson E, et al. PREVENT Investigators. Long-term, low-intensity warfarin therapy for the prevention of recurrent venous thromboembolism. N Engl J Med 2003;348:1425–1434.
7. Kearon C, Ginsber JS, Kovacs MJ, et al. Extended Low-Intensity anticoagulation for Thrombo-Embolism Investigators. Comparison of low-intensity warfarin therapy with conventional-intensity warfarin therapy for long-term prevention of recurrent venous thromboembolism. N Engl J Med 2003;349:631–639.
8. Kearon C, Gent M, Hirsh J, et al. A comparison of three months of anticoagulation with extended anticoagulation for a first episode of idiopathic venous thromboembolism. N Engl J Med 1999;340:901–907.
9. Lindmarker P, Schulman S, Sten-Linder M, et al. The risk of recurrent venous thromboembolism in carriers and non-carriers of the G1691A allele in the coagulation factor V gene and the G20210A allele in the prothrombin gene. Thromb Haemost 1999;81:684–689.
10. Büller HR, Agnelli G, Hull RD, et al. Antithrombotic therapy for venous thromboembolic disease: the seventh ACCP antithrombotic conference on antithrombotic and thrombolytic therapy. Chest 2004;126:401–428.
11. Ansell J, Hirsh J, Poller L, et al. The pharmacology and management of the vitamin K antagonists: the seventh ACCP conference on antithrombotic and thrombolytic therapy. Chest 2004;126:204–233.
12. Hansten P, Wittkowsky A. Warfarin drug interactions. In: Ansell JE, Wittkowsky AK, Oertel LB, eds. Managing Oral Anticoagulation Therapy: Clinical and Operational Guidelines. St. Louis, MO, Facts and Comparisons, 2003;35:1–35:14.

18

ISCHEMIC STROKE

Different Strokes for Different Folks. . . . . Level II

Alexander J. Ansara, PharmD, BCPS

Julia M. Koehler, PharmD

LEARNING OBJECTIVES

After completing this case study, the reader should be able to:

- Identify risk factors for ischemic stroke, and counsel a patient on cardiovascular risk reduction strategies.

- Discuss the role of thrombolytics in the management of acute ischemic stroke.

- Formulate an appropriate patient-specific drug regimen for the treatment of an acute ischemic stroke.

- Discuss the approach to multi-disease state management for the secondary prevention of ischemic stroke, including the management of hypertension, hyperlipidemia, and the use of antiplatelet agents.

PATIENT PRESENTATION

▧ Chief Complaint

"My right arm feels like it's frozen. I can barely move it."

▧ HPI

Carson Johnson is a 67-year-old African-American man who presents to the emergency room at 8:45 AM after noticing a sudden onset of weakness in his right arm. He woke up at 7:15 AM and went to the bathroom to brush his teeth. While walking from the bathroom to the kitchen, he noticed general weakness and had trouble saying "good morning" to his son, Willis, with whom he lives. His son immediately brought him to the ER. While in the ER, he started experiencing some dysarthria and began to have a right-sided facial droop. He denied any dizziness, vomiting, or headache.

▧ PMH

Hypertension, diagnosed 10 years ago
Hyperlipidemia
Two different TIAs in the past, last in 2002

▧ FH

Father passed away at age 87 from a stroke; mother passed away from "old age" at age 82. Brother, age 61, also has HTN. Son, age 34, has DM.

▧ SH

Denies ETOH use, admits to occasional cocaine use, quit smoking 20 years ago. Lives with son.

▧ Meds

Ramipril 5 mg po daily
Atorvastatin 10 mg po daily
Atenolol 50 mg po daily
Aspirin EC 81 mg po daily

▧ All

PCN (rash), adhesive tape

▧ ROS

Denies headache. Vision is blurry.

▧ Physical Examination

Gen

WD AAM lying in bed, responsive but sluggish; looks tired. Speech is slurred.

VS

BP 172/92, P 92, RR 21, T 98.6°, O₂ Sat 94% on room air; Wt 90 kg, Ht 5'8"

Skin

Warm, dry

HEENT

PERRLA, EOMI; no nystagmus, exudates, hemorrhages, or papille-dema; right-sided facial droop

Neck

(+) carotid bruits on the left side, (−) lymphadenopathy

Chest

Lungs clear to auscultation bilaterally

CV

RRR, S_1 & S_2 normal, no S_3 or S_4

Abd

Soft, non-tender, non-distended, (+) BS

GU

Deferred

MS/Ext

RUE: 2/5; RLE 4/5; LUE: 5/5; LLE: 5/5
Good pulses, no CCE; DTR: 2+ throughout, normal Babinski reflex

Neuro

A & O × 3; (+) dysarthria, right-sided facial droop

▓ Labs

Na 138 mEq/L	WBC $6.2 \times 10^3/mm^3$	Total Cholesterol
K 3.8 mEq/L	Hgb 16.9 g/dL	207 mg/dL
Cl 103 mEq/L	Hct 51.3%	LDL-C 114 mg/dL
CO_2 29 mEq/L	Plt $242 \times 10^3/mm^3$	Triglycerides
BUN 18 mg/dL	aPTT 26.3 sec	179 mg/dL
SCr 0.9 mg/dL		HDL-C 45 mg/dL
Glu 109 mg/dL		

Head CT scan: (−) hemorrhage, left-sided middle cerebral artery infarct (Fig. 18-1)

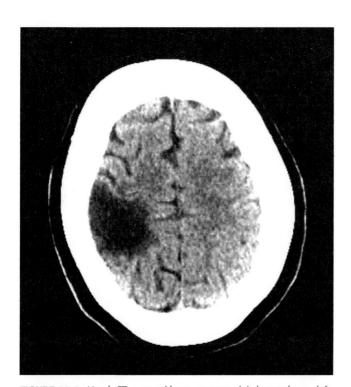

FIGURE 18-1. Head CT scan without contrast: (−) hemorrhage, left-sided middle cerebral artery infarct.

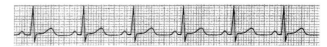

FIGURE 18-2. EKG showing sinus tachycardia.

Carotid dopplers: reduced flow, moderate to severe carotid stenosis; 65% stenosis of right carotid, 50% stenosis of left carotid
Echocardiogram: no evidence of LV thrombus, ejection fraction 55–60%; overall unremarkable
EKG: Tachycardic sinus rhythm (Fig. 18-2)

▓ Assessment

Acute ischemic stroke secondary to carotid atherosclerosis and ischemic disease in a patient with hypertension, hyperlipidemia, and a prior history of TIAs

▓ Clinical Course

It is now 2 hours later (10:45 AM), and you are seeing the patient with the rest of the stroke team.

QUESTIONS

Problem Identification

1.a. Create a list of the patient's drug therapy problems.

1.b. Identify the non-modifiable, modifiable, and Framingham risk factors for CHD present in this patient.

1.c. Which signs, symptoms, and other tests indicate the presence of an acute ischemic stroke?

Desired Outcome

2.a. What are the initial goals of pharmacotherapy in this patient?

2.b. What are the long-term goals of pharmacotherapy in this patient?

Therapeutic Alternatives

3.a. What nondrug therapies might be useful for this patient?

3.b. What feasible pharmacotherapeutic alternatives are available for the treatment of acute ischemic stroke?

Optimal Plan

4.a. What is your recommendation for the acute use of antihypertensives in this patient?

4.b. What pharmacotherapeutic regimen would you recommend for the acute treatment of stroke in this patient (include drug, dose, route, frequency, and duration)?

Outcome Evaluation

5. What clinical and laboratory parameters are necessary to evaluate the therapy for achievement of the desired therapeutic outcome(s) and to detect or prevent adverse effects?

Patient Education

6. What information should be provided to Mr. Johnson to enhance adherence, ensure successful therapy, and minimize adverse effects?

■ CLINICAL COURSE

Mr. Johnson is currently 3 days post-stroke and will be discharged home tomorrow morning. He has regained most strength in his extremities, and his speech has improved significantly. A mild facial droop is still present when prompted to show his teeth.

Follow-Up Questions

1. What antiplatelet regimen would you recommend for the secondary prevention of acute ischemic stroke in Mr. Johnson (include drugs, dose and dosage form, schedule, and duration)?

2. Which parameters related to Mr. Johnson's treatment should be monitored to ensure optimal secondary prevention?

3. What recommendations would you make to Mr. Johnson's home drug regimen to optimally manage his hypertension and hyperlipidemia?

■ SELF-STUDY ASSIGNMENTS

1. Explain which patients are candidates to receive aspirin instead of warfarin for the prevention of stroke in the setting of atrial fibrillation.

2. Summarize the role of HMG Co-A reductase inhibitors in the primary and secondary prevention of ischemic stroke.

3. Read the CURE and MATCH trials and explain when and why patients should be treated with the combination of aspirin and clopidogrel. Explain what the MATCH results tell us about the use of combination antiplatelet therapy for the prevention of ischemic stroke.

4. Review the ESPS-2 trial and write a one-page report summarizing the findings with aspirin/dipyridamole (Aggrenox) in this clinical study.

CLINICAL PEARL

Hypoglycemia results in a clinical presentation similar to ischemic stroke and therefore should be excluded as a diagnosis before treatment for an acute stroke is initiated.

REFERENCES

1. National Institute of Neurological Disorders and Stroke rt-PA Stroke Study Group. Tissue plasminogen activator for acute ischemic stroke. N Engl J Med 1995;333:1581–1587.

2. del Zoppo GJ, Higashida RT, Furlan AJ, et al. PROACT. A phase II randomized trial of recombinant pro-urokinase by direct arterial delivery in acute middle cerebral artery stroke. Stroke 1998;29:4–11.

3. Chinese Acute Stroke Trial Collaborative Group (CAST). Randomized placebo-controlled trial of early aspirin use in 20,000 patients with acute ischemic stroke. Lancet 1997;349:1641–1649.

4. International Stroke Trial Collaborative Group (IST). A randomized trial of aspirin, subcutaneous heparin, both, or neither among 19435 patients with acute ischaemic stroke. Lancet 1997;349:1569–1581.

5. Adams Jr HP, del Zoppo G, Alberts MJ, et al. Guidelines for the Early Management of Adults with Ischemic Stroke: A Guideline From the American Heart Association/American Stroke Association Stroke Council, Clinical Cardiology Council, Cardiovascular Radiology and Intervention Council, and the Atherosclerotic Peripheral Vascular Disease and Quality of Care Outcomes in Research Interdisciplinary Working Groups: The American Academy of Neurology affirms the value of this guideline as an educational tool for neurologists. Circulation 2007;115:e478–e534.

6. Matherne CA, Albright KC, Allison TA, et al. LOAD: examining the safety of loading of aspirin and clopidogrel in acute ischemic stroke and TIA. Neurology 2006;66(suppl 2):A315.

7. Bath PM, Iddenden R, Bath FJ. Low-molecular-weight heparins and heparinoids in acute ischemic stroke: a meta-analysis of randomized controlled trials. Stroke 2000;31:1770–1778.

8. CAPRIE Steering Committee. A randomized, blinded, trial of Clopidogrel Versus Aspirin in Patients at Risk of Ischemic Events (CAPRIE): CAPRIE Steering Committee. Lancet 1996;348:1329–1339.

9. Yusuf S, Zhao F, Mehta SR, et al. for the Clopidogrel in Unstable Angina to Prevent Recurrent Events Trial Investigators. Effects of clopidogrel in addition to aspirin in patients with acute coronary syndromes without ST-segment elevation. N Engl J Med 2001;345:494–502.

10. Diener HC, Cunha L, Forbes C, et al. European Stroke Prevention Study 2: dipyridamole and acetylsalicylic acid in the secondary prevention of stroke. J Neurol Sci 1996;143:1–13.

11. Chobanian AV, Bakris GL, Black HR, et al. for the National Heart, Lung, and Blood Institute Joint National Committee on Prevention, Detection, Evaluation, and Treatment of High Blood Pressure; National High Blood Pressure Education Program Coordinating Committee. The Seventh Report of the Joint National Committee on Prevention, Detection, Evaluation, and Treatment of High Blood Pressure: the JNC 7 Report. JAMA 2003;289:2560–2571.

19

HYPERLIPIDEMIA: PRIMARY PREVENTION

Ignorance Is Bliss . . . . Level II

Laurajo Ryan, PharmD, MSc, BCPS, CDE

LEARNING OBJECTIVES

After completing this case study, the reader should be able to:

• Identify patients who require screening for elevated cholesterol.

• Stratify individual patients for risk of coronary heart disease (CHD) and stroke.

• Determine appropriate LDL, HDL, triglyceride, total cholesterol, and non-HDL goals based on individual risk factors.

• Recommend a cholesterol management strategy that includes therapeutic lifestyle changes (TLC), drug therapy, patient education, and monitoring parameters.

PATIENT PRESENTATION

■ Chief Complaint

"I'm here for my yearly visit, I'm not sick!"

■ HPI

Ima Ferguson is a 56-year-old woman who presents to the clinic for her yearly follow-up. The patient states that she feels fine and has been in her usual state of health since last clinic visit. She also states she is not sure why she has to come to clinic every year, indicating; "There is nothing wrong with me." The patient's former primary care provider has transferred to a different facility.

■ PMH

Morbid obesity (BMI 35.6 kg/m^2)

HTN for 24 years
IFG diagnosed 1 year ago
Osteoarthritis bilateral knees
Leg cramping >three blocks walking
Seasonal rhinitis since childhood
Perimenopausal—has OB/GYN screening yearly

■ FH

Father; age 71 with Type 2 diabetes, COPD, hypertension
Mother; age 71 with advanced Parkinson's, "heart disease" diagnosed at age 66
Patient does not have contact with her two younger brothers, their medical history is unknown
Of her children, the only significant medical history is one daughter with epilepsy

■ SH

Patient is a widow; she has four adult children, one of whom lives with her in her home along with his three children
Completed the 9th grade and provides day-care in her home
Denies alcohol, tobacco, or illicit drug use

■ Meds

Enalapril 10 mg po BID
OTC potassium gluconate 595 mg po PRN for leg cramps
Diphenhydramine 25–50 mg po PRN rhinitis
Ibuprofen 200 mg, 4 tabs po PRN HA, knee pain

■ All

NKDA

■ ROS

Patient states that she is in her normal state of health. She denies unilateral weakness, numbness/tingling, or acute changes in vision (although over the course of the past year her vision prescription has changed twice). She additionally denies CP, SOB, changes in bowel habits, or po intake. She states that she has noticed more frequent leg cramps that begin after walking shorter distances than usual. In the past she was able to walk ~6 blocks without pain, but now she gets cramping/pain walking just 2–3 blocks. She has also noticed some swelling of the lower legs and feet, especially at the end of the day and has had increasingly severe AM knee pain over the past several months. She admits to taking ibuprofen most days of the week.

■ Physical Examination

Gen

Obese Caucasian woman in NAD

VS

BP 147/92, P 83, RR 16, T 37.2°C; Wt 97 kg, Ht 5'5"

Skin

Warm and moist, normal turgor, acanthosis nigricans noted in axilla bilaterally

HEENT

PERRLA; EOMI; funduscopic exam deferred; TMs intact; oral mucosa clear

Neck/Lymph Nodes

Neck supple, no lymphadenopathy, thyroid smooth and firm without nodules

Chest

CTA bilaterally, no wheezes, crackles or rhonchi

Breasts

Normal, slightly fibrotic, no lumps or discharge

CV

RRR, no MRG, normal S_1 and S_2; no S_3 or S_4

Abd

(+) BS, no hepatosplenomegaly

Genit/Rect

Deferred

Ext

1+ pedal edema, pulses 2+ throughout

Neuro

No gross motor–sensory deficits present

■ Labs (fasting)

Na 142 mEq/L	Ca 8.6 mg/dL	WBC $5.3 \times 10^3/mm^3$	*Lipid Profile:*
K 4.9 mEq/L	Mg 2.1 mEq/L	Hemoglobin 11.5 g/dL	TC 259 mg/dL
Cl 104 mEq/L	AST 34 U/L	Hematocrit 34.6%	HDL 37 mg/dL
CO_2 24 mEq/L	ALT 31 U/L	Platelets $151 \times 10^3/mm^3$	LDL 167 mg/dL
BUN 21 mg/dL	T. bili 0.5 mg/dL		TG 280 mg/dL
SCr 1.3 mg/dL	T. prot 7.1 g/dL		
Glucose 121 mg/dL			

■ UA

Yellow, clear, SG 1.003, pH 5.3, (–) protein, (–) glucose, (–) ketones, (–) bilirubin, (–) blood, (–) nitrites, RBC 0/hpf, WBC 1/hpf, no bacteria, 1–5 epithelial cells

■ Assessment

Ms. Ferguson is an obese woman who presents to primary care clinic for her yearly exam. Patient has OA and seasonal rhinitis, both of which she self-treats with OTC medications. She also has uncontrolled HTN, which is currently treated with an ACE inhibitor. IFG was diagnosed last year. Patient has new onset anemia, hyperlipidemia, renal insufficiency, and symptoms suggestive of possible PAD. When questioned about exercise and dietary habits, the patient immediately became very defensive about her weight and stated that she is just "big boned" and has a "slow metabolism."

QUESTIONS

Problem Identification

1.a. What drug-related problems does this patient have?

1.b. What laboratory values indicate the presence and severity of hyperlipidemia in this patient?

1.c. This patient has been diagnosed with hyperlipidemia. What are her risk factors (both modifiable and non-modifiable) for CV disease?

1.d. What is this patient's risk classification for cardiovascular disease, and how does this relate to her individual lipid goals?

Desired Outcome

2.a. What are the pharmacologic and nonpharmacologic goals of treatment in this patient?

2.b. Does this patient have any disease states that may modify treatment goals? It yes, please describe how the treatment goals would be modified.

Therapeutic Alternatives

3.a. What nonpharmacologic therapies are necessary for this patient to achieve and maintain target cholesterol values?

3.b. What pharmacotherapeutic options are available for controlling this patient's hyperlipidemia?

Optimal Plan

4.a. Design a plan that details specific lifestyle modifications for this patient.

4.b. Develop a specific pharmacotherapeutic regimen for this patient's untreated dyslipidemia and uncontrolled HTN. This regimen should include drug, dosage, and duration of therapy.

4.c. What options are available if the pharmacotherapy regimen you chose fails, or if she develops an adverse drug reaction?

Outcome Evaluation

5. Based on your treatment regimen, what are the monitoring parameters for each pharmacologic agent selected?

Patient Education

6.a. Based on your recommendations, provide appropriate education to this patient regarding pharmacologic and nonpharmacologic treatments.

6.b. What steps can you take to ensure that patient is successful in implementing nonpharmacologic measures?

■ FOLLOW-UP QUESTION

1. For questions on the use of garlic and fish oil for the treatment of hyperlipidemia, please see Section 20 of this Casebook.

■ SELF-STUDY ASSIGNMENTS

1. Review the guidelines associated with this patient's disease states unrelated to hyperlipidemia, and develop a pharmacotherapy regimen and management plan for this patient. Determine how this patient's other drug/disease interactions issues that are unrelated to hyperlipidemia should be managed.

2. Delineate the changes, if any, you would make to the pharmacotherapeutic regimen for this patient if she had presented at the initial visit with each of the following characteristics:

   • Childbearing age
   • Cirrhosis of the liver

CLINICAL PEARL

Intake of saturated fat is the primary dietary source of serum cholesterol, followed by ingestion of cholesterol itself from food. While saturated fats are present in both animal (e.g., meat, dairy, eggs) and processed (e.g., crackers, cookies, chips) food sources, dietary cholesterol is only found in animal products.

REFERENCES

1. Third Report of the National Cholesterol Education Program (NCEP) Expert Panel on Detection, Evaluation, and Treatment of High Blood Cholesterol in Adults (Adult Treatment Panel III) Final Report. Circulation 2002;106:3143–3421.

2. Grundy SM, Cleeman JI, Merz CNB, et al. Implications of recent clinical trials for the National Cholesterol Education Program Adult Treatment Panel III Guidelines. Circulation 2004;110:227–239.

3. Lichtenstein AH, Appel LJ, Brands M, et al. Diet and lifestyle recommendations revision 2006: a scientific statement from the American Heart Association Nutrition Committee. Circulation 2006;114:82–96.

4. Pearson TA, Blair SN, Daniels SR, et al. AHA Guidelines for Primary Prevention of Cardiovascular Disease and Stroke: 2002 Update: Consensus Panel Guide to Comprehensive Risk Reduction for Adult Patients Without Coronary or Other Atherosclerotic Vascular Diseases. Circulation 2002;106:388–391.

5. Fletcher B, Berra K, Ades P, et al. Managing abnormal blood lipids: a collaborative approach. Circulation 2005;112:3184–3209.

6. Mosca L, Banka CL, Benjamin EJ, et al. Evidence-based guidelines for cardiovascular disease prevention in women: 2007 update. Circulation 2007;115:1481–1501.

20

HYPERLIPIDEMIA: SECONDARY PREVENTION

So—Fix It! . . . . .Level II

Laurajo Ryan, PharmD, MSc, BCPS, CDE

LEARNING OBJECTIVES

After completing this case study, the reader should be able to:

• Identify patients who require treatment for elevated cholesterol.

• Stratify individual patients for risk of coronary heart disease (CHD) and stroke.

• Determine appropriate LDL, HDL, triglyceride, total cholesterol, and non-HDL goals based on individual risk factors.

• Recommend a cholesterol management strategy that includes therapeutic lifestyle changes (TLC), drug therapy, patient counseling, and monitoring parameters.

PATIENT PRESENTATION

■ Chief Complaint

"I just fell down—I don't know what happened, just fix it!"

■ HPI

Michael Gonzalez is a 67-year-old Hispanic man who has just been transferred to the medicine unit from the ICU. Last week he was transported by ambulance to the emergency department after his sister found him unresponsive on the floor. He was down for an unknown length of time. A CT scan at admission was negative for hemorrhage but verified a small left subcortical infarct. There was also ECG evidence of a prior MI.

■ PMH

Type 2 diabetes
Hypertension

▨ FH

Father had Type 2 diabetes and hypertension; deceased from MI age 54
Mother (deceased) had Alzheimer's disease
Sister has Type 2 diabetes, hypertension

▨ SH

Unmarried, lives with his sister
ETOH: patient admits to ~12 pack beer each day
TOB: 2 ppd × 52 years
Denies illicit drug use

▨ Meds

None

▨ OTC/Herbal

None

▨ All

NKDA

▨ ROS

Patient refuses to answer questions and tells the medicine team to "get out of my room." His sister, who is his medical power of attorney, apologizes to the team for her brother's behavior, and states that "he hates doctors" and has not received any health care that she is aware of since their father died over 30 years ago. The only reason that he is still in the hospital is that he is too weak to walk out. She states she was unaware that the patient had had an MI in the past, and when she asked him about it, he said it was "none of your business." The physical exam and laboratory information are from 2 days ago when patient was transferred from the critical care unit—he has refused all labs since his transfer to the medicine floor.

▨ Physical Examination

Gen

Unpleasant, thin, agitated Hispanic man

VS

BP 163/104, P 77, RR 18, T 37.1°C; Wt 54 kg, Ht 5'7"

Skin

Warm and dry, normal turgor

HEENT

PERRLA; EOMI; funduscopic exam deferred; TMs intact; oral mucosa clear

Neck/Lymph Nodes

Neck supple, no lymphadenopathy, thyroid smooth and firm without nodules

Chest

CTA bilaterally, no wheezes, crackles, or rhonchi

CV

RRR, no MRG, normal S_1 and S_2; no S_3 or S_4

Abd

(+) BS, no hepatosplenomegaly

Genit/Rect

Deferred

Ext

No pedal edema, pulses 2+ throughout

Neuro

No gross motor–sensory deficits present

▨ Labs (fasting)

Na 142 mEq/L	Ca 8.3 mg/dL	*Lipid Profile:*
K 4.9 mEq/L	Mg 2.2 mEq/L	TC 232 mg/dL
Cl 103 mEq/L	AST 31 U/L	HDL 32 mg/dL
CO_2 22 mEq/L	ALT 38 U/L	LDL 138 mg/dL
BUN 27 mg/dL	T. bili 0.5 mg/dL	TG 310 mg/dL
SCr 1.4 mg/dL	T. prot 7.0 g/dL	
Glucose 387 mg/dL	A1C 12.7%	

Head CT: Negative for hemorrhage; evidence suggestive of small left subcortical infarct
Carotid Dopplers: 50% stenosis RCA, 55% stenosis LCA

▨ Assessment

Mr. Gonzalez is a thin, elderly, Hispanic man who appears older than his stated age. His sister states that although he has diabetes and hypertension, he does not take any medications that she has ever seen, and he does not monitor his blood glucose. Patient has uncontrolled diabetes, hypertension, hyperlipidemia, and history of MI (as determined by ECG reading), and is now S/P ischemic stroke, likely secondary to carotid artery disease.

QUESTIONS

Problem Identification

1.a. What drug-related problems does this patient have?

1.b. What laboratory values indicate the presence and severity of hyperlipidemia in this patient?

1.c. What are the patient's risk factors (both modifiable and non-modifiable) for cardiovascular disease?

1.d. How would you categorize this patient's coronary heart disease (CHD) risk, and based on this categorization, what is the patient's target LDL goal?

Desired Outcome

2. What are the pharmacologic and nonpharmacologic goals of treatment in this patient?

Therapeutic Alternatives

3.a. What nonpharmacologic therapies are necessary for this patient to achieve and maintain target cholesterol values?

3.b. What pharmacotherapeutic options are available for controlling this patient's hyperlipidemia and preventing future CHD-related events?

Optimal Plan

4.a. Design a plan that details specific lifestyle modifications for this patient.

4.b. Develop a specific pharmacotherapeutic regimen for this patient. This regimen should include drug, dosage, and duration of therapy.

4.c. What options are available if the pharmacotherapy regimen you chose fails or if he develops an adverse drug reaction?

Outcome Evaluation

5. Based on your treatment regimen, what are the monitoring parameters for each pharmacologic agent selected?

Patient Education

6.a. Based on your recommendations, provide appropriate counseling to this patient regarding pharmacologic and nonpharmacologic recommendations.

6.b. What steps can you take to ensure that the patient is successful in implementing nonpharmacologic measures?

■ FOLLOW-UP QUESTION

1. For questions on the use of garlic and fish oil for the treatment of hyperlipidemia, please see Section 20 of this Casebook.

■ SELF-STUDY ASSIGNMENTS

1. Detail how this patient's other drug/disease interactions and issues unrelated to hyperlipidemia should be managed.

2. List what changes, if any, you would make to the pharmacotherapeutic regimen for this patient if he had presented at the initial visit with each of the following characteristics:

   • Woman of childbearing age
   • Cirrhosis of the liver

CLINICAL PEARL

Patients with diabetes have a small, dense form of LDL cholesterol that differs from the general population. This form of LDL is more atherogenic and therefore, at comparable LDL levels, patients with diabetes have a higher risk for cardiovascular events.

REFERENCES

1. Third Report of the National Cholesterol Education Program (NCEP) Expert Panel on Detection, Evaluation, and Treatment of High Blood Cholesterol in Adults (Adult Treatment Panel III) Final Report. Circulation 2002;106:3143–3421.

2. Grundy SM, Cleeman JI, Merz CNB, et al. Implications of recent clinical trials for the National Cholesterol Education Program Adult Treatment Panel III Guidelines. Circulation 2004;110:227–239.

3. Smith SC, Jr., Allen J, Blair SN, et al. AHA/ACC guidelines for secondary prevention for patients with coronary and other atherosclerotic vascular disease: 2006 update: endorsed by the National Heart, Lung, and Blood Institute. Circulation 2006;113:2363–2372.

4. Lichtenstein AH, Appel LJ, Brands M, et al. Diet and lifestyle recommendations revision 2006: a scientific statement from the American Heart Association Nutrition Committee. Circulation 2006;114:82–96.

5. Fletcher B, Berra K, Ades P, et al. Managing abnormal blood lipids: a collaborative approach. Circulation 2005;112:3184–3209.

21

PERIPHERAL ARTERIAL DISEASE

Cold Feet? . . . . Level II

Tracy L. Bottorff, PharmD, BCPS

LEARNING OBJECTIVES

After completing this case study, the reader should be able to:

• Identify risk factors for peripheral arterial disease (PAD).

• Describe the symptoms and diagnosis of PAD.

• Recommend appropriate nonpharmacologic strategies for PAD, including risk factor modification, exercise, and revascularization.

• Design an appropriate pharmacologic treatment plan for a patient with PAD.

PATIENT PRESENTATION

■ Chief Complaint

"I am having pain in both legs and in my left foot."

■ HPI

Debbie Houston is a 57-year-old woman with a history of hypertension, hyperlipidemia, TIA, and a history of bilateral leg pain for the previous 2 years. She reports to the family medicine clinic today with increased "burning pain in my left foot that radiates up to my ankles" when she walks. She reports numbness in her feet when she lies down. She reports that it is painful to walk even for 4–5 minutes and that her legs are often weak and "give out." She is having trouble "keeping up" with her 4-year-old granddaughter whom she cares for every day. She was told by her cardiologist that she might need to have Doppler studies of her legs.

■ PMH

CAD
HTN
Hyperlipidemia
TIA

■ FH

Mother died of a stroke at age 67, father died of pneumonia at the age of 62

■ SH

Retired; has one child; cares for granddaughter at home; lives with husband; smokes $1/2$ ppd × 35 years; denies ETOH and illicit drug use; has one dog in home

■ Meds

Tramadol 50–100 mg po Q 4–6 h PRN pain
Amitriptyline 50 mg po Q HS
Clopidogrel 75 mg po daily
Ezetimibe/simvastatin 10/40 mg po daily
Trazodone 50 mg po Q HS for sleep
Hydrochlorothiazide 25 mg po daily
Atenolol 50 mg po daily

■ All

NKDA

■ ROS

Complains of dyspnea on exertion. Denies chest pains, palpitations, syncope, orthopnea. Denies nausea, vomiting, diarrhea, constipation, change in bowel habits, abdominal pain, or melena. Denies joint swelling, muscle cramps, and muscle weakness. Denies transient paralysis, seizures, syncope, and tremors.

■ Physical Examination

Gen

The patient is a pleasant woman in NAD. She appears older than her stated age.

VS

BP 152/87, P 83, RR 16, T 99.2°C; Wt 78 kg, Ht 5'7"

HEENT

PERRLA; conjunctivae and lids normal; TM intact; normal dentition, no gingival inflammation, no labial lesions; tongue normal, posterior pharynx without erythema or exudate

Neck/Lymph Nodes

Supple, no masses, trachea midline; no carotid bruit; no lymphadenopathy or thyromegaly

Lungs/Thorax

No rales, rhonchi, or wheezes; no intercostal retractions or use of accessory muscles

CV

RRR, S_1, S_2 normal; no murmurs, rubs, or gallops; no thrill or palpable murmurs, no displacement of PMI

Abd

Soft, nontender, no masses, bowel sounds normal; no enlargement or nodularity of liver or spleen

Genit/Rect

Deferred

MS/Ext

Normal gait; no clubbing, cyanosis, petechiae, or nodes; normal ROM and strength, good stability and no joint enlargement or tenderness; pedal pulses 1+, symmetric

Neuro

CN II–XII grossly intact; DTRs 2+, no pathologic reflexes; sensory and motor levels intact

■ Labs

Na 141 mEq/L	Hgb 11.7 g/dL	WBC $7.4 \times 10^3/mm^3$
K 3.8 mEq/L	Hct 33.5%	CPK 71 IU/L
Cl 101 mEq/L	RBC $4.53 \times 10^6/mm^3$	
CO_2 24 mEq/L	Plt $313 \times 10^3/mm^3$	
BUN 17 mg/dL	TC 203 mg/dL	
SCr 1.0 mg/dL	TG 165 mg/dL	
Glu 99 mg/dL	LDL 140 mg/dL	
A1C 6.3%	HDL 30 mg/dL	

Lower extremity arterial Doppler; ankle/brachial index (ABI): Right: 0.63; Left: 0.47

■ Assessment

1. Intermittent claudication (IC)
2. Hyperlipidemia
3. Hypertension
4. (+) Smoking

QUESTIONS

Problem Identification

1.a. Create a list of this patient's drug-related problems.

1.b. What information presented in this case supports the diagnosis of IC? Also identify the patient's risk factors for PAD.

Desired Outcome

2. What are the goals of therapy for IC in this case?

Therapeutic Alternatives

3.a. Does this patient have any modifiable risk factors for PAD? If so, what are your recommendations for these conditions?

3.b. What pharmacologic options are available for the treatment of this patient's PAD?

3.c. What treatment options are available to patients who have severe disease or fail pharmacologic therapy?

Optimal Plan

4. What drug, dose, and schedule would be most appropriate for treating this patient's IC?

Outcome Evaluation

5. Based on your recommendations, what clinical and laboratory parameters are necessary to evaluate the therapy for achievement of the desired therapeutic outcome and to detect or prevent adverse effects?

Patient Education

6. What information should be provided to the patient to enhance adherence, ensure successful therapy, and minimize adverse effects?

■ SELF-STUDY ASSIGNMENTS

1. Review the guidelines for the treatment of patients with heart failure. How would your recommendation for treatment of this patient's PAD change if she developed heart failure?

2. Review the literature on the use of herbal medications in the treatment of PAD? What are your recommendations to a patient inquiring about their use?

3. Perform a literature search to determine the role of warfarin for the management of PAD.

CLINICAL PEARL

Previously it was thought that β-blockers should be avoided in patients with peripheral arterial disease due to worsening claudication. Current treatment guidelines state that β-blockers are effective antihypertensive agents and are not contraindicated in patients with PAD.

REFERENCES

1. Chobanian AV, Bakris Gl, Black HR, et al. The Seventh Report of the Joint National Committee on Prevention, Detection, Evaluation, and Treatment of High Blood Pressure: the JNC 7 report. JAMA 2003;289:2560–2572.
2. Hirsch AT, Haskal ZJ, Hertzer NR, et al. ACC/AHA Guidelines for the management of patients with peripheral arterial disease (lower extremity, renal, mesenteric, and abdominal aortic): executive summary a collaborative report from the American Association for Vascular Surgery, Society for Cardiovascular Angiography and interventions, Society of Interventional Radiology, Society for Vascular Medicine and Biology, and the ACC/AHA Task Force on Practice Guidelines. J Am Coll Cardiol 2006;47:1239–1312.
3. White C. Intermittent claudication. N Engl J Med 2007;356:1241–1250.
4. Gornick HL, Creager MA. Contemporary management of peripheral arterial disease: cardiovascular risk-factor modification. Cleve Clin J Med 2006;73:S30–S37.

5. CAPRIE Steering Committee. A randomized, blinded, trial of clopido-grel vs. aspirin in patients at risk of ischaemic events (CAPRIE). Lancet 1996;348:1329–1339.

6. Dawson DL, Butler BS, Meissner MH, et al. Cilostazol has beneficial effects in treatment of intermittent claudication: results from a multi-center, randomized, prospective, double-blind trial. Circulation 1998; 98:678–686.

22

HYPOVOLEMIC SHOCK

A Glass Half Full . . . . Level II

Brian L. Erstad, PharmD, FCCP, FCCM, FASHP

LEARNING OBJECTIVES

After completing this case study, the reader should be able to:

- Develop a plan for implementing fluid or medication therapies for treating a patient in the initial stages of shock.

- Outline the major parameters used to monitor hypovolemic shock and its treatment.

- List the major disadvantage of using isolated hemodynamic recordings, such as blood pressure measurements, for monitoring the progression of shock.

- Compare and contrast fluids and medications used for treating hypovolemic shock.

PATIENT PRESENTATION

▓ Chief Complaint

"I have diarrhea and I've felt very tired lately even though I'm only 47 years old."

▓ HPI

Five days PTA, Mr. Hobbs had become nauseated and did not feel like eating. Although the nausea resolved after a couple of days, he began to have diarrhea, which led him to continue his avoidance of food intake. Mr. Hobbs purchased a commercially available rehydration solution from his local pharmacy and attempted to drink the small but frequent volumes recommended by his pharmacist, but he could not keep up with fluid losses. The diarrhea, in conjunction with increasing fatigue and lack of substantial fluid intake for 2 days, prompted his physician to hospitalize him for further evaluation and to temporarily stop his tacrolimus therapy (10 mg po BID); other medications were continued.

▓ PMH

S/P orthotopic liver transplantation 6 months PTA for sarcoidosis involving the liver; the transplant was complicated by an adrenal vein hemorrhage that required reoperation for ligation
Diabetes mellitus posttransplant
Moderate cellular rejection on recent biopsy

▓ FH

Noncontributory

▓ SH

Does not smoke, drink ETOH, or use illicit drugs

▓ Meds

Prednisone 5 mg po daily
Mycophenolate mofetil 250 mg po once daily
Fluconazole 50 mg po every M, W, F
Acyclovir 400 mg po BID
Famotidine 20 mg po BID
Spironolactone 200 mg po once daily

▓ All

NKDA

▓ ROS

Patient has had a recent increase in weight over the past month (6 kg), although this has decreased by 2 kg in the past few days. Hearing is intact with no vertigo. No dizziness or fainting episodes. Colorless sputum. No chest pain or dyspnea, but heart has been "racing." Has had diarrhea for 3 days; no vomiting, abdominal pain, or cramping. No musculoskeletal pain or cramping.

▓ Physical Examination

Gen

WDWN, but somewhat anxious man in mild distress

VS

BP 84/58 (baseline 135/85), but possible orthostatic changes not determined, HR 132 (baseline 80), RR 16, T 38.2°C; admission Wt 78 kg, Ht 6'3"

Skin

Pale color (including nail beds) and dry, but not cyanotic; no lesions

HEENT

Normal scalp/skull; conjunctivae pale and dry with clear sclerae; PERRLA, dry oral mucosa; remainder of ophthalmologic exam not performed

Neck/Lymph Nodes

Supple, no lymphadenopathy or thyromegaly

Lungs/Thorax

Decreased breath sounds since last exam

CV

RRR; S_1 and S_2 normal; apical pulse difficult to palpate; no MRG

Abd

Symmetric with bulging flanks as a result of recent marked increase in ascites; palpable fluid wave; bowel sounds present; no tenderness or masses; scar from transplant evident

Genit/Rect

Normal male genitalia; prostate smooth, not enlarged; no hemorrhoids noted; stool heme (−)

MS/Ext

No deformities with normal ROM; 2–3+ leg edema; no ulcers or tenderness

Neuro

Mild muscular atrophy with weak grip strength; CN II–XII intact; 2+ reflexes throughout; Babinski downgoing

■ Labs

Na 133 mEq/L	Hgb 11.9 g/dL	Phos 6.3 mg/dL
K 5.3 mEq/L	Hct 34.3%	AST 86 IU/L
Cl 98 mEq/L	Plt 51 × 10³/mm³	ALT 59 IU/L
CO_2 20 mEq/L	WBC 13 × 10³/mm³	T. bili 1.6 mg/dL
BUN 66 mg/dL	PT 12.1 sec	Alk phos 83 IU/L
SCr 1.4 mg/dL[a]	PTT 33 sec	
Glu 237 mg/dL	Albumin 2.3 g/dL	
[a]baseline SCr 1.1 mg/dL.		

■ Other Test Results

I/O 1,260/350 (urinary catheter) for first 14 hours of hospitalization.
Ultrasound of abdomen ordered with possible paracentesis planned.
Results pending for gastroenteric pathogens on stool culture, O & P, and *Clostridium difficile* titer.
Normal response to synthetic ACTH adrenal stimulation testing.

■ Assessment

Volume depletion, possible infectious process, hyperglycemia

QUESTIONS

Problem Identification

1.a. Create a list of the patient's drug-related problems.

1.b. What information (signs, symptoms, laboratory values) indicates the presence or severity of hypovolemic shock?

Desired Outcome

2. What are the goals of pharmacotherapy in this case?

Therapeutic Alternatives

3.a. What nondrug therapies might be useful for this patient?

3.b. What feasible pharmacotherapeutic alternatives are available for treatment of shock and the associated laboratory alterations?

Optimal Plan

4. What drug, dosage form, dose, schedule, and duration of therapy are best for this patient?

Outcome Evaluation

5. What clinical and laboratory parameters are necessary to evaluate the therapy for achievement of the desired therapeutic outcome and to detect or prevent adverse events?

Patient Education

6. What information should be provided to the patient to enhance compliance, ensure successful therapy, and minimize adverse effects?

■ CLINICAL COURSE

No evidence of infection was found, including a negative titer for *Clostridium difficile*. All cultures were negative, and the elevated temperature abated within 12 hours of admission. However, the patient had a complicated clinical course since inadequate fluids were given because of concerns about fluid overload. Paracenteses were performed every few days to remove accumulated ascitic fluid; this led to further vascular depletion with decreased renal perfusion. After approximately 10 days, the patient had to be admitted to the ICU for renal failure precipitated by inadequate vascular expansion. However, there was no evidence of progressive organ rejection after resolution of the renal failure, and the tacrolimus was eventually restarted.

■ FOLLOW-UP QUESTION

1. Why might this patient have changes in urine output, heart rate, and other parameters that are consistent with volume depletion even though he has edema on physical examination and his admission weight was indicative of volume overload?

■ SELF-STUDY ASSIGNMENTS

1. Search the literature and be able to discuss the results of comparative trials involving crystalloids and colloids for plasma expansion.

2. Write a two-page report that compares the advantages and limitations of each type of fluid for the plasma expansion indication.

CLINICAL PEARL

Although interstitial fluid accumulation in the lungs possibly leading to pulmonary edema is a concern, other sites of fluid accumulation, such as the legs, should not preclude adequate intravascular expansion, which is necessary to avoid organ hypoperfusion and subsequent dysfunction.

REFERENCES

1. Fox DL, Vermeulen LC. UHC Technology Assessment: Albumin, Nonprotein Colloid, and Crystalloid Solutions. Oak Brook, IL, University Health System Consortium, May 2000.
2. Choi PT, Yip G, Quinonez LG, et al. Crystalloids vs. colloids in fluid resuscitation: a systematic review. Crit Care Med 1999;27:200–210.
3. Finfer S, Bellomo R, Boyce N, et al. SAFE Study Investigators. A comparison of albumin and saline for fluid resuscitation in the intensive care unit. N Engl J Med 2004;350:2247–2256.

23

ACUTE ASTHMA

Snotty Nose, Coughing Fits, Asthma Attack... Level II

Jennifer A. Donaldson, PharmD

LEARNING OBJECTIVES

After completing this case study, the reader should be able to:

- Recognize the signs and symptoms of an acute asthma exacerbation.

- Formulate therapeutic endpoints based on the initiation of a pharmacotherapy plan used to treat the acute asthma symptoms.

- Identify appropriate dosage form selection based on the patient's age, ability to take medication, or adherence to technique.

- Determine an appropriate home pharmacotherapy plan, including discharge counseling, as the patient nears discharge from a hospital setting.

PATIENT PRESENTATION

■ Chief Complaint

"My boy has trouble breathing and he keeps coughing. His albuterol isn't helping."

■ HPI

Peyton Harrison is a 3-year-old African-American boy who presents to the emergency department with a 3-day history of cough and congestion. The mother was giving him albuterol, 2.5 mg via nebulization twice a day since the cough started. She was also giving him an allergy medicine. He did have a fever 3 days prior to admission, and he was given ibuprofen. The previous night before admission, he seemed to be gasping for air and during the day today, he has had an increased work of breathing. Mother also notes that he has been fussy, not eating well, and has had only two to three urinations in the past 24 hours. His assessment in the emergency department revealed him to have labored breathing that was more difficult with activities. He had mild retractions with tachypnea at 52 breaths per minute. His other vital signs were a heart rate of 137 beats per minute, blood pressure of 100/68, temperature of 38.9°C, and a weight of 14.4 kg. The initial oxygen saturation was 88%, and he was started on oxygen at 1.5 liter/min via nasal cannula. His breath sounds were noted to have fair air exchange but with expiratory wheezes. His chest x-ray revealed patchy infiltrates consistent with pneumonia. Peyton was complaining of a runny nose and sore throat. He did not have any ear pain. While in the emergency department, he was given three albuterol/ipratropium nebulizations and one dose of prednisolone 15 mg orally. He received one dose of acetaminophen 210 mg. His breath sounds and oxygenation did not improve so he was started on hourly albuterol nebulizations at 5 mg. Peyton was then transferred to the Pediatric Intensive Care Unit for further treatment and monitoring.

■ PMH

Asthma, unknown if previous hospitalizations
S/P tonsillectomy/adenoidectomy at 2 years of age

■ FH

Unknown

■ SH

Lives with foster mother and two siblings. Birth mother has visitations. Unclear as to reason for foster placement. Positive tobacco exposure in current home.

■ Meds

Albuterol 2.5 mg via nebulizer as needed
Phenylephrine/chlorpheniramine/methscopolamine (Dallergy®), dose unknown

■ All

NKA

■ ROS

(+) Fever, cough, congestion, increased work of breathing

■ Physical Examination

Gen

NAD, moderate increase in work of breathing

VS

BP 103/55, P 154, T 36.4°C, R 29, O$_2$ sat 94% at 1.5 L/min nasal cannula

Skin

No rashes, no bruises

HEENT

NC/AT, PERRLA

Neck/Lymph Nodes

Soft, supple, no cervical lymphadenopathy

Chest

Slight decrease in breath sounds bilaterally, minimal wheezing

CV

RRR, no MRG

Abd

Soft, NT/ND

Ext

No clubbing or cyanosis

Neuro

A & O, no focal deficits

■ Labs

Na 134 mEq/L	WBC $6.5 \times 10^3/mm^3$
K 3.0 mEq/L	RBC $3.84 \times 10^6/mm^3$
Cl 103 mEq/L	Hgb 10 g/dL
CO_2 19 mEq/L	Hct 34%
BUN 6 mg/dL	Plt $252 \times 10^3/mm^3$
SCr 0.4 mg/dL	
Glu 140 mg/dL	

Respiratory viral panel nasal swab: positive for parainfluenza 3

■ Chest X-Ray

Patchy infiltrates throughout lung fields

■ Assessment

Asthma exacerbation with pneumonia and dehydration

QUESTIONS

Problem Identification

1.a. Create a list of the patient's drug-related problems.

1.b. What information (signs, symptoms, laboratory values) indicates the severity of the acute asthma attack?

Desired Outcome

2. What are the acute goals of pharmacotherapy in this case?

Therapeutic Alternatives

3.a. What nondrug therapies might be useful for this patient?

3.b. What feasible pharmacotherapeutic alternatives are available for the treatment of acute asthma?

Optimal Plan

4.a. What drug, dosage form, dose, schedule, and duration of therapy are best for this patient's acute asthma exacerbation?

4.b. What other pharmacotherapy would you recommend in the acute treatment of this patient?

■ CLINICAL COURSE

Within 72 hours of initiation of the treatment plan for management of the acute exacerbation, Peyton was stable enough to transfer to the general pediatric floor. His vital signs were BP 111/67, P 108, R 26, T 36.7°C, O_2 sat 99% on 0.5 L/min nasal cannula. Mother states that he is more like his normal self and doesn't seem to have much trouble breathing now.

4.c. What drug, dosage form, dose, schedule and duration of therapy are best for this patient's discharge plan?

Outcome Evaluation

5.a. Once the patient has transferred to the general medical floor and his vitals have improved (see Clinical Course), what clinical and laboratory parameters are necessary to evaluate the therapy for achievement of the desired therapeutic outcome

and to detect or prevent adverse effects at that point in the patient's care?

5.b. What clinical parameters are necessary to evaluate the efficacy of the patient's asthma therapy after hospital discharge?

Patient Education

6.a. Describe the information that should be provided to the family regarding nebulization technique, the differences between quick-relief and controller medications, and possible asthma triggers.

6.b. What should the family monitor for regarding the potential adverse effects from the drug therapy?

■ FOLLOW-UP QUESTIONS

1. Should any cough and cold products be used for asthma symptoms? Why or why not?

2. What methods could be used to help a pediatric patient and the family to be compliant with nebulization treatments?

3. What information can be given to families who are concerned about giving their child "steroids" for asthma treatment (either in an acute asthma exacerbation or for controller therapy)?

■ SELF-STUDY ASSIGNMENTS

1. Research the efficacy of systemic corticosteroids for treatment of acute asthma exacerbation when given intravenously versus orally (enterally).

2. Discuss the differences in acute asthma exacerbation symptoms in an adult patient versus a pediatric patient, and describe when you would refer a patient (or family) to the physician or emergency department based on his or her asthma action plan.

3. Discuss the appropriate use of ipratropium bromide in an acute asthma exacerbation.

CLINICAL PEARL

For proper treatment of an acute asthma exacerbation, the patient (or family) needs to be aware of the first symptoms of an exacerbation and possible triggers. At this point, the patient (family) should initiate his or her asthma action plan to minimize the symptoms, duration of drug therapy, and severity of the exacerbation. This in turn, should decrease the number of severe exacerbations and hospital admissions.

REFERENCES

1. National Asthma Education and Prevention Program Expert Panel Report 3: Guidelines for the Diagnosis and Management of Asthma. Bethesda, MD, National Institutes of Health, 2007. *http://www.nhlbi.nih.gov/guidelines/asthma/asthgdln.htm*. Accessed September 4, 2007.

2. Aldington S, Beasley R. Asthma exacerbations 5: assessment and management of severe asthma in adults in hospital. Thorax 2007; 62:447–458.

3. Hardasmalani MD, DeBari V, Bithoney WG, et al. Levalbuterol versus racemic albuterol in the treatment of acute exacerbation of asthma in children. Pediatr Emerg Care 2007;21:415–419.

4. Rodrigo GJ, Castro-Rodriguez JA. Anticholinergics in the treatment of children and adults with acute asthma: a systematic review with meta-analysis. Thorax 2005;60:740–746.

5. Hendeles L. Selecting a systemic corticosteroid for acute asthma in young children. J Pediatr 2003;142:S40–S44.

6. Khetsuriani N, Kazerouni NN, Erdman DD, et al. Prevalence of viral respiratory tract infections in children with asthma. J All Clin Immunol 2007;119:314–321.

7. Szefler SJ, Eigen H. Budesonide inhalation suspension: a nebulized corticosteroid for persistent asthma. J All Clin Immunol 2002;109:730–742.

24

CHRONIC ASTHMA

Cat Got Your Tongue? . . . . Level I

Julia M. Koehler, PharmD

Carrie Maffeo, PharmD, BCPS, CDE

LEARNING OBJECTIVES

After completing this case study, the reader should be able to:

- Recognize signs and symptoms of uncontrolled asthma.

- Identify potential causes of uncontrolled asthma.

- Formulate a patient-specific therapeutic plan (including drugs, route of administration, and appropriate monitoring parameters) for management of a patient with chronic asthma.

- Develop a self-management action plan for improving control of asthma.

PATIENT PRESENTATION

Chief Complaint

"I can't...breathe...and my albuterol...doesn't seem to be helping!"

HPI

Madison Bradley is a 29-year-old woman who presents to the ED for an acute visit due to shortness of breath. She reports feeling especially short of breath since awakening this morning. She states that she has been using her albuterol every hour for the past 6 hours and that it doesn't seem to be helping. Her peak flows have been running between 180 L/min and 200 L/min today (personal best = 400 L/min). In addition to her albuterol MDI, which she uses PRN, she also has a fluticasone MDI, which she uses "most days of the week." She reports having to use her albuterol inhaler approximately 3–4 times per week over the past 2 months, but over the past week she admits to using albuterol almost daily. She reports being awakened by a cough three times over the past month. She states she especially becomes short of breath when she exercises; although she admits that her shortness of breath is not always brought on by exercise and sometimes occurs when she is not actively exercising. She indicates that her morning peak flows have been running around 300 L/min (personal best = 400 L/min) over the past several weeks.

PMH

Asthma (previously documented as "mild persistent") since childhood; no prior history of intubations; hospitalized twice in the past year for poorly controlled asthma; three visits to the ED in the past 6 months; treated with oral systemic corticosteroids during both hospitalizations and at each ED visit.

Migraine headache disorder (diagnosed at age 21); currently taking prophylactic medication; has had only one migraine attack in the past year.

FH

Both parents living; mother 52-years-old with HTN, osteoporosis; father 54-years-old with COPD (33 pack-year smoking history) and Type 2 DM; brother, age 34 (smoker); sister, age 32 (non-smoker)

SH

No alcohol or tobacco use. Married, sexually active. Lives with husband (cabinetmaker; non-smoker) and two cats.

Meds

Fluticasone HFA 110 mcg, 2 puffs BID
Albuterol HFA 2 puffs Q 4–6 h PRN shortness of breath
Ortho-Tri-Cyclen 1 po daily
Propranolol 80 mg po BID
Maxalt-MLT 5 mg po PRN acute migraine

All

Sulfa (rash)

Physical Examination

Gen

Anxious-appearing Caucasian female; moderate respiratory distress with audible wheezing noted; unable to speak in complete sentences; suprasternal muscle retractions noted; hunched forward

VS

BP 134/78, HR 110, RR 22, T 37°C; Wt 68 kg, Ht 5'5"; Pulse Ox 88% on RA

HEENT

PERRLA; mild oral thrush; TMs intact

Neck/Lymph Nodes

Supple; no lymphadenopathy or thyromegaly

Lungs/Thorax

High-pitched, diffuse expiratory wheezes bilaterally, two-thirds of the way up

Breasts

Nontender without masses

CV

Tachycardia; Regular rhythm; no MRG

Abd

Soft, NTND; (+) BS

Genit/Rect

Deferred

Ext

Normal ROM; peripheral pulses 3+; no CCE

Neuro

No motor deficits; CN II–XII grossly intact; A & O × 3

Labs

Na 134 mEq/L	Hgb 12 g/dL	WBC $8.0 \times 10^3/mm^3$
K 3.0 mEq/L	Hct 36%	PMNs 56%
Cl 99 mEq/L	RBC $5.0 \times 10^6/mm^3$	Bands 1%
CO_2 28 mEq/L	MCH 28 pg	Eosinophils 3%
BUN 22 mg/dL	MCHC 34 g/dL	Basophils 2%
SCr 0.7 mg/dL	MCV 90 μm^3	Lymphocytes 33%
Glu 117 mg/dL	Plts $192 \times 10^3/mm^3$	Monocytes 5%
Ca 9.3 mg/dL		

Chest X-Ray

Hyperinflated lungs; no infiltrates

■ Assessment

29 yo woman with moderate to severe exacerbation of asthma; uncontrolled chronic asthma

■ Clinical Course

The patient is admitted overnight for treatment with oxygen, inhaled bronchodilators, and oral prednisone 60 mg daily. She is discharged home with her previous regimen plus nebulized albuterol 2.5 mg every 8 hours for 5 days and prednisone 60 mg orally once daily to complete a 10-day burst. She was also given nystatin swish and swallow for treatment of her oral thrush infection. On follow-up at day 4 in the clinic, her lungs are clear without wheezing; her respiratory rate is 16 breaths per minute; and her pulse oximetry is 97% on room air. Her peak flow readings have improved to 300 L/min.

QUESTIONS

Problem Identification

1.a. Create a list of the patient's drug therapy problems.

1.b. What information indicates the presence of uncontrolled chronic asthma and an acute asthma exacerbation?

1.c. What factors may have contributed to this patient's poorly controlled asthma and acute exacerbation?

1.d. How would you classify this patient's level of asthma control (well controlled, not well controlled, or very poorly controlled), according to NIH guidelines?

Desired Outcome

2. What are the goals of pharmacotherapy in this case?

Therapeutic Alternatives

3.a. What nonpharmacologic therapies might be useful for this patient?

3.b. What feasible pharmacotherapeutic alternatives are available for treatment of this patient's chronic asthma?

Optimal Plan

4.a. Outline an optimal plan of treatment for this patient's chronic asthma.

4.b. What alternatives would be appropriate if the initial therapy fails?

Outcome Evaluation

5. What clinical parameters are necessary to evaluate the therapy for achievement of the desired therapeutic effect and to detect or prevent adverse effects?

Patient Education

6. What information should be provided to the patient regarding the use of her asthma medications and how she can use her peak-flow readings to better manage her disease?

■ SELF-STUDY ASSIGNMENTS

1. Review the NIH guidelines on the management of asthma during pregnancy, and develop a pharmacotherapeutic treatment plan for this patient's asthma if she were to become pregnant.

2. Review the literature on the impact of chronic inhaled corticosteroid use on the risk for development of osteoporosis, and write a two page paper summarizing the available published literature on this topic.

CLINICAL PEARL

Patients with asthma who report that taking aspirin makes their asthma symptoms worse may respond well to leukotriene modifiers. Aspirin inhibits prostaglandin synthesis from arachidonic acid through inhibition of cyclooxygenase. The leukotriene pathway may play a role in the development of asthma symptoms in such patients, as inhibition of cyclooxygenase by aspirin may shunt the arachidonic acid pathway away from prostaglandin synthesis and toward leukotriene production. Although inhaled corticosteroids are still the preferred anti-inflammatory medications for patients with asthma and known aspirin sensitivity, leukotriene modifiers may also be useful in such patients based on this theoretical mechanism.

REFERENCES

1. National Asthma Education and Prevention Program. Executive summary of the NAEPP expert panel report 3: guidelines for the diagnosis and management of asthma. Bethesda, MD: U.S. Department of Health and Human Services, Public Health Service, National Institutes of Health, National Heart, Lung, and Blood Institute, Full Report 2007. Available at http://www.nhlbi.nih.gov/guidelines/asthma/index.htm.

2. Global Initiative for Asthma (GINA). Global strategy for asthma management and prevention (updated 2006). Available at http://www.ginasthma.org; 2006.

3. Greening AP, Ind PW, Northfield M, et al. Added salmeterol versus high-dose corticosteroid in asthma patients with symptoms on existing inhaled corticosteroid. Lancet 1994;344:219–224.

4. Busse W, Raphael GD, Galant S, et al. Fluticasone Propionate Clinical Research Study Group. Low-dose fluticasone propionate compared with montelukast for first-line treatment of persistent asthma: a randomized clinical trial. J Allergy Clin Immunol 2001;107:461–468.

5. Busse W, Nelson H, Wolfe J, et al. Comparison of inhaled salmeterol and oral zafirlukast in patients with asthma. J Allergy Clin Immunol 1999;103:1075–1080.

6. Humbert M, Beasley R, Ayres J, et al. Benefits of omalizumab as add-on therapy in patients with severe persistent asthma who are inadequately controlled despite best available therapy (GINA 2002 step 4 treatment): INNOVATE. Allergy 2005;60:309–316.

7. Food and Drug Administration (FDA) 2007. FDA alert: Omalizumab (marketed as Xolair) information 2/2007. Available at: http://www.fda.gov/cder/drug/infopage/omalizumab/default.htm.

25

CHRONIC OBSTRUCTIVE PULMONARY DISEASE

Quick Fix, Lifetime Risk . . . . Level II

Joel C. Marrs, PharmD, BCPS

LEARNING OBJECTIVES

After completing this case study, the reader should be able to:

• Recognize modifiable and nonmodifiable risk factors for the development of COPD.

- Interpret spirometry readings to evaluate and appropriately stage the severity of COPD for an individual patient.

- Identify the importance of nonpharmacologic therapy in patients with COPD.

- Develop an appropriate medication regimen for a patient with COPD based on disease severity.

- Evaluate the role of inhaled and/or oral corticosteroids in the management of COPD.

- Educate patients on the proper use of inhaled medications and determine which patients may benefit from spacers and/or holding chambers.

- Describe the relationship between α_1-antitrypsin deficiency and the development of emphysema.

PATIENT PRESENTATION

■ Chief Complaint

"Why can't I just take prednisone every day? It always works when I get admitted to the hospital."

■ HPI

Thomas Jones is a 66-year-old man with COPD who is presenting to the family medicine clinic today to have a 1-month follow-up appointment from his last hospital admission for an acute exacerbation of COPD. This last COPD exacerbation is the second hospital admission in the last 6 months related to TJ's COPD instability. After TJ's hospitalization, his discharge COPD regimen was changed to include tiotropium, 1 inhalation daily in addition to salmeterol 50 mcg, 1 inhalation Q 12 h, and an albuterol MDI as needed. TJ had pulmonary function tests (PFTs) while he was in the hospital 1 month ago but has yet to have them reassessed after the change in his COPD regimen. He wants to start taking prednisone every day because he believes this would prevent him from being readmitted to the hospital. The patient states that his respiratory symptoms are better than when he was admitted 1 month ago, but he still has shortness of breath every day and a decreased exercise capacity (e.g., he becomes very short of breath after walking a couple of blocks). He states that he is adherent to the new medication regimen that was changed on discharge from the hospital. No other medications were changed at that time that he can recall. His daughter, who is at the appointment today, states that she makes sure he uses his inhalers but often wonders if he is using them correctly because he still has daily symptoms.

■ PMH

COPD × 12 years
GERD × 5 years
HTN × 20 years
CAD (MI 5 years ago)

■ FH

Mother died from emphysema 4 years ago at the age of 82. Father has a history of coronary artery disease.

■ SH

He lives with his daughter and her family. His wife died 10 years ago from breast cancer. He has a 35 pack-year history of smoking. He quit smoking approximately 3 months ago but has had occasional relapses. He states he has not smoked for approximately a week. He drinks one to two beers every evening.

■ Meds

Metoprolol tartrate 50 mg po BID
Salmeterol (Serevent Diskus) 1 inhalation (50 mcg) BID
Tiotropium (Spiriva) 1 capsule (18 mcg) inhaled once daily
Lisinopril 20 mg po once daily
Esomeprazole (Nexium) 20 mg po once daily
Albuterol MDI 1–2 puffs Q 6 h PRN
Aspirin 81 mg po once daily

■ All

NKDA

■ ROS

(+) Shortness of breath with chronic nonproductive cough; (+) fatigue; (+) exercise intolerance

■ Physical Examination

Gen

WDWN man appearing in mild respiratory distress after walking to the end of the hall to reach the exam room

VS

BP 138/88, P 85, RR 26, T 37.5°C; Wt 95 kg, Ht 5'11"

Skin

Warm, dry; no rashes

HEENT

Normocephalic; PERRLA, EOMI; normal sclerae; mucous membranes are moist; TMs intact; oropharynx clear

Neck/Lymph Nodes

Supple without lymphadenopathy

Lungs

Tachypnea with prolonged expiration; decreased breath sounds; no rales, rhonchi, or crackles

CV

RRR without murmur; normal S_1 and S_2

Abd

Soft, NT/ND; (+) bowel sounds; no organomegaly

Genit/Rect

No back or flank tenderness; normal male genitalia

MS/Ext

No clubbing, cyanosis, or edema; pulses 2+ throughout

Neuro

A & O × 3; CN II–XII intact; DTRs 2+; normal mood and affect

■ Labs

Na 135 mEq/L	Hgb 12.1 g/dL	AST 40 IU/L	Ca 8.9 mg/L
K 4.2 mEq/L	Hct 38.5%	ALT 19 IU/L	Mg 3.6 mg/L
Cl 108 mEq/L	Plt 195 × 10³/mm³	T. bili 1.1 mg/dL	Phos 2.9 mg/dL
CO₂ 26 mEq/L	WBC 6.4 × 10³/mm³	Alb 3.1 g/dL	
BUN 19 mg/dL		Pulse Ox 93% (RA)	
SCr 1.1 mg/dL			
Glu 109 mg/dL			

■ Pulmonary Function Tests (during Hospital Admission 1 Month Ago)

Prebronchodilator FEV_1 = 1.1 L (predicted is 3.1 L)

Prebronchodilator FVC = 3.2 L
Postbronchodilator FEV_1 = 1.6 L

■ **Pulmonary Function Tests (during Clinic Visit Today)**

Prebronchodilator FEV_1 = 1.3 L (predicted is 3.1 L)
Prebronchodilator FVC = 3.2 L
Postbronchodilator FEV_1 = 1.47 L

■ **Assessment**

This is a normal-appearing 66 yo man presenting to the clinic with mild respiratory distress for follow-up on his COPD medication regimen that was changed 1 month ago on hospital discharge. He also has a history of GERD, HTN, CAD, and a chronic cough.

QUESTIONS

Problem Identification

1.a. Create a list of this patient's drug-related problems.

1.b. What signs, symptoms, and laboratory data provide evidence that this patient is not yet optimally managed to reach a stable COPD status? Based on the evidence, is his history more consistent with emphysema or chronic bronchitis?

Desired Outcome

2. What are the desired goals for the treatment of COPD?

Therapeutic Alternatives

3.a. What nonpharmacologic therapies would be useful to improve this patient's COPD symptoms?

3.b. What feasible pharmacotherapeutic alternatives are available for the treatment of COPD in this patient based on his response to the current medication regimen and the most recent GOLD guideline recommendations?

3.c. Should home oxygen therapy be considered for the patient at this time?

3.d. Is this patient a candidate for α_1-antitrypsin (Prolastin) therapy?

Optimal Plan

4. Evaluate the patient's current COPD regimen and develop recommendations to continue or change the current COPD medications at his clinic visit today. Make sure to include specific doses, route, frequency, and duration of therapy.

Outcome Evaluation

5.a. What clinical parameters will you monitor to assess the COPD pharmacotherapy regimen in this patient?

5.b. What will need to be monitored to assess any possible medication side effects?

5.c. What laboratory tests can be performed and how often should they be performed to assess the efficacy of the current COPD regimen as well as progression of the patient's lung disease?

Patient Education

6. What information should be provided to the patient to enhance adherence, ensure successful therapy, and minimize adverse effects?

■ SELF-STUDY ASSIGNMENTS

1. Describe and compare the expectations for deterioration in pulmonary function in normal healthy adults and smokers with emphysema. In particular, emphasis should be placed on expected patterns of change in DLco, FEV_1, and FVC, and general health over time in years.

2. Why would additional phenotyping be necessary if this patient were to have an abnormally low serum α_1-antitrypsin level? What are the implications of the results if the patient were designated as homozygous ZZ, heterozygous MZ, or heterozygous SZ at the α_1-antitrypsin allele?

3. Research and describe the evidence-based medicine approach to the management of an acute exacerbation of COPD and discuss the process of how to transition a COPD patient back to his or her chronic COPD regimen and/or adjust this regimen after an acute exacerbation of COPD.

CLINICAL PEARL

A pulmonary rehabilitation program including mandatory exercise training of the muscles used in respiration is recommended for patients with COPD because of the established benefit related to improvements seen in dyspnea symptoms, health-related quality of life, and reduced number of hospital days secondary to exacerbations.

REFERENCES

1. Global Initiative for Chronic Obstructive Lung Disease. Global strategy for the diagnosis, management, and prevention of chronic obstructive pulmonary disease: executive summary. Updated 2006. Available at *http://www.goldcopd.com*. Accessed March 28, 2007.

2. American Thoracic Society/European Respiratory Society Task Force. Standards for the diagnosis and management of patients with COPD [Internet]. Version 1.2. New York, American Thoracic Society, 2004. Updated Sept. 8, 2005. Available at *http://www.thoracic.org/go/copd*.

3. Callahan CM, Dittus RS, Katz BP. Oral corticosteroid therapy for patients with stable chronic obstructive pulmonary disease: a meta-analysis. Ann Intern Med 1991;114:216–223.

4. Anzueto A. Clinical course of chronic obstructive pulmonary disease: review of therapeutic interventions. Am J Med 2006;119:546–553.

5. MacDonald JL, Johnson CE. Pathophysiology and treatment of alpha 1-anti-trypsin deficiency. Am J Health Syst Pharm 1995;52:481–489.

6. Nichols J. Combination inhaled bronchodilator therapy in the management of chronic obstructive pulmonary disease. Pharmacotherapy 2007;27:447–454.

7. Toogood JH. Helping your patients make better use of MDIs and spacers. J Respir Dis 1994;15:151–166.

8. Package insert. Spiriva (tiotropium bromide). New York, Boehringer Ingelheim Pharmaceuticals Inc., October 2006.

9. Package insert. Advair (fluticasone propionate/salmeterol). Research Triangle Park, NC, GlaxoSmithKline, February 2007.

10. Ries AL, Bauldoff GS, Carlin BW, et al. Pulmonary rehabilitation: joint ACCP/AACVPR evidence-based clinical practice guidelines. Chest 2007;131:4S–42S.

26

PULMONARY ARTERIAL HYPERTENSION

The Windy Cindy. . . . . Level II

Brian C. Sedam, PharmD

LEARNING OBJECTIVES

After completing this case study, the reader should be able to:

- Determine risk factors for developing pulmonary arterial hypertension.

- Discuss common signs and symptoms associated with pulmonary arterial hypertension.

- List the pharmacologic agents used to treat pulmonary arterial hypertension.

- List the nonpharmacologic agents used to treat pulmonary arterial hypertension.

- Recommend appropriate pharmacologic and nonpharmacologic education for a patient with pulmonary arterial hypertension.

PATIENT PRESENTATION

▨ Chief Complaint

"A few hours ago, I felt really dizzy and short of breath, and I suddenly passed out on the bathroom floor."

▨ HPI

Cindy Price is a 32-year-old woman who presents to the ED complaining of episodes of dyspnea and dizziness. While stepping out of the shower this morning, she became very weak and experienced a syncopal episode. She remembers falling to the floor and hitting her head but remembers nothing after that. She was brought to the ED this morning by her sister.

▨ PMH

Hypertension × 4 years
GERD × 6 years
Possible asthma

▨ FH

Father died of heart failure at age of 62. Mother is 57 and was diagnosed with pulmonary hypertension 4 years ago. She is single and lives with her sister (her only sibling).

▨ SH

Denies tobacco or alcohol use. Admits to heavy cocaine use in her late 20's. Has tried various fad diets (including prescription amphetamines) since she was in college.

▨ Meds

Hydrochlorothiazide 12.5 mg po Q AM
Albuterol MDI 1–2 puffs Q 4–6 h PRN SOB
Famotidine 10 mg po once daily PRN

▨ All

NKDA

▨ ROS

Today, Cindy says she is comfortable at rest but complains of having experienced increased dyspnea, fatigue, and dizziness with her everyday activities for the past 6 months. She says that these symptoms only mildly limit her physical activity and denies experiencing these symptoms at rest. Over the past 2–3 months, she has developed palpitations and noticeable swelling in her ankles. She denies episodes of syncope before this acute incident. Approximately 9 months ago, Cindy was seen by her family doctor for increasing shortness of breath. Her physician believed that her increasing dyspnea was attributed to asthma, so he prescribed an albuterol inhaler for her to use. The patient says that the albuterol inhaler did not improve her shortness of breath.

▨ Physical Examination

Gen

Patient is lying in ED bed and appears to be in moderate distress

VS

BP 130/84, P 120, RR 26, T 37°C; Wt 128 kg, Ht 5′6″, O_2 sat 88% on room air

Skin

Cool to touch; no diaphoresis

HEENT

PERRLA; EOMI; dry mucous membranes; TMs intact

Neck/Lymph Nodes

(+) JVD; no lymphadenopathy; no thyromegaly; no bruits

Lungs/Thorax

Clear without wheezes, rhonchi, or rales

Breasts

Deferred

CV

Split S_2, loud P_2, S_3 gallop

Abd

Soft; (+) HJR; liver slightly enlarged; normal bowel sounds; no guarding

Genit/Rect

Deferred

MS/Ext

Full range of motion; 2+ edema to both lower extremities; no clubbing or cyanosis; pulses palpable

Neuro

A & O × 3; normal DTRs bilaterally

▨ Labs

Na 138 mEq/L	Hgb 14 g/dL	WBC 8.8×10^3/mm³	Mg 2.1 mg/dL
K 3.8 mEq/L	Hct 40%	Neutros 62%	Ca 8.4 mg/dL
Cl 98 mEq/L	RBC 5.1×10^6/mm³	Bands 2%	BNP 60 pg/mL
CO_2 28 mEq/L	Plt 311×10^3/mm³	Eos 1%	
BUN 12 mg/dL	MCV 84 μm^3	Lymphs 32%	
SCr 0.9 mg/dL	MCHC 34 g/dL	Monos 3%	
Glu 88 mg/dL			

ECG

Sinus tachycardia (rate 120 bpm); right-axis deviation; ST-segment depression in right precordial leads; tall P waves in leads 2, 3, and aVF

Chest X-Ray

Cardiomegaly; prominent main pulmonary artery; no apparent pulmonary edema

Two-Dimensional Echocardiography

Right ventricular and atrial hypertrophy; tricuspid regurgitation; estimated mPAP 55 mm Hg

Ventilation/Perfusion Scan

Negative for pulmonary embolism

Pulmonary Function Tests

FEV_1 = 1.87 L (61% of predicted)
FVC = 2.10 L (57% of predicted)
FEV_1/FVC = 0.89

Assessment

A 32 yo female presents with signs/symptoms of pulmonary arterial hypertension (likely familial)

QUESTIONS

Problem Identification

1.a. What potential risk factors does this patient have for developing pulmonary arterial hypertension?

1.b. What subjective and objective clinical evidence is suggestive of pulmonary arterial hypertension?

Desired Outcome

2. What are the initial and long-term goals of therapy in this case?

Therapeutic Alternatives

3.a. What pharmacologic alternatives are available for the treatment of pulmonary arterial hypertension? Include each medication's role in disease state management/indication, mechanism of action, dose, potential adverse effects, contraindications, significant drug interactions, and monitoring parameters.

3.b. What nonpharmacologic alternatives are available for the treatment of pulmonary arterial hypertension?

■ CLINICAL COURSE

After admission into the ED, the patient underwent a right-heart catheterization for vasoreactivity testing. The results indicated that after receiving the short-acting vasodilator epoprostenol, the patient had significant reductions in mean pulmonary arterial pressure (mPAP) and increased cardiac output. The results indicated that the patient's mPAP was reduced by 20 mm Hg to a final mPAP of 35 mm Hg.

Optimal Plan

4.a. Design a treatment plan for the initial management of this patient's pulmonary arterial hypertension. Include patient-specific information, including dosage form, dose, and schedule.

4.b. What alternatives would be appropriate if the initial therapy fails or cannot be used?

Outcome Evaluation

5. How should the recommended therapy be monitored for efficacy and adverse effects?

Patient Education

6. What information should be provided to the patient to enhance compliance, ensure successful therapy, and minimize adverse effects?

■ SELF-STUDY ASSIGNMENTS

1. Perform a literature search to determine which medications used for the treatment of PAH have been shown to be safe in pregnancy. Identify the risks associated with pregnancy in female patients with PAH.

2. Use primary and tertiary literature to identify the potential visual side effects associated with sildenafil therapy. Identify the visual side effect that is a medical emergency.

3. Review primary and tertiary literature to compare the advantages and disadvantages of using the vasodilators epoprostenol, treprostinil, and iloprost for PAH.

CLINICAL PEARL

Calcium channel blockers should only be used in patients with PAH who respond favorably to short-acting vasodilators during right-heart catheterization.

REFERENCES

1. Badesch DB, Abman SH, Simonneau G, et al. Medical therapy for pulmonary hypertension: ACCP evidence-based clinical practice guidelines. Chest 2007;131:1917–1928.
2. Raiesdana A, Loscalzo J. Pulmonary arterial hypertension. Ann Med 2006;38:95–110.
3. Rubin LJ, Badesch DB. Evaluation of the patient with pulmonary arterial hypertension. Ann Intern Med 2005;143:282–292.
4. McLaughlin VV, McGoon M. Pulmonary arterial hypertension. Circulation 2006;114:1417–1431.
5. Nagaya N. Drug therapy of primary pulmonary hypertension. Am J Cardiovasc Drugs 2004;4:75–85.
6. Humbert M, Sitbon O, Simonneau G. Treatment of pulmonary arterial hypertension. N Engl J Med 2004;351:1425–1436.
7. Johnson SR, Granton JT, Mehta S. Thrombotic arteriopathy and anticoagulation in pulmonary hypertension. Chest 2006;130:545–552.
8. Badesch DB, Abman SH, Ahearn GS, et al. Medical therapy for pulmonary hypertension: ACCP evidence-based clinical practice guidelines. Chest 2004;126:35S–62S.

27

CYSTIC FIBROSIS

Blood, Sweat, Lungs, and Gut . . . . Level II

Kimberly J. Novak, PharmD

LEARNING OBJECTIVES

After completing this case study, the reader should be able to:

- Identify signs and symptoms of common problems in patients with cystic fibrosis (CF).

- Develop an antimicrobial therapy plan and appropriate monitoring strategy for treatment of acute pulmonary exacerbation in CF.

- Devise treatment strategies for common complications of drug therapy in patients with CF.

- Provide education on aerosolized medications to patients with CF, including appropriate instructions for dornase alfa and inhaled tobramycin.

PATIENT PRESENTATION

Chief Complaint

As reported by patient's mother: "Shortness of breath, increasing cough and sputum production, and decreased energy."

HPI

Eric Smith is a 9-year-old boy with a long history of CF; he was diagnosed with CF at 4 weeks of age. He had been doing well until 3 weeks ago, when he developed cold-like symptoms, with a runny nose, dry cough, sore throat, and subjective fever. He was seen at his local pediatrician's office and prescribed a 10-day course of amoxicillin 400 mg/5 mL 1 teaspoon BID (35 mg/kg/day) for possible pneumonia. After completing the antibiotic course, Eric was not feeling any better. Mother called the pulmonary clinic regarding his symptoms, and his pulmonologist called in a prescription to a local pharmacy for ciprofloxacin 500 mg po BID (~40 mg/kg/day). Mother was also instructed to perform three chest physiotherapy sessions per day and increase his prednisone dose from 5 mg to 10 mg po once daily. The patient now presents to the pulmonary clinic for a follow-up to his outpatient treatment course. He describes worsening shortness of breath, lung and sinus congestion, and severe fatigue. Mother reports increasing cough productive of very dark-colored sputum but no fever. The patient has had a decreased appetite and has lost 3 pounds since his last clinic visit. His oxygen saturation is 88% in clinic on room air.

PMH

Significant for 11 hospitalizations for acute pulmonary exacerbations of CF since his diagnosis; last hospitalization was 6 months ago
Allergic bronchopulmonary aspergillosis (ABPA), recently under control with corticosteroid treatment
Sinus surgery 2 years ago
Pancreatic insufficiency

Pulmonary changes c/w long-standing CF with bronchiectasis and two episodes of hemoptysis
Broken arm previous summer while playing baseball
Attention-deficit/hyperactivity disorder

FH

Both parents are alive and well. Eric has one younger sister with CF who had a recent cold and upper respiratory infection. Two maternal uncles died at ages 13 and 17 from CF.

SH

Eric is in third grade but has been home schooled the last 2 months. Lives with his mother, father, and sister approximately 60 miles from the nearest CF center. They have city water and no pets; father smokes but only outside of the home. Family recently lost health insurance due to job layoff.

Meds

Ciprofloxacin tab 500 mg po BID
Aerosolized tobramycin (TOBI) 300 mg BID via nebulizer (every other month, currently "on")
Albuterol 0.083% 3 mL (1 vial) BID via nebulizer
Dornase alfa (Pulmozyme) 2.5 mg via nebulizer once daily
Fluticasone (Flovent HFA) 110 mcg, 2 puffs BID
Prednisone 10 mg po once daily
Azithromycin 250 mg po Q M, W, F
Creon 10 two caps with meals (880 units of lipase/kg/meal) and one cap with snack (440 units of lipase/kg/snack)
Lansoprazole 15 mg po once daily
Ferrous sulfate 324 mg po once daily
ADEK one tablet po once daily
Children's multivitamin one tablet po once daily
Atomoxetine 25 mg po once daily
Ibuprofen 200 mg po 3–4 times daily as needed for chest pain
Pediasure 2 cans per day

All

Codeine (itching), strawberries (anaphylaxis)

ROS

Patient complains of severe back pain, especially when coughing. Reduced ability to perform usual daily activities because of SOB. No current hemoptysis, vomiting, or abdominal pain. Reports having three to four loose or partially formed stools each day. Patient has a large appetite.

Physical Examination

Gen

A pleasant, thin, cooperative, 9 yo boy who has shortness of breath with his oxygen cannula removed during the examination

VS

BP 110/70, P 144, RR 44, T 37.4°C; Wt 23 kg, Ht 4'2"
Oxygen saturation 95% with 1.5 L of oxygen; 88% on room air

Skin

Normal tone and color

HEENT

EOMI, PERRLA; nares with dried mucus in both nostrils; no oral lesions, but secretions noted in the posterior pharynx

Neck/Lymph Nodes

Supple; no lymphadenopathy or thyromegaly

Lungs

Crackles heard bilaterally in the upper lobes greater than in the lower lobes

CV

RRR without murmurs

Abd

Ticklish during examination; (+) bowel sounds; abdomen soft and supple; mild bloating noted, with palpable stool

Genit/Rect

Deferred

MS/Ext

Clubbing noted, with no cyanosis; capillary refill <2 seconds

Neuro

Eric is alert and awake; CNs intact; somewhat uncooperative with the full neurologic examination

▉ Labs

Na 138 mEq/L	Hgb 15.4 g/dL	WBC 20.1 × 10^3/mm^3	AST 24 IU/L
K 4.5 mEq/L	Hct 45.2%	61% Segs	ALT 22 IU/L
Cl 102 mEq/L	MCV 81 μm^3	26% Bands	LDH 330 IU/L
CO$_2$ 34 mEq/L	MCH 31.1 pg	6% Lymphs	GGT 42 IU/L
BUN 10 mg/dL	MCHC 34 g/dL	1% Monos	T. Prot 7.3 g/dL
SCr 0.5 mg/dL	Ca$_i$ 4.6 mEq/L^a	6% Eos	Alb 3.3 g/dL
Glu 188 mg/dL	Phos 4.6 mEq/L	Mg 2.1 mg/dL	IgE 750 IU/mL

^{a}Ca$_i$ = ionized calcium.

▉ Sputum Culture Results

Organism A: *Pseudomonas aeruginosa*
Organism B: *Stenotrophomonas maltophilia*
Organism C: *P. aeruginosa*, mucoid strain
Organism D: *Staphylococcus aureus*
Organism E: *Aspergillus* species
Respiratory viral antigen panel: negative

▉ PFTs

FEV$_1$ 56% of predicted (baseline 70%); FVC$_1$ 80% of predicted (baseline 90%)

▉ Chest X-Ray

Bronchiectatic and interstitial fibrotic changes consistent with CF

▉ High-Resolution Chest CT (HRCT)

Interval worsening of bronchiectasis in all lobes; increased mucus plugging in left lower lobe

▉ Sinus CT

Panopacification of ethmoid and maxillary sinuses

▉ Assessment

A 9 yo CF patient with failed outpatient management of acute pulmonary exacerbation, also with nutritional failure

QUESTIONS

Problem Identification

1.a. Identify this patient's drug-related problems.

1.b. What information indicates the disease severity and the need to treat his CF pharmacologically?

1.c. Could any of his problems be caused by drug therapy?

Desired Outcome

2. What are the goals of pharmacotherapy in this case?

Therapeutic Alternatives

3.a. What nonpharmacologic therapies might be useful for this patient?

3.b. What pharmacotherapeutic alternatives are available for treatment of this patient's acute pulmonary exacerbation?

3.c. What economic and psychosocial considerations are important in this patient's acute and chronic CF management?

Optimal Plan

4.a. What drugs, dosage forms, doses, schedules, and durations of therapy are best for this patient?

4.b. During the clinical course, serum tobramycin concentrations were drawn around the fourth dose of tobramycin 115 mg (5 mg/kg/dose) IV Q 12 h. Levels are reported as follows:

- Peak: 10.5 mcg/mL collected 1 hour after the end of the 30-minute infusion

- Trough: 0.5 mcg/mL collected 30 minutes before the next scheduled dose

Based on this new information, evaluate his drug therapy. Calculate the true peak (30 minutes after the end of infusion), true trough, elimination rate, half-life, volume of distribution, and clearance (standardized for BSA) of his tobramycin therapy. If necessary, suggest modifications. Assume that the previous doses were administered on time.

Outcome Evaluation

5. What clinical and laboratory parameters are necessary to evaluate the efficacy and safety of therapy for CF exacerbations?

Patient Education

6. What information should you provide the patient regarding the administration of aerosolized drug therapy? The patient will be going home on aerosolized dornase alfa, tobramycin, and albuterol.

7. Where can you obtain information about the patient assistance programs that are available for children, adolescents, and adults with CF on a national and state/local level?

▉ SELF-STUDY ASSIGNMENTS

1. Research the potential problems associated with the use of very-high-dose pancreatic enzymes in patients with CF. What dosage guidelines should be followed to minimize any potential risk?

2. Analyze the role of azithromycin in the chronic medical management of CF. What is/are the proposed mechanism(s) of action of azithromycin in CF management?

3. Review the recommendations for the administration of high-dose ibuprofen in patients with CF. When would you suggest that serum concentrations be drawn, and what levels are thought to be necessary to optimize therapy in a patient with CF?

4. Review the recommendations for use of fluoroquinolones in children. What data support these recommendations?

5. Perform a literature search to determine the progress of gene therapy in CF.

6. Investigate the preferred treatment of acute bronchopulmonary aspergillosis (ABPA) in patients with CF. What long-term therapy is indicated?

7. Evaluate studies using aerosolized 7% hypertonic saline in CF. What role does it play in chronic and acute CF respiratory management? How can it be dispensed or prepared by the patient?

CLINICAL PEARL

Low doses of ibuprofen may increase the migration of neutrophils and inflammatory mediators in the lung and exacerbate the progression of lung disease. Care should be taken to evaluate the use of PRN ibuprofen in CF patients.

REFERENCES

1. Konstan MW, Butler SM, Wohl ME, et al. Growth and nutritional indexes in early life predict pulmonary function in cystic fibrosis. J Pediatr 2003;142:624–630.
2. Elkins MR, Robinson M, Rose BR, et al. A controlled trial of long-term inhaled hypertonic saline in patients with cystic fibrosis. N Engl J Med 2006;54:229–240.
3. Yee CL, Duffy C, Gerbino PG, et al. Tendon or joint disorders in children after treatment with fluoroquinolones or azithromycin. Pediatr Infect Dis J 2002;21:525–529.
4. Moss RB. Long-term benefits of inhaled tobramycin in adolescent patients with cystic fibrosis. Chest 2002;121:55–63.
5. Stevens DA, Moss RB, Kurup VP, et al. Allergic bronchopulmonary aspergillosis in cystic fibrosis—state of the art: Cystic Fibrosis Foundation Consensus Conference. Clin Infect Dis 2003;37(Suppl 3):S225–S264.
6. Saiman L, Marshall BC, Mayer-Hamblett N, et al. Azithromycin in patients with cystic fibrosis chronically infected with *Pseudomonas aeruginosa*: a randomized controlled trial. JAMA 2003;20:1749–1756.
7. Konstan MW, Byard PJ, Hoppel CL, et al. Effect of high-dose ibuprofen in patients with cystic fibrosis. N Engl J Med 1995;332:848–854.

28

GASTROESOPHAGEAL REFLUX DISEASE

A Burning Question. Level II

Brian A. Hemstreet, PharmD, BCPS

LEARNING OBJECTIVES

After completing this case study, students should be able to:

- Describe the clinical presentation of gastroesophageal reflux disease (GERD), including typical, atypical, and alarm symptoms.

- Discuss appropriate diagnostic approaches for GERD, including when patients should be referred for further diagnostic evaluation.

- Recommend appropriate nonpharmacologic and pharmacologic measures for treating GERD.

- Develop a treatment plan for a patient with GERD, including both nonpharmacologic and pharmacologic measures and monitoring for efficacy and toxicity of selected drug regimens.

- Effectively counsel patients with GERD on the proper use of their drug therapy.

PATIENT PRESENTATION

■ Chief Complaint

"I'm having a lot of heartburn, especially after eating. These pills and liquids I've tried seem to work for a little while, but then they wear off."

■ HPI

George Anderson is a 58-year-old man who presents to the community pharmacy with complaints of heartburn four to five times a week over the last 4 months. This also includes episodes of regurgitation, after which he is left with an acidic taste in his mouth. The heartburn and regurgitation often occur after meals, but there are times when he experiences these symptoms between meals. These symptoms wake him up at night approximately once a week. He reports no difficulty swallowing food or liquids. He tried Extra Strength Maalox liquid first and then Pepcid AC tablets, both of which were recommended by his coworkers. The Maalox provided some relief, but he had to take it several times a day. He took the Pepcid AC 10 mg twice daily for 1 week. This worked intermittently but didn't provide enough relief.

■ PMH

HTN × 12 years
CKD × 2 years
Type 2 DM × 5 years

■ SH

Patient is married with two children. He works as an information technology specialist for a large corporation. He drinks one to two beers a day after work, 4–5 days per week. He has a 25 pack-year history of tobacco use and currently smokes 1 ppd.

■ Meds

Amlodipine 5 mg once daily
Glyburide 5 mg twice daily
Aspirin 81 mg daily
Ibuprofen 200–400 mg PRN for headaches and pain

■ All

Penicillin (rash)

■ ROS

Reports occasional tension headaches but no visual changes, aura, or dizziness; (–) SOB, cough, or hoarseness; (+) frequent episodes of a burning pain that starts in his stomach area and travels up his chest but does not radiate to his back or arms; this is usually associated with an acidic taste in his mouth; (–) N/V; (–) BRBPR or dark/tarry stools; (–) dysuria, nocturia, or frequency; reports some mild ankle swelling in both ankles; he has gained approximately 8 pounds over the last 6 months.

■ Physical Examination

Gen

Well-developed African-American man in NAD

VS

BP 149/89, P 87, RR 17, T 36°C; Wt 99 kg, Ht 5'10"

Skin

No lesions or rashes

HEENT

PERRLA; EOMI; moist mucous membranes; intact dentition; oropharynx clear

Neck/Lymph Nodes

Trachea midline; (–) thyromegaly; (–) lymphadenopathy; (–) JVD

Lungs/Thorax

CTA bilaterally

CV

RRR; no MRG

Abd

Obese; NT/ND; (+) BS; (−) HSM

Genit/Rect

Prostate size WNL; (−) tenderness
Heme (−) brown stool

MS/Ext

No CVA tenderness; 1+ pitting LE edema bilaterally

Neuro

A & O × 3, CNs II–XII intact, 5/5 upper- and lower-extremity strength bilaterally

■ Labs

Na 138 mEq/L	Hgb 14 g/dL	WBC 8.7 ×	AST 21 IU/L
K 4.8 mEq/L	Hct 42%	$10^3/mm^3$	ALT 24 IU/L
Cl 108 mEq/L	RBC 4.6 × $10^6/mm^3$	Neutros 60%	Alk Phos 55 IU/L
CO_2 21 mEq/L	Plt 400 × $10^3/mm^3$	Bands 1%	*Fasting Lipid Panel:*
BUN 18 mg/dL		Eos 2%	TC 230 mg/dL
SCr 1.9 mg/dL		Lymphs 32%	LDL 146 mg/dL
Fasting Glu 200 mg/dL		Monos 5%	TG 187 mg/dL
Ca 8.9 mg/dL		A1C 8.6%	HDL 39 mg/dL
Phos 4.1 mg/dL			

■ Assessment

A 58 yo man presenting with uncontrolled GERD symptoms despite self-treatment with OTC H_2RA and antacid therapy

QUESTIONS

Problem Identification

1.a. Develop a list of this patient's drug therapy problems.

1.b. Classify the GERD symptoms this patient is experiencing. Are they typical or atypical in nature? Are any alarm symptoms present?

1.c. What factors could be contributing to the development of GERD symptoms in this patient?

1.d. What factors would cause you to refer this patient for immediate diagnostic evaluation versus recommending empiric drug therapy?

1.e. What diagnostic approaches could be used to evaluate and confirm a diagnosis of GERD?

Desired Outcome

2. Develop a list of pharmacotherapeutic goals for this patient.

Therapeutic Alternatives

3.a. What lifestyle modifications or nonpharmacologic therapies may improve this patient's GERD symptoms?

3.b. What drug therapies could be used to treat this patient's GERD symptoms?

Optimal Plan

4. Develop a complete treatment plan for managing this patient's GERD symptoms.

Outcome Evaluation

5. What parameters should be monitored to assess both the efficacy and toxicity of your selected drug regimen?

Patient Education

6. How will you educate the patient about his GERD therapy to enhance compliance, minimize adverse effects, and promote successful therapeutic outcomes?

■ CLINICAL COURSE

Six months later, Mr. Anderson is hospitalized for a severe case of pancreatitis secondary to gallstones. On admission, he is made NPO and a nasogastric tube is placed. Two peripheral IV catheters are also placed to administer fluids and electrolytes. He is expected to be NPO for at least 2–3 more days; however, the medical team wishes to continue his current GERD regimen.

■ FOLLOW-UP QUESTIONS

1. What options are available for administering GERD therapy via a nasogastric tube or IV catheter?

2. Should this patient be tested for *Helicobacter pylori*? Please explain your answer.

3. What would be the preferred pharmacologic approach if this patient develops erosive esophagitis?

4. What is the role of maintenance therapy for controlling this patient's continued GERD symptoms?

■ SELF-STUDY ASSIGNMENTS

1. Surgical intervention is a well-accepted option for treating GERD in certain patients. Conduct a primary literature search and identify two articles that compare surgery with drug therapy for treatment of GERD. What conclusions can you draw from the results of these articles? When is surgery indicated in patients with GERD?

2. Pharmacy practice involves providing care to diverse patient populations. Identify and review tertiary drug references and Internet websites that provide educational materials about GERD or its treatment in languages other than English.

CLINICAL PEARL

PPIs may cause false-negative results in patients undergoing urease-based *H. pylori* testing, such as with the urea breath test or rapid urease test, or stool antigen tests. These drugs should be discontinued 2 weeks before performing these diagnostic tests.

REFERENCES

1. Peterson WL. Improving the management of GERD: evidence-based therapeutic strategies. Bethesda, MD, American Gastroenterological Association, 2002. Available at *http://www.gastro.org/user-assets/documents/GERDmonograph.pdf*. Accessed March 21, 2008.

2. Devault KR, Castell DO. Updated guidelines for the diagnosis and treatment of gastroesophageal reflux disease. Am J Gastroenterol 2005;100:190–200.

3. Numans ME, Lau J, de Wit NJ, et al. Short-term treatment with proton-pump inhibitors as a test for gastroesophageal reflux disease: a meta-analysis of diagnostic test characteristics. Ann Intern Med 2004;140:518–527.

4. Kahrilas PJ, Pandolfino JE. Review article: oesophageal pH monitoring-technologies, interpretation and correlation with clinical outcomes. Aliment Pharmacol Ther 2005;22(Suppl 3):2–9.

5. Chang JT, Katzka DA. Gastroesophageal reflux disease, Barrett esophagus, and esophageal adenocarcinoma. Arch Intern Med 2004;164:1482–1488.

6. Vakil N, Fennerty MB. Systematic review: direct comparative trials of the efficacy of proton-pump inhibitors in the management of gastroesophageal reflux disease and peptic ulcer disease. Aliment Pharmacol Ther 2003;18:559–568.

7. Williams C, McColl KE. Review article: proton pump inhibitors and bacterial overgrowth. Aliment Pharmacol Ther 2006;23:3–10.
8. Vakil N. Review article: new pharmacological agents for the treatment of gastroesophageal reflux disease. Aliment Pharmacol Ther 2004;19:1041–1049.
9. Chey WD, Wong BC, Practice Parameters Committee of the American College of Gastroenterology. American College of Gastroenterology guideline on the management of *Helicobacter pylori* infection. Am J Gastroenterol 2007;102:1808–1825.

29

PEPTIC ULCER DISEASE

The Pain of It All . . . . Level II

John W. Devlin, PharmD, BCPS, FCCP, FCCM

LEARNING OBJECTIVES

After completing this case study, students should be able to:

- Devise an algorithm for evaluation and treatment of a patient with signs and symptoms suggestive of peptic ulcer disease (PUD).
- Identify desired therapeutic outcomes for patients with PUD.
- Identify factors that guide selection of a *Helicobacter pylori* eradication regimen and improve adherence with these regimens.
- Given patient-specific information and the prescribed drug treatment regimen, formulate a monitoring plan for a patient who is receiving drug therapy for PUD.

PATIENT PRESENTATION

▓ Chief Complaint

"My stomach has been hurting for the past few weeks. Over the weekend, I noticed my bowel movements were black and tarry."

▓ HPI

William Smith is a 62-year-old man who presents to the emergency department on Sunday evening complaining of intermittent burning epigastric pain for more than 2 months. His pain is non-radiating and occurs to the right of his epigastrium. This pain changes in intensity and is worse with meals. He also has noticed intermittent belching, being bloated, being weak when walking, and complains of nausea after eating. Since last Friday, he has been having black, tarry bowel movements. He does not have any history of PUD or GI bleeding and has not experienced anorexia or vomiting.

▓ PMH

COPD × 10 years
Type 2 DM × 10 years
Osteoarthritis × 15 years in the right shoulder

▓ FH

His father died at age 55 of an acute MI and his mother died at age 66 from lung CA. He has three siblings who are alive and well.

▓ SH

Presently employed as an accountant. He is married and has three daughters. He still smokes a cigar occasionally despite his COPD, and he drinks a case of beer per week.

▓ Meds

Metformin 500 mg po twice daily
EC aspirin 325 mg po once daily
Ipratropium MDI 2 puffs 4 times daily
Albuterol MDI 2 puffs PRN
Ibuprofen 200 mg 2 tablets PRN shoulder pain
Maalox 1 tablespoonful PRN stomach pain

▓ All

Penicillin—hives

▓ ROS

Unremarkable except for complaints noted above

▓ Physical Examination

Gen

Overweight man in moderate distress

VS

BP 120/62 right arm (seated), P 109, RR 18 reg, T 37.9°C; Wt 102 kg, Ht 5'9"

Skin

Warm and dry

HEENT

PERRLA; EOMI; discs flat; no AV nicking, hemorrhages, or exudates

Chest

Bilateral rhonchi, faint wheezes

CV

S_1 and S_2 normal; no MRG

Abd

Normal bowel sounds and mild epigastric tenderness; liver size normal; no splenomegaly or masses observed

Rect

Nontender; melenic stool found in rectal vault; stool heme (+)

Ext

Normal ROM except for restricted right shoulder movement

Neuro

CN II–XII intact, DTRs 2 + throughout

▓ Labs

Na 144 mEq/L	Hgb 9.2 g/dL	Ca 9.2 mg/dL
K 3.9 mEq/L	Hct 26.2%	Mg 2.0 mEq/L
Cl 98 mEq/L	Plt 230 × 10³/mm³	Phos 4.0 mg/dL
CO₂ 30 mEq/L	WBC 8.4 × 10³/mm³	Albumin 3.9 g/dL
BUN 10 mg/dL	MCV 74 μm³	
SCr 1.1 mg/dL	Retic 0.3%	
FBG 154 mg/dL	Fe 49 mcg/dL	

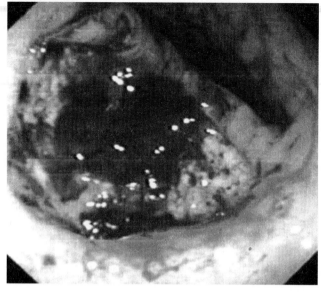

FIGURE 29-1. Endoscopy showing a 6-mm ulcer in the gastric antrum. *(Photo courtesy of the Division of Gastroenterology, Tufts-New England Medical Center, Boston, MA.)*

■ Peripheral Blood Smear

Positive for microcytic anemia

QUESTIONS

Problem Identification

1.a. Identify this patient's drug therapy problems.

1.b. What information (signs, symptoms, diagnostic tests, and laboratory values) indicates the presence of peptic ulcer disease?

■ CLINICAL COURSE (PART 1)

An EGD revealed a 6-mm ulcer in the gastric antrum (Fig. 29-1). The ulcer base is clear and without evidence of active bleeding. In addition, inflammation of the antrum was detected and biopsied. Refer to Table 29-1 for the characteristics of common causes of PUD.

Desired Outcome

2. What are your treatment goals for treating this patient's PUD?

Therapeutic Alternatives

3.a. Considering the patient's presentation, what nonpharmacologic alternatives are available to treat his PUD?

3.b. In the absence of information about the presence of *H. pylori*, what pharmacologic alternatives are available to treat gastric ulcers?

Optimal Plan

4. Based on the patient's presentation and the current medical assessment, design a pharmacotherapeutic regimen to treat his gastric ulcer, anemia, and osteoarthritis.

Outcome Evaluation

5. What clinical and laboratory parameters are necessary to evaluate therapy for achievement of the desired therapeutic outcomes and to detect or prevent adverse effects?

Patient Education

6. What information should be provided to the patient to ensure successful therapy, enhance compliance, and minimize adverse effects?

■ CLINICAL COURSE (PART 2)

At the time of endoscopy, a biopsy of the gastric mucosa was taken and indicated the presence of inflammation and abundant *H. pylori*–like organisms (Fig. 29-2).

■ FOLLOW-UP QUESTIONS

1. What is the significance of finding *H. pylori* in the gastric biopsy?

2. Based on this new information, how would you modify your goals for treating this patient's PUD?

3. What pharmacotherapeutic alternatives are available to achieve the new goals?

4. Design a pharmacotherapeutic regimen for this patient's ulcer that will accomplish the new treatment goals.

5. How should the PUD therapy you recommended be monitored for efficacy and adverse effects?

6. What information should be provided to the patient about his therapy?

7. How should his osteoarthritis-related shoulder pain now be treated?

■ SELF-STUDY ASSIGNMENTS

1. Describe the advantages and limitations of both endoscopic and nonendoscopic diagnostic tests to detect *H. pylori*.

2. After performing a literature search on *H. pylori* eradication therapy, compare the efficacy of two-drug, three-drug and four-

TABLE 29-1 Characteristics of Common Causes of Peptic Ulcer Disease			
	H. pylori	**NSAID**	**SRMD**
Onset	Chronic	Chronic	Acute
Primary location of damage	Duodenum	Stomach	Stomach
Presence of symptoms	Frequent	Rare	Rare
Primary mechanism for ulceration	Infection resulting in inflammatory state	Loss of defense mechanisms	Loss of defense mechanisms
Depth of ulcers	Superficial	Deep	Superficial
Dependence on acid for mucosal damage	Greater	Lesser	Lesser
Characterization of GI bleeding	Minor	Major	Major
Responsiveness to acid suppressive therapy	No	Yes	Yes

GI, gastrointestinal; *H. pylori, Helicobacter pylori;* NSAID, nonsteroidal anti-inflammatory drug; SRMD, stress-related mucosal damage.
Reprinted with permission from Fong JJ, Devlin JW. Peptic ulcer disease. In: Chisholm MA, Well BG, Schwinghammer TL, et al. eds. Pharmacotherapy Principles & Practice. New York, McGraw-Hill, 2007.

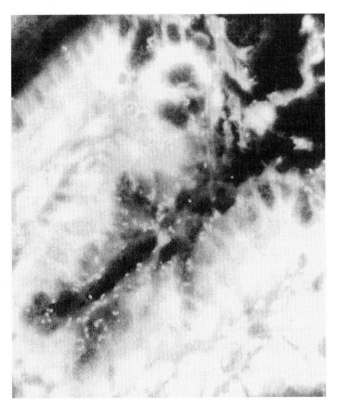

FIGURE 29-2. *Helicobacter pylori* organisms fluoresce above gastric epithelial cells.

drug regimens and whether *H. pylori* therapy should be continued for 7–14 days.

3. Describe the role of pharmacists and nurse practitioners in treating patients with PUD.

CLINICAL PEARL

Reliance on conventional antiulcer drug therapy as an alternative to *H. pylori* eradication is discouraged because it is associated with a higher incidence of ulcer recurrence and side effects.

REFERENCES

1. Suerbaum S, Micchetti P. *Helicobacter pylori* infection. N Engl J Med 2002;347:1175–1186.
2. Howden CW, Hunt RH. Guidelines for the management of *Helicobacter pylori* infection. Ad hoc Committee on Practice Parameters of the American College of Gastroenterology. Am J Gastroenterol 1998;93:2330–2338.
3. Laheij RJ, Rossum LG, Jansen JB, et al. Evaluation of treatment regimens to cure *Helicobacter pylori* infection: a meta analysis. Aliment Pharmacol Ther 1999;13:857–864.
4. ASHP Commission on Therapeutics. ASHP therapeutic position statement on the identification and treatment of *Helicobacter pylori*-associated peptic ulcer disease in adults. Am J Health-Syst Pharm 2001;58:331–337.
5. Soll AH. Consensus conference. Medical treatment of peptic ulcer disease. Practice guidelines. JAMA 1996;275:622–629.

30

NSAID-INDUCED ULCER DISEASE

To Protect and Serve . . . . .Level II

Craig Williams, PharmD

LEARNING OBJECTIVES

After completing this case study, the student should be able to:

• Debate the role of aspirin therapy in development of peptic ulcer disease (PUD).

• Identify the hallmark signs and symptoms of NSAID-induced PUD.

• Recommend appropriate therapy for the treatment of NSAID-induced PUD while taking into account *Helicobacter pylori* infection and its appropriate diagnosis and follow-up.

• Recommend alternative therapies besides traditional NSAIDs for treatment of pain and inflammation in patients with PUD.

• Educate patients effectively on treatment options for NSAID-induced PUD.

PATIENT PRESENTATION

Chief Complaint

"I have had some black stools and stomach pain in the past 2 weeks. I am worried that my ulcers have come back."

HPI

Joan Davis is a 66-year-old retired police officer who presents to her PCP with complaints of black, tarry stools, and epigastric pain for 2 weeks. She stated that she started taking bismuth subsalicylate for the stomach upset with partial relief but the symptoms persisted. They are consistent with those she experienced 4 months ago when she was diagnosed empirically with bleeding gastric ulcers. When questioned, she states that she was diagnosed with bacteria in her stomach but never had a tube inserted down her throat. She recalls being given antibiotics including clarithromycin, but she developed an odd taste in her mouth and did not complete the antibiotic course. She also says that acetaminophen has failed to provide much symptom relief from her osteoarthritis so she currently uses a variety of OTC NSAID products. Additional review of her pharmacy records shows that she was prescribed a 2-week course of clarithromycin and omeprazole 4 months ago.

PMH

Osteopenia diagnosed with bone densitometry of left ankle 5 years ago
H/O PUD with *H. pylori* eradication
GERD with hiatal hernia
Osteoarthritis primarily in right wrist and hand
HTN
Type 2 DM
S/P appendectomy after appendicitis in the 1970s
MI 6 years ago

■ FH

Father died of MI at age 70; mother died of cervical CA in her forties

■ SH

Retired local police officer; smokes 1–2 packs per week down from 2 packs per day 6 years ago; drinks one alcoholic drink per day; exercises on treadmill 30 minutes 3 times per week

■ Meds

ASA 81 mg po once daily
Lisinopril 20 mg po once daily
Alendronate 10 mg po once daily
Gemfibrozil 600 mg po twice daily
Glyburide 5 mg, $^1/_2$ tablet po twice daily
OTC naproxen (Aleve) 200 mg 1–2 tablets po 1–3 times daily for OA pain
OTC bismuth subsalicylate 262 mg, 1 tablet 2–3 times daily for epigastric pain

■ All

Codeine; bee pollen; PCN: rash/hives

■ ROS

Denies headache or chest pain. Occasional SOB. No heartburn, weakness, joint pain, polyphagia, polydipsia, or polyuria. Gait slow but steady.

■ Physical Examination

Gen

The patient is a pleasant woman in mild distress

VS

BP 130/60, P 80, RR 12, T 36.3°C; Wt 74.8 kg, Ht 5'8"

HEENT

PERRLA; funduscopic exam without hemorrhages, exudates, or papilledema; mild cataracts bilaterally

Neck/Lymph Nodes

Supple; no JVD or thyromegaly; no carotid bruits

Lungs

CTA

Cor

RRR, normal S_1, S_2

Abd

Normal BS, moderate epigastric pain on palpation

Genit/Rect

FOBT positive × 3

MS/Ext

No CCE; no skin breakdown or ulcers; mild weakness of RUE; mild deformity of right first finger at MCP joint and swelling of DIP joints on first and second finger

Neuro

A & O × 3; CN II–XII intact; negative Babinski. Normal sensation in hands bilaterally, decreased pain and vibratory sensation in right foot, normal in left.

■ Labs

Na 141 mEq/L	Hgb 7.2 g/dL	*Fasting Lipid Profile:*
K 4.6 mEq/L	Hct 21%	T. Chol 195 mg/dL
Cl 107 mEq/L	Plt 390 × 10³/mm³	LDL-C 125 mg/dL
CO₂ 27 mEq/L	WBC 7.0 × 10³/mm³	HDL-C 39 mg/dL
BUN 21 mEq/L	Retic 1.8%	TG 195 mg/dL
SCr 1.1 mg/dL	A1C 6.9%	TSH 2.93 μIU/mL
Glu 119 mg/dL		

■ *Helicobacter pylori* Testing

Serology positive but assay test of gastric biopsy negative. Urea breath test not performed.

■ UA

SG 1.005; straw-colored; pH 4.9; trace protein; glucose negative; ketones negative

■ EGD

Two small gastric ulcers approximately 6 mm in diameter, trace blood seen but no obvious active bleeding

QUESTIONS

Problem Identification

1.a. Create a list of the patient's drug therapy problems.

1.b. What signs, symptoms, and laboratory values indicate the presence of PUD in this patient?

1.c. What other diagnostic test could be ordered to assess the patient's current *H. pylori* status?

1.d. What are the strengths and weaknesses of the different methods available for *H. pylori* diagnosis?

Desired Outcome

2. What are the goals of pharmacotherapy in this case?

Therapeutic Alternatives

3.a What pharmacologic alternatives are available for treating the gastric ulcers in this patient?

3.b. What feasible pharmacotherapeutic options are available for preventing future gastric ulcers in this patient?

Optimal Plan

4.a. What is the optimal pharmacotherapeutic regimen for treating this patient's gastric ulcers?

4.b. What pharmacotherapeutic regimen is best for treating this patient's osteoarthritis?

4.c. Is this patient a candidate for prophylaxis of future NSAID-induced ulcers? If so, what drug and regimen would you recommend?

Outcome Evaluation

5. What measures would you implement for monitoring the efficacy and toxicity of the treatment regimen for gastric ulcers in this patient?

Patient Education

6. What information should be shared with this patient about management of her gastric ulcers to enhance adherence, assure successful therapy, and minimize adverse effects?

■ SELF-STUDY ASSIGNMENTS

1. Perform a literature search and assess current information on the efficacy of various agents in the secondary prevention of NSAID-induced ulcers.

2. Review the large studies examining the cardiac benefits of low-dose ASA and document the risk of gastric bleeding in this situation.

3. Perform a literature search and assess the cost effectiveness of *H. pylori* screening in patients on chronic NSAID therapy.

CLINICAL PEARL

Documented or undocumented use of NSAIDs plays a role in 60% of peptic ulcers that occur in patients who are *H. pylori* negative.

Risk factors for developing NSAID-induced ulcer disease include: 1) prior history of peptic ulcer disease; 2) age >60 years; 3) higher NSAID doses; and 4) concomitant use of anticoagulants, antiplatelet agents, and corticosteroids or other immunosuppressants.

REFERENCES

1. Suerbaum S, Michetti P. *Helicobacter pylori* infection. N Engl J Med 2002;347:1175–1186.

2. Lanza FL. A guideline for the treatment and prevention of NSAID-induced ulcers. Members of the Ad Hoc Committee on Practice Parameters of the American College of Gastroenterology. Am J Gastroenterol 1998;93:2037–2046.

3. Bannwarth B, Dorval E, Caekert A, et al. Influence of *Helicobacter pylori* eradication therapy on the occurrence of gastrointestinal events in patients treated with conventional nonsteroidal anti-inflammatory drugs combined with omeprazole. J Rheumatol 2002;29;1975–1980.

4. Chan FK, To KF, Wu JC, et al. Eradication of *Helicobacter pylori* and risk of peptic ulcers in patients starting long-term treatment with nonsteroidal anti-inflammatory drugs: a randomised trial. Lancet 2002;359:9–13.

5. ASHP Commission on Therapeutics. ASHP therapeutic position statement on the identification and treatment of *Helicobacter pylori*–associated peptic ulcer disease in adults. Am J Health Syst Pharm 2001:58:331–337.

6. Hawkey CJ, Karrasch JA, Szczepanski L, et al. Omeprazole compared with misoprostol for ulcers associated with nonsteroidal anti-inflammatory drugs. N Engl J Med 1998;338:727–734.

7. Cullen D, Bardhan KD, Eisner M, et al. Primary gastroduodenal prophylaxis with omeprazole for non-steroidal anti-inflammatory drug users. Aliment Pharmacol Ther 1998;12:135–140.

8. Graham DY, Agrawal NM, Campbell DR, et al. NSAID-Associated Gastric Ulcer Prevention Study Group. Ulcer prevention in long-term users of nonsteroidal anti-inflammatory drugs: results of a double-blind, randomized, multicenter, active- and placebo-controlled study of misoprostol vs. lansoprazole. Arch Intern Med 2002;162:169–175.

9. Silverstein FE, Faich G, Goldstein JL, et al. Gastrointestinal toxicity with celecoxib vs nonsteroidal anti-inflammatory drugs for osteoarthritis and rheumatoid arthritis: the CLASS study. JAMA 2000;284:1247–1255,

10. Schnitzer T, Bone HG, Crepaldi G, et al. Therapeutic equivalence of alendronate 70 mg once-weekly and alendronate 10 mg daily in the treatment of osteoporosis. Alendronate Once-Weekly Study Group. Aging (Milano) 2000;12:1–12.

11. Eisman JA, Rizzoli R, Roman-Ivorra J, et al. Upper gastrointestinal and overall tolerability of alendronate once weekly in patients with osteoporosis: results of a randomized, double-blind, placebo-controlled study. Curr Med Res Opin 2004;20:699–705.

12. Derry S, Loke YK. Risk of gastrointestinal haemorrhage with long term use of aspirin: meta-analysis. BMJ 2000;321:1183–1187.

13. Ridker PM, Cook NR, Lee IM, et al. A randomized trial of low-dose aspirin in the primary prevention of cardiovascular disease in women. N Engl J Med. 2005;352:1293–1304.

14. Quan C, Talley NJ. Management of peptic ulcer disease not related to *Helicobacter pylori* or NSAIDs. Am J Gastroenterol 2002;97:2950–2961.

31

STRESS ULCER PROPHYLAXIS/UPPER GI HEMORRHAGE

Prophylaxis Offers No Guarantee . . . . Level I

Kristie C. Reeves-Cavaliero, PharmD, BCPS

Henry J. Mann, PharmD, FCCP, FCCM, FASHP

LEARNING OBJECTIVES

After completing this case study, students should be able to:

- Identify risk factors associated with stress gastritis/ulceration and determine which critically ill patients should receive pharmacologic prophylaxis.

- Recommend appropriate pharmacologic alternatives including agent, route of administration, and dose for the prevention of stress-induced gastritis/ulceration.

- Identify and implement monitoring parameters for the recommended stress gastritis/ulceration prophylactic regimens.

- Discuss the pharmacologic approaches to the management of stress ulcer–induced bleeding.

PATIENT PRESENTATION

▓ Chief Complaint

"Terrible pain everywhere around my stomach."

▓ HPI

BJ is a 75-year-old man who presents to the ED complaining of increasing abdominal pain over the last 24 hours. He noticed diffuse abdominal pain yesterday that was initially relieved by oxycodone 5 mg/acetaminophen 325 mg (Percocet) that he had left over from a previous prescription. This morning he rated his pain as a 10 on a 1–10 scale, with radiation to his back. He reports several vomiting episodes (yellow-green in color) in the last day, and that his last BM was about 48 hours ago.

▓ PMH

HTN × approximately 20 years
CAD; S/P MI 8 years ago; S/P CABG × 3
CHF; EF 15–20% by transesophageal echocardiogram 4 years ago; currently experiences symptoms at rest
COPD
GI bleed secondary to NSAIDs 8 months ago
OA
S/P cholecystectomy
S/P appendectomy

FH

Father died of "heart attack" at age of 55 and mother is in "good health"

SH

Patient is retired. He smokes cigarettes 1 ppd, which is down from a couple of years ago. He had previously smoked 2 ppd for 25 years.

ROS

Patient is nauseated with labored breathing; some confusion is noted when speaking with him. No complaints of chest pain, increased weakness, fatigue, or recent weight gain.

Meds

Furosemide 40 mg po BID
Digoxin 0.25 mg po once daily
Amlodipine 5 mg po once daily
Enalapril 10 mg po BID
Atrovent inhaler 2 puffs Q 6 h
Albuterol inhaler PRN
Colace 100 mg po BID
Celecoxib 100 mg po BID

All

PCN (hives)

Physical Examination

Gen

Elderly gentleman in obvious distress with difficulty breathing and significant abdominal pain

VS

BP 105/65, P 120, RR 26, T 37.9°C; Wt 71 kg, Ht 5'10"

Skin

Warm, dry

Neck/Lymph Nodes

Supple; no JVD or bruits; no lymphadenopathy or thyromegaly

HEENT

PERRL, EOMI; fundi benign; nares patent; TMs intact

Lungs

Decreased breath sounds bilaterally with both inspiratory and expiratory wheezes bilaterally; no rales or rhonchi

CV

S_1, S_2 normal; sinus tachycardia with no S_3, S_4

Abd

Firm, with diffuse tenderness to light palpation; no bowel sounds appreciated

Genit/Rect

Normal male genitalia; stool heme negative

Neuro

A & O × 2; somewhat confused

Labs

Na 138 mEq/L	Hgb 14.1 g/dL
K 3.8 mEq/L	Hct 40.8%
Cl 101 mEq/L	WBC $10.7 \times 10^3/mm^3$
CO_2 28 mEq/L	Plt $203 \times 10^3/mm^3$
BUN 21 mg/dL	Digoxin 0.5 ng/mL
SCr 1.6 mg/dL	
Glu 160 mg/dL	

ABG

pH 7.26, $PaCO_2$ 59 mm Hg, PaO_2 95 mm Hg

Abdominal X-Ray

Demonstrates free air

Clinical Course

The patient was taken to the operating room for an exploratory laparotomy and was found to have a perforation of his cecum near the ileocecal valve. The surgeons noted minimal soilage, and the patient underwent a right hemicolectomy with a primary anastomosis. A central line was placed intraoperatively. He received 7 L of Ringer's Lactated solution and 2 units of whole blood during the operation. He was taken to the surgical ICU postoperatively, mechanically ventilated and hemodynamically stable. He received antibiotic prophylaxis with clindamycin 900 mg IV Q 8 h plus aztreonam 1 g IV Q 8 h beginning before surgery and continuing for 24 hours after surgery to prevent surgical wound infection. Six hours postoperatively, his vital signs are BP 120/75, P 95, and CVP 14. Breath sounds are decreased bilaterally with bilateral rales now present. His urine output has been 60–80 mL/h for the past 6 hours. His blood glucose level is 160 mg/dL.

QUESTIONS

Problem Identification

1.a. As the pharmacist in the surgical ICU, you review the patient's chronic medications and recommend which medications should be restarted postoperatively and suggest any changes to these regimens during patient rounds. What are your recommendations for this patient's chronic medications and why?

Clinical Course

Two days postoperatively, the patient is improving but remains mechanically ventilated. Faint bowel sounds are now present but he is still NPO and requiring continuous NG suction. During rounds, the critical care team decides to stop continuous NG suction and initiate enteral feeds with Isosource® VHN, starting at 10 mL/h, and advancing as tolerated by 20 mL/h every 4 hours to a goal of 80 mL/h. In addition to the medications restarted on your recommendation, he is also receiving lorazepam 1 mg IV Q 6 h, and morphine 2 mg/h by continuous IV infusion. Recorded NG aspirate pH is 2.0.

1.b. List all of the patient's drug therapy problems at this point in his hospital course (include both potential and actual drug therapy problems).

1.c. What are the risk factors for developing stress gastritis/ulceration in critically ill patients?

1.d. Do this patient's risk factors warrant prophylactic therapy to prevent stress ulceration?

Desired Outcome

2. What are the goals of pharmacotherapy for prevention of stress gastritis and ulceration?

Therapeutic Alternatives

3. Discuss the pharmacologic options available for the prophylaxis of stress ulceration in critically ill patients.

Optimal Plan

4. What would you recommend for stress ulcer prophylaxis in this patient?

Outcome Evaluation

5. What clinical parameters should be monitored to assess the effectiveness of this regimen?

■ CLINICAL COURSE

The surgical ICU team decides to use an H_2-receptor antagonist for prophylaxis. Morning labs: Na 141 mEq/L, K 4.3 mEq/L, BUN 29 mg/dL, SCr 1.9 mg/dL, Glu 180 mg/dL, WBC $11.2 \times 10^3/mm^3$, Hgb 11.4 g/dL.

■ FOLLOW-UP QUESTIONS

1. Based on your team's decision, what are the appropriate regimens for cimetidine, ranitidine, and famotidine in this patient?

■ CLINICAL COURSE

The following morning you note that the pH readings for the prior two nursing shifts (16 hours) have been 2.0 and 3.0, respectively, on the therapy you recommended. The nurse notes that the last measurement of NG residuals appeared to be blood tinged, and today's hemoglobin is 9.8 g/dL. You check the medication administration record and determine that all prescribed doses of therapy have been administered. Of note, the team thinks that he may be extubated later today with the possibility of moving him to the floor tomorrow.

2. Based on the above information, what action should be taken to improve the patient's prophylaxis regimen?

■ CLINICAL COURSE

Later that day, a drop in BP to 90/50 mm Hg is noted by the nurse. His HR is 125 bpm, but he remains in NSR. Hgb is 8.5 g/dL. Two 500-mL saline infusions were given and resulted in an increase in his BP to 115/80 mm Hg. His HR decreased to 105 bpm. After he was determined to be hemodynamically stable, an EGD was performed. The gastroenterologist visualized multiple small gastric lesions that are oozing blood.

3. What pharmacologic therapy would you suggest at this time?

■ CLINICAL COURSE

Three days later, the NG aspirate has cleared of blood but remains guaiac positive. He has received a total of 2 units of PRBC and is hemodynamically stable and extubated. Bowel sounds are detected in all four quadrants, the NG tube is removed, and orders are written to initiate an oral diet, beginning with clear liquids and advancing as tolerated. Hgb 11.3 g/dL, BP 135/85 mm Hg, HR 85–90 bpm.

4. What medication changes, if any, would you recommend at this time?

■ SELF-STUDY ASSIGNMENTS

1. Describe how to mix and store omeprazole and lansoprazole suspensions.

2. Identify commercially available GI protective products that may be administered via nasogastric or orogastric tube.

3. List the agents that are currently FDA approved for preventing stress-related mucosal damage (SRMD; also known as stress ulcer prophylaxis, SUP).

4. Discuss how to mix, store, and administer IV pantoprazole, lansoprazole, and esomeprazole.

5. Discuss the administration of sucralfate to renally compromised patients who may be at risk for aluminum accumulation.

6. Identify potential drug interactions and adverse effects with antisecretory therapy (antacids, sucralfate, H_2-receptor antagonists, and proton pump inhibitors).

7. Discuss whether or not sucralfate use for stress ulcer prophylaxis decreases the incidence of nosocomial pneumonia in comparison to the use of H_2-receptor antagonists.

8. Discuss the prognostic significance of the appearance of an ulcer at the time of the initial endoscopy.

CLINICAL PEARL

For agents administered through a nasogastric tube, check whether the patient is currently on active suction. If so, NG suction should be held for at least 30–60 minutes after the administration of any medication to prevent suctioning out significant amounts of the drug. Also, if a patient is receiving enteral feeds through a nasogastric tube, determine whether any of his/her medications interact with tube feeds and require holding of nutrition prior to and/or after administration of the medication(s) for any length of time.

REFERENCES

1. van den Berghe G, Wouters P, Weekers F, et al. Intensive insulin therapy in critically ill patients. N Engl J Med 2001;345:1359–1367.
2. van den Berghe G, Wilmer A, Hermans G, et al. Intensive insulin therapy in the medical ICU. N Engl J Med 2006;354:449–461.
3. Cook DJ, Fuller HD, Guyatt GH, et al. Risk factors for gastrointestinal bleeding in critically ill patients. Canadian Critical Care Trials Group. N Engl J Med 1994;330:377–381.
4. Cook D, Heyland D, Griffith L, et al. Risk factors for clinically important upper gastrointestinal bleeding in patients requiring mechanical ventilation. Crit Care Med 1999;27:2812–2817.
5. American Society of Health-System Pharmacists. ASHP therapeutic guidelines on stress ulcer prophylaxis. Am J Health Syst Pharm 1999; 56:347–379.
6. Levy MJ, Seelig CB, Robinson NJ, et al. Comparison of omeprazole and ranitidine for stress ulcer prophylaxis. Dig Dis Sci 1997;42:1255–1259.
7. Conrad SA, Gabrielli A, Margolis B, et al. Randomized, double-blind comparison of immediate-release omeprazole oral suspension versus intravenous cimetidine for the prevention of upper gastrointestinal bleeding in critically ill patients. Crit Care Med 2005;33:760–765.
8. Cook D, Guyatt G, Marshall J, et al. A comparison of sucralfate and ranitidine for the prevention of upper gastrointestinal bleeding in patients requiring mechanical ventilation. N Engl J Med 1998;338:791–797.
9. Mathot RA, Geus WP. Pharmacodynamic modeling of the acid inhibitory effect of ranitidine in patients in an intensive care unit during prolonged dosing: characterization of tolerance. Clin Pharmacol Ther 1999;66:140–151.
10. Laterre PF, Horsmans Y. Intravenous omeprazole in critically ill patients: a randomized, crossover study comparing 40 with 80 mg plus 8 mg/hour on intragastric pH. Crit Care Med 2001;29:1931–1935.

32

CROHN'S DISEASE

A Sense of Urgency .... Level II

Brian A. Hemstreet, PharmD, BCPS

LEARNING OBJECTIVES

After completing this case study, students should be able to:

- Describe the typical clinical presentation of active Crohn's disease, including signs, symptoms, and disease distribution and severity.

- Identify exacerbating factors and potential complications of Crohn's disease.

- Recommend appropriate pharmacologic treatment for active Crohn's disease.

- Review major toxicities of drugs commonly used for managing Crohn's disease.

- Educate a patient on the proper use of medications used to treat Crohn's disease.

PATIENT PRESENTATION

■ Chief Complaint

"I'm having a lot of diarrhea and I feel really run down."

■ HPI

John Jensen is a 38-year-old man with a 4-month history of intermittent episodes of watery diarrhea and crampy abdominal pain. He states that recently his episodes have increased in frequency, and he is now having five to six loose bowel movements a day. He reports intermittent fevers, as well as malaise and fatigue. Over the last 2 weeks, he has also noticed blood in some of his stools. These symptoms have caused significant problems with his job, as he is a sales representative for a pharmaceutical company and spends a lot of time driving. He has tried OTC ketoprofen for the abdominal pain and Pepto-Bismol for the diarrhea, both which have provided little relief. He has two children, both in daycare, who have not been sick in the last few months. He does not recall any exposure to other sick contacts. He reports no recent international travel. His PCP referred him to a gastroenterologist; a colonoscopy revealed a patchy "cobblestone" pattern of inflammation in the terminal ileum and the ascending and transverse colon. The inflammatory process extends below the intestinal mucosa, and there is evidence of mucosal friability and recent bleeding. A biopsy of the intestinal mucosa revealed leukocyte infiltration and submucosal granulomas consistent with active Crohn's disease.

■ PMH

GERD
Sinusitis (last treated with antibiotics 8 months ago)
Seasonal allergic rhinitis
Exercise-induced bronchoconstriction
ACL repair of the right knee 2 years ago

■ FH

Father with DM, mother with HTN. Older sister with Crohn's disease.

■ SH

Married with two children, ages 2 and 4. Works as a sales representative for a pharmaceutical company. Occasional alcohol use on the weekends. Smokes $1/_2$ ppd × 10 years.

■ Meds

Lansoprazole 15 mg po PRN
Cetirizine 10 mg po once daily
Fluticasone 2 sprays each nostril once daily
Maalox 2 tablespoons po PRN
Ketoprofen 12.5 mg po Q 4–6 h PRN pain
Albuterol MDI PRN prior to exercise

■ All

Codeine (GI upset)
Sulfa drugs (severe rash)

■ ROS

Reports five to six loose stools per day with intermittent blood, crampy abdominal pain, and occasional fevers. Feels very fatigued and thirsty. No recent weight loss or sick contacts. Heartburn three to four times a week and rhinorrhea one to two times a week. No cough, SOB, HA, or mental status changes. No knee or joint pain. No jaundice or rashes. No mouth sores.

■ Physical Examination

Gen

Well-developed Caucasian male in mild distress

VS

Sitting: BP 139/89, P 92; Standing: BP 136/70, P 99; RR 17, T 39°C; Wt 185 lb, Ht 5'9"

Skin

Pallor, dry flaky skin, no lesions or rashes

HEENT

PERRLA, EOMI, pale conjunctivae, dry mucous membranes, intact dentition, oropharynx clear

Neck/Lymph Nodes

Trachea midline, (–) thyromegaly, (–) lymphadenopathy, (–) JVD

Lungs/Thorax

CTA bilaterally

CV

Tachycardic, regular rhythm, no MRG

Abd

Diffuse upper and lower quadrant tenderness, non-distended; (+) BS, (–) HSM

Genit/Rect

Prostate size WNL, (–) tenderness
Heme (+) stool

MS/Ext

No CVA tenderness

Neuro

A & O × 3, CN II–XII intact, 5/5 upper and lower extremity strength bilaterally

■ Labs

Na 139 mEq/L	Hgb 11 g/dL	WBC 19.7 × 10³/mm³	AST 25 IU/L
K 2.9 mEq/L	Hct 33%	Neutros 67%	ALT 28 IU/L
Cl 100 mEq/L	RBC 286 ×	Bands 1%	Alk phos 50 IU/L
CO₂ 28 mEq/L	10⁶/mm³	Eos 2%	Total bili 1.2 mg/dL
BUN 18 mg/dL	Plt 400 × 10³/mm³	Lymphs 26%	Direct bili 0.6 mg/dL
SCr 1.2 mg/dL	MCV 72 μm³	Monos 4%	Albumin 3.8 g/L
Glu 104 mg/dL	Phos 3.9 mg/dL	Stool O & P (–)	
Ca 8.7 mg/dL	ESR 130 mm/h	Stool C. Diff toxin (–)	

■ Assessment

38 yo man presenting with new-onset Crohn's disease involving the terminal ileum and ascending and transverse colon requiring treatment

QUESTIONS

Problem Identification

1.a. Create a list of this patient's drug therapy problems.

1.b. What signs, symptoms, and laboratory alterations in this patient are consistent with Crohn's disease?

1.c. How would you classify the severity of this patient's Crohn's disease? Provide the rationale for your answer.

1.d. What factors could lead to the development or exacerbation of Crohn's disease in this patient?

1.e. What extraintestinal manifestations can develop in patients with Crohn's disease?

Desired Outcome

2. Develop a list of pharmacotherapeutic goals for this patient.

Therapeutic Alternatives

3.a. What drug therapies could be used to treat this patient's Crohn's disease?

3.b. When is surgical intervention indicated in patients with Crohn's disease?

Optimal Plan

4. Develop a complete treatment plan for managing this patient's Crohn's disease.

Outcome Evaluation

5. What parameters should be monitored to assess both the efficacy and toxicity of your selected drug regimen?

Patient Education

6. How will you educate the patient about his Crohn's disease therapy in order to enhance compliance, minimize adverse effects, and promote successful therapeutic outcomes?

■ CLINICAL COURSE

Mr. Jensen returns to his gastroenterologist for one of many follow-up visits. It is now 18 months after treatment was started. He achieved remission after 3 months of initial treatment and had only a few intermittent episodes of diarrhea and abdominal pain for the next 13 months. However, these episodes have become much more frequent over the last 2 months and appear to be increasing in severity. He has also developed two areas of skin breakdown on his right lower abdomen that are continually draining a cloudy, foul-smelling fluid. Upon further examination, these areas are determined to be enterocutaneous fistulae.

■ FOLLOW-UP QUESTIONS

1. Given this new information, how would you modify the patient's drug therapy?

2. Should this patient undergo baseline testing to prevent or detect bone loss?

■ SELF-STUDY ASSIGNMENTS

1. Search for websites containing information about local support groups in your area to which you may refer patients with Crohn's disease for help and support.

2. Construct a table outlining the major differences between Crohn's disease and ulcerative colitis.

3. Review the FDA pregnancy categories for the major drug classes used for treatment of both active Crohn's disease and maintenance of remission.

CLINICAL PEARL

Hospitalized patients with active Crohn's disease are at high risk for blood clots due to their inflammatory state and should be placed on prophylactic therapy for deep vein thrombosis.

REFERENCES

1. Hanauer SB, Sandborn W. Practice Parameters Committee of the American College of Gastroenterology. Management of Crohn's disease in adults. Am J Gastroenterol 2001;96:635–643.

2. Podolsky DK. Inflammatory bowel disease. N Engl J Med 2002;347:417–429.

3. Kethu SR. Extraintestinal manifestations of inflammatory bowel diseases. J Clin Gastroenterol 2006;40:467–475.

4. Buning C, Lochs H. Conventional therapy for Crohn's disease. World J Gastroenterol 2006;12:4794–4806.

5. American Gastroenterological Association Institute technical review on corticosteroids, immunomodulators, and infliximab in inflammatory bowel disease. Gastroenterology 2006;130:940–987.

6. Guslandi M. Antibiotics for inflammatory bowel disease: do they work? Eur J Gastroenterol Hepatol 2005;17:145–147.

7. Hancock L, Windsor AC, Mortensen NJ. Inflammatory bowel disease: The view of the surgeon. Colorectal Dis 2006;8(Suppl 1):0–14.

8. Bressler B, Sands BE. Review article: medical therapy for fistulizing Crohn's disease. Aliment Pharmacol Ther 2006;24:1283–1293.

9. Bernstein CN, Leslie WD, Leboff MS. AGA technical review on osteoporosis in gastrointestinal disease. Gastroenterology 2003;124:795–841.

33

ULCERATIVE COLITIS

How Do You Spell Relief?. . . . . Level I

Nancy S. Yunker, PharmD, BCPS

William R. Garnett, PharmD, FCCP

LEARNING OBJECTIVES

After completing this case study, students should be able to:

- Identify the common signs and symptoms of ulcerative colitis.

- Evaluate treatment options for an acute episode of ulcerative colitis and recommend a specific treatment plan for a patient that includes the medication, dosing regimen, potential side effects, and monitoring parameters.

- Develop a pharmacotherapeutic plan for an ulcerative colitis patient whose disease is in remission.

- Discuss recent advances in the pharmacotherapy of ulcerative colitis.

PATIENT PRESENTATION

▓ Chief Complaint

"I can't stand it anymore! I've got blood in my stool and feel very weak."

▓ HPI

Mary Evans is a 26-year-old woman who presents to the ED with the chief complaint of BRBPR and weakness. She presented to her primary care physician 2 weeks ago with BRBPR and an increased frequency of bowel movements (four to five each day). She describes bowel urgency and states that each bowel movement contained blood. She was started on mesalamine 800 mg po TID but continues to have five and sometimes six bloody bowel movements a day. No bleeding is noted between bowel movements. In addition, she states that she has become progressively weaker. She has not traveled outside the city, been hospitalized, or received antibiotics recently. Her last UC exacerbation occurred when she was diagnosed 2 years ago.

▓ PMH

HTN

Ulcerative colitis, diagnosed 2 years ago

▓ FH

Father has a history of ulcerative colitis, S/P colectomy 15 years ago

▓ SH

Works in retail sales; married with no children; no alcohol; quit smoking 1 year ago

▓ ROS

Negative for lightheadedness, previous episodes of rectal bleeding, N/V, or muscle stiffness/soreness. Positive for mild abdominal soreness.

▓ Meds

Hydrochlorothiazide 25 mg po once daily × 3 years

Lactinex granules × 3 days

▓ All

Sulfa drugs (rash/hives)

▓ Physical Examination

Gen

A & O, pleasant, healthy-appearing Caucasian woman in NAD; appears pale

VS

At 8 AM:

BP (lying down) 135/63 mm Hg, P 61 bpm
BP (standing) 112/65 mm Hg, P 89 bpm
RR 20 bpm, T 37.0°C, Pulse oximetry 96% on RA
Wt 63 kg (usual weight 65.0 kg), Ht 5'6"

Skin

No lesions; warm, adequate turgor

HEENT

PERRLA; EOMI; negative for iritis, uveitis, and conjunctivitis; funduscopic exam shows no AV nicking, hemorrhages, or exudates; moist mucous membranes; TMs intact

Lungs

CTA, no rales or rhonchi

CV

RRR, normal S_1 and S_2; no S_3, S_4

Abd

BS (+), soft, non-distended, tender to deep palpation but no palpable mass, no liver or spleen enlargement

Rect

Somewhat tender; no hemorrhoids, fissures, or lesions by anoscopy; heme (+) stool

MS/Ext

No CCE; pulses 2+; normal ROM; normal strength bilaterally

Neuro

A & O × 3; CN II–XII intact; DTRs 2+

▓ Labs

At 8:00 AM:

Na 139 mEq/L	Hgb 10.9 g/dL	WBC $6.8 \times 10^3/mm^3$	AST 32 IU/L
K 3.1 mEq/L	Hct 33.4%	PMNs 52%	ALT 30 IU/L
Cl 98 mEq/L	Plt $298 \times 10^3/mm^3$	Bands 5%	Alk phos 40 IU/L
CO_2 28 mEq/L	MCV 82 μm^3	Lymphs 36%	T. Bili 0.5 mg/dL
BUN 26 mg/dL	MCH 28 pg	Basos 1%	PT 12.0 sec
SCr 1.2 mg/dL	MCHC 32.6 g/dL	Monos 6%	INR 1 0
Glu 132 mg/dL			Ca 8.5 mg/dL
			PO_4 4.4 mg/dL

▓ Clinical Course

The patient received 1 L of 0.9% saline with KCl 40 mEq over 4 hours starting at 9:00 AM. Vital signs at 1:00 PM were as follows: BP (lying down) 140/74 mm Hg, P 62 bpm; BP (standing) 142/80 mm Hg, P 64 bpm. Repeat laboratory tests at 2:00 PM were as follows:

Na 137 mEq/L	Hgb 10.0 g/dL
K 3.5 mEq/L	Hct 31.3%
Cl 101 mEq/L	Plt 262 × 10³/mm³
CO_2 28 mEq/L	MCV 82 μm^3
BUN 11 mg/dL	MCH 26.2 pg
SCr 1.0 mg/dL	MCHC 32 g/dL
Glu 119 mg/dL	WBC 6.2 × 10³/mm³

■ ED Assessment

1. Lower GI bleeding with a history of ulcerative colitis; patient is stable after volume repletion.

2. D/C to home with instructions to return to ED or PCP if symptoms worsen.

3. Referral to GI clinic for colonoscopy.

■ Follow-Up Evaluation

Colonoscopy (2 days after discharge from the ED): Adequate preparation. Diagnoses: a) edema, erythema, crypt abscesses with mild oozing of blood; continuous from rectum to 5 cm beyond the splenic flexure, c/w moderate ulcerative colitis; b) small internal hemorrhoids; c) biopsy negative for cancer. Histology: distorted crypt architecture, mixed acute and chronic inflammation in the lamina propria, PMNs in the surface epithelium; no granulomas noted.

■ Assessment

Ulcerative colitis

QUESTIONS

Problem Identification

1.a. List all of the patient's drug therapy problems, including those existing at her initial presentation to the ED.

1.b. List the signs, symptoms, and laboratory values that indicate the presence and severity of ulcerative colitis; also include pertinent negative findings.

1.c. Could the manifestations of the patient's ulcerative colitis have been precipitated by an event?

Desired Outcome

2. What are the short- and long-term pharmacotherapeutic goals for this patient?

Therapeutic Alternatives

3.a. What nondrug therapies might be useful for this patient?

3.b. What feasible pharmacotherapeutic alternatives should be considered for the treatment of ulcerative colitis?

Optimal Plan

4.a. What drug, dosage form, schedule, and duration of therapy are best for this patient based on your assessment of the patient's disease severity?

4.b. What alternatives should be considered if the patient fails to respond to initial therapy?

Outcome Evaluation

5. What clinical and laboratory parameters are necessary to evaluate the therapy for achievement of the desired therapeutic outcome and to detect or prevent adverse effects?

Patient Education

6. What information should be provided to the patient to enhance adherence, ensure successful therapy, and minimize adverse effects?

■ CLINICAL COURSE

The patient successfully completed the initial course of therapy and returned to the physician 8 weeks later for follow-up. She stated adherence with the therapeutic regimen, described her bowel habits as normal, and had no complaints of weakness or abdominal/rectal tenderness. The repeat Hgb today is 13.1 g/dL.

■ FOLLOW-UP QUESTIONS

1. Considering this new information, what therapeutic intervention(s) do you recommend at this time?

2. What additional information should be provided to the patient?

■ SELF-STUDY ASSIGNMENTS

1. Review the literature comparing mesalamine, olsalazine, balsalazide, and sulfasalazine preparations regarding efficacy, adverse effects, and cost; include all currently available mesalamine dosage forms.

2. Perform a literature search to determine what new therapies are being evaluated for ulcerative colitis.

3. Review the literature regarding the currently proposed pathogenesis of ulcerative colitis, and relate your findings to the medications currently available and being investigated in clinical trials.

4. Conduct a literature search to determine how pharmacogenomics is affecting therapy of ulcerative colitis patients.

CLINICAL PEARL

Inflammatory changes in ulcerative colitis appear to be at least partly immune mediated, but protection against vaccine-preventable diseases is particularly important, especially in patients receiving immunosuppressants. In most patients with ulcerative colitis, immunization recommendations and administration schedules for the general population should be followed, including avoidance of live vaccines in patients receiving immunosuppressants.

REFERENCES

1. Podolsky DK. Inflammatory bowel disease. N Engl J Med 2002; 347:417–429.

2. Kornbuth A, Sachar DB. Ulcerative colitis practice guidelines in adults (update): American College of Gastroenterology, Practice Parameters Committee. Am J Gastroenterol 2004;99:1371–1385.

3. Sutherland L, MacDonald JK. Oral 5-aminosalicylic acid for induction of remission in ulcerative colitis Cochrane Database of Systematic Reviews 2006, Issue 2. Art. No.:CD000543.DOI:10.1002/14651858. CED000543.pub2.

4. Velayos FS, Terdiman JP, Walsh JM. Effect of 5-aminosalicylate use on colorectal cancer and dysplasia risk: a systematic review and metaanalysis of observational studies. Am J Gastroenterol 2005;100:1345–1353.

5. Regueiro M, Loftus EV, Steinhart AH, et al. Clinical guidelines for the medical management of left-sided ulcerative colitis and ulcerative proctitis: summary statement. Inflamm Bowel Dis 2006;12:972–978.

6. Regueiro M, Loftus EV, Steinhart AH, et al. Medical management of left-sided ulcerative colitis and ulcerative proctitis: critical evaluation of therapeutic trials. Inflamm Bowel Dis 2006;12:979–994.

7. Pham CQ, Efros CB, Berardi RR. Cyclosporine for severe ulcerative colitis. Ann Pharmacother 2006;40:96–101.

8. Rutgeerts P, Sandborn WJ, Feagan BG, et al. Infliximab for induction and maintenance therapy for ulcerative colitis. N Engl J Med 2005;353:2462–2476.

9. Ewaschuk JB, Dieleman LA. Probiotics and prebiotics in chronic inflammatory bowel diseases. World J Gastroenterol 2006;12:5941–5950.

10. Cuffari C, Hunt S, Bayless T. Use of erythrocyte 6-thioguanine metabolite levels to optimize azathioprine therapy in patients with inflammatory bowel disease. Gut 2001;48:642–646.

11. Sutherland L, MacDonald JK. Oral 5-aminosalicylic acid for maintenance of remission in ulcerative colitis. Cochrane Database of Systematic Reviews 2006; Issue 2. Art. No.:Cd00054/ DOI:10.1002/14651857.CD000544.pub2.

12. Holtmann MH, Krummenauer F, Claas C, et al. Long-term effectiveness of azathioprine in IBD beyond 4 years: a European multicenter study in 1176 patients. Dig Dis Sci 2006;51:1516–1524.

34

NAUSEA AND VOMITING

Not Up to Par . . . . Level II

Kelly K. Nystrom, PharmD, BCOP

Pamela A. Foral, PharmD, BCPS

LEARNING OBJECTIVES

After completing this case study, students should be able to:

- Develop a regimen of prophylactic antiemetics based on the emetogenic risk associated with cancer chemotherapeutic agents to optimize the management of nausea and vomiting.

- Design an appropriate treatment regimen for anticipatory, breakthrough, and delayed nausea and vomiting.

- Design a monitoring plan to assess the effectiveness of an antiemetic regimen.

- Discuss with patients and caregivers the reason for antiemetics, their appropriate use, and the management of side effects.

- Recommend appropriate alternative antiemetic strategies based on patient-specific conditions, such as response to multiple cycles of chemotherapy regimens and side effects.

PATIENT PRESENTATION

■ Chief Complaint

"I am here to start chemotherapy."

■ HPI

Kim Johnson is a 65-year-old woman who comes to the cancer center clinic to receive her first cycle of chemotherapy. She was diagnosed with Stage II epithelial ovarian cancer 1 month ago and underwent a total abdominal hysterectomy and bilateral salpingo-oophorectomy. The current plan is for her to receive six cycles of carboplatin and paclitaxel therapy. You receive orders for the following regimen:

Paclitaxel 175 mg/m² IV over 3 hours every 21 days
Carboplatin AUC 6 IV over 30 minutes every 21 days

Ondansetron 24 mg po 30 minutes before chemotherapy
Diphenhydramine 25 mg IV 30 minutes prior to chemotherapy
Famotidine 20 mg IV 30 minutes prior to chemotherapy

The nurse also gives you prescriptions for ondansetron 8 mg po Q 6 h PRN breakthrough nausea and vomiting, and scheduled metoclopramide and dexamethasone for 4 days to be started the following day to prevent delayed nausea and vomiting. She asks you to send them to the outpatient pharmacy so they are ready when Mrs. Johnson is finished with her treatment.

■ PMH

Seizure disorder
Dyspepsia

■ FH

Maternal grandmother with ovarian cancer

■ SH

Married. Two children, ages 35 and 32. No tobacco use. History of alcohol abuse; no alcohol × 7 years. Recently retired from office manager position. Her primary insurance is Medicare and her prescription benefits are through Medicare Part D. She volunteers at a local hospital and plays golf three times a week.

■ ROS

Denies nausea, vomiting, fever, abdominal pain, diarrhea, change in stool color (i.e., melena), GU complaints, weakness, SOB, numbness or tingling in extremities.

■ Meds

Phenytoin 300 mg po at bedtime
Famotidine 10 mg po PRN dyspepsia

■ All

Penicillin

■ Physical Examination

Gen

WDWN woman in no apparent distress

VS

BP 119/80, P 82, RR 14, T 37°C; Wt 70 kg, Ht 5'7"

Skin

Within normal limits. No rashes or petechiae.

HEENT

PERRLA, EOMI, fundi benign, TMs intact, mucous membranes dry

Neck/Lymph Nodes

Thyroid NL. No adenopathy.

Lungs/Thorax

Lungs clear to auscultation

CV

RRR, no MRG

Abd

Soft, nontender, well-healing abdominal incision

Genit/Rect

Genital exam not done. Rectal NL, stool guaiac negative.

MS/Ext

No edema. Pulses 3+ throughout.

Neuro

No visual abnormalities, cranial nerves intact, DTRs 2+

■ Labs

Na 137 mEq/L	Hgb 14.2 g/dL
K 4.2 mEq/L	Hct 44%
Cl 101 mEq/L	Plt $270 \times 10^3/mm^3$
CO_2 29 mEq/L	WBC $4.8 \times 10^3/mm^3$
BUN 25 mg/dL	48% PMNs
SCr 0.7 mg/dL	0% Bands
Glu 85 mg/dL	43% Lymphs
T. bili 1.1 mg/dL	6% Monos
Albumin 4.2 g/dL	2% Eos
AST 42 IU/L	1% Basos
ALT 64 IU/L	

■ Clinical Course

Ms. Johnson receives her first chemotherapy cycle and appears to being doing well without nausea or vomiting.

QUESTIONS

Problem Identification

1.a. Create a list of this patient's drug therapy problems.

1.b. What are this patient's risk factors for nausea and vomiting?

Desired Outcome

2. What are the goals of therapy in this case?

Therapeutic Alternatives

3.a. Assess the patient's antiemetic regimen for prophylaxis, breakthrough, and delayed nausea and vomiting, and make any changes as necessary.

3.b. What nondrug therapies may be useful to prevent nausea and vomiting?

Outcome Evaluation

4.a. State how you will determine whether the antiemetic regimen she received was effective for the prevention of acute and delayed nausea and vomiting.

4.b. Describe the information you will need to assess the efficacy and adverse effects of the prophylactic antiemetic regimen prior to each future course of chemotherapy.

Patient Education

5. How would you educate this patient on her antiemetic regimen?

■ CLINICAL COURSE

Mrs. Johnson tolerated her chemotherapy regimen well with her first and second cycle but presents to the clinic 2 days after her third cycle complaining of uncontrolled nausea and vomiting. She states that she has been taking her metoclopramide and dexamethasone as scheduled, and the prochlorperazine has not helped. A phenytoin level is checked and reported at 15 mcg/mL. Other labs are as follows:

Na 131 mEq/L	Hgb 12.4 g/dL
K 3.1 mEq/L	Hct 40%
Cl 90 mEq/L	Plt $220 \times 10^3/mm^3$
CO_2 29 mEq/L	WBC $3.4 \times 10^3/mm^3$
BUN 32 mg/dL	AST 45 IU/L
SCr 1.2 mg/dL	ALT 70 IU/L
Glu 85 mg/dL	
T. bili 1.1 mg/dL	
Albumin 2.3 g/dL	

Follow-Up Questions

1. What factors may be contributing to her nausea and vomiting?

2. What pharmacologic alternatives may be helpful for the acute treatment of this patient?

3. Design a plan for the prevention of acute nausea and vomiting in this patient for subsequent cycles.

4. Design a plan to prevent delayed nausea and vomiting in this patient for subsequent cycles.

■ CLINICAL COURSE

After treatment according to your recommendations, Mrs. Johnson reports that she has not vomited for several hours and no longer feels nauseated. She will be coming back to the clinic in 3 weeks for her next course of carboplatin and paclitaxel, and she is fearful that she will again experience severe nausea and vomiting.

Follow-Up Questions (continued)

5. Design a regimen to treat breakthrough nausea and vomiting in this patient for subsequent cycles.

6. Design a plan to prevent anticipatory nausea and vomiting in this patient for subsequent cycles.

■ CLINICAL COURSE

In response to your counseling, she states that she feels less anxious. She agrees to take the medications you have recommended to her for her nausea and vomiting. When she returns in 3 weeks, her physician follows your advice regarding antiemetics before and after her chemotherapy. Your follow-up phone call the next day confirms that she is taking her medications as instructed. She is experiencing no nausea or vomiting and no side effects from the antiemetics.

■ SELF-STUDY ASSIGNMENTS

1. Compare the indications, doses, and costs of the 5-HT_3 antagonists dolasetron, ondansetron, granisetron, and palonosetron.

2. Discern in which patients it would be appropriate to use palonosetron or aprepitant, and the advantages and limitations of each drug.

3. Perform a literature search for antiemetic options for refractory nausea and vomiting.

CLINICAL PEARL

Appropriate use of antiemetics is essential, especially with the newer, more expensive alternative antiemetics available. Antiemetic therapy decisions should be based on efficacy, patient-specific factors, and cost.

REFERENCES

1. The NCCN Antiemesis Clinical Practice Guidelines in Oncology (Version 2.2006). ©2006 National Comprehensive Cancer Network, Inc. Available

at: *http://www.ncch.org*. Accessed November 15, 2006. To view the most recent and complete version of the guideline, go online to *www.nccn.org*.

2. Kris MG, Hesketh PJ, Somerfield MR, et al. American Society of Clinical Oncology Guideline for Antiemetics in Oncology: Update 2006. J Clin Oncol 2006;24:2932–2947.

3. Prevention of chemotherapy- and radiotherapy-induced emesis: results of the 2004 Perugia International Antiemetic Consensus Conference: The Antiemetic Subcommittee of the Multinational Association of Supportive Care in Cancer (MASCC). Ann Oncol 2006;17:20–28.

4. Grunberg SM, Osoba D, Hesketh PJ, et al. Evaluation of new antiemetic agents and definition of antineoplastic agent emetogenicity—an update. Support Care Cancer 2005;13:80–84.

5. American Society of Health-System Pharmacists. Therapeutic guidelines on the pharmacologic management of nausea and vomiting in adult and pediatric patients receiving chemotherapy or radiation therapy or undergoing surgery. Am J Health Syst Pharm 1999;56:729–764.

6. Ioannidis JP, Hesketh PJ, Lau J. Contribution of dexamethasone to control of chemotherapy-induced nausea and vomiting: a meta-analysis of randomized evidence. J Clin Oncol 2000;18:3409–3422.

7. Droperidol. In: DRUGDEX® System [Internet database]. Greenwood Village, Colo: Thomson Micromedex. *www.thomsonhc.com*. Accessed December 13, 2006.

8. Srivastava M, Brito-Dellan N, Davis MP, et al. Olanzapine as an antiemetic in refractory nausea and vomiting in advanced cancer. J Pain Symptom Manage 2003;25:578–582.

9. Olanzapine. In: DRUGDEX® System [Internet database]. Greenwood Village, Colo: Thomson Micromedex. *www.thomsonhc.com*. Accessed December 13, 2006.

10. Aprepitant. In: DRUGDEX® System [Internet database]. Greenwood Village, Colo: Thomson Micromedex. *www.thomsonhc.com*. Accessed December 13, 2006.

35

DIARRHEA

Acute Diarrhea and Its Management. . . . . Level I

Marie A. Abate, BS, PharmD

Charles D. Ponte, BS, PharmD, BC-ADM, BCPS, CDE, FAPhA, FASHP, FCCP

LEARNING OBJECTIVES

After completing this case study, students should be able to:

- Identify the common causes of acute diarrhea.

- Establish primary goals for the treatment of acute diarrhea.

- Recommend appropriate nonpharmacologic therapy for patients experiencing acute diarrhea.

- Explain the place of drug therapy in the treatment of acute diarrhea and recommend appropriate products.

PATIENT PRESENTATION

Chief Complaint

"I've had the runs for a couple of days, along with vomiting. I haven't been able keep anything down and I feel awful."

HPI

Paul Stanley is a 60-year-old man who sees his family doctor at the Family Medicine Clinic with nausea, vomiting, cramping, and diarrhea. He had been well until 2 days ago, when he began to experience severe nausea that occurred about 6 hours after eating out at a Chinese food buffet. He had eaten a variety of traditional Chinese dishes but had no consumption of alcoholic beverages or milk/dairy products. He took 2 tablespoons of Maalox Plus at that time. The nausea persisted, and he subsequently vomited "several times" with some relief. As the evening progressed, he still felt "awful" and took 2 Prilosec OTC tablets to settle his stomach. He began to feel achy and warm, and his temperature at the time was 38.2°C. He has continued to have nausea, vomiting, and a mild fever. He has not tolerated solid foods nor has he been able to keep down small amounts of fluid. Since yesterday, he has had 6–8 liquid stools along with crampy abdominal pain. He has not noticed any blood or mucus in the bowel movements. His wife brought him to the clinic because he was becoming weak and dizzy when he tried to stand up. He denies antibiotic use, laxative use, or excessive caffeine intake.

PMH

Hypertension × 6 years
Hyperlipidemia × 3 years
GERD × 10 years
Gastric ulcer (*Helicobacter pylori* positive) in 2004

FH

Noncontributory

SH

No current tobacco use (50 pack-year history; quit 5 years ago); drinks wine or a mixed drink socially, usually not more than 1 glass per week; has about 2 cups of caffeinated coffee daily. He works as a driver for a local bus company. Married for 20 years.

ROS

Lightheadedness upon standing; denies headache, sore throat, ear pain, or nasal discharge. Denies coughing or congestion. Frequent bouts of nausea. Frequent loose stools associated with significant cramping. Decreased urination; no pain upon urination. Complains of generalized fatigue, mild aching, feels like his heart is pounding.

Meds

HCTZ 25 mg po daily × 6 years
Atorvastatin 10 mg po at bedtime × 3 years
Omeprazole 20 mg po daily
One-A-Day Men's Formula one po daily
Policosanol 20 mg po daily (for hyperlipidemia)
Co-Q10 (coenzyme Q10) 100 mg BID (for HTN) × 2 weeks

All

Morphine→itching, rash on legs 10 years ago
Pollen→sneezing, irritated eyes

Physical Examination

Gen

White man, appears ill, in moderate distress

VS

BP 135/92, P 80 (supine), BP 110/70, P 100 (standing), RR 16, T 38°C; Wt 95 kg, Ht 5'9"

Skin

Slightly warm to touch, fair skin turgor (mild tenting noted)

HEENT

Dry mucous membranes, non-erythematous TMs, PERRLA, some AV nicking, slight erythema in throat

Neck/Lymph Nodes

Without masses, lymphadenopathy, or thyromegaly

Chest

Clear to A & P

CV

RRR without MRG

Abd

Diffuse tenderness, no guarding or rebound, without organomegaly, non-distended, hyperactive bowel sounds

Genit/Rect

Heme (–) stool in the rectal vault; no gross blood, small internal hemorrhoids

MS/Ext

Normal muscle strength, no CCE

Neuro

A & O × 3; CN II–XII intact; normal reflexes, normal sensory and motor function

▇ Labs

Na 138 mEq/L	Hgb 12.5 g/dL	AST 35 IU/L
K 3.5 mEq/L	Hct 35%	ALT 30 IU/L
Cl 100 mEq/L	Plt 350 × 10³/mm³	Total chol 185 mg/dL
CO_2 25 mEq/L	WBC 12.0 × 10³/mm³	
BUN 20 mg/dL	50% PMNs	
SCr 1.1 mg/dL	48% Lymphs	
Glu 100 mg/dL	2% Monos	

▇ UA

Clear, dark amber; SG 1.033; pH 6.0; protein (–); glucose (–); acetone (–), bilirubin (–), blood (–); microscopic: 0–2 WBC/hpf, 0–2 RBC/hpf, several hyaline casts

▇ Assessment

Probable gastroenteritis; R/O acute infectious diarrhea
Hypertension
Hyperlipidemia
GERD
History of *H. pylori* (+) gastric ulcer

▇ Plan

Admit to observation unit for acute therapy

QUESTIONS

Problem Identification

1.a. Create a list of the patient's drug therapy problems.

1.b. What signs and symptoms indicate the presence or severity of the diarrhea?

1.c. What questions should you ask the patient or members of the medical team to obtain the additional information needed for a complete assessment of this patient?

1.d. Could any of this patient's problems have been caused by his prescription drug therapy?

1.e. What are other possible causes of this patient's diarrhea?

Desired Outcome

2. What are the goals of therapy for this patient?

Therapeutic Alternatives

3.a. What nonpharmacologic therapies should be considered for this patient?

3.b. What feasible pharmacotherapeutic alternatives are available for treatment of diarrhea in this patient?

Optimal Plan

4. What nonpharmacologic interventions and specific pharmacotherapeutic regimens would you recommend for treating this patient's diarrhea?

Outcome Evaluation

5. What clinical and laboratory parameters are necessary to evaluate the diarrhea therapy for achievement of the desired outcome and to detect or prevent adverse effects?

Patient Education

6. What information should be provided to this patient to enhance adherence, ensure successful therapy, and minimize adverse effects?

▇ FOLLOW-UP QUESTIONS

1. How should this patient's blood pressure be managed after he is rehydrated and returns home?

2. Does the patient need any changes in his hyperlipidemia therapy?

▇ CLINICAL COURSE

The treatment and monitoring plan you recommended was initiated upon admission. The patient's diarrhea slowed by the evening of day 1. The patient had no further episodes of diarrhea or vomiting after midnight. On the morning of day 2, his orthostasis had resolved, his temperature was normal, the IV fluids were stopped, and he received clear liquids by mouth for breakfast and lunch. His stool cultures were negative. The patient was discharged during the late afternoon.

▇ SELF-STUDY ASSIGNMENTS

1. Identify the infectious causes of diarrhea. Design an effective pharmacotherapy treatment regimen for each cause.

2. Provide recommendations for the prevention of traveler's diarrhea.

3. Describe whether or not antidiarrheal products can be safely recommended for use in very young children (<3 years old) and, if so, the specific products that could be used.

4. Describe when oral rehydration products should be used, and recommend a specific product and dosage for young or older patients who present with mild to moderate diarrhea and minimal dehydration.

CLINICAL PEARL

Dehydration and electrolyte imbalances are major concerns with diarrhea, particularly when accompanied by nausea and vomiting;

repletion and maintenance of body water and electrolytes are primary treatment goals.

REFERENCES

1. Cheng AC, McDonald JR, Thielman NM. Infectious diarrhea in developed and developing countries. J Clin Gastroenterol 2005;39: 757–773.

2. Aranda-Michel J, Giannella RA. Acute diarrhea: a practical review. Am J Med 1999;106:670–676.

3. DuPont HL. New insights and directions in travelers' diarrhea. Gastroenterol Clin N Am 2006;35:337–353.

4. Coenzyme Q-10. Natural Medicines Comprehensive Database. Stockton, CA; 2006. Available at www.naturalmedicinesdatabase.com. Accessed December 18, 2006.

5. Gadewar S, Fasano A. Current concepts in the evaluation, diagnosis and management of acute infectious diarrhea. Curr Opin Pharmacol 2005;5:559–565.

6. Steffen R, Gyr K. Diet in the treatment of diarrhea: from tradition to evidence. Clin Infect Dis 2004;39:472–473. Editorial.

7. Casburn-Jones AC, Farthing MJ. Management of infectious diarrhoea. Gut 2004;53:296–305.

8. Wingate D, Phillips SF, Lewis SJ, et al: Guidelines for adults on self-medication for the treatment of acute diarrhoea. Aliment Pharmacol Ther 2001;15:773–782.

9. Adachi JA, DuPont HL. Rifaximin: a novel nonabsorbed rifamycin for gastrointestinal disorders. Clin Infect Dis 2006;42:541–547.

10. NASPGHAN Nutrition Report Committee. Clinical efficacy of probiotics: review of the evidence with focus on children. J Pediatr Gastroenterol Nutr 2006;43:550–557.

36

IRRITABLE BOWEL SYNDROME

Not Moving . . . . Level II

Nancy S. Yunker, PharmD, BCPS

William R. Garnett, PharmD, FCCP

LEARNING OBJECTIVES

After completing this case study, students should be able to:

- Identify the signs and symptoms of irritable bowel syndrome (IBS) associated with abdominal discomfort, bloating, and constipation.

- Devise patient management strategies for patients with IBS, including pharmacologic and nonpharmacologic options.

- Discuss the role of antibiotics in IBS.

- Outline parameters for monitoring the safety and efficacy of therapy used in patients with IBS associated with abdominal discomfort, bloating, and constipation.

- Identify treatment options for IBS associated with abdominal discomfort, fecal urgency, and diarrhea.

- Evaluate the efficacy of treatment options for patients with IBS.

PATIENT PRESENTATION

Chief Complaint

"My stomach feels all stopped up, and I feel really uncomfortable. I read in *Parade* magazine that some new antibiotic is good for IBS. Will it help me?" The patient presents a piece of paper with the word "rifaximin" printed on it.

HPI

Sarah Smith is a 34-year-old woman who presents to her PCP with the chief complaint of a 4-month history of hard pellet-like stools and difficulty when passing stools. She states that she constantly feels bloated and has taken to wearing loose-fitting clothing because she cannot tolerate anything tight around her abdomen. She states that she was diagnosed with "spastic colon" in college and thinks she remembers hearing the physician talking about IBS as a diagnosis. She has been able to tolerate the minimal symptoms until about 6 months ago when she began to notice some bloating and a decrease in the number of bowel movements per week. She attributes the worsening symptoms to increased stress at work and her recent enrollment in an evening MBA program. Prior to 6 months ago, she states that she averaged about five stools a week. She estimates that she has had one or two bowel movements a week for the past month. She complains of straining to pass her stools and states that she has to get up 30 minutes earlier in the morning to allow for an attempt to pass a stool. She also states that the abdominal pain is not limited to when she passes a stool. She complains of abdominal pain and bloating almost continuously throughout the day for the past 2 months, although her symptoms are somewhat alleviated by passing a "good stool." She also states that the symptoms are worse when she has midterms or finals or when she needs to complete a major college writing assignment. Other than stress, she can't think of anything else that has changed in her life. She does not remember having any gastroenteritis symptoms in the past year, and she has never eaten yogurt. She resumed taking psyllium powder 3 months ago but could not stand the taste and wasn't sure how much it was helping. She thought about trying FiberCon but didn't know if it would help her symptoms since both psyllium and FiberCon are laxatives. She switched to sorbitol solution, but she says it tastes too sweet and doesn't seem to help.

PMH

Seasonal allergies
Tension headaches
Anxiety

PSH

Cholecystectomy 2 years ago

FH

Separated from husband for 6 months—question of abuse; divorce is pending. Her 11-year-old son lives with her. Mother is alive with HTN, and her father is alive with hypercholesterolemia. No siblings.

SH

No alcohol use or smoking. Recently promoted to assistant bank manager after working as a teller for 7 years. Has been told that when she finishes her MBA, she will be a candidate for a branch manager position. She states that the additional money will help her to support her son.

ROS

Occasional headaches, usually associated with stress or allergy symptoms; occasional nausea, no vomiting; (–) blood in the stool or tarry stools; (+) flatulence and bloating. States that the abdominal symptoms may improve at night before bedtime especially if she uses a heating pad; she is not awakened at night with abdominal pain.

Meds

Chlorpheniramine 4 mg po Q 6 h PRN allergy symptoms

Ibuprofen 200 mg, 2 tabs po Q 4–6 h PRN headaches, menstrual cramps

Sorbitol 70% solution 30 mL po PRN (approximately one to two times a week)

Lo-Ovral (discontinued 5 months ago)

All

NKDA

Physical Examination

Gen

A & O, WDWN, pleasant white female appearing slightly anxious

VS

BP 126/85, P 72, RR 18, T 37.1°C; Wt 59 kg, Ht 5'4"

Skin

Dry skin on lower extremities, no rashes noted

HEENT

PERRLA, EOMI, moist mucus membranes, TMs intact

Neck/Lymph Nodes

No thyromegaly, lymphadenopathy, or JVD

Lungs

CTA; no rales or rhonchi

Breasts

Symmetric; no lumps or masses detected; nipples without discharge

CV

RRR, normal S_1 and S_2; no S_3 or S_4

Abd

(+) BS, slightly tender in LLQ, no HSM

Genit/Rect

Vulva normal; no palpable rectal masses; brown stool with no occult blood; no hemorrhoids

MS/Ext

No CCE, pulses 2+, normal ROM, normal strength bilaterally

Labs

Na 140 mEq/L	WBC 5.0 × 10³/mm³
K 4.1 mEq/L	Hgb 13.9 g/dL
Cl 104 mEq/L	Hct 42.0%
CO₂ 27 mEq/L	
BUN 10 mg/dL	
SCr 1.1 mg/dL	
Glu 128 mg/dL	

Lactulose H_2 breath test: Negative
Serum pregnancy test: Negative

Assessment:

Irritable bowel syndrome associated with abdominal discomfort, bloating, and constipation

QUESTIONS

Problem Identification

1.a. Create a list of the patient's drug therapy problems.

1.b. What information (signs, symptoms, and laboratory values) indicates the presence and severity of abdominal discomfort, bloating, and constipation-associated IBS? What are the pertinent negative findings in this patient?

1.c. Could any of the patient's problems have been caused by drug therapy?

1.d. What additional information is needed to satisfactorily assess this patient?

Desired Outcome

2. Differentiate the patient's goals of therapy from those of her health care providers.

Therapeutic Alternatives

3.a. What nondrug therapies might be useful for this patient?

3.b. What feasible pharmacotherapeutic alternatives are available for the treatment of IBS associated with abdominal discomfort, bloating, and constipation?

3.c. What pharmacotherapeutic alternatives are available for the treatment of IBS associated with abdominal discomfort, fecal urgency, and diarrhea?

3.d. What psychosocial considerations are applicable to this patient?

Optimal Plan

4.a. What drug, dosage form, dose, schedule, and duration of therapy are best for this patient?

4.b. What alternatives would be appropriate if the initial therapy fails or cannot be used?

Outcome Evaluation

5. What clinical and laboratory parameters are necessary to evaluate the therapy for achievement of the desired therapeutic outcome and to detect or prevent adverse effects?

Patient Education

6. What information should be provided to the patient to enhance compliance, ensure successful therapy, and minimize adverse effects?

■ CLINICAL COURSE

The patient returns to the physician 6 weeks later and reports that her symptoms are much improved and that the abdominal pain has resolved. She is happy with her medication regimen, but her friends have suggested that herbal medications may be just as effective. She would like more information about the use of these products for IBS.

■ FOLLOW-UP QUESTIONS

1. What therapeutic regimen would you recommend for the patient at this time?

2. What information would you provide regarding the addition or substitution of alternative medications (e.g., herbal medications) to this patient's regimen?

■ SELF-STUDY ASSIGNMENTS

1. Conduct a literature search to determine what types of alternative therapies, including melatonin, have been evaluated in IBS. Include a discussion of the scientific rigor of these studies.

2. Conduct a search to identify literature that supports or refutes the role of bacterial overgrowth in the small intestine as a cause of symptoms in patients with IBS.

3. Conduct a literature search to identify clinical trials of antibiotics in IBS and evaluate the scientific rigor of these studies.

4. Conduct a search for IBS patient information available on the Internet. Select two sites and compare their scientific rigor and the usefulness of the information provided to the patient.

5. Conduct an informal survey among friends, family members, coworkers, and fellow students about the incidence of IBS and what therapeutic options they would recommend to a person suffering from IBS.

6. Conduct a literature search to identify new and emerging therapies for IBS and determine their commercial availability.

CLINICAL PEARL

Tegaserod was removed from the United States market in 2007 due to a small but statistically significant difference in adverse cardiovascular events (unstable angina, myocardial infarction, and stroke). This was based on an analysis of 29 trials including over 11,600 patients receiving tegaserod and 7,000 patients receiving placebo; 13 (0.1%) patients receiving tegaserod compared to 1 (0.01%) patient receiving placebo experienced an event.

REFERENCES

1. Drossman DA, Camilleri M, Mayer EA, et al. AGA technical review on irritable bowel syndrome. Gastroenterology 2002;123:2108–2131.
2. American Gastroenterological Association Clinical Practice Committee. American Gastroenterological Association medical position statement: irritable bowel syndrome. Gastroenterology 2002;123:2105–2107.
3. Miller S, Heck A. Irritable bowel syndrome. U.S. Pharmacist 2000;Nov (Suppl):3–13.
4. Harris LA, Chang L. Irritable bowel syndrome: new and emerging therapies. Curr Opin Gastroenterol 2006;22:128–135.
5. American College of Gastroenterology Functional Gastrointestinal Disorders Task Force. Evidence-based position statement on the management of irritable bowel syndrome in North America. Am J Gastroenterol 2002;97(11 Suppl):S1–S5.
6. Agrawal A, Whorwell PJ. Irritable bowel syndrome: diagnosis and management. BMJ 2006;332:280–283.
7. Fass R, Longstreth GF, Pimentel M, et al. Evidence- and consensus-based practice guidelines for the diagnosis of irritable bowel syndrome. Arch Intern Med 2001;161:2081–2088.
8. Brandt LJ, Bjorkman D, Fennerty MB, et al. Systematic review on the management of irritable bowel syndrome in North America. Am J Gastroenterol 2002;97(11 Suppl):S7–26.
9. Lesbros-Pantoflickova D, Michetti P, Fried M, et al. Meta-analysis: the treatment of irritable bowel syndrome. Aliment Pharmacol Ther 2004;20:1253–1269.
10. DiBaise JK. Tegaserod-associated ischemic colitis. Pharmacotherapy 2005;25:620–625.
11. Rivkin A, Chagan L. Lubiprostone: chloride channel activator for chronic constipation. Clin Ther 2006;28:2008–2021.
12. Pimentel M, Park S, Mirocha J, et al. The effect of a nonabsorbed oral antibiotic (rifaximin) on the symptoms of the irritable bowel syndrome: a randomized trial. Ann Intern Med 2006;145:557–563.
13. Sharara AI, Aoun E, Abdul-Baki H, et al. A randomized double-blind placebo-controlled trial of rifaximin in patients with abdominal bloating and flatulence. Am J Gastroenterol 2006;101:326–333.
14. Jailwala J, Imperiale TF, Kroenke K. Pharmacologic treatment of the irritable bowel syndrome: a systematic review of randomized, controlled trials. Ann Intern Med 2000;133:136–147.
15. Gallo-Torres H, Brinker A, Avigan M. Alosetron: ischemic colitis and serious complications of constipation. Am J Gastroenterol 2006;101:1080–1083.
16. Hussain Z, Quigley EM. Systematic review: complementary and alternative medicine in the irritable bowel syndrome. Aliment Pharmacol Ther 2006;23:465–471.
17. Camilleri M. Probiotics and irritable bowel syndrome: rationale, putative mechanisms, and evidence of clinical efficacy. J Clin Gastroenterol 2006;40:264–269.
18. Liu JP, Yang M, Liu YX, et al. Herbal medicines for treatment of irritable bowel syndrome. Cochrane Database Syst Rev 2006 Jan 25:CD0041162006.

37

PEDIATRIC GASTROENTERITIS

One Thing You *Can* Try at Home . . . . .Level II

William McGhee, PharmD

Christina M. Lehane, MD, FAAP

LEARNING OBJECTIVES

After completing this case study, students should be able to:

- Recognize the signs and symptoms of diarrhea with dehydration and be able to assess the severity of the problem.

- Understand the safety and efficacy of a new rotavirus vaccine and explain its potential impact on rotavirus-induced diarrhea.

- Recommend appropriate oral rehydration therapy (ORT) products and treatment regimens for varying degrees of dehydration severity.

- Properly assess the effectiveness of ORT using both clinical and laboratory parameters.

- Understand the limited role of all antidiarrheal products for the treatment of acute diarrhea in children and be able to educate parents on their appropriate use.

- Identify the signs and symptoms of severe dehydration that require referral to an ED for immediate IV volume replacement.

PATIENT PRESENTATION

■ Chief Complaint

Lydia Mason is a 9-month-old female who presented to the ED with a 3-day history of fever, vomiting, and diarrhea.

HPI

LM was in her baseline state of health, having just seen her pediatrician for her 9-month well-child check earlier that week, when 3 days before presentation, she was noted to have a tactile fever, confirmed at 100.4°F (38.0°C) axillary, as well as diminished energy. Two days before presentation, she awoke from sleep, experiencing nonbilious, nonbloody emesis. Throughout that day, she experienced five similar episodes, typically after attempts at oral intake. In addition, she continued to have intermittent low-grade fevers.

One day before presentation to the ED, her emesis had somewhat improved, occurring on only two occasions, but she developed copious watery stools. The stools, totaling five that day, were initially described as slightly formed, but as the day progressed were watery and contained small specks of blood. The patient's appetite continued to be poor, with very limited solid intake. On the pediatrician's recommendation, the family was encouraging liquid intake, including formula, water, and Pedialyte, but the patient refused, preferring cola and diluted apple juice.

On the morning of presentation to the ED, the patient had another watery stool and was noted to be fussy. In addition, she had a dry diaper that morning without urine output noted the night prior. The family was unable to clarify the number of wet diapers she had in the last 24 hours, given the difficulty distinguishing watery stool from urine. They also noted that her lips appeared dry and she had diminished tears.

PMH

LM was born at 38 weeks via spontaneous vaginal delivery without complications. She did require 1 day of phototherapy for hyperbilirubinemia but was discharged from the nursery within 3 days of birth. She has not required prior hospitalization or ED visitation but has experienced approximately six upper respiratory tract infections and two episodes of otitis media, all after introduction into daycare at 7 weeks of age.

Immunizations are up-to-date. There were no sick family contacts until the day she presented to the ED, when the patient's mother developed abdominal discomfort and loose stools. In addition, multiple infants at daycare were experiencing similar illnesses. Development is normal. No medications have been given to the patient except for a daily multivitamin.

All

No known allergies

FH

LM's mother and father are 29 years old and in good health. There are two older siblings in the home, ages 3 and 6, who have been well.

SH

LM lives with her parents and siblings. There are two pet fish in the home but no reptile or other animal exposures. The patient attends daycare three times a week. The family uses city water. Her diet consists of Enfamil Lipil and a myriad of solid foods. There has been no exposure to undercooked meats or fish.

Physical Examination

Gen

Patient is ill-appearing but nontoxic. She is irritable with the examination but consoled by her mother.

VS

BP 92/50, P 135, RR 42, T 38.4°C; Wt 8.2 kg (50–75%) (Wt 5 days earlier at well-child check 9.0 kg)

Skin

Pink, mild tenting noted, capillary refill 2–3 seconds

HEENT

TMs gray and translucent, nose with clear rhinorrhea, scant tears, lips and tongue dry, eyes moderately sunken, anterior fontanelle sunken

Neck/Lymph Nodes

Normal

Lungs/Thorax

Tachypneic; no focal findings, including wheezes, rales, or rhonchi; no retractions or grunting

Heart

Tachycardic, 1/6 flow murmur, normal pulses

Abd

Distended, hyperactive bowel sounds; no focal tenderness, masses, or hepatosplenomegaly

Genit/Rect

Normal female genitalia, mild diaper dermatitis

MS/Ext

Normal

Neuro

Sleepy but arousable; irritable when awake; no focal defects

Labs

Na 137 mEq/L	Hgb 12.8 g/dL	WBC $14.0 \times 10^3/mm^3$
K 4.4 mEq/L	Hct 41%	52% Polys
Cl 113 mEq/L	Plt $300 \times 10^3/mm^3$	5% Bands
CO_2 14 mEq/L		0% Eos
BUN 23 mg/dL		3% Basos
SCr 0.4 mg/dL		24% Lymphs
Glu 80 mg/dL		16% Monos

UA

Specific gravity 1.029; ketones 2+; otherwise negative

Assessment

1. Typical viral gastroenteritis, likely rotavirus infection
2. Dehydration with metabolic acidosis

QUESTIONS

Problem Identification

1.a. Create a list of the patient's drug therapy problems.

1.b. What information (signs, symptoms, laboratory values) indicates the presence or severity of gastroenteritis?

Desired Outcome

2. What are the goals of pharmacotherapy in this case?

Therapeutic Alternatives

3.a. What nondrug therapies might be useful for this patient?

3.b. What feasible pharmacotherapeutic alternatives are available for treating this patient's diarrhea?

Optimal Plan

4.a. What drug(s), dosage forms, schedule, and duration of therapy are best for this patient?

4.b. What is the efficacy and safety record of the new rotavirus vaccine, and what impact is it expected to have on preventing rotavirus-induced diarrhea?

Outcome Evaluation

5. What clinical and laboratory parameters should be monitored to evaluate therapy for achievement of the desired therapeutic outcome?

Patient Education

6. What information should be provided to the child's parents to enhance compliance, ensure successful therapy, and minimize adverse effects?

■ SELF-STUDY ASSIGNMENTS

1. In what circumstances would antimicrobial therapy be considered for children with diarrhea and dehydration?

2. What role does zinc supplementation have in the treatment of diarrhea in developing countries? Describe the rationale for its use and the most efficient way to administer it. What is the efficacy of drug therapy in preventing diarrhea when traveling to foreign countries? What drugs are recommended, and what are the adult and pediatric doses?

3. What barriers exist to the widespread implementation of ORT, including parents and physicians? How can these barriers be overcome? (Hint: Explore the advantages of ORT versus IV rehydration therapy, including ease of care at home versus hospitalization, insurance issues, and physician reluctance).

4. Write a two-page essay describing the role of the community-based practitioner in the care of patients with pediatric gastroenteritis and dehydration. Emphasize how you would monitor patient safety and outcome and what you would tell the parents to optimize treatment at home.

CLINICAL PEARL

ORT is equivalent to IV therapy in rehydrating children with gastroenteritis and diarrhea with mild to moderate dehydration. ORT is the standard of care in the treatment of these patients and usually can be performed at home. Antidiarrheal, antiemetic, probiotic, and antimicrobial therapies are rarely necessary. IV rehydration is necessary only in patients with severe dehydration.

REFERENCES

1. Elliot EJ. Acute gastroenteritis in children. BMJ 2007;334:35–40.
2. Duggan C, Santosham M, Glass RI. The management of acute diarrhea in children: oral rehydration, maintenance, and nutritional therapy. MMWR Morb Mortal Wkly Rep 1992;41(RR-16):1–20.
3. Snyder J. The continuing evolution of oral therapy for diarrhea. Semin Pediatr Infect Dis 1994;5:231–235.
4. Spandorfer PR, Alessandrini EA, Joffe MD, et al. Oral versus intravenous rehydration of moderately dehydrated children: a randomized, controlled trial. Pediatrics 2005;115:295–301.
5. Vanderhoof JA, Young RJ. Pediatric applications of probiotics. Gastroenterol Clin North Am 2005;34:451–463.
6. Szajewska H, Mrukowiz JZ. Probiotics in the treatment and prevention of acute infectious diarrhea in infants and children: a systematic review

of published randomized, double-blind, placebo-controlled trials. J Pediatr Gastroenterol Nutr 2001;33:S17–S25.
7. Guandalini S. Probiotics for children: use in diarrhea. J Clin Gastroenterol 2006;40:244–248.
8. Borowitz SM. Are antiemetics helpful in young children suffering from acute viral gastroenteritis? Arch Dis Child 2005;90:646–648.
9. Bhatnagar S, Bahl R, Sharma PK, et al. Zinc with oral rehydration therapy reduces stool output and duration of diarrhea in hospitalized children: a randomized controlled trial. J Pediatr Gastroenterol Nutr 2004:38:34–40.
10. Vesikari T, Matson DO, Dennedy P, et al. Safety and efficacy of a pentavalent human-bovine (WC3) reassortant rotavirus vaccine. N Engl J Med 2006;354:23–33.
11. Anonymous. Postmarketing monitoring of intussusception after Rotateq™ vaccination—United States, February 1, 2006–February 15, 2007. MMWR Morb Mortal Wkly Rep 2007;56:218–222.
12. Centers for Disease Control and Prevention. Managing acute gastroenteritis among children: Oral rehydration, maintenance, and nutritional therapy. MMWR Morb Mortal Wkly Rep 2003;52:(RR-16):1–16.

38

CONSTIPATION

Unlock the Block . . . . Level II

Michelle O'Connor, PharmD

Beth Bryles Phillips, PharmD, FCCP, BCPS

LEARNING OBJECTIVES

After completing this case study, students should be able to:

- Identify medications that can exacerbate constipation.

- Describe the advantages and disadvantages of each class of laxatives and discuss the appropriate use of each class.

- Recommend an appropriate plan for the treatment of constipation, including lifestyle modifications and drug therapy.

- Educate patients regarding laxative therapy.

PATIENT PRESENTATION

■ Chief Complaint

"I've been having increasing stomach pain."

■ HPI

Myrna Cook is a 54-year-old woman who presents to the ED complaining of increasing abdominal cramping for several days. Her last bowel movement was 6 days ago. She began "not feeling well" 4 days ago, with some mild chills, bloating, decreased appetite, and fatigue. She reports no fever, N/V, CP, or SOB. She reports that yesterday, when her cramping was at its worst, she used magnesium citrate, Miralax, and Fleet enema but still had no bowel movement. She states that she typically has daily bowel movements, with no straining, and spends less than 10 minutes, with little effort, having a bowel movement. She reports having a similar episode approximately 1 year ago; however, at that time her symptoms responded to magnesium citrate and Miralax. She does not use stool softeners on a regular basis. She reports drinking approximately 1 gallon of water daily, even before her constipation began. Her last colonoscopy, performed 6 years ago, was unremarkable.

■ PMH

Asthma
Obstructive sleep apnea
HTN
Mitral valve stenosis
Atrial fibrillation
Depression
Hypothyroidism
Iron deficiency anemia
GERD

■ FH

Her mother is in her 70's and is healthy. Her father died in his 50's from lung cancer. She has three brothers and three sisters; one brother has viral hepatitis. She has two sons who are healthy.

■ SH

She is married and works as a social worker. She quit smoking 20+ years ago. She does not drink alcohol and does not use illicit drugs.

■ ROS

(+) for constipation, lower abdominal fullness, and fatigue after not using her CPAP machine for the past two nights; (−) for N/V, SOB, CP, and fever/chills

■ Meds

Diltiazem CR 240 mg po daily
Digoxin 0.25 mg po daily
Flecainide 100 mg po BID
Atenolol 25 mg po daily
Buspirone 10 mg po BID
Duloxetine 60 mg po daily
Lansoprazole 30 mg po daily
Warfarin 2.5 mg po daily
Fluticasone/salmeterol 500/50 1 puff BID
Albuterol inhaler 90 mcg 2 puffs Q 4 h PRN
Levothyroxine 50 mcg po daily
Multivitamin 1 tablet po daily
Ferrous gluconate 324 mg po TID

■ All

NKDA

■ Physical Examination

Gen

Pleasant woman in mild distress; appears tired

VS

BP 122/60, P 57, RR 16, T 36.2°C; Wt 112.4 kg, Ht 5'5"

Skin

Normal skin turgor and color

HEENT

PERRLA and EOM full without nystagmus; no scleral icterus; oral mucosa moist; no ulcerations noted

Neck/Lymph Nodes

Supple, no lymphadenopathy or JVD; no thyromegaly or bruits

CV

Regular, S_1 and S_2 without murmur

Lungs

Normal breath sounds; no crackles, rales, or wheezes

Abd

Soft, obese, tender; decreased bowel sounds; stool palpable on left side

Rectal

External hemorrhoids noted; no stool in rectal vault; no masses felt; tone fair; push strength fair; nontender

MS/Ext

No tenderness; strength good; sensation intact; no edema

Neuro

A & O × 3; CNs II–XII symmetric and intact; DTRs 2+

■ Labs

Na 138 mEq/L	Glu 133 mg/dL	RBC 6.05 × 10⁶/mm³	RDW 15.4%
K 4.7 mEq/L	Ca 9.3 mg/dL	Hgb 15.5 g/dL	
Cl 101 mEq/L	TSH 2.70 mIU/mL	Hct 48%	
CO_2 30 mEq/L	Free T_4 1.2 ng/dL	MCV 79 fl	
BUN 14 mg/dL	TIBC 251 mcg/dL	MCH 26 pg	
SCr 0.8 mg/dL	Ferritin 85.4 ng/mL	MCHC 33%	

■ Assessment

Constipation with secondary symptoms of abdominal discomfort, etiology unknown

■ Plan

Obtain abdominal x-ray and CT scan to evaluate potential causes of the constipation; consult GI service

■ Clinical Course

A plain x-ray of the abdomen showed gas-dilated loops in the colon. An abdominal CT scan was then performed and showed a large amount of stool in the colon. The GI service was consulted, and the recommendation was made to hold warfarin for colonoscopy. The laxative regimen used for colonoscopy bowel preparation was successful in clearing her bowel for the procedure and also in relieving the patient's abdominal pain. Colonoscopy was unremarkable, and she was discharged with directions to establish a regimen to maintain regular bowel function.

QUESTIONS

Problem Identification

1.a. Develop a list of the potential therapy problems in this patient other than those related to her constipation.

1.b. What signs or symptoms are indicative of constipation in this patient?

1.c. What are some of the possible nonpharmacologic contributors to her constipation?

1.d. What are some of the possible pharmacologic contributors to constipation in this patient?

1.e. What information should be obtained from a patient who presents with a chief complaint of constipation?

Desired Outcome

2. What are the goals of pharmacotherapy in treating constipation?

Therapeutic Alternatives

3.a. What are some nonpharmacologic steps useful in treating constipation?

3.b. What are the pharmacologic options for the treatment of constipation?

3.c. Is this patient's current regimen for iron deficiency anemia appropriate? If not, what recommendations can you make to optimize this regimen?

Optimal Plan

4. After nonpharmacologic measures have been attempted, what would be the most appropriate choice of drug therapy for her, including dose and schedule? Provide the rationale for your answer.

Outcome Evaluation

5.a. How would you monitor this patient to ensure that your pharmacotherapeutic goals have been achieved? How would you follow up with her to ensure resolution of the constipation?

■ CLINICAL COURSE

The recommendations you made were implemented, and Ms. Cook returns to your clinic 1 month later. She reports that she has been using the drug therapy you recommended and has somewhat regular bowel function; however, she still feels constipated at times. She asks if there is something else she can take.

5.b. What agent would you recommend for this patient who reports only partial relief of constipation with first-line therapy?

Patient Education

6. When instructing this patient on using an osmotic laxative, what information should you convey to ensure appropriate use of this product?

■ SELF-STUDY ASSIGNMENTS

1. Suggest pharmacotherapeutic options for the treatment of external hemorrhoids.

2. What are the recommendations for bowel preparation before colonoscopy?

CLINICAL PEARL

Constipation is often a sign of an underlying problem, such as an adverse reaction to a medication or a symptom of a comorbid condition. These possibilities should always be considered when evaluating a patient complaining of constipation.

REFERENCES

1. Lembo A, Camilleri M. Chronic constipation. N Engl J Med 2003;349:1360–1368.
2. Wald A. Constipation in the primary care setting: current concepts and misconceptions. Am J Med 2006;119:736–739.
3. Corazziari E, Badiali D, Bazzocchi G, et al. Long term efficacy, safety, and tolerability of low daily doses of isosmotic polyethylene glycol electrolyte balanced solution (PMF-100) in the treatment of functional chronic constipation. Gut 2000;46:522–526.

39

ASCITES MANAGEMENT IN PORTAL HYPERTENSION AND CIRRHOSIS

Occupational Hazard . . . . Level II

Laurel Rodden Andrews, PharmD

Jeffery Evans, PharmD

LEARNING OBJECTIVES

After completing this case study, students should be able to:

- Identify signs and symptoms of cirrhosis and associated complications.

- Provide pharmacotherapeutic and lifestyle recommendations for managing ascites due to portal hypertension and cirrhosis.

- Develop a patient-specific regimen and monitoring parameters to meet the needs of a patient with ascites, spontaneous bacterial peritonitis, and hepatic encephalopathy.

- Interpret laboratory values associated with ascites.

- Provide appropriate patient education for the recommended pharmacologic and nonpharmacologic therapy to control complications of cirrhosis, as well as to prevent further complications.

PATIENT PRESENTATION

▓ Chief Complaint

"I can't breathe, and my stomach is swelling again."

▓ HPI

Priscilla Smith is a 53-year-old woman with a history of alcoholic cirrhosis who has been admitted to the hospital due to a 6-kg weight gain over the past 8 days, abdominal swelling and pain, shortness of breath, and confusion.

▓ PMH

Alcoholic cirrhosis diagnosed 6 years ago
Bleeding esophageal varices (last one occurred 6 months ago)
Multiple occurrences of ascites (last episode occurred 12 months ago)
Hepatic encephalopathy (last episode occurred 12 months ago)
Chronic sinusitis
Hypothyroidism diagnosed 2 years ago

▓ FH

Father was an alcoholic and died in an MVA 12 years ago at age 62. Mother, age 75, resides in a nursing home and suffers from Alzheimer's disease.

▓ SH

Lives alone, husband died 2 years ago. Works part-time at a convenience store; was a bartender for 15 years before the cirrhosis diagnosis. History of alcohol abuse; quit 6 years ago. While abusing alcohol, drank between four and six 4-oz. glasses of wine per day on the weekdays and added two or three 1.5-oz. shots of whiskey to that on the weekends.

Meds

Triamcinolone acetonide (Nasacort AQ), 2 sprays per nostril once daily
Propranolol LA 80 mg po once daily
Levothyroxine 25 mcg po once daily
Lactulose 15 mL po BID

All

NKDA

ROS

Abdominal discomfort described as occurring throughout the abdomen, shortness of breath, and mild confusion. Patient denies chills or fevers.

Physical Examination

Gen

Pleasant, chronically ill Caucasian woman appearing to be in mild distress and fatigued

VS

BP 121/74, P 82, RR 27, T 36.9°C; Wt 73.2 kg, Ht 5'4"

Skin

(+) palmar erythema, (+) spider angiomata, otherwise normal color

HEENT

PERRL, EOMI, clear sclerae, TMs normal, mucous membranes moist

Neck/Lymph Nodes

Supple, no thyroid nodules

Lung/Thorax

Mild bilateral rales, decreased breath sounds in right lower lobe due to enlarged liver and ascites

Breasts

Nontender without masses

CV

RRR, S_1 and S_2 are normal, no MRG

Abd

Bulging, tender abdomen; hepatomegaly; (+) fluid wave; bowel sounds normal

Genit/Rect

Guaiac negative

MS/Ext

1+ pitting edema in both LE, palmar erythema; no clubbing or cyanosis

Neuro

Mildly confused, forgetful, A & O × 2 (oriented to person and place but not time)

Labs

Na 133 mEq/L	Hgb 13 g/dL	AST 108 IU/L	Alb 2.8 g/dL
K 3.9 mEq/L	Hct 38%	ALT 120 IU/L	Ca 9.2 mg/dL
Cl 103 mEq/L	Plt 79 × 10³/mm³	LDH 152 IU/L	Mg 2.0 mEq/L
CO₂ 26 mEq/L	WBC 7.0 × 10³/mm³	T. bili 2.9 mg/dL	Phos 3.2 mg/dL
BUN 22 mg/dL	PT 14.9 sec	D. bili 0.8 mg/dL	TSH 5.2 mIU/L
SCr 0.8 mg/dL	PTT 46 sec	HIV (−)	NH₃ 102 mcg/dL
Glu 85 mg/dL	INR 1.42	T. prot 6.1 g/dL	

Assessment

Worsening alcohol-induced cirrhosis; Child-Pugh score—10, grade C; now presenting with recurrent ascites and encephalopathy
Perform diagnostic and therapeutic paracentesis
R/O spontaneous bacterial peritonitis (SBP)

Clinical Course

After removal of 5 liters of fluid by paracentesis, an analysis of the fluid was performed. The analysis reported a protein level of 0.8 g/dL, PMN 333 cells/mm³, and SAG 1.5 g/dL. The culture results are pending.

The patient's mental status began to improve after paracentesis and the lactulose dose was increased to 30 mL po BID.

QUESTIONS

Problem Identification

1.a. Create a list of the patient's drug therapy problems.

1.b. What information (signs, symptoms, lab values) indicates the presence of ascites in this patient? (See Fig. 39-1.)

1.c. What information (signs, symptoms, lab values) indicates the presence of hepatic encephalopathy and SBP in this patient?

Desired Outcome

2. What are the goals of pharmacotherapy for managing ascites and related complications of cirrhosis?

Therapeutic Alternatives

3.a. What nonpharmacologic therapies might be considered for this patient?

3.b. What pharmacologic therapies should be considered for this patient?

Optimal Plan

4.a. Outline a suitable pharmaceutical care plan for the acute management of this patient. Include drug, dosage form, dose, dosing schedule, and duration of therapy.

4.b. Outline a suitable pharmacologic care plan for the chronic management of this patient. Include drug, dosage form, dose, dosing schedule, and duration of therapy.

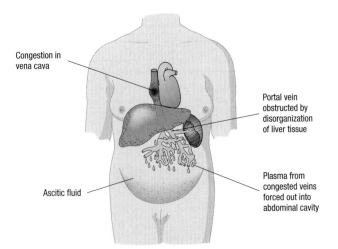

FIGURE 39-1. Development of ascites with portal hypertension due to cirrhosis. *(Reprinted with permission from Mulvihill ML. Human Diseases: A Systemic Approach, 4th ed. Norwalk, CT, Appleton & Lange, 1995:203.)*

4 c. If the initial therapy fails or is intolerable for the patient, what pharmacologic alternatives should be considered?

Outcome Evaluation

5. How should the recommended therapy be monitored for efficacy and adverse effects?

Patient Education

6. On discharge from the hospital, what information should be provided to the patient to enhance compliance, ensure successful treatment, and minimize or prevent adverse effects?

■ ADDITIONAL CASE QUESTIONS

1. What other diseases should the patient be tested for that could impact her liver function?

2. What vaccinations should she receive upon discharge, assuming that she has not had any vaccinations for over 20 years?

■ SELF-STUDY ASSIGNMENTS

1. Identify which pain medications may be used safely in patients with cirrhosis and ascites.

2. Based on this patient's history, what 1-, 2-, and 5-year survival rates would be expected if the patient does not receive a liver transplant?

CLINICAL PEARL

Ascites that does not respond to high-dose diuretics or that persists in patients unable to tolerate high-dose diuretics is referred to as *refractory ascites*. This complication requires the patient to undergo frequent large-volume paracenteses (one to two times per month) and indicates a poor prognosis.

REFERENCES

1. Dib N, Oberti F, Cales P. Current management of the complications of portal hypertension: variceal bleeding and ascites. CMAJ 2006;174:1433–1443.
2. Garcia-Tsao G. Current management of cirrhosis and portal hypertension: variceal hemorrhage, ascites, and spontaneous bacterial peritonitis. Gastroenterology 2001;120:726–748.
3. Gines P, Cardenas A, Arroyo V, et al. Management of cirrhosis and ascites. N Engl J Med 2004;350:1646–1654.
4. Han M, Hyzy R. Advances in critical care management of hepatic failure and insufficiency. Crit Care Med 2006;34(9 Suppl):S225–S231.
5. Moore KP, Aithal GP. Guidelines on the management of ascites in cirrhosis. Gut 2006;55(Suppl 6):vi1–vi12.
6. Runyon BA, Practice Guidelines Committee, American Association for the Study of Liver Diseases (AASLD). Management of adult patients with ascites due to cirrhosis. Hepatology 2004;39:841–856.

40

ESOPHAGEAL VARICES

Veins under Pressure . . . . Level I

Cesar Alaniz, PharmD

LEARNING OBJECTIVES

After completing this case study, students should be able to:

- List nonpharmacologic options for managing patients with bleeding esophageal varices.

- Recommend appropriate pharmacologic therapy for controlling bleeding esophageal varices and adjunctive therapy in the setting of acute variceal bleed.

- Provide appropriate education for patients receiving therapy for portal hypertension.

PATIENT PRESENTATION

■ Chief Complaint

"I'm throwing up blood, and my stools are black."

■ HPI

Sean Smith is a 39-year-old man who presents to the emergency room with a complaint of black stools. He was in his usual state of health until approximately 4 months ago, when he had one episode of vomiting a large volume of blood followed by a second episode 1 month later. He reports not seeking medical attention at the time. Subsequently, he did fine until approximately 3–4 weeks ago, when he had several more similar episodes. He still did not seek treatment but states that he stopped drinking and smoking at that time. Four days ago, he experienced four episodes of vomiting blood. Yesterday, he began to feel weak and was becoming lightheaded on standing. Today, he reports having two more episodes of vomiting blood, which prompted his coming to the hospital. He reports that during his vomiting episodes, he also has black stools. On initial presentation to the ER, he suffered a near syncopal episode that was witnessed by the ER staff. He occasionally takes ibuprofen, most recently 2 days ago.

■ PMH

Atypical pneumonia 5 years ago
Diverticulosis diagnosed 4 years ago

■ FH

Father died of colon cancer

■ SH

He drinks 3–12 beers a day and has been drinking for 20 years; quit 2 weeks ago, except for 2 days ago when he had 3 beers. Lives with wife and does not have any children. He works as a patio furniture salesman. He does not use any illicit drugs.

■ ROS

Negative except for complaints noted above

■ Meds

Ibuprofen (occasionally)

■ All

NKDA

■ Physical Examination

Gen

Ill-appearing male who looks older than his stated age and is pale and diaphoretic; awake but looks very sleepy

VS

BP 90/55 (unable to get orthostatic BP due to patient's lethargic condition), P 140, RR 20 (shallow breathing), T 37.5°C

Skin

Pale; diaphoretic; normal skin turgor; no palmar erythema

HEENT

PERRLA; icteric sclerae; dried blood on lips

Neck/Lymph Nodes

Neck supple; no masses

Lungs/Thorax

Clear to auscultation

CV

Reg S_1, S_2; no S_3; no mitral regurgitation appreciated

Abd

Soft, nontender, (+) bowel sounds; no palpable or pulsatile masses

Rect

Heme positive with obvious melena

Ext

Cool

Neuro

Sleepy, but A & O × 3; CNs II–XII intact; no asterixis

◾ Labs (on Admission)

Na 139 mEq/L	Hgb 4.9 g/dL	AST 92 IU/L	Protein 5.0 g/dL
K 4.2 mEq/L	Hct 14.0%	ALT 43 IU/L	Alb 2.0 g/dL
Cl 102 mEq/L	WBC 6.8 × 10³/mm³	Alk phos 114 IU/L	Ca 8.5 mg/dL
CO_2 22 mEq/L	Plt 191 × 10³/mm³	T. bili 5.9 mg/dL	Phos 5.4 mg/dL
BUN 39 mg/dL	aPTT 28.1 sec		
SCr 0.9 mg/dL	PT 15.5 sec		
Glu 158 mg/dL	INR 1.6		

◾ ECG

NSR; no ST changes; no Q waves

◾ EGD

After gastric lavage and hemodynamic resuscitation, an EGD is performed, which reveals grade III varices with nipple sign (plug of platelet fibrin, a sign of recent bleed) in lower esophagus.

◾ Assessment

This is a 39-year-old male with a history of alcohol abuse who presents to the emergency department acutely ill after hematemesis secondary to bleeding esophageal varices. Laboratory values show severe anemia, hypoalbuminemia, increased serum aminotransferases, and coagulopathy. History of significant alcohol consumption suggests that the patient likely has varices secondary to alcoholic liver disease. The patient should be admitted to an intensive care unit for further management.

QUESTIONS

Problem Identification (Figure 40-1)

1.a. Create a list of the patient's drug therapy problems.

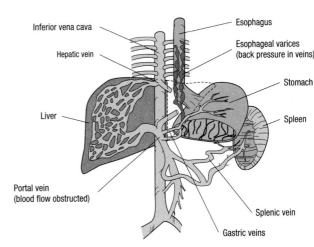

FIGURE 40-1. Anatomic relationships among intestinal veins affected by alcoholic cirrhosis. (Reprinted with permission from Mulvihill ML. Human Diseases: A Systemic Approach, 4th ed. Norwalk, CT, Appleton & Lange, 1995:202.)

1.b. What information supports the diagnosis of bleeding esophageal varices, and what indicates the relative severity of disease?

Desired Outcome

2. What are the goals for managing this patient's clinical condition?

Therapeutic Alternatives

3.a. What nonpharmacologic interventions should be considered for this patient?

3.b. What pharmacologic interventions should be considered for this patient?

Optimal Plan

4.a. What pharmacotherapeutic plan should be implemented for managing the patient's current problems?

4.b. How might the pharmacotherapeutic plan change if the etiology of the bleed is yet to be determined?

Outcome Evaluation

5. What clinical and laboratory parameters should be followed to evaluate the therapeutic interventions and to minimize the risk of adverse effects?

Patient Education

6. What information should be provided to the patient about his medication therapy?

CLINICAL PEARL

Use of continuous infusion proton pump inhibitor therapy is appropriate before performing EGD in patients being evaluated for an upper GI bleed. However, once the source of bleeding is determined to be variceal, the continuous infusion should be stopped because there are no data to support its use in this setting.

◾ SELF-STUDY ASSIGNMENTS

1. Evaluate the relative efficacy of medications used for treating bleeding varices.

2. Describe the benefits of antibiotic therapy for preventing infections in the setting of acute variceal bleeding.

3. Describe the role of primary prophylaxis in patients presenting with a diagnosis of esophageal varices.

REFERENCES

1. Avgerinos A, Armonis A, Stefanidis G, et al. Sustained rise of portal pressure after sclerotherapy, but not band ligation, in acute variceal bleeding in cirrhosis. Hepatology 2004;39:1623–1630.

2. Gotzsche PC, Hrobjartsson A. Somatostatin analogues for acute bleeding oesophageal varices. Cochrane Database Syst Rev 2005;1: CD000193.

3. Longacre AV, Garcia-Tsao G. A common sense approach to esophageal varices. Clin Liver Dis 2006;10:613–625.

4. Groszmann RJ, Garcia-Tsao G, Bosch J, et al. Portal Hypertension Collaborative Group. Beta-blockers to prevent gastroesophageal varices in patients with cirrhosis. N Engl J Med 2005;353:2254–2261.

5. Shaheen NJ, Stuart E, Schmitz SM, et al. Pantoprazole reduces the size of post-banding ulcers after variceal band ligation: a randomized controlled trial. Hepatology 2005;41:588–594.

41

HEPATIC ENCEPHALOPATHY

Dazed and Confused . . . . Level I

Carrie A. Sincak, PharmD, BCPS

LEARNING OBJECTIVES

After completing this case study, students should be able to:

- Identify and correct the precipitating factors associated with the development of hepatic encephalopathy in a cirrhotic patient.

- Recommend appropriate nonpharmacologic and pharmacologic intervention for a cirrhotic patient who develops hepatic encephalopathy.

- Design a plan for monitoring the efficacy and adverse effects of recommended treatments for hepatic encephalopathy.

- Provide patient education for those receiving treatment for hepatic encephalopathy.

PATIENT PRESENTATION

■ Chief Complaint (from Wife)

"My husband has been confused and disoriented for the past 2 days."

■ HPI

Luke Mytlund is a 50-year-old man who was brought to the ED by his wife because of confusion and disorientation. Patient was discharged from the hospital 6 days ago for increased lower-extremity edema and worsening renal function. The wife states that he was doing fine at home, adjusting to all the medication changes since last admission, and getting caught up on day-to-day house-

hold activities. Two days ago, she noticed that her husband, who is typically very sharp about his illnesses, was now confused and continually asking where his dress was for the party. His wife also noted that he has had difficulty sleeping.

■ PMH

Liver cirrhosis diagnosed 1 year ago secondary to chronic granulomatous hepatitis; last admission included uncontrolled ascites and portal hypertension
Chronic kidney disease, stage IV
CVID (common variable immunodeficiency)
Chronic right femoral osteomyelitis currently treated with doxycycline (therapy started 3 weeks ago)
Pain secondary to osteomyelitis

■ FH

Not attainable at this time

■ SH

Unemployed; lives with his wife; they have two daughters who are both away at college

■ ROS

Constitutional: confused; weight gain
Eyes: no vision loss or pain
Ears, nose, mouth, throat: no hearing loss, nasal discharge, mouth or throat problems
Cardiovascular: no chest pains or palpitations
Respiratory: no shortness of breath or cough
Gastrointestinal: no abdominal pain or change in bowel habits
Genitourinary: no discharge or pain
Musculoskeletal: no joint pain or weakness
Neurologic: no weakness or headache
Psychiatric: no anxiety or depression
Endocrine: no diabetes or thyroid disease
Hematologic: no enlarged lymph nodes

■ Meds

Doxycycline 100 mg po Q 12 h
Torsemide 100 mg po Q 12 h
Hydrochlorothiazide 25 mg po daily
Immune globulin 40 g IV Q 14 days
Oxycodone CR 10 mg po Q 12 h
MVI 1 tablet po once daily
Folic acid 1 mg po once daily
Docusate sodium 200 mg po daily PRN
Zinc sulfate 224 mg po daily
Lactulose 30 mL po daily

■ All

Aspirin—reaction unknown

■ Physical Examination

Gen

Middle-aged man in no apparent distress who is disoriented to time and place

VS

BP 110/78, P 96, RR 18, T 36.2°C; Wt 91 kg, Ht 6'0" (per patient's wife)

Skin

Erythema on the right lower extremity; decreased skin turgor

HEENT

PERRLA; dry mucous membranes; TMs intact; EOMI; fundi benign; icteric sclerae; no sinus tenderness

Lungs

Chest symmetric; lungs CTA bilaterally; normal percussion

CV

Tachycardic; S_1 and S_2 normal; 3/6 systolic murmur

Abd

Obese; nontender; distended abdomen; (+) splenomegaly; liver palpable 4 cm below the costal margin; spider angiomata more pronounced compared with previous admission; hypoactive bowel sounds

Rect

Heme (–) stool; no masses

Ext

2+ LE edema with right LE ulceration at anterior tibial region

Neuro

Confused; oriented only to person; CNs II–XII intact; DTRs 2+; (+) asterixis

▓ Labs

Na 130 mEq/L	Hgb 10.4 g/dL	WBC 4.5 ×	AST 63 IU/L	Ca 10.4 mg/dL
K 3.1 mEq/L	Hct 33%	$10^3/mm^3$	ALT 35 IU/L	Mg 2.5 mg/dL
Cl 100 mEq/L	MCV 83 μm^3	75% PMNs	Alk Phos	Phos 5.8 mg/dL
CO_2 25 mEq/L	MCHC 34 g/dL	6% Bands	401 IU/L	PT 15.4 sec
BUN 98 mg/dL	Retic 1.1%	4% Eos	T. bili 1.4 mg/dL	aPTT 32.9 sec
SCr 4.1 mg/dL	Plt 94 × $10^3/mm^3$	8% Lymphs	D. bili 0.4 mg/dL	INR 1.4
Glu 131 mg/dL		7% Monos	Alb 3.1 g/dL	
			Ammonia	
			176 mcg/dL	

▓ Assessment

Hepatic encephalopathy

QUESTIONS

Problem Identification

1.a. Create a list of the patient's drug therapy problems.

1.b. What information indicates the presence of hepatic encephalopathy in this patient?

1.c. What precipitating factors in this patient could potentially cause hepatic encephalopathy?

1.d. What additional information is needed to satisfactorily assess the hepatic encephalopathy of this patient?

Desired Outcome

2. What are the general principles for the management of hepatic encephalopathy and desired therapeutic outcomes?

Therapeutic Alternatives

3.a. What nondrug interventions are important before initiating pharmacotherapeutic agents for the treatment of hepatic encephalopathy?

3.b. What pharmacotherapeutic alternatives are available for the treatment of hepatic encephalopathy? Include the mechanism of action of each drug in your answer.

Optimal Plan

4. Outline a pharmacotherapeutic plan for this patient's drug therapy problems. Include the drugs, dosage forms, doses, schedules, and duration of treatment for each problem.

Outcome Evaluation

5. How would you monitor the efficacy and adverse effects of the treatment you recommended? (See Fig. 41-1.)

Patient Education

6. What medication-related information should be provided to the patient about his therapy on discharge?

■ CLINICAL COURSE

Three days after beginning treatment with the regimen you recommended, the patient is responding positively, and the dose has been titrated appropriately. He is oriented to time, place, and person, and no asterixis is detected. The plan is to discharge the patient home tomorrow.

■ SELF-STUDY ASSIGNMENTS

1. Perform a literature search to assess the efficacy and the potential role of rifaximin in the treatment of hepatic encephalopathy.

Number Connection Test 1.

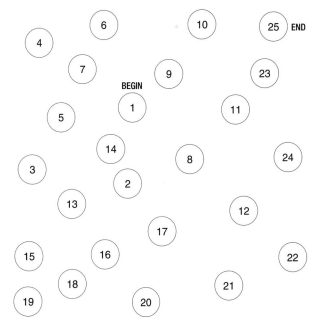

FIGURE 41-1. Number Connection Test part A (NCT-A), which measures cognitive motor abilities. Subjects have to connect the numbers printed on paper consecutively from 1 to 25, as quickly as possible. Errors are not counted, but patients are instructed to return to the preceding correct number and then carry on. The test score is the time the patient needs to perform the test, including the time needed to correct all errors. A low score represents a good performance. *(Reprinted with permission from Quero JC, Schalm SW. Subclinical hepatic encephalopathy. Semin Liver Dis 1996;16:321–328.)*

2. List the potential advantages and disadvantages of using antibiotics for the treatment of hepatic encephalopathy.

3. List the amino acid contents in the commercially available oral and parenteral formulations of branched-chain amino acid products; determine the cost of these products in your area.

CLINICAL PEARL

Sedatives, tranquilizers, and other CNS depressants can precipitate acute hepatic encephalopathy. A careful medication history is important in patients presenting with the disorder to eliminate reversible causes.

REFERENCES

1. Blei AT, Cordoba J. Practice Parameters Committee of the American College of Gastroenterology. Hepatic encephalopathy. Am J Gastroenterol 2001;96:1968–1976.
2. Blei AT. Diagnosis and treatment of hepatic encephalopathy. Baillieres Best Pract Res Clin Gastroenterol 2000;14:959–974.
3. Gerber T, Schomerus H. Hepatic encephalopathy in liver cirrhosis: pathogenesis, diagnosis and management. Drugs 2000;60:1353–1370.
4. Mas A. Hepatic encephalopathy: from pathophysiology to treatment. Digestion 2006;73(Suppl 1):86–93.
5. Festi D, Vestito A, Mazzella G, et al. Management of hepatic encephalopathy: focus on antibiotic therapy. Digestion 2006;73(Suppl 1):94–101.
6. Mas A, Rodes J, Sunyer L, et al. Comparison of rifaximin and lactitol in the treatment of acute hepatic encephalopathy: results of a randomized, double-blind, double-dummy, controlled clinical trial. J Hepatol 2003;38:51–58.
7. Miglio F, Valpiani D, Rossellini SR, et al. Rifaximin, a non-absorbable rifamycin, for the treatment of hepatic encephalopathy. A double-blind, randomised trial. Curr Med Res Opin 1997;13:593–601.
8. Williams R, James OFW, Warnes TW, et al. Evaluation of the efficacy and safety of rifaximin in the treatment of hepatic encephalopathy: a double-blind, randomized, dose-finding multi-centre study. Eur J Gastroenterol Hepatol 2000;12:203–208.

42

DRUG-INDUCED LIVER DISEASE: ACETAMINOPHEN TOXICITY

What a Pain . . . . Level II

Elizabeth J. Scharman, PharmD, DABAT, BCPS, FAACT

LEARNING OBJECTIVES

After completing this case study, students should be able to:

• Determine when a potentially toxic acetaminophen exposure exists.

• Monitor a patient for signs and symptoms associated with acetaminophen toxicity.

• Recommend appropriate antidotal therapy for acetaminophen poisoning.

• Describe the time frame in which N-acetylcysteine is most likely to be effective after acetaminophen poisoning.

PATIENT PRESENTATION

■ Chief Complaint

Nausea and vomiting (as per physician report)

■ HPI

The poison center receives a telephone call at 2:15 AM from a physician at an ED regarding a 41-year-old woman named Marsha Gray who reported that between 6:30 PM and 8:30 PM she ingested 14 acetaminophen extra-strength tablets. When that failed to treat her backache, she started taking ibuprofen and naproxen. She estimates that she ingested 12 ibuprofen tablets and 4 naproxen tablets between 9 PM and midnight. She states that she did not intend to harm herself; she was just treating a bad back. She denies ingestion of alcohol. The physician asks whether this is a toxic dose of acetaminophen and whether any specific therapies are recommended. The poison specialist is able to obtain the following information from the physician:

■ PMH

Hypertension

■ FH

Not available

■ SH

Significant for an overdose 2 months earlier; details not available

■ Meds

Diltiazem, unknown dose, po daily

■ All

Not available

■ Physical Examination

Gen

The patient appears drowsy. There are no external signs of trauma. The patient has vomited twice since arrival in the ED. The vomitus was not bloody. Her breath smells like alcohol.

VS

BP 159/88, HR 88, RR 15, O$_2$ sat 98–99% on room air, T 37°C; Wt 65 kg

Skin

Mucous membranes are moist

HEENT

Pupil size is normal

Abd

Bowel sounds are present

Neuro

Patient is oriented to time and place; reflexes are normal

■ Labs (Drawn at 01:30)

Na 142 mEq/L	Hgb 12.9 g/dL	Aspirin <2.0 mg/dL
K 3.3 mEq/L	Hct 38%	Acetaminophen 139.1 mcg/mL
Cl 96 mEq/L	AST 52 U/L	Ethanol (ETOH) 88 mg/dL
CO$_2$ 23 mEq/L	ALT 28 U/L	β-HCG (–)
BUN 20 mg/dL	T. bili 0.8 mg/dL	
SCr 1.0 mg/dL	INR 1.0	
Glucose 86 mg/dL		

ECG
Normal sinus rhythm

Assessment
Possible acetaminophen poisoning

QUESTIONS

Problem Identification

1.a. Is the amount of acetaminophen the patient states she took consistent with the potential for acetaminophen toxicity? Why or why not?

1.b. What factors should be considered when evaluating this patient's history for accuracy?

1.c. Which signs, symptoms, and laboratory values indicate that acetaminophen toxicity is present?

1.d. What are possible causes of the nausea and vomiting in this patient?

1.e. Does toxicity from any other drug(s) need to be considered in this patient? If so, which one(s) and why?

Desired Outcome

2. What are the goals of pharmacotherapy in this case?

Therapeutic Alternatives

3. What feasible pharmacotherapeutic alternatives are available for treating acetaminophen toxicity in this patient?

Optimal Plan

4.a. What medication dose, schedule, and duration of therapy are best for this patient?

4.b. If the physician asks the pharmacy to make an IV containing the exact dose of IV N-acetylcysteine (Acetadote) for this patient, instead of rounding to the nearest dose designated in the prescribing information dosing table, how many milliliters of N-acetylcysteine should this patient receive? Show all calculations including how the total dose needed was obtained and how the amount of N-acetylcysteine in each milliliter of Acetadote was calculated.

4.c. If this patient were to refuse treatment, should she be allowed to refuse or should other steps be taken to ensure that treatment is provided?

4.d. If the laboratory test had shown that the patient was β-HCG (+), would recommendations for N-acetylcysteine therapy change? Why or why not?

Outcome Evaluation

5. What clinical and laboratory parameters are necessary to evaluate the therapy for achievement of the desired therapeutic outcome and to detect adverse effects?

Patient Education

6. What should the patient be told about the effectiveness of N-acetylcysteine therapy?

■ CLINICAL COURSE

At 3:00 the next morning, the poison center calls the hospital for additional follow-up information. Ms. Gray was started on N-acetylcysteine therapy per the recommendations given. The poison specialist determines that the correct dosage was administered and that no adverse effects occurred. Vital signs are BP 139/82, HR 65, and RR 14. Physical examination is normal, although she was complaining of a severe headache the previous evening. She has not vomited since she arrived in ICU. She is noted to be depressed and tearful. Lab results from 19:00 the previous evening were as follows:

Na 144 mEq/L
K 3.7 mEq/L
Cl 98 mEq/L
CO_2 24 mEq/L
BUN 11 mg/dL
SCr 0.9 mg/dL
Glucose 92 mg/dL

Hgb 12.8 g/dL
Hct 38%
AST 51 U/L
ALT 35 U/L
T. bili 0.9 mg/dL
INR 1.4

The poison specialist asks the nurse what therapies, if any, the patient received for her headache.

Follow-Up Questions

1. Explain the cause of any abnormal laboratory findings on day 2.

2. Which pain medications would the poison specialist want to make sure are not being administered to this patient?

3. Given Ms. Gray's history of drug overdoses, should other medications be considered for the management of her hypertension? Why or why not?

■ SELF-STUDY ASSIGNMENTS

1. Defend the argument that all patients with an intentional drug overdose, no matter what their stated history, should have an acetaminophen level drawn to rule out acetaminophen toxicity.

2. Provide a detailed description of the differences between anaphylactoid reactions (as reported with IV N-acetylcysteine administration) and anaphylactic reactions.

3. Write a recommendation to the hospital formulary committee justifying the need to begin stocking the FDA-approved IV N-acetylcysteine in addition to the oral N-acetylcysteine currently on formulary.

CLINICAL PEARL

When evaluating patients with drug overdoses, consider all aspects of the patient's history and initial medical evaluation; do not assume that the initial history provided is accurate.

REFERENCES

1. Dart RC, Erdman AR, Olson KR, et al. Acetaminophen poisoning: an evidence-based consensus guideline for out-of-hospital management. Clin Toxicol (Phila) 2006;44:1–18.

2. Rowden AK, Norvell J, Eldridge DL, et al. Acetaminophen poisoning. Clin Lab Med 2006;26:49–65.

3. Kao LW, Kirk MA, Furbee RB, et al. What is the rate of adverse events after oral N-acetylcysteine administered by the intravenous route to patients with suspected acetaminophen poisoning? Ann Emerg Med 2003;42:741–750.

4. Dribben WH, Porto SM, Jeffords DK. Stability and microbiology of inhalant N-acetylcysteine used as an intravenous solution for the treatment of acetaminophen poisoning. Ann Emerg Med 2003;42:9–13.

5. Acetadote package insert. Nashville, TN, Cumberland Pharmaceuticals Inc. 2006.

6. Bromberg S, Cassel CK. Suicide in the elderly: the limits of paternalism. J Am Geriatr Soc 1983;31:698–703.

7. Wilkes JM, Clark LE, Herrera JL. Acetaminophen overdose in pregnancy. South Med J 2005;98:1118–1122.

8. Payen C, Dachraoui A, Pulce C, et al. Prothrombin time prolongation in paracetamol poisoning: a relevant marker of hepatic failure? Hum Exp Toxicol 2003;22:617–621.

43

ACUTE PANCREATITIS

Friday Night Plight . . . . Level II

Robert MacLaren, BSc, PharmD, FCCM, FCCP

LEARNING OBJECTIVES

After completing this case study, students should be able to:

- Identify precipitating factors associated with acute pancreatitis.

- Recognize signs, symptoms, and laboratory abnormalities commonly associated with acute pancreatitis.

- Describe potential systemic complications associated with acute pancreatitis.

- Recommend appropriate pharmacologic and nonpharmacologic therapies for patients with acute pancreatitis.

- Outline monitoring parameters to assist in realization of desired therapeutic outcomes.

PATIENT PRESENTATION

Chief Complaint

"I've got a really bad pain in my stomach."

HPI

Bill Jones is a 48-year-old man who presents to the ED shortly after midnight on a Friday night because of intense mid-epigastric pain radiating to his back. He states that the pain started shortly after dinner the night before but has progressively worsened, and he began vomiting around midnight tonight.

PMH

Alcohol withdrawal seizures 8 months ago during which he suffered a small subdural hematoma.

FH

Father died at age of 56 from an MVA; mother is 72 years old and has Type 2 DM and "cholesterol issues," for which she is taking an unknown medication. One sister, also with "cholesterol issues," taking an unknown medication. The sister has a remote history of pancreatitis as well.

SH

Divorced with three children. Employed as a groundskeeper at a golf course. Denies any smoking. He states that he used to consume six beers per day until 8 months ago when he had a withdrawal seizure but now drinks only on weekends a total of about six beers; he reports sharing a couple of pitchers with two friends last night with dinner. Drinks at least two cups of coffee each morning.

Meds

Valproic acid 250 mg twice daily since his seizure
Advil 200 mg OTC several doses per day PRN

All

Phenytoin makes his "heart pound."

ROS

He states that he has been feeling well until last night. He hurt his back 2 weeks ago at work but the Advil has helped relieve the pain. He has vomited approximately six times since midnight tonight. No complaints of diarrhea or blood in the stool or vomit. No knowledge of any prior history of uncontrolled blood sugars or cholesterol.

Physical Examination

Gen

The patient is restless and in moderate distress but otherwise is a well-appearing, well-nourished male who looks his stated age.

VS

BP 98/55, P 122, RR 30, T 38.9°C; Wt 89 kg, Ht 5'10"

HEENT

PERRLA; EOMI; oropharynx pink and clear; oral mucosa dry

Skin

Dry with poor skin turgor

Neck/Lymph Nodes

Supple; no bruits, lymphadenopathy, or thyromegaly

Cor

Sinus tachycardia; no MRG

Lungs

Bilateral basilar rales

Abd

Moderately distended with active but diminished bowel sounds; (+) guarding; pain is elicited on light palpation of left upper and mid-epigastric region. No rebound tenderness, masses, or hepatosplenomegaly.

Ext

Extremities are warm and well perfused. Good pulses present in all extremities. No clubbing, palmar erythema, or spider angiomata.

Rect

Normal sphincter tone; no BRBPR or masses; stool is guaiac negative; prostate normal size.

Neuro

A & O × 3; neuro exam benign; CN II–XII intact; strength is equal bilaterally in all extremities. Normal tone and reflexes. No asterixis.

■ Labs

Na 128 mEq/L	Hgb 17 g/dL	AST 342 IU/L	Ca 7.2 mg/dL
K 3.4 mEq/L	Hct 50%	ALT 166 IU/L	Mg 1.7 mEq/L
Cl 105 mEq/L	WBC 15.2 × 10³/mm³	Alk phos 285 IU/L	Phos 2.2 mg/dL
CO₂ 18 mEq/L	Neutros 72%	LDH 255 IU/L	Trig 982 mg/dL
BUN 35 mg/dL	Bands 4%	T. bili 0.6 mg/dL	Repeat Trig 1,010 mg/dL
SCr 1.5 mg/dL	Eos 1%	Alb 3.2 g/dL	PT 12.8 sec
Glu 375 mg/dL	Basos 1%	Prealb 25 mg/dL	INR 1.1
	Lymphs 20%	Amylase 1,555 IU/L	aPTT 19.3 sec
	Monos 2%	Lipase 2,220 IU/L	VPA 51 mg/L
			BAC 4 mg/dL

■ Other Tests

Negative for serum ketones, ASA, acetaminophen, all alcohols, viral hepatitis titers, and HIV

■ Arterial Blood Gases

pH 7.31, PCO₂ 38 mm Hg, PO₂ 88 mm Hg, HCO₃⁻ 17 mEq/L, O₂ sat 98% on room air

■ UA

Color yellow; turbidity clear; SG 1.010; pH 7.2; glucose >1,000 mg/dL; bilirubin (–); ketones (–); Hgb (–); protein (–); nitrite (–); crystals (–); casts (–); mucous (–); bacteria (–); urobilinogen: 0.25 EU/dL; WBC 0–5/hpf; RBC 0/hpf; epithelial cells: 0–10/hpf

■ Chest X-Ray

AP view of chest shows the heart to be normal in size. The lungs are clear without any infiltrates, masses, effusions, or atelectasis. No notable abnormalities.

■ Abdominal Ultrasound

Non-specific gas pattern; no dilated bowel. Questionable opacity/abnormality of common bile duct. Cannot rule out gallstone/obstruction.

■ ECG

Sinus tachycardia; rate 140 bpm

■ Assessment

Acute pancreatitis precipitating hyperglycemia, hypocalcemia, and non-anion gap metabolic acidosis
R/O choledocholithiasis

QUESTIONS

Problem Identification (Fig. 43-1)

1.a. What factors may have precipitated acute pancreatitis in this case?

1.b. What signs, symptoms, and laboratory tests are consistent with the diagnosis of acute pancreatitis?

1.c. Construct a drug therapy problem list for this patient.

Desired Outcome

2. What are the goals of therapy for this patient?

Therapeutic Alternatives

3. What therapies may be instituted to achieve the goals outlined above? Provide a rationale for each therapy.

Optimal Plan

4. Develop a pharmacotherapeutic care plan for this patient, including duration of therapy.

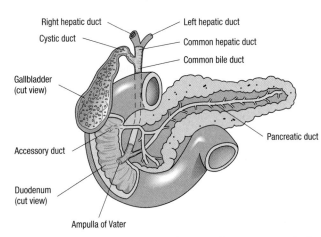

FIGURE 43-1. Anatomic relationship between the pancreas and other digestive organs. *(Reprinted with permission from Mulvihill ML. Human Diseases: A Systemic Approach, 4th ed. Norwalk, CT, Appleton & Lange, 1995:209.)*

Outcome Evaluation

5. Outline the monitoring parameters for efficacy and adverse effects of therapy for pain management.

Patient Education

6. When this patient is stable, what information should be provided to him to reduce the likelihood of recurrent pancreatitis?

■ CLINICAL COURSE

IV morphine is initiated for pain control. Partial parenteral nutrition (without lipids) is instituted after 24 hours and oral nutrition is started 24 hours later, at which time parenteral nutrition is discontinued. However, after several days of improvement in the hospital, the patient develops a WBC count of 23.4 × 10³/mm³ with neutrophils 77%, bands 15%, eosinophils 1%, basophils 0%, lymphocytes 3%, and monocytes 4%. He has a temperature of 39.8°C and is noted to be orthostatic (BP 128/76 sitting, 98/60 standing) with a glucose of 480 mg/dL. He has also experienced several episodes of diarrhea and steatorrhea.

Because of these setbacks in the patient's progress, a contrast-enhanced CT scan is obtained. The results demonstrate peripancreatic and retroperitoneal edema. The pancreas itself appears relatively normal with the exception of small non-enhancing areas around the neck of the pancreas, which are suggestive of necrosis.

■ FOLLOW-UP QUESTIONS

1.a. What potential etiologies might explain this patient's fever and relapsing acute pancreatitis?

1.b. What are the new treatment goals for this patient?

1.c. Given this new information, what therapeutic interventions should be considered for this patient?

1.d. How should these new therapies be monitored for efficacy and adverse effects?

■ SELF-STUDY ASSIGNMENTS

1. Describe the pathophysiology of autodigestion during acute pancreatitis.

2. Describe the controversies of early enteral nutrition, prophylactic antibiotics, and octreotide for management of acute pancreatitis.

3. Summarize published information regarding opioid effects on the sphincter of Oddi.

4. Review the Ranson scoring method for predicting the severity of acute pancreatitis, and outline its advantages and disadvantages when clinically applied.

5. Compose a list of drugs believed to aggravate or cause pancreatitis and assess the level of association for each agent.

CLINICAL PEARL

More expensive microencapsulated pancreatic enzyme products have not consistently been shown to be superior to standard therapeutic doses of the less expensive, non-enteric coated dosage forms.

REFERENCES

1. Whitcomb DC. Acute pancreatitis. N Engl J Med 2006;354:2142–2150.
2. Kingsnorth A, O'Reilly D. Acute pancreatitis. BMJ 2006;332:1072–1076.
3. Mitchell RM, Byrne MF, Baillie J. Pancreatitis. Lancet 2003;361:1447–1455.
4. Nathens AB, Curtis JR, Beale RJ, et al. Management of the critically ill patient with severe acute pancreatitis. Crit Care Med 2004;32:2524–2536.
5. Koizumi M, Takada T, Kawarada Y, et al. JPN guidelines for the management of acute pancreatitis: diagnostic criteria for acute pancreatitis. J Hepatobiliary Surg 2006;13:25–32.
6. Meier R, Ockenga J, Pertkiewicz M, et al. ESPEN guidelines on enteral nutrition: pancreas. Clin Nutr 2006;25:275–284.
7. Thomson A. Enteral versus parenteral nutritional support in acute pancreatitis: a clinical review. J Gastroenterol Hepatol 2006;21(1 Pt 1):22–25.
8. McClave SA, Chang WK, Dhaliwal R, et al. Nutrition support in acute pancreatitis: a systematic review of the literature. J Parenter Enteral Nutr 2006;30:143–156.
9. Eatock FC, Chong P, Menezes N, et al. A randomized study of early nasogastric versus nasojejunal feeding in severe acute pancreatitis. Am J Gastroenterol 2005;100:432–439.
10. Isenhower HL, Mueller BA. Selection of narcotic analgesics for pain associated with pancreatitis. Am J Health Syst Pharm 1998;55:480–486.
11. Mazaki T, Ishii Y, Takayama T. Meta-analysis of prophylactic antibiotic use in acute necrotizing pancreatitis. Br J Surg 2006;93:674–684.

44

CHRONIC PANCREATITIS

Mac's Attack . . . . Level II

Joseph J. Kishel, PharmD, BCPS

LEARNING OBJECTIVES

After completing this case study, students should be able to:

- Identify subjective and objective findings consistent with chronic pancreatitis and acute exacerbations of chronic pancreatitis.

- Evaluate patient-specific data and develop a problem list for patients with acute exacerbations of chronic pancreatitis.

- Understand the rationale for "pancreatic rest" in the resolution of pain and symptoms of an acute exacerbation of pancreatitis.

- Discuss therapeutic alternatives and outline a patient-specific plan for pain management during an acute exacerbation of chronic pancreatitis.

- Recommend appropriate pancreatic enzyme replacement therapy for management of steatorrhea in a patient with chronic pancreatitis.

PATIENT PRESENTATION

■ Chief Complaint

"I have been having three to five foul-smelling, liquid, green stools per day for the past few days."

■ HPI

Macintyre Jones is a 33-year-old man who presents to his PCP complaining of an increase in loose, foul-smelling stools and has observed a fatty content and consistency to his stools. There has been an increase in the frequency of the stools, partly coincident with his return to night school, as he has been less careful about his diet. These symptoms have been present for the past week. Mr. Jones has also noticed some nausea, with vomiting, associated with increased abdominal discomfort within the past week. Mr. Jones vomited twice while in the waiting room and admits in the exam room that his pain is more than just "discomfort" and has actually been quite debilitating.

■ PMH

Has been hospitalized nearly every 6 months of his life for cystic fibrosis exacerbations. His last stay was 2 months ago, which lasted 4 weeks and included 10 days in the MICU for respiratory support. He has always received low-dose pancreatic enzyme supplements, but he has not had his doses titrated for several years.

■ SH

Parents are alive and healthy. One older sister died 6 years ago with CF at age 29. One younger brother is alive and healthy at age 28. Patient does not drink alcohol, smoke cigarettes, or use illicit drugs per patient report.

■ Meds

Albuterol 0.083% for nebulization inhalation Q 6 h
Ipratropium bromide 0.02% for nebulization inhalation QID
Pancrelipase (Ultrase MT 20) 1 capsule by mouth with meals
Tobramycin 300 mg inhaled BID

■ All

Sulfamethoxazole/trimethoprim → hives

■ ROS

No hematemesis or other complaints other than those described above

■ Physical Examination

Gen

Thin, ill-appearing Caucasian man, appearing anxious

VS

BP 92/60, P 105, RR 28, T 37.6°C; Wt 45 kg, Ht 5'10"

Skin

Normal skin turgor

HEENT

PERRLA, EOMI, oropharynx clear, mucous membranes moist

Neck/Lymph Nodes

Supple; (−) JVD, thyromegaly, lymphadenopathy, or bruits

Lung/Thorax

Hyperventilation; marked hyperresonance on percussion; audible breath sounds in all lung fields

CV

Regular rate and rhythm without gallops or murmur

Abd

Sparse bowel sounds, (+) rebound and guarding

Genit/Rect

No masses, guaiac (−)

MS/Ext

(+) Clubbing; proximal nail beds cyanotic, (−) edema

Neuro

A & O × 3, CN II–XII intact

■ Labs

Na 133 mEq/L	Hgb 14.2 g/dL	WBC 10.1 × 10³/mm³	T. bili 0.4 mg/dL
K 4.4 mEq/L	Hct 43%	Neutros 73%	Alk Phos 113 IU/L
Cl 93 mEq/L	RBC 4.8 × 10⁶/mm³	Bands 0%	Alb 2.6 g/dL
CO₂ 32 mEq/L	Plt 387 × 10³/mm³	Eos 1%	Pre alb 19 mg/dL
BUN 9 mg/dL	MCV 89.6 μm³	Lymphs 11%	Lipase 130 IU/L
SCr 0.7 mg/dL	MCHC 33 g/dL	Monos 15%	Amylase 358 IU/L
Glu 94 mg/dL			

■ ERCP

Changes consistent with chronic pancreatitis: presence of intra-pancreatic duct calculi

■ Assessment

1. Chronic pancreatitis
2. Cystic fibrosis
3. Dietary insufficiency

QUESTIONS

Problem Identification

1.a. Create a list of this patient's drug therapy problems.

1.b. What subjective and objective information is consistent with the diagnosis of chronic pancreatitis?

1.c. What signs, symptoms, and test results indicate that the patient is experiencing an acute exacerbation of chronic pancreatitis?

1.d. Which of the patient's problems are amenable to drug therapy?

1.e. What additional information is needed to satisfactorily assess the patient?

Desired Outcome

2. What are the goals of pharmacotherapy in this case?

Therapeutic Alternatives

3.a. What nondrug therapies could be useful in this patient?

3.b. What feasible pharmacotherapeutic alternatives are available for treating this acute exacerbation of chronic pancreatitis?

Optimal Plan

4. What drug, dosage form, and duration of therapy are best for this patient?

Outcome Evaluation

5. What clinical and laboratory parameters are necessary to evaluate the therapy for achievement of the desired therapeutic outcome and to detect or prevent adverse effects?

Patient Education

6. Mr. Jones is ready to be discharged from hospital. As the floor-based pharmacist, what information will you provide him to enhance compliance with his new medication regimen, maximize the chance of success, and minimize adverse effects?

■ SELF-STUDY ASSIGNMENTS

1. Analyze the association between mutations of the cystic fibrosis transmembrane regulator gene and clinical manifestations of disease in CF, such as: pulmonary disease, pancreatic disease, and effects on reproduction.

2. Explain why this patient with pancreatic insufficiency has developed chronic pancreatitis and what other consequences may manifest in the future.

3. Non-enteric pancreatic enzyme supplements can be destroyed by the low pH of the stomach. What medications can help minimize this effect?

CLINICAL PEARL

Cystic fibrosis is classically associated with pulmonary disease, diagnosis during childhood, and a lifespan generally not exceeding age 30. However, genetic mutations and symptoms vary widely; some patients have symptoms predominantly in the GI tract without pulmonary manifestations. As a result, some patients are not diagnosed until they have reached adulthood.

REFERENCES

1. Robertson MB, Choe KA, Joseph PM. Review of the abdominal manifestations of cystic fibrosis in the adult patient. Radiographics 2006;26:679–690.

2. Witt H. Chronic pancreatitis and cystic fibrosis. Gut 2003;52(Suppl 2):ii31–ii41.

3. DiMagno MJ, Dimagno EP. Chronic pancreatitis. Curr Opin Gastroenterol 2006;22:487–497.

4. Bornman PC, Marks IN, Girdwood AW, et al. Pathogenesis of pain in chronic pancreatitis: ongoing enigma. World J Surg 2003;27:1175–1182.

5. Etemad B, Whitcomb DC. Chronic pancreatitis: diagnosis, classification, and new genetic developments. Gastroenterology 2001;120:682–707.

6. Malka D, Hammel P, Sauvanet A, et al. Risk factors for diabetes mellitus in chronic pancreatitis. Gastroenterology 2000;119:1324–1332.

45

VIRAL HEPATITIS A VACCINATION

Avoiding the Spread . . . . Level II

Juliana Chan, PharmD

LEARNING OBJECTIVES

After completing this case study, students should be able to:

- Determine which patient populations are at greatest risk for contracting hepatitis A.

- Recommend hepatitis A immunization for appropriate individuals based on current guidelines of the Centers for Disease Control and Prevention (CDC).

- Assess the efficacy and adverse effects of hepatitis A vaccines.

- Counsel eligible patients on the benefits of hepatitis A vaccination and the possible adverse effects associated with its use.

PATIENT PRESENTATION

■ Chief Complaint

"I'm here today with my baby daughter for our shots before going to Mexico."

■ HPI

Samantha is a 27-year-old Mexican-American woman with a 9-month-old baby girl. She presents to the Family Medicine Clinic today for a routine annual physical exam for herself. During the history, the patient reports that she will be leaving for Mexico with her daughter in 12 months to visit her parents so that they can see their granddaughter.

■ PMH

Postpartum depression × 6 months

■ Surgical History

Tonsillectomy at the age of 5

■ FH

Mother and father are alive and well; four brothers all with a history of gout; one sister is alive and well and a second sister died at the age of 30 due to liver disease.

■ SH

Married for 3 years and lives with husband and daughter. She does not smoke or drink. She worked as a housekeeper for the past 7 years.

■ ROS

The patient is quite active. She denies any dyspnea on exertion, palpitations, fainting, cough, sputum, wheezing, abdominal pain, changes in bowel habits, melena, hematochezia, urinary urgency or frequency.

■ Meds

Multivitamin tablet po once daily
Paroxetine 10 mg po once daily

■ All

Sulfa

■ Physical Examination

Gen

The patient is a healthy Mexican-American woman in no apparent distress.

VS

BP 104/60, P 72, RR 20, T 36.9°C; Wt 56 kg, Ht 5'5"

Skin

Warm and dry

HEENT

PERRLA, EOMI; fundi normal; TMs clear

Neck/Lymph Nodes

No adenopathy or goiter

Chest

Clear without wheezes, rhonchi, or rales

CV

RRR, S_1, S_2 normal; no S_3 or S_4

Abd

(+) Bowel sounds, no masses, non-tender

Genit/Rect

No rectal masses

MS/Ext

Normal range of motion throughout; no CCE

Neuro

A & O × 3; CN II–XII intact; no focal deficits

■ Labs (Non-Fasting)

Na 139 mEq/L	Hgb 13.2 g/dL	AST 38 IU/L	T. chol 198 mg/dL
K 4.1 mEq/L	Hct 39.5%	ALT 39 IU/L	Anti-HBs (+)
Cl 107 mEq/L	WBC 5.6×10^3/mm³	Alk phos 85 IU/L	HBsAg (–)
CO₂ 26 mEq/L	Plt 181×10^3/mm³	T. bili 0.6 mg/dL	Total anti-HAV (–)
BUN 17 mg/dL		LDH 167 IU/L	
SCr 0.8 mg/dL		PT 13.7 sec	
Glu 102 mg/dL		Alb 4.5 g/dL	

■ Assessment

The patient is healthy with no complaints. She is here with her daughter to be evaluated for the hepatitis A vaccination.

QUESTIONS

Problem Identification

1.a. What patient factors make Samantha a candidate for the hepatitis A vaccination?

1.b. Is Samantha's daughter a candidate for the hepatitis A vaccination? Please explain your answer.

1.c. What other patient populations or environments present an increased risk for infection with hepatitis A?

Desired Outcome

2. What are the goals of hepatitis A vaccination?

Therapeutic Alternatives

3.a. What nonpharmacologic recommendations should be made to this patient and her daughter to minimize their risk of developing hepatitis A infection while in Mexico?

3.b. What commercial products are available for vaccination against hepatitis A, and how effective are they in providing protective efficacy?

Optimal Plan

4.a. Outline a vaccination regimen that includes dose, route of administration, and the number of doses required for Samantha.

4.b. Outline a vaccination regimen that includes dose, route of administration, and the number of doses required for Samantha's 9-month-old daughter.

Outcome Evaluation

5.a. How should the regimen you recommended be monitored for efficacy?

5.b. What adverse effects may be experienced with the regimen you recommended, and how may these events be treated?

Patient Education

6. What information should be provided to Samantha about the hepatitis A vaccine?

■ CLINICAL COURSE

It is now approximately 14 months later. Samantha and her daughter traveled to Mexico as planned and returned to the United States 30 days ago; they are both healthy with no complaints. However, her husband Jorge who also accompanied them on the trip has progressively developed severe abdominal pain and yellow skin and eyes for the past 20 days. Jorge was admitted to the hospital for medical attention. The following labs were obtained during the first day of Jorge's hospitalization.

Na 141 mEq/L	Hgb 12.1 g/dL	AST 94 IU/L	Anti-HBs (+)
K 5.0 mEq/L	Hct 36.3%	ALT 101 IU/L	HBsAg (−)
Cl 111 mEq/L	WBC 7.1×10^3/mm^3	Alk phos 201 IU/L	Total anti-HAV (+)
CO$_2$ 30 mEq/L	Plt 123×10^3/mm^3	T. bili 0.6 mg/dL	anti-HAV IgM (+)
BUN 25 mg/dL		LDH 182 IU/L	
SCr 1.3 mg/dL		PT 14.2 sec	
Glu (non-fasting)		Alb 4.5 g/dL	
98 mg/dL			

■ FOLLOW-UP QUESTIONS

1. Based on the information provided, what medical condition does Jorge have?

2. What is your treatment recommendation for Jorge?

■ SELF-STUDY ASSIGNMENTS

1. Compare and contrast the mechanism of action, immunogenicity rate, and adverse effects of the two commercially available hepatitis A vaccines.

2. Determine what other vaccines can be given simultaneously with the hepatitis A vaccine.

3. Compare the cost of administering the Havrix and Engerix-B vaccines separately versus the combination product Twinrix for an adult.

CLINICAL PEARL

According to the CDC, all children over 1 year of age should receive the hepatitis A vaccine in the United States.[1]

REFERENCES

1. Centers for Disease Control and Prevention. Prevention of hepatitis A through active or passive immunization: recommendations of the Advisory Committee on Immunization Practices (ACIP). MMWR Morb Mortal Wkly Rep 2006;55(RR07):1–23.
2. Craig AS, Schaffner W. Prevention of hepatitis A with the hepatitis A vaccine. N Engl J Med 2004;350:476–481.

46

VIRAL HEPATITIS B

Generations of Infections. . . . . Level III

Juliana Chan, PharmD

LEARNING OBJECTIVES

After completing this case study, students should be able to:

- Outline a pharmacologic and nonpharmacologic regimen for patients with chronic hepatitis B.

- Determine clinical and laboratory endpoints for treatment of chronic hepatitis B.

- Assess the efficacy and adverse effects of chronic hepatitis B treatment with interferon, pegylated interferon, lamivudine, adefovir dipivoxil, entecavir, and telbivudine.

- Recommend hepatitis B immunization for appropriate individuals based on current guidelines of the Centers for Disease Control and Prevention (CDC).

- Provide patient education on interferon, pegylated interferon, lamivudine, adefovir dipivoxil, entecavir, and telbivudine treatment.

PATIENT PRESENTATION

■ Chief Complaint

"I'm here for a follow-up visit for my hepatitis B."

■ HPI

Cindy Smith is a 39-year-old woman with no significant past medical history except for HTN. According to the patient, she is a known carrier of hepatitis B for the past 4 years and was completely free of signs or symptoms until 2 weeks ago when an abnormal transaminase level was noted during her yearly physical. She was referred to the liver clinic today for further evaluation and possible treatment.

■ PMH

HTN
Seasonal allergies
Denies any psychiatric disorders

■ Surgical History

Appendectomy 20 years ago requiring a blood transfusion

■ FH

Father died of lung cancer at age 65; mother died of hepatitis at age 62; three siblings are alive and well

■ SH

Married for 20 years and lives with her husband. She has an 18-year-old daughter and a 19-year-old son. She does smoke a half pack per day and drinks wine occasionally at social events. She has not used IV drugs. She is employed as a computer analyst.

■ Meds

Hydrochlorothiazide 25 mg, 1 tablet by mouth daily
Claritin 10 mg po daily

■ All

Penicillin ("rash all over the body")

■ ROS

Denies any symptoms. Her weight is stable with no loss of appetite. No nausea, vomiting, diarrhea, or constipation. No melena or hematochezia. No changes in urine or stool color and no history of icteric sclerae.

■ Physical Examination

Gen

The patient is a well-appearing Caucasian woman in NAD

VS

BP 128/82, P 76, RR 20, T 37.2°C; Wt 47.6 kg, Ht 5'2"

Skin

Warm and dry; no obvious icterus; no spider nevi or palmar erythema

HEENT

PERRLA, EOMI, sclerae anicteric; funduscopic exam normal; TMs intact

Cor

RRR, S_1, S_2 normal; no S_3 or S_4

Lungs

Clear to P & A

Abd

Soft, nontender; liver span 10 cm; no evidence of ascites; spleen is not palpable

Rect

Guaiac negative

MS/Ext

Normal range of motion throughout; no C/C/E

Neuro

CN II–XII intact; DTRs 2+ throughout; negative Babinski

■ Labs Today

Na 142 mEq/L	Hgb 12.8 g/dL	AST 98 IU/L	HBsAg (+)
K 4.0 mEq/L	Hct 40.3%	ALT 109 IU/L	Anti-HBs (–)
Cl 102 mEq/L	Plt 273 × 10^3/mm^3	Alk Phos 76 IU/L	HBeAg (+)
CO$_2$ 23 mEq/L	WBC 5.6 × 10^3/mm^3	T. bili 0.8 mg/dL	HBV DNA 120,432,871
BUN 13 mg/dL	TSH 1.61 μIU/mL	PT 10.8 sec	copies/mL
SCr 1.3 mg/dL	Total chol 163	Alb 3.9 g/dL	Anti-HCV (–)
Glu (non-fasting)	mg/dL		Anti-HIV (–)
113 mg/dL	Trigly 82 mg/dL		

■ Other Tests

Liver biopsy 1 week later: Active disease with moderate portal infiltrate and mild to moderate piecemeal necrosis, grade 3, with minimal evidence of cirrhosis, stage 1 fibrosis.

Abdominal CT scan: There is a tiny subcapsular enhancement in the anterior segment of the right lobe of the liver near the dome. There are no other enhancing lesions, and the spleen is normal size. There are small cysts in the right kidney, and gallstones are present with non-obstructing nephrolithiasis.

■ Assessment

Elevated hepatic enzymes with positive HBV serologies and liver biopsy consistent with chronic active hepatitis B without cirrhosis.

QUESTIONS

Problem Identification

1.a. Create a list of this patient's drug therapy problems.

1.b. In addition to the liver biopsy results, which clinical findings, laboratory values, and items in the medical history suggest the presence of chronic hepatitis B virus (HBV) infection?

Desired Outcome

2. What are the goals of treatment for chronic active HBV infection?

Therapeutic Alternatives

3.a. What nonpharmacologic measures should be considered for this patient?

3.b. What pharmacotherapeutic alternatives are available for treatment of this patient?

Optimal Plan

4. What drug, dose, dosage form, schedule, and duration of therapy should be recommended?

Outcome Evaluation

5.a. How should the therapy you recommended be monitored for efficacy and adverse effects?

5.b. Which baseline parameters suggest that this patient may have a favorable response to treatment (i.e., sustained loss of HBeAg and HBV DNA)?

Patient Education

6. What information should be provided to this patient regarding the treatment?

■ CLINICAL COURSE

The patient tolerated the initial therapy very well with minimal adverse effects. After 12 months of treatment, her physician stopped the therapy. However, 3 months post-treatment, her serum HBV DNA was detectable. Her lab results for the last few months of treatment were as follows:

Test	6 Months After Therapy Started	3 Months after Therapy Discontinued
AST	42 IU/L	55 IU/L
ALT	31 IU/L	84 IU/L
Alk phos	71 IU/L	73 IU/L
T. bili	0.9 mg/dL	0.8 mg/dL
PT	10.3 sec	10.1 sec
Alb	4.2 g/dL	4.2 g/dL
HbsAg	(+)	(+)
Anti-HBs	(−)	(−)
HBeAg	(+)	(+)
HBeAb	(−)	(−)
HBV DNA	0 copies/mL	552,411 copies/mL

Follow-Up Questions

1. Based on these results, what changes in therapy would you recommend? Include the drug name, dose, dosage form, schedule, and duration of therapy.

2. What adverse effects may occur with this new therapy, and how would you monitor for them?

3. What information should be provided to this patient about the new treatment?

■ CLINICAL COURSE

Ms. Smith's 18-year-old daughter, Mandy, just gave birth 2 hours ago to a baby girl weighing 5 pounds and 9 ounces. Mandy's HBsAg status is negative.

Follow-Up Questions (continued)

4. For the hepatitis B vaccines currently available, outline treatment regimens for each age category that include number of doses, dosage schedule, and dose in micrograms.

5. Would you recommend hepatitis B vaccination to Ms. Smith's daughter, Mandy, and the infant? If yes, include the doses, dosage schedule, and doses in micrograms for Mandy and the baby.

■ SELF-STUDY ASSIGNMENTS

1. Describe the ideal hepatitis B candidate to respond to entecavir therapy and what you would monitor for therapeutic efficacy and adverse effects.

2. Compare and contrast the mechanism of action, immunogenicity rate, and adverse effects of the two available hepatitis B vaccines.

3. Survey several pharmacies to estimate the approximate retail cost of adefovir dipivoxil, lamivudine, entecavir, telbivudine, pegylated interferon, and interferon therapy for the treatment of hepatitis B.

4. Review the time course of serologic markers after acute hepatitis B virus infection and explain their significance to one of your peers (Fig. 46-1).

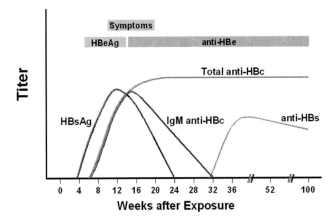

FIGURE 46-1. Typical serologic course of acute hepatitis B virus infection with recovery. *Note:* Serologic markers of infection vary depending on whether the infection is acute or chronic. *(Source: National Center for Infectious Diseases: Hepatitis B Virus. http://www.cdc.gov/ncidod/diseases/hepatitis/slideset/hep_b/slide_3.htm. Accessed March 29, 2008.)*

CLINICAL PEARL

To eliminate HBV transmission that occurs during infancy and childhood, the Immunization Practices Advisory Committee of the Centers of Disease Control and Prevention recommends that all newborn infants be vaccinated regardless of the hepatitis B status of the mothers.[3,4]

REFERENCES

1. Lok AS, McMahon BJ. Practice Guidelines Committee, American Association for the Study of Liver Diseases. Chronic hepatitis B: update of recommendations. Hepatology 2004;39:857–861.

2. Keeffe EB, Dieterich DT, Han SH, et al. A treatment algorithm for the management of chronic hepatitis B virus infection in the United States: an update. Clin Gastroenterol Hepatol 2006;4:936–962.

3. Centers for Disease Control and Prevention. Hepatitis virus B: a comprehensive immunization strategy to eliminate transmission of hepatitis B virus infection in the United States: recommendations of the Advisory Committee on Immunization Practices (ACIP) part 1: immunization of infants, children, and adolescents. MMWR Morb Mortal Wkly Rep 2005;54(RR16):1–31.

4. Centers for Disease Control and Prevention. Hepatitis virus B: a comprehensive immunization strategy to eliminate transmission of hepatitis B virus infection in the United States: recommendations of the Advisory Committee on Immunization Practices (ACIP) part II: immunization of adults. MMWR Morb Mortal Wkly Rep 2006;55(RR16):1–33.

5. Marcellin P, Chang TT, Lim SG, et al. Adefovir dipivoxil for the treatment of hepatitis B e antigen-positive chronic hepatitis B. N Engl J Med 2003;348:808–816.

6. Jones R, Nelson M. Novel anti-hepatitis B agents: a focus on telbivudine. Int J Clin Pract 2006;60:1295–1299.

7. Standring DN, Seifer M, Patty A, et al. HBV resistance determination from the telbivudine GLOBE registration trial. Presented at the 41st Annual Meeting of the European Association for the Study of Liver Diseases; Poster 514, April 26–30, 2006, Vienna, Austria.

8. ter Borg MJ, van Zonneveld M, Zeuzem S, et al. Patterns of viral decline during PEG-interferon alpha-2b therapy in HBeAg-positive chronic hepatitis B: relation to treatment response. Hepatology 2006;44:721–727.

9. Lau GK, Piratvisuth T, Luo KX, et al. Peginterferon Alfa-2a, lamivudine, and the combination for HBeAg-positive chronic hepatitis B. N Engl J Med 2005;352:2682–2695.

47

VIRAL HEPATITIS C

From Fibrosis to Cirrhosis . . . . Level I

Randolph E. Regal, BS, PharmD

LEARNING OBJECTIVES

After completing this case study, students should be able to:

- Develop a treatment plan for patients with chronic hepatitis C.

- Evaluate the clinical and laboratory endpoints for treatment of chronic hepatitis C.

- Develop a plan for monitoring efficacy and adverse effects of pharmacologic management of chronic hepatitis C.

- Provide patient education for patients with chronic hepatitis C regarding their medications.

PATIENT PRESENTATION

■ Chief Complaint

"My family doctor told me that my liver function tests were abnormal. I've been a little more tired than usual, but I thought that was because of menopause. I've also been retaining more fluid in my legs, been dizzy and lightheaded at times, and having more head-aches than I did last year. I've lost some weight lately, too, but that's good, isn't it?"

■ HPI

Linda Lane is a 49-year-old woman who has been referred by her family physician to the liver clinic for assessment of her abnormal liver enzymes. She reports remote use of recreational drugs in high school, including marijuana, alcohol, occasional ampheta-mines, and IV cocaine. She still drinks alcohol occasionally (2–4 glasses of wine once or twice a week), but otherwise has been "drug free" since her mid-twenties when she was married. She states that she feels fine much of the time, but sometimes has fatigue, fluid retention, headaches, and difficulty sleeping. She tends to get dizzy on exertion at times. She has lost about 10 pounds in the last 2 months, which she attributes to reduced appetite, since her activity level has diminished. She is perimeno-pausal and has isolated episodes of hot flashes and flushes but still menstruates on a regular 25-day cycle. She has no past history of liver problems.

■ PMH

IV drug abuse in high school
HTN
GERD
Early menopause

■ FH

No known family history of liver disease. Both parents are alive, still living independently, and doing reasonably well considering they are in their early 80's. Her father has HTN, her mother has hypothyroidism and a chronic "bathroom problem." One older brother with DM Type 2, HTN, and GERD.

■ SH

Married for 24 years; two children in college. Non-smoker; denies illicit drug or inhalant use; drinks two to four glasses of wine once or twice weekly.

■ ROS

Denies any signs or symptoms of liver diseases except for non-specific constitutional symptoms such as fatigue and headaches. No changes in urine color. Recalls having icteric sclerae and a period of severe fatigue and nausea in high school, which she had thought to be "mono."

■ Meds

MVI 1 tablet po daily × 1 year
Calcium citrate with vitamin D 1 tablet po BID × 1 year
Protonix 40 mg po once daily × 2 years
Norvasc 10 mg po once daily × 5 years
Acetaminophen 500 mg 1–2 tablets up to 3 times daily PRN for headaches and other body aches (averages 3–4 tablets per day)

■ All

No known drug or food allergies

■ Physical Examination

Gen

Well-nourished woman in NAD

VS

BP 100/63, P 72, RR 17, T 37.0°C; Wt 61 kg, Ht 5'4"

Skin

No jaundice; no spider angiomata or palmar erythema

HEENT

PERRLA; EOMI; sclerae anicteric; funduscopic exam normal; TMs intact

Neck/Lymph Nodes

Neck supple; no lymphadenopathy or thyromegaly; no carotid bruits

Lungs

Normal breath sounds

CV

RRR, S_1, S_2 normal; no S_3 or S_4

Abd

Liver span 11 cm; spleen not palpable; no evidence of ascites

MS/Ext

+1 edema in LE bilaterally; peripheral pulses 2+ throughout; nor-mal ROM

Neuro

A & O × 3; CN II–XII intact; DTRs 2+

Labs

Obtained 1 week ago from patient's PCP:

Na 140 mEq/L	Hgb 13.0 g/dL	AST 177 IU/L	HbsAg (–)
K 4.0 mEq/L	Hct 39.3 %	ALT 198 IU/L	Anti-HAV (–)
Cl 100 mEq/L	Plt 220 × 10^3/mm^3	Alk phos 86 IU/L	Anti-HCV (+)
CO_2 28 mEq/L	WBC 6.7 × 10^3/mm^3	T. bili 1.5 mg/dL	HCV RNA (bDNA assay)
BUN 11 mg/dL	67% PMNS	Alb 3.5 g/dL	4.4 million copies/mL
SCr 1.0 mg/dL	3% Bands	PT 12.3 sec	HCV genotype 1
Glu 111 mg/dL	20% Lymphs	ANA (–)	HIV (–)
TSH 2.32 μIU/	10% Monos	Serum iron: 45	Ferritin: 83 ng/mL
mL		mcg/dL	TIBC: 334 mcg/dL
			T. Sat. 13.5%

Liver Biopsy (Performed after Liver Clinic Visit)

Moderate degree of fibrosis and inflammation consistent with chronic hepatitis

Diagnosis

Chronic hepatitis C

QUESTIONS

Problem Identification

1.a. Create a list of the patient's drug therapy problems.

1.b. What physical findings, laboratory values, and medical history information suggest the presence of chronic hepatitis C virus (HCV) infection?

Desired Outcome

2. What are the goals of treatment for chronic HCV infection?

Therapeutic Alternatives

3.a. What nonpharmacologic measures should be considered for this patient?

3.b. What pharmacotherapeutic alternatives are available for treatment of this patient?

3.c. Does this patient have any medical conditions that are considered contraindications to receiving the treatments discussed in the previous question?

Optimal Plan

4.a. Design a pharmacotherapeutic plan for this patient. Include the drug, dose, schedule, and duration of therapy.

4.b. With respect to the patient's other drug therapy, are there any drug related interventions that need to be made other than acetaminophen use?

Outcome Evaluation

5.a. How should the therapy you recommended for HCV infection be monitored for efficacy and adverse effects?

5.b. Which baseline parameters of this patient have been suggested as predictors of poor response to the treatment you recommended?

5.c. What actions can be taken if the patient develops intolerable adverse effects to the treatment you recommended?

Patient Education

6. What information should be provided to this patient regarding her treatment?

■ CLINICAL COURSE

At her 12-week visit, she reports feeling about the same overall, with her AST and ALT still around 150 IU/L, but her HCV RNA value is now at less than 20,000 copies/mL. The chills and muscle aches that plagued her during the first few weeks of therapy have abated. She is beginning to exercise a bit more, taking her regular "power walks" with her neighbors as well as doing more outside work. Other labs are similar with the exception of hemoglobin 11.4 g/dL, WBC 4.5 × 10^3/mm^3, and platelets 180 × 10^3/mm^3.

Follow-Up Questions

1. Based on this information, should the therapy continue as planned? Why or why not?

2. What likely caused her "flu-like" symptoms early in therapy?

3. What is the likely cause of her anemia?

4. What other laboratory tests should be obtained to better monitor her drug therapy tolerance?

■ CLINICAL COURSE

At her 24-week visit, she is feeling much better, although she has noticed a bit more fatigue on exertion (when cutting the grass or taking "power walks" with her neighbors). Laboratory tests include: AST 90 IU/L, ALT 100 IU/L, qualitative HCV RNA test (–), hemoglobin 10.5 g/dL, WBC 4.2 × 10^3/mm^3 (ANC ~3.0 × 10^3/mm^3), and platelets 150 × 10^3/mm^3.

Follow-Up Questions (continued)

5. Based on this new information, what changes would you recommend for the treatment of chronic hepatitis C for this patient, and for how long?

6. Outline a plan for vaccination of this patient against other forms of viral hepatitis.

■ SELF-STUDY ASSIGNMENTS

1. Estimate the cost of a 12-month course of interferon and ribavirin treatment for chronic hepatitis C. Include the cost of syringes and needles, monthly clinic visits, and laboratory tests.

2. Perform a literature search to compare the differences in pharmacokinetic properties and tolerance between interferon and peginterferon.

3. Perform a literature search on efforts to develop a vaccine for hepatitis C.

CLINICAL PEARL

The course of chronic hepatitis C infection and treatment response can be adversely affected by alcohol consumption. Patients should be advised to stop all alcohol ingestion.

REFERENCES

1. Manns MP, McHutchinson JG, Gordon SC, et al. Peginterferon alfa-2b plus ribavirin compared with interferon alfa-2b plus ribavirin for initial treatment of chronic hepatitis C: a randomised trial. Lancet 2001;358:958–965.

2. Fried MW, Shiffman ML, Reddy KR, et al. Peginterferon alfa-2a plus ribavirin for chronic hepatitis C virus infection. N Engl J Med 2002;347:975–982.

3. Pawlotsky JM, Bouvier-Alias M, Hezode C, et al. Standardization of hepatitis C virus RNA quantification. Hepatology 2000;32:654–659.

4. National Institutes of Health Consensus Development Conference Statement: management of hepatitis C: 2002—June 10–12, 2002. Hepatology 2002;36(5 Suppl 1):S3–S20.

48

DRUG-INDUCED ACUTE KIDNEY INJURY

Not a Cute Consequence.................. Level II

Mary K. Stamatakis, PharmD

LEARNING OBJECTIVES

After completing this case study, students should be able to:

- Evaluate clinical and laboratory findings in a patient with acute kidney injury (AKI).

- Select pharmacotherapy for treatment of complications associated with AKI.

- Assess appropriateness of aminoglycoside serum concentrations in relation to efficacy and toxicity.

- Develop strategies to prevent drug-induced AKI, including the selection of pharmacologic alternatives that do not adverse affect kidney function.

- Adjust drug dosages based on a patient's estimated kidney function to maximize efficacy and minimize adverse events.

PATIENT PRESENTATION

Chief Complaint
Not available.

HPI

Martin James is a 73-year-old man who originally presented to the hospital with symptoms of heart failure that culminated in aortic and mitral valve replacement surgery. His surgery was complicated by a 1-hour hypotensive episode, with BP as low as 70/50. Three days post-operation, purulent drainage was noted from the surgical site, and he was subsequently diagnosed with mediastinitis. At that time, the patient was also found to have a *Serratia* bacteremia (blood cultures × 4 positive for *Serratia marcescens*, sensitive to gentamicin, piperacillin, ceftazidime, and ciprofloxacin; resistance was noted to ampicillin). Therapy was initiated with gentamicin and piperacillin. Thus far, he has completed day 25 of a 6-week course of antibiotics. A gradual increase in his BUN and serum creatinine concentration from baseline and signs of volume overload have been noted over the past 7 days (see Table 48-1).

PMH
Type 1 DM
CKD
Gout
Osteoarthritis
HTN
Atrial fibrillation

PSH
Aortic and mitral valve replacement surgery 28 days ago

FH
Father had Type 1 DM

SH
Denies smoking or alcohol; retired coal miner (11 years ago)

Current Meds
Gentamicin 180 mg IVPB Q 48 h (See Table 48-1 for previous dosages)
Ceftazidime 1 g IVPB Q 12 h × 25 days
Enalapril 5 mg po once daily
Colace 100 mg po BID
Furosemide 80 mg po Q 12 h × 2 days
Digoxin 0.25 mg po once daily
Allopurinol 100 mg po once daily
Ranitidine 150 mg po Q 12 h
Meperidine 25 mg IM Q 4–6 h PRN pain (started 3 days ago)
Ibuprofen 400 mg po Q 4–6 h PRN pain (started today for joint pain)
Sliding scale insulin

All
Bactrim (experienced rash about 10 years ago; subsided when drug discontinued)

ROS
Currently complains of trouble breathing, weakness, general malaise, and pain in joints in hands. No fever or chills.

Physical Examination
Gen
Confused-appearing man in mild distress

VS
BP 152/90, P 80, RR 26, T 37.7°C; Current Wt 87 kg (admission Wt 73 kg), Ht 5'10"

Skin
Normal skin turgor

TABLE 48-1 Serum Creatinine, BUN, and Serum Gentamicin Concentrations during Hospitalization

Postop Day	SCr (mg/dL)	BUN (mg/dL)	Gentamicin (mcg/mL) Peak[a]	Gentamicin (mcg/mL) Trough[b]	Gentamicin Dosages
3	1.4	15			160 mg × 1, then 120 mg Q 12 h
5	1.2	22	4.2	1.1	Change to 160 mg Q 12 h
7	1.4	21			
10	1.4	22	8.1	2.3	Change to 240 mg Q 24 h
14	1.2	21			
17	1.4	26	9.4	1.3	Change to 180 mg Q 24 h
21	1.7	27			
24	2.4	38	7.4	2.6	Change to 180 mg Q 48 h
26	2.9	44			
28	3.2	52			

BUN, blood urea nitrogen; SCr, serum creatinine.
[a]Serum drug concentrations drawn 30 minutes after a 30-minute infusion.
[b]Serum drug concentrations drawn immediately before a dose.

HEENT

PERRLA, EOMI, poor dentition

Neck/Lymph Nodes

(+) JVD

Chest

Basilar crackles, inspiratory wheezes

CV

S_1, S_2 normal, no S_3, irregular rhythm

Abd

Soft, nontender, (+) BS, (−) HSM

Genit/Rect

(−) Masses

MS/Ext

2+ Ankle/sacral edema

Neuro

A & O to person and place, but not to time

■ Labs (Current)

Na 138 mEq/L	Hgb 9.2 g/dL	Ca 8.5 mg/dL
K 3.9 mEq/L	Hct 28.5%	Mg 2.0 mg/dL
Cl 104 mEq/L	Plt 263 × 10³/mm³	Phos 4.7 mg/dL
CO_2 25 mEq/L	WBC 9.9 × 10³/mm³	
BUN 52 mg/dL	(BUN 17 mg/dL on admission)	
SCr 3.2 mg/dL	(SCr 1.3 mg/dL on admission)	
Glu 130 mg/dL		

■ UA

Color, yellow; character, hazy; glucose (−); ketones (−); SG 1.010; pH 5.0; protein 30 mg/dL; coarse granular casts 5–10/lpf; WBC 0–3/hpf; RBC 0–2/hpf; no bacteria; nitrite (−); osmolality 325 mOsm; urinary sodium 45 mEq/L; creatinine 33 mg/dL, FENA = 3.2%.

■ Repeat Blood Cultures Today

Negative.

■ Fluid Intake/Output and Daily Weights

Day	I/O	Wt (kg)
3 days ago	3,200 mL/1,100 mL	N/A
2 days ago	2,500 mL/1,050 mL	76
Yesterday	2,500 mL/1,250 mL	N/A
Today	N/A	80

■ Assessment

Acute kidney injury with extracellular fluid expansion

QUESTIONS

Problem Identification

1.a. Create a list of the patient's drug therapy problems.

1.b. What information (signs, symptoms, laboratory values) indicates the presence or severity of the patient's problem(s)?

1.c. Based on the patient's estimated creatinine clearance and clinical presentation, do any of his medications require dosage adjustment? If so, what adjustment would you recommend?

1.d. What additional laboratory information would assist in the assessment of this patient?

1.e. When assessing fractional excretion of sodium (FE_{NA}), what influence do previous dosages of furosemide have on interpretation of the results?

1.f. Could any of the patient's problems have been caused by drug therapy?

1.g. What risk factors did the patient have for gentamicin-induced acute kidney injury?

1.h. What therapeutic interventions could have been initiated to decrease the likelihood of developing drug-induced acute kidney injury?

Desired Outcome

2. What are the goals of pharmacotherapy in this case?

Therapeutic Alternatives

3.a. What nondrug therapies might be useful for this patient?

3.b. What feasible pharmacotherapeutic alternatives are available for treating acute kidney injury in this patient?

Optimal Plan

4. What drugs, dosage forms, doses, schedules, and duration of therapy are best for this patient?

Outcome Evaluation

5. What clinical and laboratory parameters are necessary to evaluate therapy for achievement of the desired therapeutic outcomes and to detect or prevent adverse effects?

Patient Education

6. What information should be provided to the patient to enhance compliance, ensure successful therapy, and minimize adverse effects?

CLINICAL PEARL

Equations to estimate creatinine clearance that incorporate a single creatinine concentration (e.g., the Cockcroft-Gault equation) may underestimate or overestimate kidney function, depending on whether renal function is improving or worsening.

■ SELF-STUDY ASSIGNMENTS

1. Review the literature to determine whether once-daily dosing of aminoglycosides (i.e., large dose-extended interval dosing method) may decrease the incidence of nephrotoxicity, and if this approach should have been initially recommended in this patient.

2. Recommend an appropriate dosage of digoxin for this patient given a trough digoxin concentration of 2.7 ng/mL.

3. Now that Mr. James has completed 25 days of antibiotics to treat *S. marcescens* in the blood, should single or double antibiotic coverage be recommended for the remainder of his 6-week course of therapy? Provide the rationale for your recommendation.

4. Mr. Jones' serum creatinine is 1.4 mg/dL at 1 month after discharge. At what point would you consider restarting the ACE inhibitor? Justify the use of ACE inhibitors in patients with chronic kidney disease.

REFERENCES

1. Bellomo R, Ronco C, Kellum JA, et al. Acute renal failure—definition, outcome measures, animal models, fluid therapy and information technology needed: the Second International Consensus Conference of the Acute Dialysis Quality Initiative (ADQI) Group. Crit Care 2004;8:R204–R212.
2. Jelliffe R. Estimation of creatinine clearance in patients with unstable renal function, without a urine specimen. Am J Nephrol 2002;22:320–324.
3. Triggs E, Charles B. Pharmacokinetics and therapeutic drug monitoring of gentamicin in the elderly. Clin Pharmacokinet 1999;37:331–341.
4. Schetz M. Diuretics in acute renal failure? Contrib Nephrol 2004;144:166–181.
5. Friedrich JO, Adhikari N, Herridge MS, et al. Meta-analysis: low-dose dopamine increases urine output but does not prevent renal dysfunction or death. Ann Intern Med 2005;142:510–524.

49

ACUTE KIDNEY INJURY

The Kidney Has Left the Building. . . . . Level II

Scott Bolesta, PharmD

Reina Bendayan, PharmD

LEARNING OBJECTIVES

After completing this case study, the reader should be able to:

• Assess a patient with acute kidney injury (AKI) using clinical and laboratory data.

• Classify the extent of AKI in a patient.

• Distinguish between AKI resulting from prerenal and intrinsic injury.

• Recommend changes to the pharmacotherapeutic regimen of a patient with AKI.

• Justify appropriate therapeutic interventions for a patient with AKI.

PATIENT PRESENTATION

■ Chief Complaint

"I feel really weak."

■ HPI

Everit Mitchell is a 72-year-old man who presents to the ED with complaints of severe weakness that started this morning. He was feeling normal until last night when he felt more tired than usual and went to bed early. Since waking this morning, he has not had the energy to eat or perform his normal ADLs. His wife brought him to the ED because his physician is away on vacation.

■ PMH

HTN × 25 years
CHF × 8 years
PUD (recently diagnosed)

■ FH

Father died of an acute MI; mother was diabetic

■ SH

Retired and living at home with his wife. Before retirement, the patient was employed as an accountant. No alcohol, no tobacco use.

■ Meds

Furosemide 40 mg po once daily
Metoprolol succinate 50 mg po once daily
Enalapril 20 mg po once daily
Famotidine 20 mg po BID

■ All

NKA

■ ROS

Patient complains of feeling cold but denies chills or fever. No changes in vision. Denies SOB, CP, and cough. Complains of vertigo. Has been having frequent black diarrhea over the last 2 days, but denies abdominal pain. Has noted a decrease in the frequency of urination over the last 24 hours. Denies musculoskeletal pain or cramping.

■ Physical Examination

Gen

Pale, elderly Caucasian man who appears generally weak and lethargic

VS

BP 96/48 (82/37 on standing), P 105, RR 26, T 37.1°C; Wt 78 kg, Ht 5'9"

Skin

Pale and cold with poor turgor

HEENT

PERRLA; EOMI; Fundi normal; conjunctivae pale and dry; TMs intact; tongue and mouth dry

Neck/Lymph Nodes

No JVD or HJR; no lymphadenopathy or thyromegaly

Lungs

No crackles or rhonchi

CV

Tachycardic with regular rhythm; normal S_1, S_2; no S_3; faint S_4; no MRG

Abd

Soft, NT/ND; No HSM; hyperactive BS

Genit/Rect

Stool heme (+); slightly enlarged prostate

MS/Ext

Weak pulses; no peripheral edema

Neuro

A & O × 3; CNs intact; DTRs 2+; Babinski (–)

■ Labs

Na 139 mEq/L	Ca 8.6 mg/dL
K 5.3 mEq/L	Mg 2.1 mg/dL
Cl 103 mEq/L	Phos 4.3 mg/dL
CO_2 21 mEq/L	WBC $11.3 \times 10^3/mm^3$
BUN 48 mg/dL	Hgb 9.1 g/dL
SCr 1.8 mg/dL	Hct 27.3%
Glu 113 mg/dL	Plt $128 \times 10^3/mm^3$

■ Assessment

72-year-old man with a suspected acute UGI bleed, possibly related to PUD, that has resulted in anemia and AKI from hypovolemia.

QUESTIONS

Problem Identification

1.a. Create a list of the patient's drug therapy problems as they relate to his acute kidney injury (AKI).

1.b. What information (signs, symptoms, laboratory values) indicates the presence or severity of hypovolemia and AKI in this patient?

Desired Outcome

2. What are the goals of therapy in this case?

■ CLINICAL COURSE

Upon admission, the patient was resuscitated aggressively with IV normal saline and multiple transfusions (4 units of PRBCs). His home medications were held, and he underwent an emergent EGD. During endoscopy, a large ulcer in the gastric antrum was found with an oozing vessel at the base. Endoscopic therapy was unsuccessful, and the patient was taken to the OR for surgical intervention. He was hypotensive in the OR (BP 70 mm Hg systolic on average) and was started on a norepinephrine infusion to maintain a stable BP. Postoperatively his urine output was <100 mL total over the first 12 postoperative hours despite continued aggressive IV hydration and repeated transfusions in the OR. He also remained on norepinephrine for a continued low BP. On the morning of postoperative day 1, his labs were as follows:

Na 132 mEq/L	Ca 8.2 mg/dL
K 4.9 mEq/L	Mg 2.2 mg/dL
Cl 98 mEq/L	Phos 4.7 mg/dL
CO_2 19 mEq/L	WBC $14.6 \times 10^3/mm^3$
BUN 39 mg/dL	Hgb 10.3 g/dL
SCr 2.5 mg/dL	Hct 29.8%
Glu 145 mg/dL	Plt $112 \times 10^3/mm^3$

Urinalysis also showed muddy brown casts, a urine sodium of 72 mEq/L, and specific gravity of 1.004. A diagnosis of ATN was made, and the patient was started on furosemide 80 mg IV Q 8 h. On postoperative day 2, the patient remained on norepinephrine, his urine output had not improved, and his chest radiograph showed diffuse bilateral pulmonary edema with a decrease in O_2 saturation to 86%. A femoral vein catheter was inserted and continuous venovenous hemodiafiltration (CVVH-DF) was started. On postoperative day 5, his heart failure had resolved, and the catheter was removed. His subsequent hospital course was uneventful, and his kidney function gradually improved.

Therapeutic Alternatives

3.a. What nondrug therapies were used to manage this patient's AKI? Discuss the evidence that supports their use.

3.b. What pharmacotherapeutic alternatives have been studied for the treatment of AKI?

Optimal Plan

4. Design an optimal therapeutic plan for managing this patient's AKI postoperatively.

Outcome Evaluation

5. What clinical and laboratory parameters are necessary to evaluate the therapy for achievement of the desired therapeutic outcome and to detect or prevent adverse effects?

Patient Education

6. What information should be provided to the patient to help avoid future episodes of AKI?

CLINICAL PEARL

A decrease in BUN and serum electrolytes can transiently occur during treatment of patients with AKI. This is usually due to a dilutional effect in the setting of acute hypervolemia and does not reflect an improvement in kidney function.

■ SELF-STUDY ASSIGNMENTS

1. Produce a chart that displays the RIFLE criteria (**R**isk of renal dysfunction, **I**njury to the kidney, **F**ailure of kidney function, **L**oss of kidney function, and **E**nd-stage kidney disease) in a logically organized fashion.

2. Write a brief paper that discusses the pharmacotherapeutic interventions that have been studied for the prevention of AKI from causes other than IV contrast agents.

REFERENCES

1. Lameire N, Van Biesen W, Vanholder R. Acute renal failure. Lancet 2005;365:417–430.

2. Gill N, Nally JV Jr, Fatica RA. Renal failure secondary to acute tubular necrosis: epidemiology, diagnosis, and management. Chest 2005;128: 2847–2863.

3. Mehta RL, Pascual MT, Soroko S, et al. Diuretics, mortality, and nonrecovery of renal function in acute renal failure. JAMA 2002;288: 2547–2553.

4. Uchino S, Doig GS, Bellomo R, et al. Diuretics and mortality in acute renal failure. Crit Care Med 2004;32:1669–1677.

5. Ho KM, Sheridan DJ. Meta-analysis of furosemide to prevent or treat acute renal failure. BMJ 2006 August 26;333(7565):420. Epub 2006 July 21.

6. Kellum JA, M Decker J. Use of dopamine in acute renal failure: a meta-analysis. Crit Care Med 2001;29:1526–1531.

7. Friedrich JO, Adhikari N, Herridge MS, et al. Meta-analysis: low-dose dopamine increases urine output but does not prevent renal dysfunction or death. Ann Intern Med 2005;142:510–524.

50

PROGRESSIVE RENAL DISEASE

Not to Make Matters Worse . . . . Level III

Michelle D. Furler, BSc Pharm, PhD

Reina Bendayan, PharmD

LEARNING OBJECTIVES

After completing this case study, students should be able to:

- Differentiate acute renal failure from chronic renal failure.

- Identify risk factors for progression of renal disease.

- Recognize potential comorbid or pathologic conditions that are frequently associated with chronic renal insufficiency.

- Recommend nonpharmacologic and pharmacologic interventions to alter the rate of progression of renal disease.

- Educate patients about the common medications prescribed for chronic renal insufficiency.

- Provide recommendations for renal disease therapy during pregnancy.

PATIENT PRESENTATION

▪ Chief Complaint

"I'm here to check the results of my urine test."

▪ HPI

Robin Morales is a 37-year-old woman with diabetes mellitus who visited her PCP 1 week ago for a routine physical examination. Her laboratory tests revealed a serum creatinine of 1.4 mg/dL and spot urine albumin-to-creatinine ratio (ACR) of >300 mg albumin per gram of creatinine. These values were elevated over her baseline of SCr 1.1 mg/dL and ACR 210 mg/g 1 year ago. A 24-hour urine collection was performed last week, and she was scheduled to return to clinic today for further evaluation of her kidney function. She states that she has not been checking her blood glucose at home because her machine is not working and she has difficulty getting blood. However, she asserts that she has been taking most of her medications faithfully and has recently quit smoking. The patient says that she has been trying to lose weight in the last few weeks; she has occasional dizziness and weakness that usually resolve if she skips her blood pressure medicine for a few days.

▪ PMH

Type 2 DM × 10 years
HTN × 4 years
Hypercholesterolemia × 5 years (previously noncompliant with diet)

▪ FH

Father had DM and died in an MVA 3 years ago at age 64; mother had HTN and died at age 50 secondary to MI.

▪ SH

She is a public school teacher, recently married with no children. No tobacco use but occasional alcohol (2 or 3 glasses of wine or beer on weekends or when out with friends). Previous diet included eggs and bacon for breakfast, chicken sandwiches for lunch, and pasta and salad for dinner with snacks mid-afternoon and in the evening (usually a couple diabetic treats or a muffin). Recently, she and some friends from work have started a "low-carbohydrate diet" and have cut out all breads, pastas, and rice while increasing consumption of red meats and proteins. She consumes 4–5 cups of coffee per day to alleviate fatigue but indicates that because of the diet, she no longer snacks at work and eats three high-protein, low-carbohydrate meals per day according to the diet plan.

▪ ROS

Occasional headaches, generally associated with menstruation; no c/o polyuria, polydipsia, polyphagia, sensory loss, or visual changes. No dysuria, flank pain, hematuria, pedal edema, chest pain, or SOB. Occasional dizziness, weakness, and mild diaphoresis during mid-afternoon.

▪ Meds

Metformin 1,000 mg po TID × 8 years
Glyburide 10 mg po BID × 6 years
Hydrochlorothiazide 25 mg po once daily × 2 years
Pravastatin 40 mg po once daily × $1^{1}/_{2}$ years; on current dose for 1 year
Acetaminophen 650 mg po Q 6 h PRN headaches
Oral contraceptive × 20 years; currently using Ortho Tri-Cyclen
Ferrous sulfate 300 mg po BID × 1 year; recently discontinued by patient due to constipation
Multivitamin po once daily

▪ All

Sulfa (anaphylaxis), macrolides (rash)

▪ Physical Examination

Gen

The patient is an obese Hispanic woman in NAD

VS

BP 156/94 sitting and standing in both arms, HR 76, RR 18, T 37.9°C; Wt 82.5 kg, Ht 5'2"

Skin

Warm, dry

HEENT

PERRLA, EOMI, fundi have microaneurysms consistent with diabetic retinopathy; no retinal edema or vitreous hemorrhage. TMs intact. Oral mucosa moist with no lesions.

Neck/Lymph Nodes

Supple; no cervical adenopathy or thyromegaly

Lungs/Thorax

CTA

CV

Heart sounds are normal

Abd

NT; no masses or organs palpable. No abdominal bruits.

Genit/Rect

Normal rectal exam; heme (–) stool; recent Pap smear negative

MS/Ext

No CCE

Neuro

A & O × 3; CNs intact; normal DTRs

■ Labs (2 weeks ago, fasting)

Na 145 mEq/L	Hgb 10.6 g/dL	*Fasting Lipid Profile:*
K 4.9 mEq/L	Hct 36.5%	T. chol 226 mg/dL
Cl 106 mEq/L	WBC 10.8 × 10³/mm³	Trig 134 mg/dL
CO₂ 27 mEq/L	Plt 148 × 10³/mm³	LDL 150 mg/dL
BUN 28 mg/dL	Ca 9.4 mg/dL	HDL 47 mg/dL
SCr 1.4 mg/dL	Phos 2.6 mg/dL	
Glu 192 mg/dL	Uric acid 6.9 mg/dL	
A1C 9.6%	Alb 3.4 g/dL	

■ UA (1 week ago)

1+ glucose, (+) ketones, 3+ protein, (–) leukocyte esterase and nitrite; (–) RBC; 2–5 WBC/hpf

■ 24-Hour Urine Collection

Total urine volume 2.1 L, urine creatinine 62 mg/dL, urine albumin 687 mg/24 h

■ Assessment

37-year-old woman newly diagnosed with diabetic nephropathy complicated by inadequately controlled comorbid conditions.

QUESTIONS

Problem Identification

1.a. Create a list of the patient's drug therapy problems. What other clinical conditions require intervention?

1.b. What are the signs and symptoms of renal disease (diabetic nephropathy) and comorbid illnesses (e.g., diabetes mellitus, hypertension, and dyslipidemia) in this patient?

1.c. (i) Calculate this patient's creatinine clearance (CLcr in mL/min) using the following data: 1) baseline CLcr from 1 year ago; 2) current CLcr using the SCr from 2 weeks ago; and 3) current CLcr using the data from the 24-hour urine collection.

 (ii) Discuss whether the Cockcroft-Gault equation and data from a 24-hour urine collection provide good estimates of the patient's GFR.

 (iii) Discuss other methods to calculate GFR for this patient and comment on the accuracy of these alternate measures.

 (iv) What is the role of Cockcroft-Gault CLcr calculation if there are more accurate predictors of GFR?

1.d. What degree of renal failure is shown by this patient? Compare the definition, classification, and prognosis of chronic renal failure to acute renal failure.

Desired Outcome

2. What are the goals of pharmacotherapy for the patient's current clinical conditions? Focus on renal insufficiency, diabetes, hypertension, and hypercholesterolemia.

Therapeutic Alternatives

3.a. What nonpharmacologic therapies might be useful to control this patient's medical conditions?

3.b. What are the pharmacotherapeutic alternatives for preventing renal disease progression and managing this patient's diabetes mellitus, hypertension, and dyslipidemia?

Optimal Plan

4. What drug regimens would provide optimal therapy for this patient's current medical problems?

Outcome Evaluation

5. Outline the clinical and laboratory parameters necessary to evaluate the efficacy and safety of the recommended regimens for the patient's nephropathy, diabetes mellitus, hypertension, and dyslipidemia.

Patient Education

6. What information should be provided to the patient to ensure successful therapy and minimize adverse effects of the antihypertensive and insulin therapy?

■ CLINICAL COURSE

The plan you recommended is implemented, and the patient returns to her PCP 1 month later. Her blood pressure is 148/90 mm Hg (sitting and standing) and HR is 87 bpm. She has no new complaints and reports tolerating her new medications well. She also states that she is still watching her diet and has been using a new salt substitute in her meals for the last 5 days. She indicates that she is having more fruit as snacks when she gets hungry during the day and finds she particularly likes bananas. She indicates that she and her husband are thinking of trying to get pregnant and indicates she has discontinued her birth control pill. Her laboratory results are BUN 29 mg/dL, SCr 1.6 mg/dL, Na 142 mEq/L, K 5.4 mEq/L, Cl 110 mEq/L, CO₂ 28 mEq/L, Glu 135 mg/dL. A pregnancy test is negative.

■ FOLLOW-UP QUESTIONS

1. What new or persistent drug therapy problems does this patient have?

2. What changes, if any, would you recommend in the patient's drug regimen?

3. The patient has indicated a desire to get pregnant. Is she at increased risk for complications? What would you recommend and why?

■ SELF-STUDY ASSIGNMENTS

1. Discuss the role of diuretic therapy in patients with normal renal function compared to those with creatinine clearance values <20 mL/min.

2. Review and compare the effects of antihypertensive agents on renal blood flow and glomerular filtration rate in patients with hypertension and diabetic nephropathy.

CLINICAL PEARL

Normotensive patients with type 2 diabetes and persistent microalbuminuria should be treated with an ACE inhibitor to slow the progression of diabetic nephropathy. Effective treatment must be tailored to patient needs and modified according to changes in lifestyle.

CHAPTER 51

REFERENCES

1. National Kidney Foundation. K/DOQI clinical practice guidelines for chronic kidney disease: evaluation, classification, and stratification. Am J Kidney Dis 2002;39(2 Suppl 1):S1–S266.

2. Ibrahim H, Mondress M, Tello A, et al. An alternative formula to the Cockcroft-Gault and the modification of diet in renal diseases formulas in predicting GFR in individuals with type 1 diabetes. J Am Soc Nephrol 2005;16:1051–1060.

3. Salazar DE, Corcoran GB. Predicting creatinine clearance and renal drug clearance in obese patients from estimated fat-free body mass. Am J Med 1988;84:1053–1060.

4. National Kidney Foundation. KDOQI clinical practice guidelines and clinical practice recommendations for diabetes and chronic kidney disease. Am J Kidney Dis 2007;49(Suppl 2):S1–S180. www.kidney.org/professionals/kdoqi/guidelines.cfm.

5. Gross JL, de Azevedo MJ, Silveiro SP, et al. Diabetic nephropathy: diagnosis, prevention, and treatment. Diabetes Care 2005;28:164–176.

6. American Diabetes Association. Standards of medical care in diabetes—2007. Diabetes Care 2007;30:S4–S41.

7. Chobanian AV, Bakris GL, Black HR, et al. The Seventh Report of the Joint National Committee on Prevention, Detection, Evaluation, and Treatment of High Blood Pressure: the JNC 7 Report. JAMA 2003;289:2560–2572.

8. Kidney Disease Outcomes Quality Initiative (K/DOQI). K/DOQI clinical practice guidelines on hypertension and antihypertensive agents in chronic kidney disease. Am J Kidney Dis 2004;43(5 Suppl 1):S1–S290.

9. National Kidney Foundation. Clinical practice guidelines for managing dyslipidemias in chronic kidney disease. Am J Kidney Dis 2003;41(4 Suppl 3):S1–S91.

10. Franz MJ, Bantle JP, Beebe CA, et al; American Diabetes Association. Nutrition principles and recommendations in diabetes. Diabetes Care 2004;27(Suppl 1):S36–S46.

11. National Kidney Foundation. KDOQI clinical practice guidelines and clinical practice recommendations for anemia in chronic kidney disease [published erratum Am J Kidney Dis 2006 Sep;48(3):518]. Am J Kidney Dis 2006 May;47(5 Suppl 3):S1–S145.

12. Ramin SM, Vidaeff AC, Yeomans ER, et al. Chronic renal disease in pregnancy. Obstet Gynecol 2006;108:1531–1539. Erratum in: Obstet Gynecol 2007;109:788.

Note: All NKF K/DOQI clinical practice guidelines are available online at *www.kidney.org/professionals/kdoqi/guidelines.cfm.*

51

END-STAGE KIDNEY DISEASE

Urine Trouble. . . . . Level II

Edward F. Foote, PharmD, FCCP, BCPS

LEARNING OBJECTIVES

Upon completing this case study, students should be able to:

- Identify medication-related problems in a patient with end-stage kidney disease maintained on chronic hemodialysis.

- State the desired therapeutic outcomes of each problem.

- List therapeutic alternatives for managing each problem.

- Develop a plan for managing each problem that includes plans for monitoring patient response to interventions.

- Outline a plan for helping the patient understand and effectively implement medication-related interventions.

PATIENT PRESENTATION

▧ Chief Complaint

"I feel so tired lately, and my blood pressure keeps dropping after dialysis."

▧ HPI

John Woods is a 68-year-old man who presents to the outpatient dialysis center for his routine hemodialysis treatment. He has been on dialysis for 11 months. His kidney failure is thought to be secondary to longstanding hypertension. He is dialyzed via a left forearm AV fistula.

▧ PMH

Longstanding history of hypertension
Hyperlipidemia
ESRD secondary to hypertension

▧ FH

Father died of heart disease at age 80. Mother died of "old age." No siblings. Two sons in good health.

▧ SH

Shares home with wife who is his primary caretaker. Retired accountant. Occasional social alcohol use. Minimal caffeine consumption; no tobacco use.

▧ ROS

Negative except for dry, itchy skin; feeling tired and weak over the past several weeks. Some swelling in feet and lower legs. No other complaints related to central or peripheral nervous system or cardiovascular system. Wears glasses for reading and driving.

▧ Meds

Atenolol 50 mg po daily
Paxil 10 mg $^1/_2$ tablet po once daily
Glyburide 10 mg po daily
Calcium carbonate 1,000 mg elemental calcium po TID with meals
Epoetin alfa 5,000 units IV 3 times weekly with dialysis

▧ All

NKA

▧ Physical Examination

Gen

The patient is a WDWN African-American man in NAD who appears his stated age.

VS

BP 150/92 (predialysis), 130/75 (postdialysis), P 82, RR 16, T 36.8°C; Wt 70 kg, Ht 5'10"

Skin

Dry, scaly arms and legs noted

Ext

Mild bilateral foot and ankle edema
Remainder of the PE was WNL

■ Labs

Na 142 mEq/L	Hgb 10.3 g/dL	AST 16 IU/L	*Fasting Lipid Profile:*	Iron 90 mcg/dL
K 5.3 mEq/L	Hct 30%	ALT 21 IU/L	T. chol 228 mg/dL	TIBC 500 mcg/dL
Cl 110 mEq/L	RBC 3.41 × 10⁶/mm³	LDH 371 IU/L	HDL 33 mg/dL	TSAT 18%
CO₂ 24 mEq/L	MCV 81.7 μm³	Alk phos 124 IU/L	LDL 149 mg/dL	Ferritin 120 ng/mL
Anion gap 12	MCHC 33.4 g/dL	T. bili 0.5 mg/dL	Chol/HDL 6.9	PTH 900 pg/mL
BUN 80 mg/dL	WBC 6.9 × 10³/mm³	D. bili 0.3 mg/dL	Trig 229 mg/dL	A1C 6.5
SCr 6.2 mg/dL		Alb 3.0 g/dL	Ca 8.6 mg/dL	
Glu 85 mg/dL			Phos 6.4 mg/dL	

Mr. Woods' nephrologist provided the following dialysis prescription:

Dialyze 4 hours per session, three times per week (M, W, F morning shift)

Dry weight: 67.5 kg
Dialyzer: Fresenius F80
Blood flow rate: 400 mL/min
Dialysate flow rate: 500 mL/min
Dialysate: Bicarbonate
 Na 145 mEq/L, K 2.0 mEq/L, Ca 2.5 mEq/L, HCO₃ 35 mEq/L

Heparin: 2,000 unit bolus, then 500 units/h until 1 hour before termination

QUESTIONS

Problem Identification

1.a. Create a list of this patient's drug therapy problems.

1.b. What information (signs, symptoms, laboratory values) indicates the severity of this patient's end-stage kidney disease?

Desired Outcome

2. State the goal of pharmacotherapy for each problem identified.

Therapeutic Alternatives

3. What therapeutic options are available for each of this patient's drug therapy problems? Indicate the advantages and disadvantages of each option.

Optimal Plan

4. Which of the available therapeutic options identified in question 3 would you recommend for this patient? Provide a rationale for each recommendation. Include the name, dosage form, dose, schedule, and duration of therapy for any drugs recommended.

Outcome Evaluation

5. What clinical and laboratory parameters would you recommend to evaluate the desired and undesired consequences of each of your recommended interventions?

Patient Education

6. What information should be provided to the patient to enhance compliance, ensure successful therapy, and minimize adverse effects?

■ SELF-STUDY ASSIGNMENTS

1. Assume that Mr. Woods presents as above except that his serum ferritin is 272 ng/mL and TSAT is 33%. Develop a therapeutic plan, including a monitoring plan, to treat his anemia under this scenario.

2. Compare the content and cost of a variety of water-soluble vitamin supplements appropriate for use by ESRD patients. Select the product that you would recommend for use by your patients.

3. Assume that Mr. Woods develops Gram-positive bacteremia. Develop a therapeutic plan for the use of vancomycin in this patient, including a monitoring plan.

CLINICAL PEARL

One of the most important contributors to hyperparathyroidism and bone disease is an elevated phosphorous level. Patient education regarding appropriate diet and the use of dietary phosphate-binding agents is critical!

REFERENCES

1. National Kidney Foundation. K/DOQI clinical practice guidelines and clinical practice recommendations for anemia in chronic kidney disease. Am J Kidney Dis 2006;47:S11–S145.
2. National Kidney Foundation. K/DOQI clinical practice guidelines for bone metabolism and disease in chronic kidney disease. Am J Kidney Dis 2003;42(4 Suppl 3):S1–S201.
3. Henrich WL, Mailloux LU. Hypertension in dialysis patients. In: Rose BD, ed. UpToDate. Waltham, MA, UpToDate, 2007.
4. National Kidney Foundation. Clinical practice guidelines for managing dyslipidemias in chronic kidney disease. Am J Kidney Dis 2003;41(4 Suppl 3):S1–S91.
5. Wanner C, Krane V, Marz W, et al. Atorvastatin in patients with type 2 diabetes mellitus undergoing hemodialysis. N Engl J Med 2005;353:238–248.
6. National Kidney Foundation. KDOQ Clinical practice guidelines and clinical practice recommendations for diabetes and chronic kidney disease. Am J Kidney Dis 2007;49(Suppl 2):S1–S180.
7. Fosrenol (lanthanum carbonate) package insert. Shire US Inc.; 2005.
8. Sensipar (cinacalcet HCL) package insert. Amgen Inc.; 2004.
9. Lugon JR. Uremic pruritus: a review. Hemodial Int 2005;9:180–188.
Note: All NKF K/DOQI clinical practice guidelines are available online at *www.kidney.org/professionals/kdoqi/guidelines.cfm.*

52

SYNDROME OF INAPPROPRIATE ANTIDIURETIC HORMONE RELEASE

Disturbing Behavior . . . . Level I

Jane Gervasio, PharmD, BCNSP
Maria Tsoras, PharmD

LEARNING OBJECTIVES

After completing this case study, readers should be able to:

- Identify the etiologies of hyponatremia and specifically the syndrome of inappropriate antidiuretic hormone (SIADH) release.
- Assess risk factors for developing hyponatremia and SIADH.
- Evaluate osmotic and fluid status in patients with hyponatremia.
- Recommend and monitor appropriate therapy and alternative treatments for SIADH.
- Discuss treatment options for SIADH, proper administration of selected treatments, and potential side effects.

PATIENT PRESENTATION

■ Chief Complaint

"There's nothing wrong with me, I don't know why she made me come here!"

■ HPI

Kevin Flannery is a 23-year-old man who presents to the ED after several episodes of "weird" behavior, according to his family and friends. He is accompanied by his girlfriend who stated that Kevin had been the unrestrained driver in a car accident 3 days earlier. Kevin was driving himself and four other passengers home from a party when he swerved off the road and hit a tree. His girlfriend indicated that he hit his head on the steering wheel and lost consciousness for approximately 2 minutes but appeared otherwise unharmed except for a cut on his forehead. No other passengers were injured, but they did call 911. The paramedics cleaned and bandaged the patient's lesion and noted that he was combative and disoriented but refused to go to the hospital. The girlfriend stated that Kevin has not been "acting like himself" since the accident and she had observed him displaying worsening confused and disoriented behavior in the last 24 hours.

■ PMH

Asthma

■ SH

Lives with girlfriend in an apartment. No children. Employed at a music store. Social alcohol use. Denies smoking.

■ Meds

Fluticasone/salmeterol 250/50 mcg inhaled twice daily
Albuterol inhaler PRN

■ All

NKDA

■ ROS

Difficult to obtain because of decreased mental status. Girlfriend states that he has no medical problems except asthma.

■ Physical Examination

Gen

A & O × 3 but disoriented about recent events. Patient is agitated and confused.

VS

BP 158/94, P 110, RR 26, T 35.9°C; Wt 75kg, Ht 5'9"

Skin

Diaphoretic centrally and very warm; small lesion above left eye

HEENT

NC/AT; EOMI; PERRL; TMs WNL bilaterally

Neck/Lymph Nodes

Supple without lymphadenopathy, masses, goiter, or bruits

Lung/Thorax

Clear to A & P bilaterally

CV

RRR; no MRG

Abd

Soft, NT/ND w/o masses or organomegaly; decreased bowel sounds in all four quadrants

Genit/Rect

Deferred

MS/Ext

Normal ROM; muscle strength 5/5 and equal bilaterally; pulses 2+ throughout; no CCE; capillary refill <2 sec

Neuro

CN II–XII intact; DTRs 2/4 and equal bilaterally; sensory intact; (–) Babinski

■ Labs

Na 115 mEq/L	Ca 9.2 mg/dL	T. chol 177 mg/dL
K 3.2 mEq/L	Phos 2.9 mg/dL	TG 72 mg/dL
Cl 90 mEq/L	Uric acid 3.2 mg/dL	T4 6.9 mcg/dL
CO_2 27 mEq/L	AST 87 IU/L	Serum osm 238 mOsm/kg
BUN 16 mg/dL	ALT 59 IU/L	
SCr 0.9 mg/dL	T. bili 0.7 mg/dL	
Glu 115 mg/dL	LDH 256 IU/L	

■ UA

SG 1.008, pH 6.8, leukocyte esterase (–), nitrite (–), protein (–), ketones (–), urobilinogen nl, bilirubin (–), blood (–), glucose 80 mg/dL, spot urine sodium 125 mEq/L, osmolality 420 mOsm/kg

■ CT Head

Closed head injury (head trauma)

■ Assessment

1. Closed head injury
2. SIADH
3. Electrolyte disturbances

QUESTIONS

Problem Identification

1.a. Create a list of the patient's drug therapy problems.

1.b. What information (signs, symptoms, laboratory values) indicates the presence or severity of SIADH as the cause of his hyponatremia?

1.c. Could any of the patient's problems have been caused by drug therapy?

Desired Outcome

2. What are the goals of pharmacotherapy in this case?

Therapeutic Alternatives

3.a. What nondrug therapies might be useful for this patient?

3.b. What pharmacotherapeutic alternatives are available for the treatment of hyponatremia?

Optimal Plan

4. What drug dosage form, dose, schedule, and duration of therapy are most appropriate for initial treatment of this patient?

Outcome Evaluation

5. What clinical and laboratory parameters are necessary to evaluate the therapy for achievement of the desired therapeutic outcome and to detect or prevent adverse effects?

Patient Education

6. What information should be provided to the patient to enhance compliance, ensure successful therapy, and minimize adverse effects?

■ CLINICAL COURSE

The patient received the treatment you recommended, and his serum electrolytes normalized over the next 48 hours. At that time, the patient admitted that he and his friends had been taking the drug "ecstasy" at the party before the car accident.

■ FOLLOW-UP QUESTION

1. Does this information alter your assessment of the patient's drug therapy problems?

■ SELF-STUDY ASSIGNMENTS

1. Calculate this patient's serum osmolality.

2. What are the risk factors for SSRIs to cause hyponatremia?

3. Perform a literature or Internet search to identify the vasopressin receptor antagonist agents available and those under investigation.

CLINICAL PEARL

Cerebral salt wasting (CSW) is another potential cause of hyponatremia, especially if the patient has had a head injury such at subarachnoid hemorrhage or stroke. It is often difficult to differentiate CSW from SIADH due to the overlap in their clinical features. Both CSW and SIADH present with inappropriately high urine osmolality and high urine sodium (usually >40 mEq/L). One difference is that cerebral salt wasting is associated with extracellular fluid depletion, whereas SIADH is associated with normal or slightly increased extracellular fluid volume. CSW can only be diagnosed in patients with clear evidence of volume depletion (hypotension, decreased skin turgor, elevated hematocrit). SIADH is usually corrected through fluid restriction; however, establishing euvolemia through volume repletion with normal saline usually corrects cerebral salt wasting.

REFERENCES

1. Sterns RH. Severe symptomatic hyponatremia: treatment and outcome. A study of 64 cases. Ann Intern Med 1987;107:656–664.

2. Adrogue HJ, Madias NE. Hyponatremia. N Engl J Med 2000;342:1581–1589.

3. Hillier TA, Abbott RD, Barrett EJ. Hyponatremia: evaluating the correction factor for hyperglycemia. Am J Med 1999;106:399–403.

4. Fried LF, Palevsky PM. Hyponatremia and hypernatremia. Med Clin North Am 1997;81:585–609.

5. Laureno R, Karp BI. Myelinolysis after correction of hyponatremia. Ann Intern Med 1997;126:57–62.

6. Milionis HJ, Liamis GL, Elisaf MS. The hyponatremic patient: a systematic approach to laboratory diagnosis. CMAJ 2002;166:1056–1062.

7. Siragy HM. Hyponatremia, fluid-electrolyte disorders, and the syndrome of inappropriate antidiuretic hormone secretion: diagnosis and treatment options. Endocr Pract 2006;12:446–457.

8. Munger MA. New agents for managing hyponatremia in hospitalized patients. Am J Health-Syst Pharm 2007;64:253–265.

9. Teter CJ, Guthrie SK. A comprehensive review of MDMA and GHB: two common club drugs. Pharmacotherapy 2001;21:1486–1513.

53

ELECTROLYTE ABNORMALITIES IN CHRONIC KIDNEY DISEASE

Maintaining Homeostasis on an
Individualized Basis . . . . .Level II

Mary K. Stamatakis, PharmD

LEARNING OBJECTIVES

After completing this case study, students should be able to:

• Interpret clinical and biochemical findings in patients with chronic kidney disease (CKD).

• Recommend a patient-specific therapeutic plan for treating electrolyte abnormalities and secondary hyperparathyroidism in CKD.

• Monitor the effectiveness of the pharmacotherapeutic plan for treating electrolyte abnormalities in CKD.

• Educate patients with CKD on nonprescription medications that can worsen electrolyte abnormalities in CKD.

PATIENT PRESENTATION

▓ Chief Complaint

"I'm not feeling too good."

▓ HPI

Bob Foster is a 42-year-old man with type 1 DM, HTN, and stage 5 CKD. He receives hemodialysis 3 times a week with a high-flux hemodialysis membrane (Fig. 53-1). Two days earlier, he developed fever, chills, general malaise, and SOB. This morning, he developed nausea and vomiting. He admits to missing his HD session 2 days ago.

▓ PMH

IDDM since age 18

HTN × 12 years

Stage 5 chronic kidney disease; he has been receiving HD for the past 5 years with a high-flux cellulose triacetate membrane; he has no residual renal function

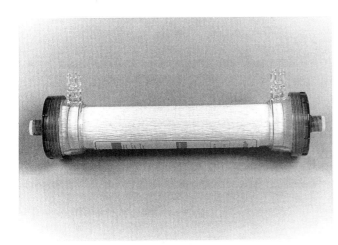

FIGURE 53-1. Example of a high-flux hemodialysis membrane.

Left arm AV graft thrombus formation with thrombectomy last month, multiple episodes of AV graft thrombus formation
AV graft infected with MRSA 2 months ago
Hyperlipidemia
Secondary hyperparathyroidism

FH

Father with CAD; no family history of DM, HTN, CA

SH

Retired from a glass factory; on disability; past history of smoking, quit 3 years ago; (−) ETOH for the past 7 years

Meds

Warfarin 2.5 mg po daily
Ranitidine 150 mg po daily
Calcium acetate 667 mg, 2 po TID
Nephrocaps, 1 po daily
Sodium ferric gluconate 62.5 mg IV once weekly with HD
Clonidine patch, TTS-2, 1 patch once weekly
Procardia XL 60 mg po daily
Lipitor 10 mg po daily
Insulin lispro 6 units SC before meals
Insulin glargine 24 unit SC at bedtime
Epogen 6,000 IU IV 3 times a week with HD
Calcijex 2 mcg IV 3 times a week with HD
Ensure nutritional supplement, 1 bottle (240 mL) po TID

All

NKDA

ROS

Decreased appetite, intermittent headache, and left arm pain

Physical Examination

Gen

Patient appears to be in mild to moderate distress

VS

BP 172/86, P 122, RR 18, T 39.0°C; dry body Wt 72 kg, Ht 5'11"

Skin

Erythematous left arm AV graft site with marked tenderness, warm to the touch

HEENT

NC/AT, PERRLA, EOMI, funduscopy WNL, oropharyngeal mucosa clear

Neck/Lymph Nodes

No JVD or lymphadenopathy, normal thyroid

Lungs

CTA bilaterally

CV

Tachycardia; normal S_1 and S_2; no S_3 or S_4; II/VI SEM at apex radiating to LSB

Abd

Soft, NT/ND, no HSM

Genit/Rect

Normal prostate, guaiac negative stool

MS/Ext

Trace bilateral pedal edema, no clubbing or cyanosis

Neuro

A & O × 3, CN II–XII intact, normal DTRs bilaterally

Labs

Na 135 mEq/L	Hgb 12.3 g/dL	Ca 10.2 mg/dL
K 5.8 mEq/L	Hct 35.5%	Mg 2.2 mg/dL
Cl 97 mEq/L	Plt 205 × 10³/mm³	Phos 7.6 mg/dL
CO_2 22 mEq/L	WBC 13.4 × 10³/mm³	AST 35 IU/L
BUN 71 mg/dL		ALT 29 IU/L
SCr 8.8 mg/dL		T. bili 0.9 mg/dL
Glu 127 mg/dL		Alk Phos 87 IU/L
		Alb 2.8 g/dL
		Intact PTH 140 pg/mL (last month 175 pg/mL)

Chest X-Ray

No infiltrates or effusions

ECG

Sinus tachycardia

Bacteriology

Blood culture from AV graft positive for coagulase-positive cocci

Assessment

42-year-old man with IDDM, CKD on HD with infected AV graft site, hyperkalemia, hyperphosphatemia, hypercalcemia, and H/O secondary hyperparathyroidism.

Plan

Patient missed HD session yesterday. Will dialyze now to correct some of the electrolyte abnormalities.
Will start vancomycin for probable MRSA-infected dialysis graft.

QUESTIONS

Problem Identification

1.a. Create a list of the patient's drug therapy problems.

Problem 1—Hyperkalemia:

1.b. What information (signs, symptoms, laboratory values) indicates the presence or severity of hyperkalemia?

1.c. Could any medications the patient is receiving be contributing to his hyperkalemia?

1.d. What is the pathophysiology of the patient's hyperkalemia?

1.e. What are the clinical consequences of hyperkalemia?

Desired Outcome

2. What are the goals for treating this patient's hyperkalemia?

Therapeutic Alternatives

3.a. What nondrug therapies are available for treating hyperkalemia?

3.b. What feasible pharmacotherapeutic alternatives are available for treating hyperkalemia?

Optimal Plan

4. What drug, dosage form, dose, schedule, and duration of therapy are best for treating hyperkalemia in this patient?

Outcome Evaluation

5. What clinical and laboratory parameters are necessary to evaluate the therapy for achievement of the desired therapeutic outcomes and to detect or prevent adverse effects?

Patient Education

6. What information should be provided to the patient regarding nonprescription medications that could reduce the risk of hyperkalemia?

Problem 2—Hyperphosphatemia, Hypercalcemia, and Secondary Hyperparathyroidism:

1.b. What information (signs, symptoms, laboratory values) indicates the presence or severity of hyperphosphatemia and hypercalcemia?

1.c. Could any of the patient's medications be contributing to his hyperphosphatemia and hypercalcemia?

1.d. What is the pathophysiology of the patient's hyperphosphatemia and hypercalcemia?

1.e. What are the clinical consequences of hyperphosphatemia and hypercalcemia?

Desired Outcome

2. What are the goals of pharmacotherapy for treating this patient's hyperphosphatemia and hypercalcemia?

Therapeutic Alternatives

3.a. What nondrug therapies might be useful for treating this patient's hyperphosphatemia and hypercalcemia?

3.b. What pharmacotherapeutic alternatives are available for treating hyperphosphatemia?

3.c. What pharmacotherapeutic options are available for treating hypercalcemia?

Optimal Plan

4. What drugs, dosage forms, schedules, and duration of therapy are best for treating this patient's hyperphosphatemia and hypercalcemia?

Outcome Evaluation

5. What clinical and laboratory parameters are necessary to evaluate the therapy for achievement of the desired therapeutic outcome and to detect or prevent adverse effects?

Patient Education

6. What information should be provided to the patient to help ensure successful therapy and prevent future complications?

■ ADDITIONAL CASE QUESTIONS

1. What is an appropriate dosage of vancomycin for treating presumed MRSA bacteremia in this patient who receives dialysis with a cellulose triacetate (high-flux) dialyzer?

2. The following laboratory values and erythropoietin dosages were available from the outpatient hemodialysis unit. Formulate a treatment plan for the patient's anemia of chronic kidney disease.

Time	Hgb (g/dL)	Ferritin (ng/mL)	% Transferrin Saturation	Erythropoietin Dosage
2 weeks ago	12.1	210	28	6,000 IU IV 3 ×/week
1 month ago	11.8	—	—	6,000 IU IV 3 ×/week

CLINICAL PEARL

Electrolyte disorders, such as hyperkalemia and hypercalcemia, can be prevented in dialysis patients by lowering dialysate potassium or calcium concentrations.

■ SELF-STUDY ASSIGNMENT

Compare the cost of a 1-month supply of calcium carbonate, calcium acetate, sevelamer, and lanthanum carbonate using usual doses for treatment of hyperphosphatemia.

REFERENCES

1. Ahmed J, Weisberg LS. Hyperkalemia in dialysis patients. Semin Dial 2001;14:348–56.
2. Noordzij M, Korevaar J, Boeschoten E, et al. Netherlands Cooperative Study (NECOSAD) Study Group. The Kidney Disease Outcomes Initiative (K/DOQI) Guideline for Bone Metabolism and Disease in CKD: association with mortality in dialysis patients. Am J Kidney Dis 2005;46:925–932.
3. National Kidney Foundation. K/DOQI clinical practice guidelines for bone metabolism and disease in chronic kidney disease. Am J Kidney Dis 2003;42(4 Suppl 3):S1–S201.
4. Sprague SM, Llach F, Amdahl M, et al. Paricalcitol versus calcitriol in the treatment of secondary hyperparathyroidism. Kidney Int 2003;63:1483–1490.
5. Ariano RE, Fine A, Sitar DS, et al. Adequacy of a vancomycin dosing regimen in patients receiving high-flux hemodialysis. Am J Kidney Dis 2005;46:681–687.
6. Phrommintikul A, Haas SJ, Elsik M, et al. Mortality and target haemoglobin concentrations in anaemia patients with chronic kidney disease treated with erythropoietin: a meta-analysis. Lancet 2007;369:381–388.

54

HYPERCALCEMIA OF MALIGNANCY

What Goes Up Must Come Down . . . . Level I

Laura L. Jung, BS, PharmD

Lisa M. Holle, PharmD, BCOP

LEARNING OBJECTIVES

After completing this case study, students should be able to:

- Recognize the signs and symptoms of hypercalcemia.

- Evaluate laboratory data and clinical symptoms for assessment and monitoring of hypercalcemia, hypercalcemia treatment, and complications of hypercalcemia.

- Recommend a pharmacotherapeutic plan for the initial treatment of cancer-related hypercalcemia.

- Recognize and develop management strategies for toxicities associated with treatment options for hypercalcemia.

PATIENT PRESENTATION

■ Chief Complaint

"I feel really goofy and I think I'm going to throw up."

■ HPI

Sandra Bentley is a 42-year-old woman who presented to her oncologist's office today with a 2-day history of confusion, somnolence, lethargy, nausea, and constipation. She states she has not felt like herself for the past 2 days. Her husband states that since yesterday she has been acting very "goofy" and is at times uncertain of her whereabouts and has difficulty recognizing family and friends. He reports that his wife's last bowel movement was 5 days ago despite administration of a stool softener and enema.

■ PMH

Stage II breast cancer of the left breast diagnosed 3 years ago; ER+/PR– and HER2-neu–. S/P left breast lumpectomy and axillary lymph node dissection with two of 22 lymph nodes positive. S/P doxorubicin/cyclophosphamide × 4 cycles and docetaxel × 4 cycles; last cycle was 2 years ago.
Hypertension × 8 years.
Tonsillectomy at age 3.

■ FH

Mother alive and healthy; father died of MI 5 years ago; brother killed in MVA 2 years ago; no history of cancer in other family members.

■ SH

No tobacco, ETOH, or recreational drug use. Former dental assistant × 15 years. Lives at home with husband of 18 years and twin daughters, age 14 years.

■ ROS

States that she is nauseated and feels very tired and goofy. However, her husband has noted that she is more tired, has constipation, and is nauseated, which he believes has affected her appetite and contributed to an unintentional weight loss of 10 pounds over the past month. Mrs. Bentley has no other complaints except a history of sharp aching pain near her left clavicle that began 2 months ago. Currently, Mrs. Bentley is not complaining of pain.

■ Medications

Tamoxifen 20 mg po once daily
Hydrochlorothiazide 25 mg po Q AM
Calcium citrate 750 mg po BID
MVI 1 po once daily
Docusate sodium 200 mg po at bedtime PRN

■ ALL

NKDA

■ Physical Examination

Gen

Patient is pale; does not appear to be in any discomfort

VS

BP 92/68, P 110, RR 20, T 37.3°C; Wt 52 kg, Ht 5'6"

Skin

Dry with tenting on the dorsal surfaces of both hands; slow capillary refill bilaterally. Lumpectomy scar present on left breast at the 2 o'clock position.

HEENT

PERRLA, EOMI, fundi benign; TMs intact; oropharynx clear; mucous membranes dry

Neck/Lymph Nodes

Palpable inguinal lymph nodes

Cor

RRR, S_1, S_2 normal; no MRG

Lungs

CTA bilaterally with normal respirations, no crackles

Abd

Firm, distended, nontender; high-pitched BS; no abdominal masses

Genit/Rect

Normal female genitalia; normal rectal tone; stool heme (–)

MS/Ext

Pronounced edema in the left arm when compared to the right

Neuro

Lethargic, oriented × 3 (self, location, and year). Speech is clear but slow. Language normal. Follows simple commands. Answers questions with prompting from husband. Cranial nerves grossly intact; moves all extremities.

Labs

Na 146 mEq/L	Hgb 12.1 g/dL	AST 32 IU/L	Ca 12.5 mg/dL
K 3.2 mEq/L	Hct 36.3%	ALT 25 IU/L	Mg 1.5 mEq/L
Cl 101 mEq/L	Plt 110 × 10³/mm³	Alk phos 200 IU/L	Phos 3.5 mEq/L
CO_2 28 mEq/L	WBC 6.5 × 10³/mm³	LDH 200 IU/L	
BUN 45 mg/dL	45% PMNs	T. bili 1.2 mg/dL	
SCr 1.5 mg/dL	2% Bands	D. bili 0.5 mg/dL	
Glu 95 mg/dL	32% Lymphs	T. prot 5.6 g/dL	
	12% Monos	Alb 2.0 g/dL	
	4% Eos		
	5% Basos		

■ Chest X-Ray

Osteolytic lesions on the left clavicle consistent with metastatic breast cancer.

■ Assessment/Plan

1. 42 yo woman S/P chemotherapy for early-stage breast cancer and currently receiving tamoxifen therapy. Presenting with first episode of possible tumor-induced hypercalcemia and associated complications.

2. Recurrence of breast cancer with metastatic bony lesions.

3. Somnolence and lethargy: R/O infection, brain metastases.

4. Admit to inpatient oncology service for further management of hypercalcemia and related complications.

QUESTIONS

Problem Identification

1.a. Create a list of this patient's drug therapy problems.

1.b. What information (signs, symptoms, laboratory values) indicates the presence or severity of hypercalcemia?

1.c. What is Mrs. Bentley's corrected serum calcium level based on her serum albumin level?

1.d. Could any of the patient's problems have been exacerbated by her current drug therapy?

1.e. What are the possible etiologies of hypercalcemia in this patient?

1.f. What additional information is needed to satisfactorily assess this patient?

Desired Outcome

2. What are the goals of pharmacotherapy in this case?

Therapeutic Alternatives

3. What are the therapeutic options for the acute and chronic treatment of hypercalcemia?

Optimal Plan

4. Outline an optimal treatment regimen for hypercalcemia in this patient. Include drug(s), dose, schedule, and duration.

Outcome Evaluation

5. How would you monitor the therapy you recommended for efficacy and adverse effects?

Patient Education

6. What information would you provide Mrs. Bentley and her family about the treatment regimen you recommended for her hypercalcemia?

■ CLINICAL COURSE

Mrs. Bentley completed the initial treatment for hypercalcemia you recommended without difficulty. She began therapy with letrozole 2.5 mg po once daily and zoledronic acid 4 mg IV every 4 weeks for treatment of metastatic breast cancer; tamoxifen was discontinued. She was discharged with morphine sulfate 15 mg po Q 4 h PRN pain. One month after discharge, Mrs. Bentley began complaining of increased left clavicle pain. Her pain was controlled with sustained-release morphine sulfate 30 mg po Q 12 h, immediate-release morphine sulfate 15 mg po Q 2 h PRN pain, and ibuprofen 600 mg po Q 6 h PRN. The sustained-release morphine sulfate was subsequently increased to 90 mg Q 12 h over the next $1\frac{1}{2}$ months to adequately control her pain.

Two months after her initial treatment for hypercalcemia, Mrs. Bentley's husband noticed that his wife was again becoming confused and lethargic. Her use of immediate-release morphine dropped from four times a day to zero over a period of 3 days. She

is due for her monthly zoledronic acid infusion next week. Upon presentation at her oncologist's office, Mrs. Bentley is found to have a serum calcium level of 13.0 mg/dL with an albumin of 2.1 g/dL and is oriented × 1 to self only. Her last bowel movement was 5 days ago. Normal saline at 150 mL/h is initiated, and she is admitted to the inpatient oncology service for further management.

Follow-Up Questions

1. Mrs. Bentley's husband is unfamiliar with the neurologic side effects of hypercalcemia and thinks his wife is "dopey" from pain medications. He requests that you stop all pain medications because his wife has no pain at this time. Outline a plan to manage Mrs. Bentley's pain until her hypercalcemia resolves.

2. What is Mrs. Bentley's corrected serum calcium level based on her serum albumin level, and what is your assessment of this value?

3. What pharmacotherapeutic regimen would you recommend for Mrs. Bentley now? State the rationale for your answer.

■ CLINICAL COURSE

Mrs. Bentley's hypercalcemia resolves with treatment and she reports that her pain is well controlled. She is discharged from the hospital on the same pain regimen she was taking prior to admission. Over the next 2 months, Mrs. Bentley experiences episodes of hypercalcemia with increasing frequency. The last two episodes were separated by 2 weeks, and both were treated by her outpatient oncologist with normal saline rehydration and zoledronic acid. One week after her last treatment with zoledronic acid, Mrs. Bentley reports to her outpatient oncologist's office with complaints of nausea, disorientation, and dehydration.

Labs

Na 147 mEq/L	Hgb 10.9 g/dL	AST 34 IU/L
K 3.7 mEq/L	Hct 33%	ALT 30 IU/L
Cl 105 mEq/L	Plt 150 × 10³/mm³	Alk phos 500 IU/L
CO_2 28 mEq/L	WBC 4.5 × 10³/mm³	T. bili 1.1 mg/dL
BUN 30 mg/dL	50% PMNs	D. bili 0.2 mg/dL
SCr 1.1 mg/dL	4% Bands	Alb 2.1 g/dL
Glu 110 mg/dL	28% Lymphs	Ca 12.5 mg/dL
	10% Monos	Mg 1.8 mEq/L
	3% Eos	Phos 4.0 mEq/L
	5% Basos	

Follow-Up Questions

4. What treatment options might be considered for Mrs. Bentley at this time and why?

5. How would you monitor the therapy you recommended for efficacy and adverse effects?

■ SELF-STUDY ASSIGNMENTS

1. What are the roles of oral bisphosphonates and intranasal calcitonin in the treatment of hypercalcemia?

2. What nonmalignant disease states can induce hypercalcemia?

3. What treatment(s) can decrease the risk of developing hypercalcemia in patients receiving calcitriol for anticancer therapy?

CLINICAL PEARL

When evaluating a patient for hypercalcemia, a corrected calcium must be used to account for the patient's albumin level.

REFERENCES

1. National Cancer Institute. Hypercalcemia (PDQ) supportive care—Health professionals. Available at: *www.cancer.gov/cancertopics/pdq/supportivecare/ hypercalcemia/healthprofessional.* Accessed March 30, 2008.
2. Leyland-Jones B. Treating cancer-related hypercalcemia with gallium nitrate. J Support Oncol 2004;2:509–516.
3. Leyland-Jones B. Treatment of cancer-related hypercalcemia: the role of gallium nitrate. Semin Oncol 2003;(2 Suppl 5)30:13–19.
4. Stewart AF. Hypercalcemia associated with cancer. N Engl J Med 2005;352:373–379.
5. Saunders Y, Ross JR, Broadley KE, et al. Systematic review of bisphosphonates for hypercalcemia of malignancy. Palliat Med 2004;18:418–431.
6. Davidson TG. Conventional treatment of hypercalcemia of malignancy. Am J Health Syst Pharm 2001;58(Suppl 3):S8–S15.
7. Tanvetyanon T, Stiff PJ. Management of the adverse effects associated with intravenous bisphosphonates. Ann Oncol 2006;17:897–907.
8. Ruggiero S, Gralow J, Marx RE, et al. Practical guidelines for the prevention, diagnosis, and treatment of osteonecrosis of the jaw in patients with cancer. J Oncol Pract 2006;2:7–14.
9. Zojer N, Keck AV, Pecherstorfer M. Comparative tolerability of drug therapies for hypercalcaemia of malignancy. Drug Saf 1999;21:389–406.
10. Major P, Lortholary A, Hon J, et al. Zoledronic acid is superior to pamidronate in the treatment of hypercalcemia of malignancy: a pooled analysis of two randomized, controlled clinical trials. J Clin Oncol 2001;19:558–567.

55

HYPOKALEMIA AND HYPOMAGNESEMIA

Back to the Lodge Meetings . . . . Level III

Denise R. Sokos, PharmD, BCPS

W. Greg Leader, PharmD

LEARNING OBJECTIVES

After completing this case study, students should be able to:

- Identify potential causes of electrolyte disorders given a patient case history.
- Select the appropriate route of administration and dose of electrolyte replacement therapy specific for a patient.
- Monitor patients receiving electrolyte replacement therapy for efficacy and toxicity.

PATIENT PRESENTATION

■ Chief Complaint

"Dad has been more confused and sleepy for the past 2 days."

■ HPI

Michael Wentz is a 56-year-old man with a history of alcoholic cirrhosis who presents to the ED with a 2-day history of increased somnolence and confusion, per his son's report. Two days ago, the patient's son noticed that Mr. Wentz was unusually sleepy during the day, and yesterday he complained of feeling weak and fatigued. This morning, he was insisting that he had to attend a lodge meeting because it was elections. The son reports that the patient has not attended a lodge meeting in 3 years.

■ PMH (Per Son and Old Medical Records)

Alcoholic cirrhosis
Encephalopathy
Ascites
Mild portal hypertensive gastropathy
Grade 1 esophageal varices
Anemia
Depression
Seizure disorder (last seizure approximately 8 months ago)

■ FH

Mother alive and father deceased per patient's son; no other information available.

■ SH

Lives with his son. Extensive alcohol history: drank up to two cases of beer/day; none in 1 year.

■ ROS

Patient is unable to answer questions but is complaining of abdominal pain. Son reports that his father has not had a bowel movement in 3 days. He did not notice his father feeling warm.

■ Meds

Spironolactone 100 mg po daily
ASA 81 mg po daily
Lactulose 30 mL po BID
Epoetin alfa 40,000 units SC once weekly
Fluoxetine 40 mg po daily
Oxcarbazepine 300 mg po BID
Ferrous sulfate 325 mg po BID
Furosemide 80 mg po BID
Ursodiol 300 mg po TID
Folic acid 1 mg po daily
Risperidone 4 mg po at bedtime
Benztropine 0.5 mg po BID

■ All

NKDA

■ Physical Examination

Gen

Appears older than stated age; cachectic; oriented to self only; confused and uncooperative; stated the year is 2002 and that he is at Al's Bar. He attempts to respond to questions and follow commands during the examination, but he cannot remain awake.

VS

P 98, RR 16, BP 122/77, T 35.8°C

Skin

Skin warm, not jaundiced, dry, tented, no spider angiomata

HEENT

PERRLA; no scleral icterus; pale conjunctivae; dry mucous membranes; tongue midline; no fasciculation

Neck/Lymph Nodes

Supple; no lymphadenopathy; thyroid smooth and not enlarged; neck veins distended to the angle of the jaw when the head is elevated 30 degrees

Lungs

CTA bilaterally

CV

RRR; normal S_1 and S_2; no murmurs, rubs, or gallops

Abd

Massive ascites; soft, tender to deep palpation in RUQ; (+) fluid wave and shifting dullness; no rebound or guarding; liver firm and palpable 2 cm below the RCM; spleen palpable; BS present in all four quadrants

Genit/Rect

Heme-negative stool

Ext

Upper and lower extremities reveal pallor in the nail beds and clubbing of the nails; lower extremities show trace edema bilaterally; upper extremities reveal (+) palmar erythema. Pulses palpable bilaterally.

Back

No CVA tenderness

Neuro

Confused and unable to cooperate with examination. DTR 2+ throughout. Plantars downgoing. Unable to perform test for asterixis. He is unable to raise his legs from the bed and cannot raise his arms for any extended period of time.

▨ Labs

Na 140 mEq/L	Hgb 9.2 g/dL	Ca 7.9 mg/dL	Alk Phos 144 IU/L
K 2.9 mEq/L	Hct 27.1%	Mg 1.0 mEq/L	GGT 117 IU/L
Cl 108 mEq/L	WBC 4.5×10^3/mm³	Phos 3.1 mEq/L	Alb 1.8 g/dL
CO₂ 25 mEq/L	PMN 76%	AST 38 IU/L	INR 2.0
BUN 40 mg/dL	Bands 4%	ALT 47 IU/L	aPTT 47 sec
SCr 1.4 mg/dL	Lymph 5%	T. bili 3.2 mg/dL	NH₃ 226 μmol/L
Glu 100 mg/dL	Plt 69×10^3/mm³		

▨ Abdominal Ultrasound

Cirrhotic liver with large ascites and no intrahepatic and extrahepatic biliary ductal dilatation; spleen enlarged at 18.6 cm; normal pancreas

▨ Diagnostic Paracentesis

Hazy, 20 WBC, 2,728 RBC, 34% PMN, 12% Lymph, 52% Mono

▨ Chest X-Ray

No abnormal findings

▨ Cultures

Blood cultures drawn × 2

▨ Assessment

Admit to inpatient bed.

1. Hepatic encephalopathy
2. Dehydration
3. Electrolyte abnormalities
4. Acute renal insufficiency—mild
5. Portal hypertension and ascites
6. Anemia/thrombocytopenia
7. Coagulopathy
8. Depression
9. Seizure disorder

QUESTIONS

Problem Identification

1.a. Create a list of the patient's drug therapy problems.

1.b. What information (signs, symptoms, laboratory values) indicates the presence and severity of the electrolyte abnormalities?

1.c. What are the potential causes of the electrolyte disorders in this patient?

1.d. What additional information is needed to satisfactorily assess this patient's electrolyte disorders?

Desired Outcome

2. What are the goals of pharmacotherapy in this patient?

Therapeutic Alternatives

3. What feasible pharmacotherapeutic alternatives are available for treatment of dehydration, hypokalemia, and hypomagnesemia?

Optimal Plan

4. Given the therapeutic alternatives outlined above, what is the most appropriate therapy?

Outcome Evaluation

5. What clinical and laboratory parameters are necessary to evaluate the therapy for the desired therapeutic outcome and prevention of adverse effects?

■ FOLLOW-UP QUESTIONS

1. What medical options are available for treating this patient's hepatic encephalopathy?

2. What changes should be made to the patient's medication regimen to prevent future electrolyte imbalances?

3. What changes should be made in the therapy for the patient's other medical conditions?

4. What vaccinations should this patient receive?

■ SELF-STUDY ASSIGNMENTS

1. Outline a therapeutic plan for the treatment of portal hypertension in this patient.

2. Describe how a patient's acid–base status can affect serum electrolyte concentrations.

CLINICAL PEARL

Hypokalemia and hypomagnesemia often coexist. In patients refractory to potassium replacement, magnesium concentrations should be evaluated, and any magnesium deficit must be corrected before potassium can be appropriately replaced.

REFERENCES

1. Weiner ID, Wingo CS. Hypokalemia—consequences, causes and correction. J Am Soc Nephrol 1997;8:1179–1188.
2. Gennari FJ. Hypokalemia. N Engl J Med 1998;339:451–458.
3. Agus ZS. Hypomagnesemia. J Am Soc Nephrol 1999;10:1616–1622.
4. Kruse JA, Carlson RW. Rapid correction of hypokalemia using concentrated intravenous potassium chloride infusions. Arch Intern Med 1990;150:613–617.
5. Hamill RJ, Robinson LM, Wexler HR, et al. Efficacy and safety of potassium infusion therapy in hypokalemic critically ill patients. Crit Care Med 1991;19:694–699.
6. Blei AT, Cordoba J, Practice Parameters Committee of the American College of Gastroenterology. Hepatic encephalopathy. Am J Gastroenterol 2001;96:1968–1976.
7. Runyon BA, Practice Guidelines Committee, American Association for the Study of Liver Diseases (AASLD). Management of adult patients with ascites due to cirrhosis. Hepatology 2004;39:841–856.

56

METABOLIC ACIDOSIS

Oh, My Aching Acidosis . . . . Level II

Brian M. Hodges, PharmD, BCPS, BCNSP

LEARNING OBJECTIVES

After completing this case study, students should be able to:

- Recognize the clinical and laboratory manifestations of metabolic acidosis.

- Differentiate among different causes of metabolic acidosis.

- Develop a patient-specific pharmacotherapeutic plan for treating chronic metabolic acidosis.

- Provide medication education for patients with chronic metabolic acidosis.

PATIENT PRESENTATION

Chief Complaint

"I just feel so weak all the time."

HPI

Sue Rider is a 67-year-old woman with progressively declining renal function, due to hypertension, who is being seen in the nephrology clinic for management of fatigue, dyspnea, somnolence, and lethargy. She further reports that over the last few months she has experienced a decrease in appetite and occasionally feels nauseated without vomiting. She reports frequent nonadherence to her antihypertensive regimen "when I feel good." She also reports no history of diarrhea.

PMH

HTN
Declining renal function due to HTN
Seasonal allergic rhinitis

SH

She is a retired schoolteacher who lives with her husband of 38 years and has three grown children. She denies alcohol use. There is no history of tobacco habituation or recreational drug use.

FH

History of CAD in her mother's family

ROS

As per HPI

Meds

Amlodipine 5 mg po daily
Lisinopril 20 mg po daily
Metolazone 2.5 mg po daily, taken intermittently for lower extremity edema (reports that she has not taken any for the last few months)

All

NKDA

Physical Examination

Gen

Pleasant African-American woman in NAD

VS

BP 145/85, P 78, RR 22, T 37.2°C; Wt 75 kg, Ht 5'4"

HEENT

No hemorrhages or exudates on funduscopic examination

Neck/Lymph Nodes

JVP was 5 cm; carotid pulses were 2+ bilaterally; no thyromegaly or lymphadenopathy

Lungs

CTA and P

CV

Unable to palpate PMI; regular rate and rhythm; normal S_1 and S_2; no murmurs

Abd

Obese, soft, nontender; normoactive bowel sounds; no organomegaly

MS/Ext

Minimal sternal and quadriceps tenderness

Neuro

No focal cranial nerve deficits; strength 5/5 in all extremities. DTRs are 1+ brachioradialis, 2+ biceps, 2+ quadriceps, 1+ ankle jerks, toes downgoing bilaterally

Labs

Na 132 mEq/L	Hgb 12.2 g/dL	AST 13 IU/L
K 4.4 mEq/L	Hct 37%	ALT 7 IU/L
Cl 98 mEq/L	Plt 225 × 10³/mm³	Alk phos 113 IU/L
CO₂ 16 mEq/L	WBC 7.6 × 10³/mm³	GGT 14 IU/L
BUN 37 mg/dL	Ca 7.4 mg/dL	T. bili 0.4 mg/dL
SCr 2.9 mg/dL	Mg 2.2 mg/dL	Alb 3.6 g/dL
Glu 89 mg/dL	Phos 4.3 mg/dL	

■ ABG on RA

pH 7.28; pCO$_2$ 34 mm Hg; pO$_2$ 106 mm Hg; bicarbonate 15.5 mEq/L

■ UA

SG 1.025; pH 5.0

■ KUB

No nephrocalcinosis

■ Assessment

1. Acidosis

2. Chronic kidney disease

3. Hypertension

4. Hyponatremia

5. Hypocalcemia

QUESTIONS

Problem Identification

1.a. Identify the type of acidosis (metabolic versus respiratory) this patient exhibits, calculate the anion gap, and identify the potential causes.

1.b. What medical conditions present in this patient are either untreated or inadequately treated?

1.c. Which information obtained from the patient's symptoms, physical examination, and laboratory analysis indicates the presence of a chronic metabolic acidosis due to chronic kidney disease (CKD)?

1.d. What are the proposed mechanisms of metabolic acidosis in patients with chronic kidney disease?

1.e. What are the complications associated with prolonged acidosis in patients with chronic kidney disease?

Desired Outcome

2. What are the pharmacotherapeutic goals for this patient?

Therapeutic Alternatives

3. What treatment alternatives are available to achieve the desired therapeutic outcomes?

Optimal Plan

4. Design a pharmacotherapeutic plan for the management of metabolic acidosis and its complications in this patient.

Outcome Evaluation

5. Outline a clinical and laboratory monitoring plan to assess the patient's response to the pharmacotherapeutic regimen you recommended.

Patient Education

6. How should the patient be counseled about the drug therapy to treat chronic metabolic acidosis?

■ CLINICAL COURSE

At the patient's 3-month clinic visit, 2+ pedal edema is noted. During the patient interview, she states that her adherence to her medications has improved. Labs are as follows:

Na 135 mEq/L
K 3.9 mEq/L
Cl 101 mEq/L
CO$_2$ 22 mEq/L
BUN 36 mg/dL
SCr 3.0 mg/dL
Glu 99 mg/dL

Ca 8.6 mg/dL
Mg 1.9 mg/dL
Phos 5.0 mg/dL
Alb 3.0 g/dL

■ FOLLOW-UP CASE QUESTIONS

1. How might the patient's buffer therapy requirement change if she is started on sevelamer to prevent dietary phosphorus absorption?

2. What clinical and laboratory parameters should be monitored to assess the adequacy of the patient's ACE inhibitor dosing to slow the progression of her CKD?

■ SELF-STUDY ASSIGNMENTS

1. Differentiate between the bone disease of metabolic acidosis versus that associated with chronic renal failure and osteoporosis.

2. Discuss the types of metabolic acidoses that may be present in patients with CKD and how they may be differentiated.

CLINICAL PEARL

The metabolic acidosis associated with CKD is associated with a subnormal, but typically stable, plasma bicarbonate concentration. Unlike many other types of elevated anion gap metabolic acidoses, it does not appear to be progressive unless the patient's renal function worsens.

REFERENCES

1. Uribarri J. Acidosis in chronic renal insufficiency. Semin Dial 2000; 13:232–234.
2. Kraut JA, Kurtz I. Metabolic acidosis of CKD: diagnosis, clinical characteristics, and treatment. Am J Kidney Dis 2005;45:978–993.
3. Mandayam S, Mitch WE. Dietary protein restriction benefits patients with chronic kidney disease. Nephrology (Carlton) 2006;11:53–57.
4. National Kidney Foundation. K/DOQI clinical practice guidelines on hypertension and antihypertensive agents in chronic kidney disease. Am J Kidney Dis 2004;43(Suppl 1):S1–S290.
5. Mathur RP, Dash SC, Gupta N, et al. Effects of correction of metabolic acidosis on blood urea and bone metabolism in patients with mild to moderate chronic kidney disease: a prospective randomized single blind controlled trial. Ren Fail 2006;28:1–5.
6. National Kidney Foundation. K/DOQI clinical practice guidelines for bone metabolism and disease in chronic kidney disease. Am J Kidney Dis 2003;42(Suppl 3):S1–S201.
Note: All NKF K/DOQI clinical practice guidelines are available online at *www.kidney.org/professionals/kdoqi/guidelines.cfm.*

57

METABOLIC ALKALOSIS

Debugging Metabolic Alkalosis . . . . Level I

Stephanie D. Vail, PharmD

Thomas D. Nolin, PharmD, PhD

LEARNING OBJECTIVES

After completing this case study, students should be able to:

- Recognize the signs and symptoms of metabolic alkalosis.
- Describe patient-specific factors that contribute to the development of metabolic disorders.
- Recommend appropriate therapeutic alternatives for the treatment of metabolic alkalosis.
- Formulate a patient-specific pharmacotherapeutic plan for the treatment and monitoring of metabolic alkalosis.

PATIENT PRESENTATION

▨ Chief Complaint

"I can't stop throwing up."

▨ HPI

Henry Greene is a 43-year-old African-American man who presents to the ED with complaints of uncontrolled vomiting, fatigue, generalized weakness, and myalgias over the past 24 hours. He also reports a fever of 102°F (38.9°C) from this morning.

▨ PMH

Hypertension × 20 years
Hyperlipidemia
Chronic kidney disease (SCr 2.2 mg/dL 1 year ago); has never been on dialysis

▨ FH

Father is alive with a history of HTN, CAD, and MI. Mother is deceased × 3 years. She had a history of breast cancer and type 1 diabetes mellitus. Brother is alive with HTN.

▨ SH

"Social" alcohol use reported. Further questioning reveals consumption of four to six beers on weekend days. There is no history of tobacco or illicit drug use reported. He is a computer software engineer and lives at home with his wife and two children. He has not seen a doctor in almost one year.

▨ ROS

The patient denies recent weight gain or loss, but he reports a 24-hour history of fever, chills, sore throat, cough, N/V, nasal congestion, and severe headache. He also reports uncharacteristic fatigue and weakness. No reported chest pain, palpitations, or diaphoresis. He denies diarrhea, constipation, or change in bowel habits or color of stool. Urine output has decreased over the past 24 hours since he reports last taking his medication or anything else by mouth. He reports increased thirst.

▨ Meds

Furosemide 40 mg po daily
Lisinopril 20 mg po daily
Calcium carbonate 500 mg po TID with meals
Atorvastatin 20 mg po daily

▨ All

PCN—hives (cephalexin used in the past with no allergic reaction)

▨ Physical Examination

Gen

The patient is ill-appearing and feels warm to the touch

VS

BP 155/89, HR 82, RR 19, T 39.8°C; Wt 80 kg, Ht 5'9"; O_2 sat 97% on RA

Skin

Soft, intact, warm, dry

HEENT

EOMI; PERRLA; sclerae anicteric; funduscopic exam shows AV nicking; no sinus tenderness; dry mucous membranes; no oral lesions; nasal congestion present

Neck/Lymph Nodes

No JVD or bruits; no lymphadenopathy or thyromegaly

Chest

Lungs CTA bilaterally

CV

RRR; normal S_1, S_2, no S_3, or S_4; no murmurs, rubs, gallops

Abd

Soft, NTND; (+) bowel sounds

GU

Noncontributory

Ext

Distal pulses 2+ bilaterally; femoral pulses 2+ bilaterally

Neuro

A & O × 3. UE strength 3/5, LE strength 3/5. CNs II–XII intact. Babinski negative bilaterally.

▨ Labs

Na 150 mEq/L	Hgb 11.9 g/dL	AST 38 IU/L
K 3.0 mEq/L	Hct 37.1%	ALT 33 IU/L
Cl 89 mEq/L	Plt 361 × 10³/mm³	Alk phos 109 IU/L
CO2 38 mEq/L	WBC 11 × 10³/mm³	T. bili 0.4 mg/dL
BUN 99 mg/dL	Mg 2.5 mEq/L	PT 12.1 sec
SCr 4.2 mg/dL	Phos 4.5 mg/dL	PTT 21.9 sec
Glu 113 mg/dL		

▨ ABG

pH 7.51, pCO_2 48 mm Hg, pO_2 85 mm Hg on RA

▨ UA

Urine sodium 13 mEq/L; potassium 10 mEq/L; chloride 9 mEq/L

▨ Chest X-Ray

Unremarkable

▨ ECG

Normal

▨ Assessment

Admit patient for flu-like symptoms, acute-on-chronic kidney disease, electrolyte abnormalities, and metabolic alkalosis.

QUESTIONS

Problem Identification

1.a. Identify the type of acid–base disturbance present in this patient. Explain how the patient's arterial blood gas results and medical history support your response.

1.b. Create a list of this patient's drug therapy problems.

1.c. Describe the clinical findings that are consistent with metabolic alkalosis and those that are inconsistent with this acid–base disorder.

1.d. Explain how severe vomiting can result in metabolic alkalosis.

1.e. Explain how diuretics such as furosemide can result in metabolic alkalosis.

Desired Outcome

2. What are the desired therapeutic outcomes for this patient?

Therapeutic Alternatives

3. What pharmacologic and nonpharmacologic alternatives should be considered for the treatment of metabolic alkalosis in this patient?

Optimal Plan

4.a. What drug, dosage form, dose, schedule, and duration of therapy are best for this patient?

4.b. What other modifications to the patient's current drug regimen are warranted? Include your rationale.

Outcome Evaluation

5.a. What clinical and laboratory parameters are necessary to evaluate the therapy for achievement of the desired outcome and prevention of adverse effects?

■ CLINICAL COURSE

The patient was started on IV fluids for metabolic alkalosis. Urine output improved from 15 mL/h during the first 2 hours after admission to 50 mL/h. Total fluid intake was 3.3 L, and urine output was 1.2 L for the first 24 hours. Laboratory values 24 hours after the initiation of therapy are as follows:

Na 142 mEq/L	BUN 40 mg/dL	ABG
K 3.6 mEq/L	SCr 3.6 mg/dL	pH 7.46
Cl 99 mEq/L	Mg 2.3 mEq/L	pCO_2 43 mm Hg
CO_2 31 mEq/L		pO_2 92 mm Hg

5.b. What is your assessment of the patient's response to the IV fluid therapy initiated for treatment of metabolic alkalosis? Is a modification of therapy warranted?

Patient Education

6. What information should be provided to the patient regarding the use of lisinopril and any other antihypertensive medications the patient may require?

■ SELF-STUDY ASSIGNMENTS

1. Prepare a paper on the use of hydrochloric acid for treatment of metabolic alkalosis. Include indications, dosing, infusion preparation, and safe administration technique in your discussion.

2. Describe how urine electrolytes play a role in the diagnosis and treatment of metabolic alkalosis.

CLINICAL PEARL

It is important to identify the cause of metabolic alkalosis and correct it. However, correcting the underlying cause does not always reverse the alkalosis, and additional therapy may be required.

REFERENCES

1. Bakris GL, Williams M, Dworkin L, et al. Preserving renal function in adults with hypertension and diabetes: a consensus approach. National Kidney Foundation Hypertension and Diabetes Executive Committees Working Group. Am J Kidney Dis 2000;36:646–661.

2. Ostermann ME, Girgis-Hanna Y, Nelson SR, et al. Metabolic alkalosis in patients with renal failure. Nephrol Dial Transplant 2003;18:2442–2448.

3. Khanna A, Kurtzman NA. Metabolic alkalosis. J Nephrol 2006;(Suppl 9):S86–S96.

4. Galla JH. Metabolic alkalosis. J Am Soc Nephrol 2000;11:369–375.

5. Mazur JE, Devlin JW, Peters MJ, et al. Single versus multiple doses of acetazolamide for metabolic alkalosis in critically ill medical patients: a randomized, double-blind trial. Crit Care Med 1999;27:1257–1261.

6. Cochran EB, Kamper CA, Phelps SJ, et al. Parenteral nutrition in the critically ill patient. Clin Pharm 1989;8:783–799.

58

MULTIPLE SCLEROSIS

White Dots and Black Holes . . . . Level I

Jacquelyn L. Bainbridge, BS Pharm, PharmD, FCCP

John R. Corboy, MD

LEARNING OBJECTIVES

After completing this case study, students should be able to:

- Describe the signs and symptoms of multiple sclerosis (MS) that often mimic those of other neurologic diseases.

- Design a pharmacotherapeutic regimen for treating an acute exacerbation of MS.

- Identify patients for whom disease-modifying therapy would be appropriate and recommend the most appropriate alternative for an individual patient.

- Implement a pharmacotherapeutic plan for a patient with worsening MS.

- Educate a patient on the proper dosing, self-administration, adverse effects, and storage of interferon β-1a (Avonex, Rebif), interferon β-1b (Betaseron), glatiramer acetate (Copaxone), mitoxantrone, and natalizumab.

PATIENT PRESENTATION

Chief Complaint

"My left leg and arm are numb, and I'm having trouble walking."

HPI

Cathy Olson is a 24-year-old woman who was in excellent health until 10 months ago, when she developed progressive sensory loss on her right face, distorted hearing in the right ear, and intense vertigo. These symptoms intensified over 10 days, at which time she was hospitalized. A brain MRI showed an enhancing lesion in her right pons and a total of six other lesions, three of which are periventricular. CSF evaluation revealed elevated IgG index and oligoclonal bands. During that time, she elected to start glatiramer acetate 20 mg SC daily. She presents to clinic today indicating that she has had progressive left-sided sensory loss, resulting in a left footdrop, left arm weakness, and difficulty ambulating that began approximately 10 days ago, when she had a mild URI and was experiencing increased stress at work.

PMH

Frequent migraine headaches since adolescence that have been difficult to control despite therapy with acetaminophen, aspirin, and caffeine (Excedrin) and sumatriptan

Mild recurrent bouts of depression that have not been treated pharmacologically

FH

The patient is of Norwegian descent. She was born in Arizona and moved at the age of 12 to Ohio. She has no siblings, and both parents are alive and well. There is no family history of neurologic disease.

SH

The patient is married and is employed as an accountant. She has not smoked for 3 years; before that she smoked 1 ppd. Her use of alcohol is limited to an occasional glass of wine or beer on weekends.

Meds

Acetaminophen, aspirin, and caffeine (Excedrin) 2 tablets po PRN headache

Sumatriptan 50 mg po PRN migraine

Glatiramer acetate (Copaxone) 20 mg SC daily

All

NKDA

ROS

Unremarkable except that she reports feeling run down and tired. Also reports past difficulty with urinary control (incontinence) and a subjective feeling of weakness in hot weather. No previous history of visual disturbance (e.g., pain, blurred or double vision) or motor disturbance.

Physical Examination

Gen

The patient is a white woman who appears to be slightly anxious but is otherwise in NAD.

VS

BP 120/72, P 88 and regular, RR 20, T 36.6°C; Wt 55 kg, Ht 5'5"

Skin

Normal turgor; no obvious lesions, tumors, or moles

HEENT

NC/AT, TMs clear

Neck/Lymph Nodes

Supple, without lymphadenopathy or thyromegaly

CV

RRR; S_1, S_2 normal; no MRG

Lungs

Clear to A & P

Abd

NTND

Genit/Rect

Deferred

MS/Ext

Normal ROM; pulses 2+ throughout

Neuro

The patient is alert, oriented, and cooperative.

CNs II–XII: Mild subjective sense of auditory distortion and tinnitus in right ear despite intact auditory acuity. PERRLA; visual acuity is 20/20 both eyes. Funduscopic examination is normal. EOMs are full in extent. Slight nystagmus present.

Motor tone and strength are 5/5 on the right upper and lower extremities and 4/5 on the left upper and lower extremities. DTRs are hyperactive throughout. Sensory examination reveals moderate diminution in the subjective intensity of light touch and pinprick on the left, with maximal deficits noted in the left foot. Coordination testing is normal except for modest unsteadiness on performing tandem walking and casual gate. Romberg maneuver is positive.

▓ Labs

Na 145 mEq/L	AST 12 IU/L
K 4.1 mEq/L	ALT 40 IU/L
Cl 99 mEq/L	GGT 33 IU/L
CO_2 23 mEq/L	Wintrobe ESR 20 mm/h
BUN 11 mg/dL	TSH 1.0 μIU/mL
SCr 0.9 mg/dL	ANA negative
Glu 109 mg/dL	CRP 1.0 mg/dL
	Lyme serology negative

▓ Brain MRI

Multiple areas of increased periventricular white matter signal (plaque); see Figure 58-1.

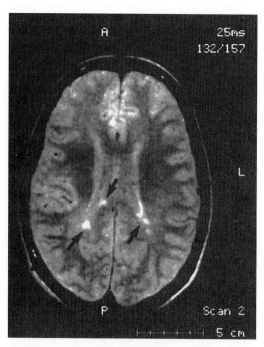

FIGURE 58-1. Brain MRI scan. Arrows highlight typical periventricular white matter lesions seen in multiple sclerosis.

QUESTIONS

Problem Identification

1.a. Which clinical information (patient demographics, signs, symptoms, lab values) suggests the diagnosis of multiple sclerosis in this patient?

1.b. What additional information (laboratory tests, diagnostic procedures) may be useful in assessing this patient?

Desired Outcome

2. What are the goals of therapy for this patient?

Therapeutic Alternatives

3.a. What pharmacotherapeutic options are available to treat this patient's acute exacerbation, and which one would you recommend?

3.b. What adjunctive treatments may be indicated for this patient?

3.c. What adverse effects might be anticipated for both first-line and adjunctive treatments?

▓ CLINICAL COURSE

The patient was treated with the regimen you recommended, with gradual resolution of her symptoms. Two years after the initial presentation, she returns to clinic with complaints of increased difficulty walking and some blurring of her vision. Her muscle strength is intact in the upper extremities, but there is marked weakness in the lower extremities, especially the left side. DTRs are hyperactive in the lower extremities, and tone is slightly spastic. The patient's gait is slow, but she is able to walk without assistance. Her affect is sad, and she is tearful during the examination. She states that she is concerned about the progression of her disease.

3.d. What therapeutic options are available to modify this patient's disease course?

Optimal Plan

4. Design an optimal pharmacotherapeutic plan for reducing the frequency of MS exacerbations in this patient.

Outcome Evaluation

5. Which clinical and laboratory parameters are necessary for assessment of both efficacy and toxicity?

Patient Education

6. What information would you provide to this patient about her long-term MS therapy?

▓ SELF-STUDY ASSIGNMENTS

1. Identify recent clinical trials assessing the efficacy and toxicity of mitoxantrone, IV immune globulin (IVIG), and natalizumab for MS. Considering the data available, define the potential role(s) of these agents for patients with MS.

2. Review the clinical studies evaluating glatiramer acetate for MS. How does this agent compare to interferon β-1b and interferon β-1a in terms of both efficacy and toxicity?

3. Outline a plan for providing patient counseling on the dosing, administration, monitoring, and storage of interferon β-1b, interferon β-1a, and glatiramer acetate.

4. Obtain relevant information and formulate an opinion on the role of plasmapheresis in the treatment of MS.

CLINICAL PEARL

Many patients do not feel better with interferon therapy and may experience unpleasant adverse effects. It is important to reinforce that the ABC-R (Avonex, Betaseron, Copaxone, Rebif) medications do not alter ongoing symptoms of the disease but will reduce attacks and progression of disability over time. Adequate counseling about the potential benefits and expected side effects is essential to ensuring adherence to the therapy.

REFERENCES

1. Schapiro RT. Symptom management in multiple sclerosis. Ann Neurol 1994;36(Suppl):S123–S129.
2. The INFB Multiple Sclerosis Study Group and the British Columbia MS/MRI Analysis Group. Interferon beta-1b in the treatment of multiple sclerosis. Final outcome of the randomized controlled trial. Neurology 1995;45:1277–1285.
3. Jacobs LD, Cookfair DL, Rudick RA, et al. Intramuscular interferon beta-1a for disease progression in relapsing multiple sclerosis. The Multiple Sclerosis Collaborative Research Group. Ann Neurol 1996;39:285–294.
4. Jacobs LD, Beck RW, Simon JH, et al. Intramuscular interferon beta-1a therapy initiated during a first demyelinating event in multiple sclerosis. CHAMPS Study Group. N Engl J Med 2000;343:898–904.
5. Corboy JR, Goodin DS, Frohman EM. Disease-modifying therapies for multiple sclerosis. Curr Treat Options Neurol 2003;5:35–54.
6. Johnson KP, Brooks BR, Cohen JA, et al. Extended use of glatiramer acetate (Copaxone) is well tolerated and maintains its clinical effect on multiple sclerosis relapse rate and degree of disability. Copolymer 1, Multiple Sclerosis Study Group. Neurology 1998;50:701–708.
7. PRISMS (Prevention of Relapses and Disability by Interferon beta-1a Subcutaneously in Multiple Sclerosis) Study Group and the University of British Columbia MS/MRI Analysis Group. PRISMS-4. Long-term efficacy of interferon-beta-1a in relapsing MS. Neurology 2001;56:1628–1636.
8. Goodin DS, Frohman EM, Garmany GP, et al. Disease modifying therapies in multiple sclerosis. Report of the therapeutics and technology assessment subcommittee of the American Academy of Neurology and the MS Council for Clinical Practice Guidelines. Neurology 2002;58:169–178.
9. Miller DH, Khan OA, Sheremata WA, et al. A controlled trial of natalizumab for relapsing multiple sclerosis. N Engl J Med 2003;348:15–23.
10. Polman CH, O'Connor PW, Havrdova E, et al. A randomized, placebo-controlled trial of natalizumab for relapsing multiple sclerosis. N Engl J Med 2006;354:899–910.

ACKNOWLEDGMENT

The author gratefully acknowledges the following PharmD candidates for their contributions to this chapter: Khaloud Alsilmi, RPh; Kai Davids; and Christien Paynter.

59

COMPLEX PARTIAL SEIZURES

An Overdue Visit to a Neurology Clinic . . . . Level I

James W. McAuley, RPh, PhD

LEARNING OBJECTIVES

After completing this case study, students should be able to:

• Identify necessary data to collect for patients with complex partial seizures.

• Define potential drug related problems for established and new antiepileptic drugs.

• List desired therapeutic outcomes for patients with complex partial seizures.

• Based on patient characteristics, choose appropriate pharmacotherapy for treatment of partial seizures and develop a suitable care plan.

PATIENT PRESENTATION

■ Chief Complaint

"My family doctor told me I should see a neurologist about my seizures."

■ HPI

Peggy Livingston is a 36-year-old woman referred to the neurology clinic by her PCP for evaluation of her seizures and anticonvulsant therapy. She is enduring quite a heavy seizure burden. Her last seizure was 10 days ago, which resulted in her falling down her basement stairs. Her seizures started at a very early age, and she said no one has been able to identify why she started having seizures. She remembers having them in grade school and being confused a lot throughout her schooling. She was briefly tried on phenobarbital initially but has been on phenytoin most of her life. She has poor seizure control with no extended seizure-free periods. She has not seen a neurologist for years, if ever. She has not had any neuroimaging studies and provides no previous EEG results.

Upon speaking with the patient and her husband of $2^{1}/_{2}$ years, most of her events involve "blackouts" and losing track of time. Occasionally, she has "grand mal" seizures. She is more likely to have a seizure if she gets overly tired or stressed. She has no history of severe head injury with loss of consciousness, or other significant risk factors for seizures. She states that at some time in her past, she "felt really bad, almost drunk" on higher doses of phenytoin. She states that she is very adherent, although she has run out of medication more than once. Because she is having seizures, she does not drive and therefore must rely on others for transportation.

Data gathered from reviewing her seizure calendar over the last two months (Figure 59-1) suggest that she is experiencing approximately eight "small" seizures per month (complex partial seizures with no secondary generalization) and one "big" seizure per month (a secondarily generalized tonic-clonic seizure). Her interview details and her overall score on her responses to the Quality of Life in Epilepsy Inventory (QOLIE-89) show a significant impact of the seizures on her quality of life. Her scores on the energy/fatigue, pain, and social support domains are especially low in comparison with a cohort of other patients with epilepsy. Upon asking if there is anything else the patient would like to discuss, Ms. Livingston and her husband state they desire to start a family in the near future.

■ PMH

Noncontributory, except as described previously

■ FH

Both parents deceased; one younger brother in good health; no seizure disorder, cancer, or CV disease

Patient Instructions: Please record the number and type of seizures you have each day.

Patient: P. Livingston

April 2008

Sunday	Monday	Tuesday	Wednesday	Thursday	Friday	Saturday
		1	2	3	4	5 S
6	7	8	9	10	11 S	12 S
13	14 S → B	15	16	17	18 S	19
20	21	22 S, S	23 S	24	25 S	26
27	28	29	30 S			

May 2008

Sunday	Monday	Tuesday	Wednesday	Thursday	Friday	Saturday
				1	2	3
4	5 S	6	7 S	8 S	9	10
11	12	13	14	15	16 S	17 S, S → B
18	19	20 S	21	22	23	24
25	26 ? S	27	28	29	30 S	31

FIGURE 59-1. Seizure calendar (S, small; B, big; ?, possible seizure).

SH

Married; works in a local restaurant; denies tobacco and alcohol use; finished high school with a "C" average; no children

ROS

Tired a lot, but no problems with balance or double vision

Meds

Phenytoin (Dilantin) 300 mg po at bedtime

All

NKDA

Physical Examination

Gen

Pleasant woman showing some anxiety during this initial visit

VS

BP 132/87, P 72, RR 18, T 36.2°C; Wt 66.8 kg, Ht 5'1"

Skin

Normal color, hydration, and temperature

HEENT

Mild hirsutism; (+) gingival hyperplasia

Neck/Lymph Nodes

(–) JVD; (–) lymphadenopathy

Lungs/Thorax

CTA

Breasts

Deferred

CV

Normal S_1 and S_2, RRR, NSR, normal peripheral pulses

Abd

NTND, (+) BS, no HSM

Genit/Rect

Deferred

MS/Ext

Significant burn on palm of right hand. This happened within the last week or so, when she had a seizure while frying eggs on the stovetop. She evidently put her hand directly on the frying pan.

Neuro

CNs II–XII intact; slight lateral gaze nystagmus noted. Motor: 4/5 muscle strength on left side, 5/5 on right side. DTRs: 2+ RUE, 1+ LUE, 0 RLE, 0 LLE. Sensory: normal light touch and pinprick. Station: normal.

Labs

Na 137 mEq/L	Hgb 14.5 g/dL	AST 31 IU/L
K 4.1 mEq/L	Hct 41.7%	ALT 22 IU/L
Cl 100 mEq/L	RBC 4.71 × 10⁶/mm³	Alk phos 187 IU/L
CO_2 29 mEq/L	MCV 88.6 μm^3	GGT 45 IU/L
BUN 9 mg/dL	MCHC 34.7 g/dL	Ca 7.3 mg/dL
SCr 0.6 mg/dL	Plt 212 × 10³/mm³	Alb 3.9 g/dL
Glu 107 mg/dL	WBC 5.4 × 10³/mm³	

EEG

Abnormal for bitemporal slowing, which is more significant in the left temporal region, as characterized by polymorphic and epileptiform discharges consistent with a history of seizure disorder

Assessment

Uncontrolled complex partial seizures, with occasional secondary generalization

QUESTIONS

Problem Identification

1.a. Create a list of the patient's drug therapy problems.

1.b. Which information (signs, symptoms, laboratory values) indicates the presence or severity of complex partial seizures?

Desired Outcome

2. What are the goals of pharmacotherapy in this case?

Therapeutic Alternatives

3.a. What nonpharmacologic therapies might be useful for this patient?

3.b. What feasible pharmacotherapeutic alternatives are available for treatment of complex partial seizures in this patient?

Optimal Plan

4. What drug, dosage form, dose, schedule, and duration of therapy are best for this patient?

Outcome Evaluation

5. Which clinical and laboratory parameters are necessary to evaluate the therapy for achievement of the desired therapeutic outcome and to detect or prevent adverse effects?

Patient Education

6. What information should be provided to the patient to enhance adherence, ensure successful therapy, and minimize adverse effects?

■ CLINICAL COURSE

A collective decision was made among the health care practitioners, the patient, and her husband to add one of the newer antiepileptic drugs to her current drug regimen and to see her back in 6 weeks. She was given written and verbal information on this new drug and instructed to call with any questions, problems, or concerns. She and her husband verbalized an understanding. At her next visit, the patient reported that there had been an initial response to the addition of the new antiepileptic drug (i.e., fewer seizures), but she still has some "small" seizures and one "big" seizure per month. There are no recent laboratory data. Her neurologic examination is unchanged. She and her husband would like to discuss further their desire to start a family.

Follow-Up Question

1. What is known about long-term effects on cognition and behavior in children exposed to antiepileptic drugs *in utero*?

■ SELF-STUDY ASSIGNMENTS

1. Outline a plan for assessing this patient's compliance with her

medication regimen.

2. What risk factors does this patient have for osteoporosis? What interventions should be made?

3. Would switching this patient from brand Dilantin to generic phenytoin be an appropriate alternative? What are the ramifications of making this change?

CLINICAL PEARL

Although epilepsy affects men and women equally, there are many women's health issues in epilepsy, including menstrual cycle influences on seizure activity, contraceptive–antiepileptic drug interactions, teratogenicity of antiepileptic drugs, and influence of hormone replacement therapy in postmenopausal women with epilepsy.

REFERENCES

1. Schachter SC. Quality of life for patients with epilepsy is determined by more than seizure control: the role of psychosocial factors. Expert Rev Neurother 2006;6:111–118.

2. Mohanraj R, Brodie MJ. Measuring the efficacy of antiepileptic drugs. Seizure 2003;12:413–443.

3. Elliott JO, Jacobson MP. Bone loss in epilepsy: barriers to prevention, diagnosis, and treatment. Epilepsy Behav 2006;8:169–175.

4. McAuley JW, Anderson GD. Treatment of epilepsy in women of reproductive age: pharmacokinetic considerations. Clin Pharmacokinet 2002;41:559–579.

5. Shneker BF, McAuley JW. Pregabalin: a new neuromodulator with broad therapeutic indications. Ann Pharmacother 2005;39:2029–2037.

6. Meador KJ, Baker GA, Finnell RH, et al. In utero antiepileptic drug exposure: fetal death and malformations. Neurology 2006;67:407–412.

7. Motamedi GK, Meador KJ. Antiepileptic drugs and neurodevelopment. Curr Neurol Neurosci Rep 2006;6:341–346.

60

GENERALIZED TONIC-CLONIC SEIZURES

Jessica Is Not a Little Girl Anymore . . . . Level II

Sharon M. Tramonte, PharmD

LEARNING OBJECTIVES

After completing this case study, students should be able to:

• Define epilepsy and differentiate seizure types based on clinical presentation and description.

• Recommend drugs of choice and alternative therapies for different types of seizures.

• Identify gender-specific concerns in caring for women with epilepsy.

• Discuss key topics in educating women with epilepsy about their treatment plans.

• Develop an appropriate pharmaceutical care plan for a woman with epilepsy.

PATIENT PRESENTATION

Chief Complaint

Jessica is here for her routine follow-up.

HPI

Jessica Taylor is a 16-year-old female brought into the epilepsy clinic for routine follow-up by her mother. Mrs. Taylor describes her daughter's seizures as involving her whole body. "Jessica generally yells out or grunts; then she falls to the ground and her whole body begins to shake. Her arms and legs are going every which way. It really is very scary! She will do this for a minute or two then she is kind of out of it for about 15 minutes. Then she will spend the rest of day kind of out of it; you know, in kind of a daze."

Jessica experienced a "black out spell" at age 11 years, and phenobarbital was started. Evaluation included a skull radiograph and brain CT that were normal. An EEG demonstrated 6 Hz bioccipital and central phantom spike waves. (*Note:* Although there is some controversy regarding their clinical significance, the presence of spike waves over the anterior hemisphere and recorded during wakefulness may have a high correlation with seizures. Spike waves over the occipital area occur during drowsiness and have no correlation with epileptic seizures.) Phenobarbital was discontinued after 2 weeks of therapy because her evaluation was normal. Seizures did not recur for 16 months. Evaluation performed after seizure recurrence included a brain CT and EEG that were normal. A course of carbamazepine was then initiated. One and one-half years ago, a trial of levetiracetam was attempted for approximately 6 weeks but had to be discontinued secondary to agitation and feelings of restlessness.

Seizure control has been fair with 1–2 seizures per month for the last 4 years in the following pattern: 4 years ago—15 seizures, 3 years ago—20 seizures, 2 years ago—18 seizures. A summary of her medication regimen and the number of seizures per month for the last year are included in the following table:

Number of Months Ago	Number of Seizures	Carbamazepine Dose (po)	Carbamazepine Plasma Conc.
11	1	200 mg TID + 400 mg at bedtime	7.3 mcg/mL
10	1	200 mg TID + 400 mg at bedtime	
9	2	200 mg TID + 400 mg at bedtime	
8	1	200 mg TID + 400 mg at bedtime	
7	2	200 mg TID + 400 mg at bedtime	
6	2	200 mg TID + 400 mg at bedtime	
5	1	200 mg TID + 400 mg at bedtime	
4	1	200 mg TID + 400 mg at bedtime	
3	1	200 mg TID + 400 mg at bedtime	
2	1	200 mg TID + 400 mg at bedtime	
1	2	200 mg TID + 400 mg at bedtime	
Current	1	200 mg TID + 400 mg at bedtime	8.0 mcg/mL

PMH

Term birth after a normal pregnancy with prenatal care. Jessica experienced typical childhood illnesses without sequelae. Immunizations are current. Medical history is significant for epilepsy and seasonal allergic rhinitis. Menarche was at approximately 11.5 years.

FH

Negative for seizures. Jessica is the second of three children. Both parents are alive and well. The parents, brother, and sister have no significant medical illnesses.

SH

Attends local public school where she performs at grade level. She began to date last year although denies having a "boyfriend." Patient denies alcohol and tobacco use and reports that she is not sexually active.

Meds

Mometasone nasal spray two sprays each nostril once daily
Carbamazepine 200 mg po TID + 400 mg at bedtime
Erythromycin/benzoyl peroxide gel applied to face BID
Ibuprofen 400 mg po PRN dysmenorrhea

All

NKDA

Adverse Drug Effect History
Levetiracetam (agitation, restlessness)

ROS

Negative except for symptoms described in the HPI section

Physical Examination

Gen

Exam reveals a 16-year-old girl in NAD

VS

BP 112/72, P 86, RR 20, T 36.3°C; Wt 118 lb, Ht 5'2"

Skin

Smooth, warm, and dry. Facial acne well controlled without scarring.

HEENT

Head normocephalic, atraumatic; PERRL

Neck/Lymph Nodes

Supple without thyromegaly or lymphadenopathy

Lungs/Thorax

Chest is symmetric without deformities or scars; lungs CTA

Breasts

Breasts are symmetric, supple and without masses; nipples show no inversion, retraction, or deviation

CV

RRR, no MRG

Abd

Soft, nontender; no HSM; (+) BS

Genit/Rect

Deferred

MS/Ext

Muscles well developed, strength is 5/5 and symmetrical, ROM WNL

Neuro

CN II–XII intact, reflexes 2+ and symmetric throughout

Labs

Na 140 mEq/L	Hgb 13.7 g/dL	AST 28 IU/L	T. protein 7.1 g/dL
K 4.5 mEq/L	Hct 41.3%	ALT 18 IU/L	Albumin 3.9 g/dL
Cl 103 mEq/L	RBC 4.14×10^6/mm^3	T. bili 0.6 mg/dL	Calcium 9.4 mg/dL
CO_2 26 mEq/L	WBC 5.8×10^3/mm^3	Alk Phos 72 IU/L	TSH 2.46 μIU/mL
BUN 6 mg/dL	Diff WNL	GGT 136 IU/L	Carbamazepine 8.0 mcg/mL
SCr 0.5 mg/dL	MCV 90.6 μm^3		
Glu 75 mg/dL	RDW 13.8%		

EEG

This is a 16-channel EEG with a 10–20 system of electrode lead placement. (*Note:* This internationally accepted system is called the 10–20 system because the electrodes are placed at sites that are 10% or 20% of a measured length from known landmarks on the skull.) Both referential and background montages were used, and ECG monitoring was performed. The background activity is in Alpha frequency at 10–11 Hz. No focal changes or epileptiform activity was present. Photic stimulation failed to produce any changes. Hyperventilation was not performed. ECG rate regular at 90 per minute.

Assessment

A 16-year-old adolescent female whose seizures are fairly well controlled on carbamazepine monotherapy presents to clinic for routine follow up.

QUESTIONS

Problem Identification

1.a. List the drug therapy problems for this patient.

1.b. What information would be helpful in fully assessing this patient's problems related to epilepsy or her drug therapy?

1.c. List the gender-specific management issues for this patient.

Desired Outcome

2.a. What are the goals of pharmacotherapy in this case?

2.b. What are the goals of patient education in this case?

Therapeutic Alternatives

3.a. What nonpharmacologic interventions may be helpful for this patient?

3.b. What pharmacotherapeutic options are available to treat her epilepsy?

Optimal Plan

4. What is the best pharmacotherapeutic plan for this patient?

Outcome Evaluation

5. Which clinical and laboratory parameters are needed to evaluate the therapy to ensure the best possible outcome and minimize adverse events?

Patient Education

6. What information should be discussed with the patient to ensure successful therapy and to minimize adverse effects?

■ SELF-STUDY ASSIGNMENTS

1. Write a concise paper outlining the current recommendations for assisting a person who is having a seizure.

2. Perform a literature search to identify articles that concluded that seizure medications can be withdrawn after a certain seizure-free interval.

3. List the advantages and disadvantages of using a vagus nerve stimulator (VNS) to control seizures.

4. Perform a literature search to identify articles that outline the advantages and disadvantages of the ketogenic diet to prevent seizures.

CLINICAL PEARL

Every state regulates driver license eligibility for persons with many medical conditions. State-specific driving laws for individuals with epilepsy can be found at *www.epilepsyfoundation.org*. If requirements for a regular license are not met, many states allow individuals with seizures to hold a restricted license, which would allow driving under certain conditions, such as only during daytime, only to and from work within a certain distance from home, or only during an emergency.

REFERENCES

1. Commission on Classification and Terminology of the International League Against Epilepsy. Proposal for revised classification of epilepsies and epileptic syndromes. Epilepsia 1989;30:389–399.

2. Garnett WR. Antiepileptic drug treatment: outcomes and adherence. Pharmacotherapy 2000;20(8 Pt 2):191S–199S.

3. Liporace J, D'Abreu A. Epilepsy and women's health: family planning, bone health, menopause, and menstrual-related seizures. Mayo Clin Proc 2003;78:497–506.

4. Tatum WO, Liporace J, Benbadis SR, et al. Updates on the treatment of epilepsy in women. Arch Intern Med 2004;164:137–145.

5. Practice parameter: management issues for women with epilepsy (summary statement). Report of the Quality Standards Subcommittee of the American Academy of Neurology. Neurology 1998;51:944–948.

6. Shafer PO. Counseling women with epilepsy. Epilepsia 1998;39(Suppl 8):S38–S44.

7. Glauser T, Ben-Menachem E, Bourgeois B, et al. ILAE Treatment Guidelines: evidence-based analysis of antiepileptic drug efficacy and effectiveness as initial monotherapy for epileptic seizures and syndromes. Epilepsia 2006;47:1094–1120.

8. Jallon P, Picard F. Bodyweight gain and anticonvulsants: a comparative review. Drug Saf 2001;24:969–978.

9. Aldenkamp AP, De Krom M, Reijs R. Newer antiepileptic drugs and cognitive issues. Epilepsia 2003;44(Suppl 4):21–29.

61

STATUS EPILEPTICUS

Calming the Storm . . . . Level I

Sharon M. Tramonte, PharmD

LEARNING OBJECTIVES

After completing this case study, students should be able to:

- Define status epilepticus and its precipitating causes.

- Identify measures that should be taken in the ED for a patient in status epilepticus.

- Recommend appropriate drug treatment for status epilepticus.

- Recommend an appropriate pharmaceutical care plan for a patient with status epilepticus.

PATIENT PRESENTATION

■ Chief Complaint

As per the patient's attendant: "Mary has had a bunch of seizures this morning."

■ HPI

Mary Sanchez is a 53-year-old woman who was transported via ambulance from a local long-term care facility for individuals with mental retardation and developmental disabilities. An attendant and her medical record accompanied the patient. The attendant reported that Mary had a 27-second seizure at 6:30 this morning while she was being bathed. She had a second seizure at about 9:00 this morning that lasted about 45 seconds. The facility nurse gave Mary her dose of lorazepam after the second seizure. About a half hour ago, Mary had two brief seizures, and the doctor told the staff to take her to the ER. Mary normally responds to her name and will follow activity with her eyes. After the last few seizures, the staff were unable to get Mary to respond.

■ PMH

Medical records accompanying the patient detail a PMH of profound mental retardation, quadriparesis, generalized tonic-clonic seizures and neurogenic swallowing disorder secondary to tuberous sclerosis and Dandy Walker variant. Her history is also significant for recurrent aspiration pneumonia, chronic bacteriuria, and chronic intermittent ileus. She has been institutionalized since age 7. Over the years, she has experienced progressive physical deterioration and is presently unable to sit, stand, or walk and is totally dependent on others for all of her needs. Seizures have been present since an early age, but the exact date of onset is unknown. These seizures have always been difficult to control. Anticonvulsants used in the past include phenobarbital (withdrawn due to ineffectiveness), carbamazepine (withdrawn due to hyponatremia), valproic acid (withdrawn due to abnormal liver enzymes), and topiramate (withdrawn due to ineffectiveness). She currently receives phenytoin, lamotrigine, and clonazepam. She receives all of her nutrition and medication via a gastrostomy tube that was placed secondary to her neurogenic swallowing disorder and subsequent numerous aspiration pneumonias.

■ FH

Negative for epilepsy; the patient has three siblings, all alive and well and without significant medical illnesses. Both parents are deceased. No other family history is available.

■ SH

Patient has resided in an MR/DD institution for the majority of her life.

■ Meds

Calcium carbonate suspension 1,250 mg GT twice daily
Chlorpheniramine 4 mg GT 4 times daily
Clonazepam 3.5 mg GT 3 times daily
Ergocalciferol 400 IU GT daily
Lamotrigine 125 mg GT Q AM and 100 mg GT at bedtime
Metoclopramide 10 mg GT Q 8 h

Multivitamins/minerals GT daily

Phenytoin $2^1/_2$ 50-mg chewable tablets (125 mg) GT Q 8 h

Lorazepam 2 mg buccally as needed for more than 1 seizure/24 hours or a seizure lasting more than 1 minute

All

NKDA

Adverse Drug Effect History

Valproic acid (abnormal liver enzymes); carbamazepine (severe hyponatremia with sodium 119 mEq/L)

ROS

Unobtainable

Physical Examination

Gen

Nonresponsive female, 52-second tonic-clonic seizure during examination

VS

BP 135/85, P 115, RR 22, T 37.8°C

Skin

Warm, dry; nail beds are pale; hyperpigmented nevi over chest and back

HEENT

Mucous membranes are dry; (+) gingival hyperplasia; moderate hirsutism on her chin, upper lip, and eyebrows

Neck/Lymph Nodes

Neck supple without thyromegaly or lymphadenopathy

Lungs/Chest

Chest expansions symmetric, lungs CTA

CV

RRR, no MRG

Abd

Soft, no HSM, BS absent, gastrostomy tube in situ

Genit/Rect

Rectal vault empty, no mass, no stool

MS/Ext

Poorly developed musculature; spastic upper extremities; extremities flexed at elbows and knees

Neuro

Unarousable, DTR 4+, Babinski (+)

Labs

Sodium 138 mEq/L	Hgb 11.9 g/dL
Potassium 4.3 mEq/L	Hct 35.3%
Chloride 101 mEq/L	RBC $3.61 \times 10^6/mm^3$
CO_2 32 mEq/L	Plt $190 \times 10^3/mm^3$
BUN 6 mg/dL	WBC $11.3 \times 10^3/mm^3$
SCr 0.4 mg/dL	Neutros 92.5%
Glu 74 mg/dL	Eos 0.1%
	Basos 0%
	Lymphs 3.6%
	Monos 3.8%

Urinalysis

Color yellow; appearance slightly cloudy; glucose (–); bilirubin (–); ketones trace; specific gravity 1.020; blood (–), pH 8.0; protein (–); nitrate (+); leukocyte esterase—large. Microscopic: WBC 10–15/hpf; RBC 1–2/hpf; epithelial cells—few squamous, transitional, and renal; bacteria—heavy; crystals—moderate amorphous urates.

Urine Culture & Sensitivity

Pending

Blood Cultures

Pending

Phenytoin Level

Pending

Head CT

Baseline from medical record demonstrates multiple bilateral intracranial calcifications and dilated 4th ventricle

Assessment:

53-year-old medically fragile woman with a history of difficult-to-control tonic-clonic seizures now in status epilepticus

QUESTIONS

Problem Identification

1.a. What are this patient's drug therapy problems?

1.b. What steps should be taken when the patient is first seen in the ED?

Desired Outcome

2. What are the goals of pharmacotherapy in this case?

Therapeutic Alternatives

3. What pharmacotherapeutic options are available to treat status epilepticus?

Optimal Plan

4. What is the best pharmacotherapeutic plan for this patient to treat status epilepticus?

Outcome Evaluation

5. What clinical and laboratory parameters are needed to evaluate the therapy to ensure the best possible outcome?

Patient Education

6. What patient-specific factors can interfere with phenytoin levels, and what can the patient (or those who care for her) do to minimize them?

■ SELF-STUDY ASSIGNMENTS

1. Identify the advantages of using lorazepam in status epilepticus, and perform a literature search to identify articles that support its use over diazepam.

2. Write a concise paper outlining the proper procedure for administering Diastat to a person in status epilepticus.

3. Prepare a short paper summarizing the hematologic adverse effects of all of the antiepileptic drugs.

4. Women with epilepsy who take antiepileptic drugs may consider self-discontinuing their medication when they become (or want

to become) pregnant. Describe the potential risks to the mother and baby from antiepileptic drugs and from uncontrolled seizures. What can be done to minimize these risks?

CLINICAL PEARL

Status epilepticus in patients receiving anticonvulsants for epilepsy often resolves if the medication that had been withdrawn is restarted.

REFERENCES

1. Lowenstein DH, Alldredge BK. Status epilepticus. N Engl J Med 1998;338:970–976.
2. Weise KL, Bleck TP. Status epilepticus in children and adults. Crit Care Clin 1997;13:629–646.
3. Bone RC, ed. Treatment of convulsive status epilepticus. Recommendations of the Epilepsy Foundation of America's Working Group on Status Epilepticus. JAMA 1993;270:854–859.
4. Lowenstein DH. Treatment options for status epilepticus. Curr Opin Pharmacol 2005;5:334–339.
5. Sinha S, Naritoku DK. Intravenous valproate is well tolerated in unstable patients with status epilepticus. Neurology 2000;55:722–724.
6. Kumar A, Bleck TP. Intravenous midazolam for the treatment of refractory status epilepticus. Crit Care Med 1992;20:483–488.

62

ACUTE MANAGEMENT OF THE BRAIN INJURY PATIENT

Pipe Dreams . . . . Level III

Denise H. Rhoney, PharmD, FCCP, FCCM

Dennis Parker, Jr., PharmD

LEARNING OBJECTIVES

After completing this case study, students should be able to:

- Discuss the goals of cerebral resuscitation.

- Interpret parameters beneficial in assessing the severity of the brain injury.

- Discuss the therapeutic management of traumatic brain injury and increased intracranial pressure associated with acute brain injury.

- Recommend appropriate therapy to prevent medical complications after brain injury.

PATIENT PRESENTATION

▓ Chief Complaint

Not available—the patient was brought in by EMS as a trauma code.

▓ HPI

Tony Carter is a 61-year-old 80-kg man who was reportedly struck several times in the head with a lead pipe during an assault.

Witnesses report that he was initially lethargic and in severe pain at the scene and has become progressively less responsive since the incident.

▓ PMH

Unknown

▓ FH

Unknown

▓ SH

Unknown

▓ ROS

Unobtainable

▓ Meds

Unknown

▓ All

Unknown

▓ Physical Examination

Gen

Well-developed elderly male who does not speak, open his eyes, or move upon verbal stimuli. Upon painful stimuli, he does not speak or open his eyes but does exhibit extensor posturing. Mood and affect are not assessable.

VS

BP 80/50, P 145, RR 40, T 38.4°C; Wt 80 kg, Ht 6'2"

Skin

Facial lacerations noted

HEENT

The patient has obvious soft tissue and bone deformities on the left side. The left pupil is 6 mm and nonreactive, and the right pupil is 3 mm and slowly reactive. EOMs are not reactive and not moving. External inspection of ears and nose reveals no acute abnormalities. There is some dried blood in both nares and mouth. Inspection and palpation around the eyes reveal multiple orbital fractures with crepitus. The head has an open 4-cm scalp laceration over the left frontal region of the skull with some swelling. Neck is in a cervical collar, therefore movement was not attempted. There are no gross masses in the neck.

Lungs

Increased respiratory effort with retractions and rhonchi noted diffusely

Heart

Auscultation reveals a tachycardic rhythm with no abnormal sounds

Abd

Soft with no masses or tenderness but decreased bowel sounds. There is no gross hepatosplenomegaly.

Ext

No non-traumatic edema is noted

Neuro

There is no response other than extensor posturing to pain

▥ Labs

Na 132 mEq/L	Hgb 13.4 g/dL	Ca 8.7 mg/dL	ABG
K 3.8 mEq/L	Hct 40.7%	Mg 1.2 mg/dL	pH 7.5
Cl 109 mEq/L	Plt 101 × 10³/mm³	Phos 1.4 mEq/L	HCO_3 18 mEq/L
CO_2 21 mEq/L	WBC 16.0 × 10³/mm³	Alb 2.4 g/dL	pCO_2 28 mm Hg
BUN 15 mg/dL	Diff N/A		pO_2 71 mm Hg
SCr 1.2 mg/dL			O_2 sat 80% on RA
Glu 235 mg/dL			

▥ Portable Chest X-Ray

No evidence of pneumothorax, hemothorax, or rib fractures; the ET tube is above the carina

▥ Head CT

There is a left open depressed skull fracture with tripod orbital fracture. There is an area of hemorrhagic contusion in the left-frontal region. There is evidence of subarachnoid blood within the sulci of the frontal and parietal regions.

▥ Assessment

1. S/P assault

2. Skull fracture and cerebral contusion with traumatic subarachnoid hemorrhage

3. Coma

4. Respiratory distress

5. Electrolyte disturbance

▥ Clinical Course

Upon arrival in the ED, IV access was initiated, and the patient was intubated orally using a rapid sequence intubation technique (vecuronium 10 mg IV followed by lidocaine 100 mg IV, midazolam 2 mg IV, and succinylcholine 100 mg IV). The patient received methylprednisolone 30 mg/kg loading dose then 5.4 mg/kg/hour × 48 hours and nimodipine 60 mg po Q 4 h. A ventriculostomy was placed for monitoring of ICP with an initial ICP reading of 28 mm Hg. The patient was then transferred to the neurotrauma unit for monitoring.

Over the next 48 hours, ICP values ranged from 18 to 30 mm Hg. Other pertinent labs include serum sodium 128 mEq/L, serum osmolality 280 mOsm/L, urine osmolality 465 mOsm/L, urine sodium 40 mEq/L, and CVP measurements ranging from 7 to 11 mm Hg.

QUESTIONS

Problem Identification

1.a. What information (signs, symptoms, laboratory values) indicates the severity of this patient's brain injury?

1.b. What is the Glasgow coma score for this patient?

1.c. Does this patient have any factors that may complicate assessment of the neurologic examination?

1.d. What poor prognostic indicators does this patient exhibit?

Desired Outcome

2.a. What are the goals of therapy for this patient?

2.b. What are the goals of fluid resuscitation and hemodynamic monitoring for this patient?

2.c. What are the goals of neuroprotection?

Therapeutic Alternatives

3.a. What therapeutic alternatives are available for fluid resuscitation, and which would be the most appropriate for this patient?

3.b. What is the role of corticosteroids and nimodipine as neuroprotective therapies in patients with traumatic brain injury?

3.c. What nondrug therapies may be useful for preventing or treating increased intracranial pressure (ICP)?

3.d. What pharmacotherapeutic alternatives are available for treating increased ICP?

Optimal Plan

4.a. Develop an optimal pharmacotherapeutic plan to treat the patient's increased ICP.

4.b. Outline a pharmacotherapeutic plan for prevention of medical complications that may occur in this patient.

Outcome Evaluation

5. What monitoring parameters should be instituted to ensure efficacy and prevent toxicity for the therapy recommended for treating increased ICP and hyponatremia?

Patient Education

6. What medication education should this patient receive if he is discharged on phenytoin?

▥ SELF-STUDY ASSIGNMENTS

1. Review the different types of neurologic monitoring devices that are available and how drug therapy might influence these monitoring parameters.

2. Review cerebral autoregulation in the normal brain and injured brain and discuss the potential use of hypertensive cerebral perfusion pressure as a treatment modality for increased ICP.

3. Evaluate the role of serum biomarkers in predicting outcome after traumatic brain injury.

4. Review the guidelines for managing the neurobehavioral sequelae of traumatic brain injury.

CLINICAL PEARL

There are only three standards of care for severe brain injury patients: 1) use of corticosteroids is not recommended for improving outcome or reducing ICP; 2) in the absence of increased ICP, chronic prolonged hyperventilation ($Paco_2$ <25 mm Hg) should be avoided; and 3) prophylactic use of antiepileptic drugs is not recommended for preventing late post-traumatic seizures (>7 days).

REFERENCES

1. The Brain Trauma Foundation. Early indicators of prognosis in severe traumatic brain injury. J Neurotrauma 2000;1(6–7, Pt 2):557–627.

2. Clifton GL, Miller ER, Choi SC, et al. Fluid thresholds and outcome from severe brain injury. Crit Care Med 2002;30:739–745.

3. Roberts I, Yates D, Sandercock P, et al. Effect of intravenous corticosteroids on death within 14 days in 10,008 adults with clinically significant head injury (MRC CRASH trial): randomised placebo-controlled trial. Lancet 2004;364:1321–1328.

4. Vergouwen MD, Vermeulen M, Roos YB. Effect of nimodipine on outcome in patients with traumatic subarachnoid haemorrhage: a systematic review. Lancet Neurol 2006;5:1029–1032.

5. The Brain Trauma Foundation. Guidelines for the management of severe head injury. J Neurotrauma 2000;17(6–7, Pt 1):453–556.

6. Kelly DF, Goodale DB, Williams J, et al. Propofol in the treatment of moderate and severe head injury: a randomized, prospective double-blinded pilot trial. J Neurosurg 1999;90:1042–1052.

7. Doyle JA, Davis DP, Hoyt DB. The use of hypertonic saline in the treatment of traumatic brain injury. J Trauma 2001;50:367–383.

8. Vespa P, Boonyaputthikul R, McArthur DL, et al. Intensive insulin therapy reduces microdialysis glucose values without altering glucose utilization or improving the lactate/pyruvate ratio after traumatic brain injury. Crit Care Med 2006;34:850–856.

9. Temkin NR, Dikmen SS, Wilensky AJ, et al. A randomized, double-blind study of phenytoin for the prevention of post-traumatic seizures. N Engl J Med 1990;323:497–502.

10. Rhoney DH, Parker D Jr. Considerations in fluids and electrolytes after traumatic brain injury. Nutr Clin Pract 2006;21:462–478.

11. Juul N, Morris GF, Marshall SB, et al. Intracranial hypertension and cerebral perfusion pressure: influence on neurological deterioration and outcome in severe head injury. The Executive Committee of the International Selfotel Trial. J Neurosurg 2000;92:1–6.

12. Mascia L, Andrews PJ, McKeating EG, et al. Cerebral blood flow and metabolism in severe brain injury: the role of pressure autoregulation during cerebral perfusion pressure management. Int Care Med 2000;26:202–205.

13. Riker RR, Fraser GL, Wilkins ML. Comparing the bispectral index and suppression ratio with burst suppression of the electroencephalogram during pentobarbital infusions in adult intensive care patients. Pharmacotherapy 2003;23:1087–1093.

63

PARKINSON'S DISEASE

Stuck and Slow . . . . Level II

Mary Louise Wagner, PharmD, MS

Margery H. Mark, MD

LEARNING OBJECTIVES

After completing this case study, students should be able to:

- Recognize motor and non-motor symptoms of Parkinson's disease (PD).

- Develop an optimal pharmacotherapeutic plan for a patient with PD.

- Recommend alterations in therapy for a patient experiencing adverse drug effects.

- Educate patients with PD about the disease and its drug therapy.

PATIENT PRESENTATION

■ Chief Complaint

"I have trouble getting myself started, and it takes me longer to do things."

■ HPI

Joan Miller is a 58-year-old, right-handed woman who presents to the neurology clinic because of stiffness on her right side over the last 6 months. It takes her longer to do things because it takes more effort to get movement started, and her muscles feel stiff. For the last year, she feels that she does not think as quickly and it takes her longer to remember things. She also complains of constipation and

decreased libido for over a year. Recently, it has become difficult to read because the words occasionally look blurry. These symptoms have affected her job performance as a high-school gym teacher, resulting in her contemplating early retirement.

■ PMH

None

■ FH

Mother died at age 94 of complications associated with Alzheimer's disease; father died of colon cancer; two daughters and husband are alive and in good health

■ SH

(–) Alcohol, (–) tobacco, married for 25 years

■ ROS

No complaints other than those noted in the HPI. She denies any other symptoms of autonomic dysfunction such as problems with swallowing, urination, sweating episodes, drooling, or dizziness. She also denies any psychological problems such as depression, panic attacks, vivid dreams, hallucinations, or paranoia.

■ Meds

None

■ All

None

■ Physical Examination

Gen

The patient is a Caucasian woman who appears to be her stated age

VS

BP 118/76 sitting, 114/70 standing; P 70; RR 13; T 36.8°C; Wt 55 kg, Ht 5'3"

Skin

Small amount of dry yellow scales in her eyebrows

HEENT

Decreased volume of speech, decreased facial expression, decreased eye blinking; PERRLA; EOMI

Neck/Lymph Nodes

Supple, no masses, normal thyroid, no bruits

Lungs/Thorax

Clear, normal breath sounds, CTA

CV

RRR, no murmurs, no bruits

Abd

Soft, nontender, no palpable masses

Genit/Rect

No nodules palpated; no rectal polyps

MS/Ext

Mild rigidity in right arm. Decreased fine motor coordination on the right. Normal peripheral pulses and postural stability. No CCE.

Neuro

General neurologic exam intact, Folstein MMSE 30/30, Hamilton Depression Scale 4/21.

Unified Parkinson's Disease Rating Scale (UPDRS):

Part 1: Mentation, Behavior, and Mood score 0/16.

Part 2: ADL score 3/52 (Mild trouble with dressing—putting on nylon stockings and small buttons. No problems with salivation, swallowing, cutting food, hygiene, turning in bed, falling, freezing, walking, or sensory effects).

Part 3: Motor Exam 10/108 (Mild problems with facial expression, rigidity in right limbs, rapid alternating movements in right hand, and bradykinesia. No problems with tremor, arising from a chair, posture, gait, or postural stability).

Handwriting sample: Somewhat slow and progressively smaller in size indicating signs of micrographia.

■ Labs

Na 136 mEq/L	Hgb 13.5 g/dL	AST 20 IU/L
K 4.3 mEq/L	Hct 40.5%	ALT 24 IU/L
Cl 101 mEq/L	RBC 4.42×10^6	Alk phos 80 IU/L
CO_2 23 mEq/L	WBC $5.0 \times 10^3/mm^3$	GGT 18 IU/L
BUN 8 mg/dL	Plt $395 \times 10^3/mm^3$	Ferritin 100 ng/mL
SCr 1.0 mg/dL	Homocysteine 16.0 μmol/L	TSH 2.0 mIU/L
Glu 95 mg/dL		T4 total 7.5 mcg/dL

■ Assessment

Based on the HPI and UPDRS, the patient's symptoms are consistent with early, mild Parkinson's disease.

QUESTIONS

Problem Identification

1.a. List and assess each one of the patient's complaints.

1.b. Assess the potential problems observed in the physical examination and laboratory findings.

1.c. List the cardinal motor and non-motor symptoms of PD, and describe which signs and symptoms of PD are present in this patient.

1.d. According to the Hoehn–Yahr Scale, what stage is the patient's disease?

Desired Outcome

2. What are the goals of therapy for patients with PD?

Therapeutic Alternatives

3.a. What nonpharmacologic alternatives may be beneficial for the treatment of PD in this patient?

3.b. Based on the patient's signs and symptoms, what pharmacotherapeutic alternatives are viable options for her at this time?

Optimal Plan

4. What drug, dosage form, dose, schedule, and duration of therapy are best for this patient's current problems?

Outcome Evaluation

5. Which monitoring parameters should be used to evaluate the patient's response to medications and to detect adverse effects?

Patient Education

6. What information should be provided to the patient to ensure successful therapy, enhance compliance, and minimize adverse effects?

■ CLINICAL COURSE–6 MONTHS LATER

Six months later, Ms. Miller returns to the clinic. Her medications include multivitamin daily, eye emollient ointment (Refresh PM), Metamucil 1 tablespoon twice daily, pramipexole 1 mg 3 times daily, and rasagiline 1 mg daily in the morning. Her libido, slowness, stiffness, and thinking have improved. She is better able to perform her job, enjoys the work, and is no longer planning her retirement. Her constipation has improved marginally. She continues to complain of blurred vision but has not been to the ophthalmologist. She now complains of itchy eyebrows and scalp. The patient reports no side effects from the medicine. However, her husband complains that her personality has changed because she shops excessively, often buying duplicates of things, which is straining their budget.

Follow-Up Questions

1. Was the initial treatment plan reasonable? Why or why not?

2. What side effects from therapy does the patient now manifest?

3. What adjustments in drug therapy do you recommend at this time?

4. How would you educate this patient to ensure successful therapy, enhance compliance, and minimize adverse effects?

■ CLINICAL COURSE–10 YEARS LATER

Ms. Miller returns to the neurology clinic for a routine follow-up visit. She is now 68 years old and retired because she is less able to handle activities of daily living. She no longer has trouble with compulsive behaviors. Her constipation has improved with a bowel regimen. Her blurred vision improved after cataract surgery. Her PD medication does not last as long as it used to and she is having "off" periods. Her symptoms are now bilateral and include tremor, rigidity, stiffness, and gait problems (dragging right foot). She also reports that she is slower and clumsier in almost all activities but especially when driving, handling utensils, dressing, turning in bed, and getting out of a chair. She still has good postural stability without falls. There are no difficulties with autonomic symptoms or hallucinations.

She reports mild depression, sleep problems, and forgetfulness. She complains that it is hard for her to make decisions and has lost her initiative to do activities and participate in social events. She denies changes in her appetite, self-esteem, anxiety, guilt, or suicidal thoughts. She tends to feel worse as her PD medication wears off. She sometimes takes more than 30 minutes to fall asleep because she feels restless and is worrying about her condition. She often wakes up around 3:00 AM because she is unable to move in bed. She complains of being off when she awakens again at 7:00 AM.

Her medications include multivitamin daily, Benefiber 1 tablespoonful twice daily with meals, docusate sodium 100 mg daily, magnesium hydroxide (milk of magnesia) 1 tablespoonful 1–2 times per month, and carbidopa/levodopa 25/100 mg 3 times daily with meals (7:00 AM, noon, and 5:30 PM). Her 7 AM dose starts working by 7:30 and lasts until about 11 AM. She has bad tremors until her noon dose starts to work around 12:30 PM. Her noon dose lasts until 4:30 or 5:00 PM, so she takes her last dose at 5:30 PM. The 5:30 dose does not start to work until about 7:00 PM.

UPDRS scores while "on" are: Mood 3, ADL 12, and Motor 43. She has a positive glabellar reflex (Myerson's sign). Hamilton Psychiatric

Rating Scale for Depression 18/53. MMSE 28/30. There are no changes in vital signs or weight. All laboratory values are normal.

Follow-Up Questions

1. List the patient's problems at this visit.

2. What adjustments in drug therapy do you recommend at this time?

3. For questions related to the use of coenzyme Q10 in treatment of Parkinson's disease, please see section 20 of the Casebook.

■ SELF-STUDY ASSIGNMENTS

1. Review the pharmacology and efficacy reports of investigational drugs for PD.

2. Investigate the use of over-the-counter medications for treatment of PD.

CLINICAL PEARL

As Parkinson's disease progresses, the timing of medication needs to coincide with symptoms. Evaluate the onset and duration of each dose and make modifications accordingly. Symptoms may worsen when patients are forced to receive medications at predetermined dosing times such as those used in hospitals and nursing homes. Thus, let the patient's symptoms guide the dosing times.

REFERENCES

1. Samii A, Nutt JG, Ransom BR. Parkinson's disease. Lancet 2004;363:1783–1793.

2. Nutt JG, Wooten GF. Diagnosis and initial management of Parkinson's disease. N Engl J Med 2005;353:1021–1027.

3. Golbe LI, Mark MH, Sage JI, et al., eds. Parkinson's Disease Handbook (revised ed.). New York, American Parkinson Disease Association, 2007.

4. Suchowersky O, Gronseth G, Perlmutter J, et al. Practice parameter: neuroprotective strategies and alternative therapies for Parkinson's disease (an evidence-based review). Report of the Quality Standards Subcommittee of the American Academy of Neurology. Neurology 2006;66:976–982.

5. Anonymous. Treatment Guidelines from the Medical Letter. Drugs for Parkinson's disease. 2004;2:41–46.

6. Lang AE. Clinical rating scales and videotape analysis. In: Koller WC, Paulson G, eds. Therapy of Parkinson's Disease, 2nd ed. New York, Marcel Dekker, 1995:21–46.

7. Pahwa R, Factor SA, Lyons KE, et al. Practice parameter: treatment of Parkinson's disease with motor fluctuations and dyskinesia (an evidence-based review). Report of the Quality Standards Subcommittee of the American Academy of Neurology. Neurology 2006;66:983–995.

8. Miyasaki JM, Shannon K, Voon V, et al. Practice parameter: evaluation and treatment of depression, psychosis, and dementia in Parkinson disease (an evidence-based review). Report of the Quality Standards Subcommittee of the American Academy of Neurology. Neurology 2006;66:996–1002.

64

ACUTE PAIN

No Pain, Much Gain . . . . Level I

Gina M. Carbonara, PharmD

Charles D. Ponte, BS, PharmD, BC-ADM, BCPS, CDE, FAPhA, FASHP, FCCP

LEARNING OBJECTIVES

After completing this case study, students should be able to:

• Differentiate acute pain from chronic pain.

• Describe the typical clinical findings associated with acute pain.

• Describe the subjective and objective assessment of pain.

• Identify appropriate non-opioid and opioid analgesics for selected patients with acute pain.

• Choose suitable drug and nondrug therapy for the management of common opioid analgesic side effects.

• Develop an appropriate therapeutic plan (including monitoring parameters) for a patient with acute pain.

PATIENT PRESENTATION

■ Chief Complaint

"My belly hurts, and I can't stand the sight of food."

■ HPI

Charles Porter is a 68-year-old man who presents to the Family Practice Center with a 2-day history of nausea, vomiting, and RUQ abdominal pain. The patient states that the pain began several hours after eating a double-sized cheeseburger, french fries, and a chocolate milkshake at a local fast food restaurant. The pain intensified and was associated with escalating nausea followed by several episodes of vomiting. The vomiting finally ceased but the abdominal pain has persisted and is made worse after meals. The pain is now dull and achy in nature. Since the initial episode, his appetite has decreased and he has been avoiding fried or fatty foods. He denies any change in stool color or consistency.

■ PMH

Hypertension since 1992; poorly controlled
Type 2 DM since 1987; under fair control
History of gout; last attack in 1995
Hyperlipidemia; since 1987

■ FH

Father deceased (CVA), age 76; mother deceased (MI), age 83; brother alive and well, age 65; sister with breast cancer and gallbladder disease, age 58

■ SH

Is a retired bar owner. He lives with his wife (married for 45 years) on a 10-acre farm. He has two dogs and a cat. He has a 50 pack-year history of smoking and a history of binge drinking. He quit drinking 5 years ago.

■ ROS

As per HPI; otherwise negative

■ Meds

Atorvastatin 20 mg po once daily
Hydrochlorothiazide 25 mg po once daily
Lisinopril 20 mg po once daily
Glipizide 10 mg po BID
Metformin 500 mg po BID
Aspirin 81 mg po once daily
Insulin glargine 10 units SC at bedtime
Maalox TC 30 mL po PRN heartburn
MVI 1 po once daily

▨ All

Erythromycin–abdominal pain (1997)
Codeine—nausea and itching (1987)

▨ Physical Examination

Gen

A pleasant, elderly white male in mild to moderate acute distress; appears his stated age

VS

BP 145/89 (sitting), P 84, RR 20, T 37°C, pain 4/10, dull, somewhat achy; Wt 78 kg, Ht 5'10"

HEENT

PERRLA, fundi with mild AV nicking; TMs WNL; mucous membranes moist

Chest

Clear to A & P

Heart

Normal S_1 and S_2; without murmur, rub or gallop

Abd

Normal bowel sounds, without organomegaly, moderate RUQ pain with deep palpation with mild guarding

Genit/Rect

Normal prostate; guaiac (–) stool

Ext

Good strength throughout, reflexes intact, mild decreased pinprick sensation to both lower extremities; no CCE

▨ Labs

Na 138 mEq/L	Hgb 12.6 g/dL	AST 78 U/L
K 3.3 mEq/L	Hct 36%	ALT 67 U/L
Cl 97 mEq/L	Platelets 340 × 10³/mm³	Alk Phos 180 U/L
CO_2 23 mEq/L	WBC 12.0 × 10³/mm³	T. bili 3.4 mg/dL
BUN 15 mg/dL	Neutros 76%	D. bili 2.6 mg/dL
SCr 1.3 mg/dL	Bands 4%	Amylase 130 U/L
Glu 100 mg/dL	Eos 2%	Lipase 50 U/L
	Lymphs 18%	

▨ Assessment

Acute RUQ abdominal pain; R/O cholelithiasis, acute cholecystitis, ascending cholangitis, acute pancreatitis

QUESTIONS

Problem Identification

1.a. Create a list of the patient's drug therapy problems.

1.b. What clinical information indicates the presence of an acute pain syndrome?

1.c. What is the pathophysiologic basis for the development of acute pain?

1.d. Could the patient's problem have been caused by drug therapy?

Desired Outcome

2. What are the goals of pharmacotherapy in this case?

Therapeutic Alternatives

3.a. What feasible pharmacotherapeutic alternatives are available for the treatment of acute pain?

3.b. What economic, psychosocial, and ethical considerations are applicable to this patient?

Optimal Plan

4.a. What drug, dosage form, dose, schedule, and duration of therapy are best for this patient?

4.b. What alternatives would be appropriate if the initial therapy fails or cannot be used?

Outcome Evaluation

5. What clinical and laboratory parameters are necessary to evaluate the therapy for achievement of the desired therapeutic outcome and to detect or prevent adverse effects?

Patient Education

6. What information should be provided to the patient to enhance adherence, ensure successful therapy, and minimize adverse effects?

▨ CLINICAL COURSE

The patient was admitted to the inpatient service for presumed cholecystitis/acute pancreatitis and pain control. A right upper quadrant ultrasound and abdominal CT were ordered. Blood cultures were obtained. Gastroenterology and general surgery services were consulted. The patient was made NPO except for his home medications. A sliding scale insulin regimen was also ordered.

The drug therapy regimen that you recommended for the patient was initiated. At the end of the first hospital day, the patient states that the medication "eases the pain some" but the pain is inadequately controlled, with each dose lasting only last about 2 hours. The pain is rated as an 8/10 using a single-dimension pain scale. The patient also complains of some nausea and urinary hesitancy.

▨ FOLLOW-UP QUESTIONS

1. What is the most likely cause of this patient's inadequate pain control?

2. What are the revised management goals for this patient?

3. What therapeutic alternatives would be appropriate for this patient?

4. What clinical and laboratory parameters are necessary to evaluate the therapy for achievement of the desired therapeutic outcome and to detect or prevent adverse effects?

5. What is the role of the pharmacist in the management of patients with acute pain?

▨ SELF-STUDY ASSIGNMENTS

1. Describe the role of NMDA antagonists in the management of pain.

2. Describe the pathophysiology and management of opioid-induced respiratory depression.

3. What types of pain do *not* typically respond to opioid analgesics?

4. Explain the pathophysiology behind the development of opioid tolerance.

5. Explain the concepts of equianalgesic doses and relative analgesic potency.

6. Explain the WHO analgesic ladder and list representative analgesic classes (or individual agents) associated with each step of the ladder.

7. Describe the advantages and disadvantages of single and multi-dimensional pain assessment instruments.

CLINICAL PEARL

Tolerance to constipation does not develop with chronic opioid use as it does with other side effects and analgesic effects; therefore, therapy with a stimulant with or without a stool softener will be necessary.

REFERENCES

1. American Pain Society. Pain: current understanding of assessment, management, and treatments. The American Pain Society, 2006. Available at: *www.ampainsoc.org/ce/downloads/npc/npc.pdf*. Accessed June 28, 2007.

2. American Medical Association. Pain management: pathophysiology of pain and pain assessment. Module 1. American Medical Association, 2003. Available at: *www.ama-cmeonline.com/pain_mgmt/module01/03patho/index.htm*. Accessed January 28, 2007.

3. Institute for Clinical Systems Improvement (ICSI) Healthcare Guideline. Assessment and management of acute pain. Bloomington MN, Institute for Clinical Systems Improvement (ICSI); 2006 Mar. 67 p. Available at: *www.icsi.org/guidelines_and_more/guidelines__order_sets___protocols/musculoskeletal/pain_acute/pain_acute__assessment_and_management_of__2.html*. Accessed January 28, 2007.

4. National Institutes of Health. Pathophysiology of alcohol and drug-induced pancreatitis. Available at: *www.grants.nih.gov/grants/guide/rfa-files/RFA-DK-94-022.html*. Accessed January 28, 2007.

5. Standards of Medical Care in Diabetes–2007. American Diabetes Association. Diabetes Care 2007;30(S1):S4–S41. Available at: *http://care.diabetesjournals.org*. Accessed July 2, 2007.

6. Principles of Analgesic Use in the Treatment of Acute Pain and Cancer Pain. American Pain Society, 5th ed. Glenview IL, American Pain Society, 2003.

7. Thompson DR. Narcotic analgesic effects on the sphincter of Oddi: a review of the data and therapeutic implications in treating pancreatitis. Am J Gastroenterol 2001;96:1266–1272.

8. Carroll JK, Herrick B, Gipson T, et al. Acute pancreatitis: diagnosis, prognosis, and treatment. Am Fam Physician 2007;75:1513–1520.

9. Spiegel B. Meperidine or morphine in acute pancreatitis? Am Fam Physician 2001:64:219–220.

65

CHRONIC PAIN MANAGEMENT

A Different Kind of Pain . . . . Level I

Christine K. O'Neil, PharmD, BCPS, FCCP, CGP

LEARNING OBJECTIVES

After completing this case study, students should be able to:

- Define the goals for pain management in a patient with chronic nonmalignant pain.

- Define a pharmacotherapeutic pain management plan.

- Understand the use of NSAIDs, other non-opioids, and opioid analgesics in the treatment of chronic nonmalignant pain.

- Establish monitoring parameters for safety and efficacy when managing analgesic therapy.

PATIENT PRESENTATION

Chief Complaint

"The pain in my hips was bad, but this pain in my feet is really different. The medication doesn't seem to make a difference."

HPI

Olivia Adams is 75-year-old woman who has had a 15-year history of osteoarthritis, primarily affecting her hips and knees. She has frequent complaints of joint pain after walking or other activities and experiences stiffness in the morning when she awakes or after sitting during bridge games. Recently, she has had difficulty walking and has had several near falls. She states that her feet feel very heavy and feel numb and tingly. She describes the feeling as like pins and needles.

PMH

Type 2 diabetes mellitus × 10 years
HTN × 15 years
Osteoarthritis × 15 years

SH

Ms. Adams is a retired university professor. She lives at a retirement community that has multiple levels of care, from independent living to skilled nursing care. She lives alone in an apartment. She is independent but has assistance with housekeeping and laundry. She enjoys cooking for herself but frequently participates in social events and dining at the community's social center. She has two sisters and one brother and numerous nieces and nephews. She volunteers at the local library as a storyteller.

FH

Noncontributory

Meds

Aspirin 325 mg po once daily
Lisinopril 20 mg po once daily
Glyburide 10 mg po BID × 2 years
Acetaminophen 500 mg 2 tablets po BID

All

Meperidine→bronchospasm, hives; PCN→allergy as a child; flurbiprofen→GI intolerance

ROS

Positive for mild to moderate hip pain. Tingling and numbness in feet—reports 8 out of 10 level of discomfort. No other complaints.

Physical Examination

Gen

Patient is a 75-year-old woman in no obvious distress.

VS

BP 104/72, P 72, RR 15, T 37.4°C; Wt 68 kg, Ht 5'0"

HEENT

PERRLA, EOMI, TMs intact

Neck

Supple, no JVD, no bruits

Resp

CTA and P; no crackles or wheezes

CV

NSR without MRG

Breasts

Negative

Abd

Soft, NT, liver and spleen not palpable, (+) BS

Genit/Rect

Heme (−) stool, pelvic exam deferred

MS/Ext

Both hips tender to palpation; right hip pain with flexion >90° and with internal and external rotation >45°; diminished hair growth on toes, and reduced peripheral pulses in lower extremities

Neuro

CN II–XII intact, A & O × 3; diminished ankle and knee jerks, decreased sensation to monofilament testing and decreased vibratory sensation

▓ Labs

Na 144 mEq/L	CBC and diff: WNL	AST 30 IU/L
K 3.9 mEq/L	A1C 7.0%	ALT 15 IU/L
Cl 103 mEq/L	Ca 9.8 mg/dL	Alk phos 182 IU/L
CO_2 31 mEq/L	T. bili 0.2 mg/dL	
BUN 16 mg/dL	T. prot 8.1 g/dL	
SCr 1.6 mg/dL	Alb 3.8 g/dL	
Glu 53 mg/dL (fasting)		

▓ MRI of Spine

Slight degenerative disc disease; no evidence of spinal stenosis or herniated disc

▓ DEXA Scan

Lumbar spine T score: −0.8
Left hip T score: −0.5

▓ Assessment

Diabetic peripheral neuropathy
Chronic mild–moderate hip pain due to osteoarthritis
Type 2 diabetes mellitus
HTN—controlled

QUESTIONS

Problem Identification

1.a. Create a list of the patient's drug therapy problems.

1.b. What information indicates the presence or severity of chronic nonmalignant pain?

1.c. Could any of the patient's problems have been caused by drug therapy?

1.d. What additional information is needed to satisfactorily assess this patient's pain?

Desired Outcome

2. What are the goals of pharmacotherapy in this case?

Therapeutic Alternatives

3.a. What nondrug therapies might be useful for this patient?

3.b. Compare the pharmacotherapeutic alternatives available for treatment of this patient's pain.

Optimal Plan

4.a. What drug, dosage, form, schedule, and duration of therapy are best for treating this patient's pain?

4.b. What alternatives would be appropriate if the initial therapy fails or cannot be used?

Outcome Evaluation

5. What clinical and laboratory parameters are necessary to evaluate the therapy for achievement of the desired therapeutic outcome and to detect or prevent adverse effects?

Patient Education

6. What information should be provided to the patient to enhance compliance, ensure successful therapy, and minimize adverse effects?

▓ CLINICAL COURSE

The physician elected to use gabapentin at the recommended initial dosing of 300 mg po TID. At her 2-week follow-up appointment the patient reported some pain relief but new complaints of dizziness. She describes the pain in her feet as 6 on scale of 1–10. Her hip pain is bearable and does not affect her activities.

▓ FOLLOW-UP QUESTIONS

1. Based on this new information, how would you alter your treatment plan?

2. Considering that she describes her pain as 6 out of 10, would you alter your treatment plan?

3. If this patient were to require an alternative therapy for osteoarthritis, what would you recommend?

4. What changes or additions to her diabetes regimen would you suggest?

▓ SELF-STUDY ASSIGNMENTS

1. Prepare a list of opioids and their corresponding equianalgesic dosing.

2. Prepare a set of guidelines for managing chronic malignant cancer pain.

CLINICAL PEARL

Antidepressants, particularly tricyclic antidepressants, are effective first-line therapy for neuropathic pain.

REFERENCES

1. American Geriatrics Society Panel on Persistent Pain in Older Persons. The management of persistent pain in older persons. J Am Geriatr Soc 2002;50:1–20.

2. American College of Rheumatology Subcommittee on Osteoarthritis. Recommendations for the medical management of osteoarthritis of the hip and knee. Arthritis Rheum 2000;43:1905–1915.

3. U.S. Food and Drug Administration. FDA Public Health Advisory: FDA announces important changes and additional warnings for COX-2 selective and non-selective non-steroidal anti-inflammatory drugs (NSAIDs). Available at: *www.fda.gov/cder/drug/advisory/COX2.htm*. Accessed January 30, 2007.

4. Agency for Health Care Policy and Research. Management of cancer pain: adults. Am J Hosp Pharm 1994;51:1643–1656.

5. Portenoy RK. Opioid therapy for chronic nonmalignant pain: a review of critical issues. J Pain Symptom Manage 1996;11:203–217.

6. McCarberg BH, Barkin RL. Long-acting opioids for chronic pain: pharmacotherapeutic opportunities to enhance compliance, quality of life, and analgesia. Am J Ther 2001;8:181–186.

7. Rowbotham MC, Twilling L, Davies PS, et al. Oral opioid therapy for chronic peripheral and central neuropathic pain. N Engl J Med 2003;348:1223–1232.

8. Collins SL, Moore RA, McQuay HJ, et al. Antidepressants and anticonvulsants for diabetic neuropathy and postherpetic neuralgia: a quantitative systematic review. J Pain Symptom Manage 2000;20:449–458.

9. Maizels M, McCarberg B. Antidepressants and antiepileptic drugs for chronic non-cancer pain. Am Fam Physician 2005;71:483–490.

10. Dworkin RH, Backonja M, Rowbotham MC, et al. Advances in neuropathic pain: diagnosis, mechanisms, and treatment recommendations. Arch Neurol 2003;60:1524–1534.

66

HEADACHE DISORDERS

The Migraineur . . . . Level II

Susan R. Winkler, PharmD, BCPS

Sandra L. Kim, PharmD

LEARNING OBJECTIVES

After completing this case study, students should be able to:

- Develop pharmacotherapeutic goals for treating and preventing migraine headaches.

- Make recommendations regarding pharmacotherapeutic regimens for an individual patient based on information concerning the patient's headache type and severity, medical history, previous drug therapy, concomitant problems, and pertinent laboratory data.

- Provide information to patients on the use of abortive and prophylactic agents for migraine headaches.

- Describe the appropriate use of a headache diary and how it may be used to refine headache treatment.

PATIENT PRESENTATION

■ Chief Complaint

"This new medication is not working for my headaches, and I have been gaining weight!"

■ HPI

Caroline Parker is a 30-year-old woman who presents to the Neurology Clinic for follow-up of migraine headaches. She states that she used to get about two migraines every month; however, she recently got divorced and started a new job. Since then, the frequency of her migraines has increased to about four to five per month. She states her migraines usually occur in the morning, and there is no identifiable relationship with her menses. Her typical headache evolves quickly (within 1 hour) and involves severe throbbing pain, which is unilateral and temporal in distribution and preceded by an aura, which consists of nausea and pastel lights flashing throughout her visual field. It frequently involves photophobia as well. Vomiting may occur with an extreme headache. She reports experiencing severe migraine attacks that cause her to miss 2 days of work each month. She is not able to complete household chores for the 2 days she has severe migraine attacks, and she misses working out at the gym. She also complains of having mild migraine attacks lasting 3 days per month during which her productivity at work and at home is reduced by half. She typically has to retreat to a dark room and avoid any noise, or the severity of the migraine increases. She rates her migraines as 7–8 on a headache scale of 1–10, with 10 being the worst. At her previous visit to the Neurology Clinic 2 months ago, she was prescribed naratriptan 2.5 mg orally to be taken at the onset of headache. However, naratriptan has not been effective for half of the migraines she has had in the last 2 months. During two of the attacks, she experienced partial pain relief, with the pain returning later in the day. She mentions that she was prescribed naratriptan when the Cafergot she was taking stopped working. She states she has taken her medications exactly as advised. She prefers to use medications that can be taken orally. She was also started on valproic acid at her last clinic visit for prophylaxis and has noticed a 10-pound weight gain since then. She inquires about switching from valproic acid to another medication.

■ PMH

Migraine with aura since age 27; previous medical work-up, including an EEG and a head MRI, demonstrated no PVD, CVA, brain tumor, infection, cerebral aneurysm, or epileptic component. Drug therapies have included the following:

- Abortive therapies

  1. Simple analgesics, NSAIDs, and Cafergot (good efficacy until 2 months ago)

  2. Narcotics (good efficacy, but puts her "out of commission for days")

  3. Midrin (no efficacy)

  4. Naratriptan (minimal efficacy)

- Prophylactic therapies

  1. Valproic acid 500 mg daily (weight gain)

  2. Propranolol 20 mg BID (increased episodes of dizziness and lightheadedness; patient self-discontinued medication)

- Mild depression for 8 months, treated with

  1. Phenelzine 15 mg po TID (minimal efficacy, discontinued 1 month ago)

  2. Sertraline 50 mg po at bedtime (recently started 2 weeks ago)

■ FH

Positive for migraines (both parents); hypertension and Type 2 diabetes (mother)

SH

Secretary. Recently divorced; mother of two boys, ages 3 and 2. Denies tobacco or alcohol use. Occasional caffeine intake.

ROS

Complains of increased frequency of headaches starting about 6 months ago and limited efficacy with naratriptan; no nausea, vomiting, diarrhea, or flashing lights at present

Meds

Naratriptan 2.5-mg tablets, 1 tablet po at onset of migraine, repeat dose of 2.5 mg po in 4 hours if partial response or if headache returns. Maximum dose 5 mg per 24 hours.
Metoclopramide 10 mg po at onset of migraine.
Valproic acid 500 mg po at bedtime.
Sertraline 50 mg po at bedtime.

All

NKDA

Physical Examination

Gen

WDWN woman in mild distress

VS

BP 132/86, HR 76, RR 18, T 37.2°C; Wt 70 kg, Ht 5'0"

Skin

Normal skin turgor; no diaphoresis

HEENT

PERRLA; EOMI; no funduscopic exam performed

Neck

Supple; no masses, thyroid enlargement, adenopathy, bruits, or JVD

Chest

Good breath sounds bilaterally; clear to A & P

CV

RRR, S_1, S_2 normal, no MRG

Abd

Soft, NT/ND, no hepatosplenomegaly, (+) BS

Genit/Rect

Deferred

MS/Ext

UE/LE strength 5/5 with normal tone; radial and femoral pulses 3+ bilaterally; no edema; no evidence of thrombophlebitis; full ROM

Neuro

A & O × 3; no dysarthria or aphasia; memory intact; no nystagmus; no fasciculations, tremor, or ataxia; (−) Romberg; CN II–XII intact; sensory intact; DTRs: 2+ throughout; Babinski (−) bilaterally

Labs

Na 138 mEq/L	Hgb 13 g/dL	AST 23 IU/L
K 4.5 mEq/L	Hct 40%	ALT 25 IU/L
Cl 101 mEq/L	Plt 302 × 10³/mm³	Alk Phos 35 IU/L
CO_2 23 mEq/L	WBC 8 × 10³/mm³	Urine pregnancy test (−)
BUN 8 mg/dL	Differential WNL	
SCr 0.6 mg/dL		
Glu 95 mg/dL		

Assessment

1. Increase in frequency of migraines related to an increase in stress.

2. Minimal efficacy of naratriptan 2.5 mg po as an abortive treatment.

3. Previous prophylactic treatments have been unsuccessful and cause unwanted adverse effects.

QUESTIONS

Problem Identification

1.a. Create a list of the patient's drug therapy problems at this clinic visit.

1.b. Calculate the patient's MIDAS score and describe the severity of her migraine headaches. (See Fig. 66-1 for MIDAS questionnaire.)

1.c. What clinical information is consistent with a diagnosis of migraines in this patient?

1.d. Could any of the patient's problems have been caused or exacerbated by her drug therapy?

Desired Outcomes

2. What are the goals of therapy for this patient?

Therapeutic Alternatives

3.a. What pharmacotherapeutic alternatives are available for treatment of the patient's nausea, and how will they impact potential abortive therapies?

3.b. What pharmacotherapeutic alternatives are available for the abortive treatment of this patient's migraine attacks?

3.c. What pharmacotherapeutic alternatives are available for prophylaxis of this patient's migraine attacks?

Optimal Plan

4.a. Considering this patient's past successes and failures in treating her migraine attacks, design an optimal pharmacotherapeutic plan for aborting her migraine headaches.

4.b. Design an optimal pharmacotherapeutic plan for prophylaxis of her migraine headaches.

Outcome Evaluation

5. Which clinical and/or laboratory parameters should be assessed regularly to evaluate the therapy for achievement of the desired therapeutic outcome and to detect or prevent adverse effects?

Patient Education

6. What information should be provided to the patient regarding her new abortive and prophylactic therapies?

FOLLOW-UP QUESTIONS

1. Describe how a headache diary could help the treatment of this patient's migraine headaches (Fig. 66-2).

SELF-STUDY ASSIGNMENTS

1. Review the literature regarding IV agents (e.g., dihydroergotamine, valproate sodium) that are used for aborting migraines.

2. Familiarize yourself with different strategies (stratified and step-care) used for treating migraine.

INSTRUCTIONS: Please answer the following questions about ALL the headaches you have had over the last 3 months. Write your answer in the box next to each question. Write zero if you did not do the activity in the last 3 months.

Days

1. How many days in the last 3 months did you miss work or school because of your headaches?

2. How many days in the last 3 months was your productivity at work or school reduced by half or more because of headaches? *(Do not include days you counted in question 1 where you missed work or school.)*

3. How many days in the last 3 months did you NOT do household work because of your headaches?

4. How many days in the last 3 months was your productivity in household work reduced by half or more because of your headaches? *(Do not include days you counted in question 3 where you did not do household work.)*

5. On how many days in the last 3 months did you miss family, social, or leisure activities because of your headaches?

MIDAS Score: Add the total number of days from questions 1–5.   **Total**

NOTE: Scores from A and B below are not included in the MIDAS score, but are used to assess frequency and intensity of pain.

A. How many days in the last 3 months did you have a headache? *(If a headache lasted more than 1 day, count each day.)*

B. On a scale of 0–10, on average how painful were these headaches? *(0 = no pain, and 10 = pain as bad as it can be.)*

Interpretation

The MIDAS questionnaire is scored in units of lost days. Depending on the MIDAS score, patients are assigned to 1 of 4 grades:

MIDAS Grade	Definition	Score
I	Minimal or infrequent disability	0–5
II	Mild or infrequent disability	6–10
III	Moderate disability	11–20
IV	Severe disability	≥ 21

FIGURE 66-1. Migraine Disability Assessment (MIDAS) Questionnaire. *(Reprinted with permission from: Bigal ME, Lipton RB, Krymchantowski AV. The medical management of migraine. Am J Ther 2004;11:130–140. Lippincott Williams & Wilkins, www.lww.com.)*

Name: _____   Month: _____   Year: _____

Date of Headache														
Headache Intensity														
Excruciating pain	10	10	10	10	10	10	10	10	10	10	10	10	10	10
	9	9	9	9	9	9	9	9	9	9	9	9	9	9
Severe pain	8	8	8	8	8	8	8	8	8	8	8	8	8	8
	7	7	7	7	7	7	7	7	7	7	7	7	7	7
Severe pain	6	6	6	6	6	6	6	6	6	6	6	6	6	6
	5	5	5	5	5	5	5	5	5	5	5	5	5	5
Moderate pain	4	4	4	4	4	4	4	4	4	4	4	4	4	4
	3	3	3	3	3	3	3	3	3	3	3	3	3	3
Mild pain	2	2	2	2	2	2	2	2	2	2	2	2	2	2
Aura only	1	1	1	1	1	1	1	1	1	1	1	1	1	1
Headache Duration (hours)														
Level of Disability														
Hospitalized														
Treatment by health care professional														
Bedrest required														
Decrease in activity by 50%														
Decrease in activity by 25%														
Normal activity														
Other (comment below)														
Associated Symptoms														
Nausea														
Vomiting														
Visual disturbances														
Menstrual period														
Neurological														
Other (comment below)														
Medications Taken														
1.														
2.														
3.														
4.														
5.														
Treatment Results														
Complete relief														
75% relief														
50% relief														
25% relief														
No relief														
Other (comment below)														
General Comments														

Note: A normal diary includes space to record a full month of headache activity. This form has been truncated for space purposes.

FIGURE 66-2. A headache diary.

3. Prepare a report highlighting antiepileptic drugs used for the prophylaxis of migraines.

CLINICAL PEARL

Migraines are three times more prevalent in women and are associated with estrogen levels. Sixty percent of women migraineurs report menstrually associated migraines, and 7–14% have migraines exclusively with menses.

REFERENCES

1. Bigal ME, Lipton RB, Krymchantowski AV. The medical management of migraine. Am J Ther 2004;11:130–140.

2. Mannix LK. Relieving migraine pain: sorting through the options. Cleve Clin J Med 2003;70:8–28.

3. Eadie MJ. Clinically significant drug interactions with agents specific for migraine attacks. CNS Drugs 2001;15:105–118.

4. Tepper SJ. Drug interactions and the triptans. CNS News 2001;3:43–46.

5. Silberstein SD, Lipton RB, Dodick DW, et al. Efficacy and safety of topiramate for the treatment of chronic migraine: a randomized, double-blind, placebo-controlled trial. Headache 2007;47:170–180.

6. Modi, S, Lowder DM. Medications for migraine prophylaxis. Am Fam Physician 2006;73:72–78.

7. Schrader H, Stovner LJ, Helde G, et al. Prophylactic treatment of migraine with angiotensin converting enzyme inhibitor (lisinopril): randomised, placebo controlled, crossover study. BMJ 2001;322:19–22.

8. Tronvik, E, Stovner LJ, Helde G, et al. Prophylactic treatment of migraine with an angiotensin II receptor blocker: a randomized controlled trial. JAMA 2003;289:65–69.

9. Ferrari MD, Roon KI, Lipton RB, et al. Oral triptans (serotonin 5-HT 1B/1D agonists) in acute migraine treatment: a meta-analysis of 53 trials. Lancet 2001;358:1668–1675.

10. Silberstein SD. Practice parameter: evidence-based guidelines for migraine headache (an evidence-based review): report of the Quality Standards Subcommittee of the American Academy of Neurology. Neurology 2000;55:754–762.

67

ATTENTION-DEFICIT HYPERACTIVITY DISORDER

He Keeps Going and Going and . . . . .Level I

Darin C. Ramsey, PharmD, BCPS

Jasmine D. Gonzalvo, PharmD

LEARNING OBJECTIVES

After completing this case study, the reader should be able to:

- Recognize and describe the signs and symptoms of attention-deficit hyperactivity disorder (ADHD) as defined by DSM-IV.

- Apply the diagnostic criteria for ADHD and differentiate between symptoms of inattention and hyperactivity/impulsivity.

- Differentiate treatment options for ADHD with regard to effectiveness, tolerability, safety, monitoring parameters, and potential for drug interactions.

- Compare the advantages and disadvantages of once-daily stimulant preparations to immediate-release stimulants.

- Develop useful dosing schedule strategies that may be employed in the management of patients with ADHD to enhance medication adherence.

- Perform patient assessment to determine efficacy with selected therapy and appropriate monitoring for any adverse effects.

PATIENT PRESENTATION

Chief Complaint

"I need some help with my son."

HPI

Ethan Abeln is an 8-year-old boy who was referred to the psychiatrist 3 months ago by his pediatrician. He is accompanied by his mother, who reports "I can no longer control my child." She states that she has always noticed that Ethan has more energy compared to most kids his age, but assumed that it was due to his excess caffeine intake at home. Ethan's disruptive classroom behavior resulted in his having to repeat the first grade, and after a recent parent-teacher conference, it was suggested that Ethan would benefit from repeating the second grade. Academically, he has difficulty concentrating at school and at home. Ethan finds his

video games more stimulating than studying for his spelling tests. He has difficulty staying focused in the classroom and is constantly squirming and fidgeting in his seat. At times, he will burst into uncontrollable laughter for no apparent reason. At school, he is somewhat of a loner and isolates himself from other children. Currently, he plays basketball on weekends, but is often found daydreaming on the court and not paying attention to which team has the ball. At his first pediatrician visit 3 months ago, it was decided that Ethan would initially be started on Adderall 10 mg twice a day, and a referral was placed for him to follow-up with a psychiatrist. At that time, his mother was reluctant to start medication but admitted "I don't want him to get involved with the wrong crowd . . . I just don't know what to do."

Today at his initial visit with the psychiatrist, his behavior is found to be controlled in the morning, but by the afternoon he is once again "out of control." His mother reports that yesterday, Ethan was found throwing paper wads at his substitute teacher and also at his bus driver. At home, he has resorted to his old behavior of not completing his homework. Currently, his mother gives the initial dose of Adderall in the morning before he gets on the bus at approximately 7:00 AM and the second dose is to be given by the school nurse during lunch around noon. Because Ethan is easily distracted, he doesn't always remember to stop by the nurses' station to take his second dose of the day. Mrs. Abeln has talked with the nurse on several occasions, but the school policy is that the child must be responsible to pick up any medication that is to be taken during school hours.

PMH

Asthma × 3 years
ADHD × 2 years

FH

Both mother and maternal uncle have a history of hyperactivity and are currently receiving treatment as adults.

SH

Lives with mother and stepfather in the suburbs

Meds

Adderall 10 mg po BID
Albuterol inhaler 2 puffs Q 4 h PRN shortness of breath
Singulair 5 mg po daily

All

NKDA

ROS

Physical assessment was difficult to assess in Ethan as he could not sit still for more than 30 seconds and was jumping off of the exam table. Asthma symptoms appear controlled with PRN inhaler use at bedtime only.

■ Physical Examination

Gen

Well-nourished, healthy-appearing male child, normal physical development

VS

BP 108/62, P 82, RR 25, T 37.5°C; Wt 29.5 kg, Ht 4'5"

Skin

No signs of rash, cuts, scrapes, skin irritation, or bruising noted

HEENT

Unable to assess

Neck/Lymph Nodes

Unable to assess

Lungs/Thorax

No rales, rhonchi, or wheezing

CV

Normotensive, RRR

Abd

Deferred

Genit/Rect

Deferred

MS/Ext

Unable to assess

Neuro

A & O × 3; no underlying tics noted

■ Labs

Na 138 mEq/L	Hgb 14 g/dL	WBC $9 \times 10^3/mm^3$	Mag 1.8 mg/dL
K 3.8 mEq/L	Hct 44.5%	Neutros 66%	Serum Iron 95 mcg/dL
Cl 106 mEq/L	RBC $4.6 \times 10^6/mm^3$	Bands 2%	TSH 3.6 mIU/L
CO_2 23 mEq/L	Plt $278 \times 10^3/mm^3$	Eos 3%	
BUN 18 mg/dL	MCV 85 μm^3	Lymphs 24%	
SCr 0.8 mg/dL	MCHC 33 g/dL	Monos 5%	
Glu 110 mg/dL			

■ Assessment

1. ADHD
2. Mild-intermittent asthma; well-controlled with PRN albuterol

QUESTIONS

Problem Identification

1.a. Create a list of the patient's drug therapy problems.

1.b. What information (signs, symptoms, laboratory values) indicates the presence or severity of ADHD?

Desired Outcome

2. What are the goals of treatment (pharmacotherapy and nonpharmacotherapy) for a patient diagnosed with ADHD?

Therapeutic Alternatives

3.a. What nondrug therapies might be beneficial for patients diagnosed with ADHD?

3.b. What pharmacotherapeutic agents are available that might benefit this patient with ADHD?

Optimal Plan

4.a. What drug, dosage form, dose, schedule, and duration of therapy are best for this patient?

4.b. What therapeutic alternatives would be appropriate if the patient fails to respond to initial therapy?

Outcome Evaluation

5. What clinical and laboratory parameters are necessary to evaluate the therapy for achievement of the desired therapeutic outcome and to detect or prevent adverse effects?

Patient Education

6. What information should be provided to the patient and to the patient's family to enhance compliance, ensure successful therapy, and minimize adverse effects?

■ SELF-STUDY ASSIGNMENTS

1. Many parents are apprehensive about starting stimulants in children with the fear of the potential for stimulant abuse when they become older. After performing a literature search, prepare an educational brochure addressing the question, "Does Stimulant Treatment of ADHD Increase the Risk for Drug Abuse?"

2. Prepare a one-page summary that addresses the long-term effect stimulants have on growth and appetite.

3. Review the "black box" warning that the Drug Safety and Risk Management Advisory Committee of the FDA recommended to be added to the product labeling of stimulants used to treat ADHD. What patient population does this "black box" warning affect, and what events prompted this recommendation by the FDA?

4. Develop an appropriate recommendation for product conversion in a patient who is switching from oral methylphenidate (Concerta) 36 mg po daily to methylphenidate (Daytrana) Transdermal Patch.

5. Perform a literature search and defend or refute the role of modafinil, selective serotonin reuptake inhibitors, and atypical antipsychotics in the treatment of ADHD.

CLINICAL PEARL

Stimulant medications are considered first-line therapy in children with ADHD. If a patient does not respond adequately to initial therapy, a second or even third stimulant should be tried before initiating a non-stimulant medication. Most patients will be successfully treated by an alternative stimulant.

REFERENCES

1. American Academy of Pediatrics, Subcommittee on Attention-Deficit/Hyperactivity Disorder and Committee on Quality Improvement. Clinical practice guideline: treatment of the school-aged child with attention-deficit/hyperactivity disorder. Pediatrics 2001;108:1033–1044.

2. Institute for Clinical Systems Improvement. Health care guideline: diagnosis and management of attention deficit hyperactivity disorder in primary care for school-age children and adolescents, 7th ed. March 2007. Available at: *http://www.icsi.org/adhd/adhd_2300.html.* Accessed April 9, 2008.

3. Rappley MD. Attention deficit-hyperactivity disorder. N Engl J Med 2005;352:165–173.

4. Abramowicz M, Zuccotti G, Pflomm JM, et al. Drugs for treatment of ADHD. Treatment Guidelines from The Medical Letter. 2006;4:77–82.

5. Culpepper L. Primary care treatment of attention-deficit/hyperactivity disorder. J Clin Psychiatry 2006;67:51–58.

6. Allen AJ, Kurlan RM, Gilbert DL, et al. Atomoxetine treatment in children and adolescents with ADHD and comorbid tic disorders. Neurology 2005;65:1941–1949.

68

EATING DISORDERS: ANOREXIA NERVOSA

Frail Featherweight . . . . .Level III

Jasmine D. Gonzalvo, PharmD

Darin C. Ramsey, PharmD, BCPS

LEARNING OBJECTIVES

After completing this case study, the reader should be able to:

- Define anorexia nervosa according to DSM-IV criteria, and classify the disorder as either restrictive or binge-eating/purging.

- Recognize and assess signs and symptoms commonly associated with the presentation of longstanding, relapsing anorexia nervosa.

- Name effective pharmacologic and nonpharmacologic treatment options for the management of anorexia nervosa.

- Recommend a therapeutic treatment plan for comprehensive inpatient management and outpatient interdisciplinary follow-up of anorexia nervosa.

- Specify monitoring parameters and counseling points for a patient with anorexia nervosa.

PATIENT PRESENTATION

Chief Complaint

"How long am I going to need to be in the hospital? I'd like to get back to exercising as soon as possible."

HPI

Rachel Townsend is a 24-year-old woman who was brought to the ED after fracturing her leg while running. She states that there was suddenly a sharp pain in her leg while she was on the treadmill after about 1 hour. Her roommate heard Rachel calling for help and subsequently brought her to the ED.

She has fractured her left femur two times in the past 2 years while exercising. After her second fracture last year, a DXA scan revealed that she was osteopenic with a T-score of −1.7. At that time, she was placed on a calcium and vitamin D supplement. She has a history of anorexia nervosa for the past 6 years, but now claims that she has recovered and "eats all the time." Rachel seems defensive when asked about her eating habits but states that she has always

counted calories and exercised to "stay fit." She reports that her antidepressant did not seem to be helping anymore and she subsequently stopped taking it about 3 months ago. She complains of being tired all the time but still exercises for at least 1 hour two times daily. She denies suicidal thoughts or ideation at this time. She says that she drinks heavily on the weekends to "forget about all the problems" in her life.

During a separate interview, Rachel's roommate of 4 years reports that Rachel's daily caloric intake is probably only about 700 calories. The roommate reveals that Rachel maintains a notebook in which she records the daily amount of calories she consumes and the exact amount of calories she burns with exercise. Her normal diet consists mainly of iceberg lettuce salads, sugar-free foods, diet sodas, and water. Rachel reportedly binge drinks during the week and on the weekends and commonly does not consume any food until late at night when she gets home and eats heavily. Rachel's roommate reports that she can hear Rachel vomiting in the bathroom after her late-night food binges. The roommate states that she first noticed Rachel relapsing about 2 years ago shortly after her parents divorced.

PMH

Anorexia nervosa × 6 years
Two femur fractures to left leg in past 2 years
Osteopenia × 1 year
Suicide attempt at 19 years old
Depression × 6 years

FH

Parents divorced 2 years ago. Father is an alcoholic. Father does not currently receive treatment or counseling. Mother lives out of state.

SH

Denies tobacco use
Drinks seven to eight mixed drinks 3 to 4 days weekly (prefers whiskey and diet cola)

Meds

Fluoxetine 20 mg daily (admits noncompliance × 3 months)
Calcium 500 mg—1 tablet three times daily
Vitamin D 400 IU daily

All

NKDA

ROS

Rachel expresses feelings of hopelessness and frustration with her life in general. She seems to be craving attention from anyone who will listen. She rates her fracture pain as 4 out of 10. She reports baseline fatigue and cold intolerance. She states that she is also concerned that she has not had her period for the past year. She denies being sexually active.

Physical Examination

Gen

Pale, thin, depressed Caucasian female

VS

BP 98/72, P 52, RR 20, T 36.4°C; Wt 40.9 kg, BMI 15.4, Ht 5'4"

Skin

Dry, positive skin tenting, decreased skin turgor, lanugo hair present

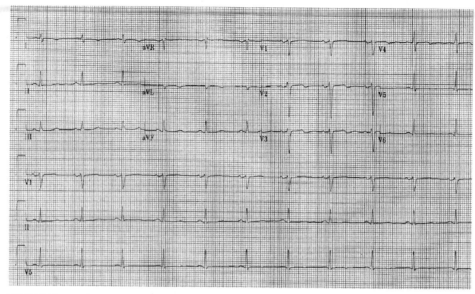

FIGURE 68-1. Admission EKG showing QT prolongation.

HEENT

Normocephalic; brittle/coarse hair; PERRLA, EOMI; no JVD; mild parotid gland enlargement

Neck/Lymph Nodes

Unremarkable

Lungs/Thorax

Lungs CTA; No rales, rhonchi, wheezes

Breasts

Atrophic; nontender

CV

Hypotensive; bradycardic

Abd

Nondistended, nontender, +BS

Genit/Rect

Unremarkable

MS/Ext

No cyanosis, clubbing, edema; abrasions on palmar surface of hands (Russell's sign)

Neuro

A & O × 3

■ Labs

Na 132 mEq/L	Hgb 11 g/dL	WBC 7.3 × 10³/mm³	AST 59 IU/L
K 2.9 mEq/L	Hct 33%	Neutros 55%	ALT 42 IU/L
Cl 82 mEq/L	RBC 5 × 10⁶/mm³	Bands 3%	*Blood Gases:*
HCO₃ 36 mEq/L	Plt 147 × 10³/mm³	Eos 2%	pH 7.50
BUN 17 mg/dL	MCV 83 fL	Lymphs 31%	pCO₂ 48 mm Hg
SCr 1.5 mg/dL	MCHC 34 g/dL	Monos 4%	pO₂ 86 mm Hg
Glu 69 mg/dL	Ferritin 110 ng/mL	ANC 1,628/mm³	Albumin 4.1 g/dL
Ca 8.9 mg/dL	Serum Iron 96 mcg/dL		hCG 1.1 mIU/mL
Mg 1.2 mg/dL	Folic acid 9.3 ng/mL		
PO₄ 2.2 mg/dL	B₁₂ 570 pg/mL		

X-ray confirming femur fracture
DXA Scan of the hip: T-score –2.3

12-lead EKG on admission reveals QT prolongation (Fig. 68-1) Follow-up EKG during inpatient stay reveals bradycardia and U waves (Fig. 68-2).

■ Assessment

1. Relapsing anorexia nervosa, complicated by dehydration, electrolyte abnormalities, and metabolic alkalosis
2. Pain secondary to femur fracture (recurrent); known osteopenia
3. Anemia
4. Amenorrhea
5. History of depression and reported nonadherence to treatment
6. Alcohol abuse

QUESTIONS

Problem Identification

1.a. Create a list of the patient's drug therapy problems.

1.b. What signs, symptoms, and laboratory values indicate the severity of the anorexia nervosa, secondary complications, and depression?

Desired Outcome

2.a. What are the goals of inpatient management of this patient as well as the long-term, follow-up treatment goals for appropriate management of this patient?

Therapeutic Alternatives

3.a. What nonpharmacologic, psychotherapy treatment strategies would be beneficial for this patient?

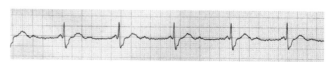

FIGURE 68-2. Follow-up EKG showing bradycardia and U waves.

3.b. What pharmacologic treatment strategies would be implemented during this patient's inpatient stay and continued or initiated after discharge?

3.c. What economic considerations apply to inpatient versus outpatient management for this patient?

Optimal Plan

4.a. What drug, dosage form, route, schedule, and duration of therapy are best for comprehensive management of this patient?

4.b. What pharmacologic alternatives would be appropriate if initial treatment interventions fail or are insufficient to achieve desired outcomes?

Outcome Evaluation

5. What clinical and laboratory parameters are necessary to evaluate the therapy for achievement of the desired therapeutic outcome and to detect or prevent adverse effects?

Patient Education

6. What information should be provided to the patient to enhance compliance, ensure successful therapy, and minimize adverse effects?

■ CLINICAL COURSE

Rachel successfully reaches a healthy weight after 2 months of refeeding and psychological counseling as an inpatient. On discharge, she seemed genuinely committed to maintaining a healthy weight and appropriate exercise regimen.

One year following this hospital discharge, she has kept her regular outpatient, follow-up visits with her primary care physician, nutritionist, and psychiatrist. She has been compliant with daily fluoxetine, calcium, and vitamin D therapy. A recent DXA scan of the hip reveals the same T-score from the previous year of –2.3. She follows a healthy diet and exercise regimen as determined by her physician and nutritionist. She still drinks heavily on the weekends, but is not in the habit of binge-eating and purging following nights of excessive alcohol intake. She is not interested in complete avoidance of alcohol at this time, because she feels that she is "still young" and should be allowed to "have fun." She says she gets depressed some days, but she reports the symptoms of depression do not seem as noticeable lately.

■ FOLLOW-UP QUESTIONS

1. Should the dose of fluoxetine be increased from 20 mg at this point, 1 year after hospital discharge?

■ SELF-STUDY ASSIGNMENTS

1. Design an appropriate TPN regimen taking into account the patient's electrolyte imbalances and nutritional status.

2. Prepare a one-page patient information handout to aid in counseling the patient on various pharmacologic treatment options if she were diagnosed with osteoporosis.

3. Modify relevant lab parameters to represent a patient presenting with acidosis from laxative abuse instead of alkalosis from excessive purging.

4. Provide a chart containing dosage conversions for commonly used opioid medications.

CLINICAL PEARL

Comprehensive management of longstanding, relapsing anorexia nervosa involves intensive pharmacologic and nonpharmacologic treatment of complications such as metabolic alkalosis with respiratory compensation, electrolyte imbalances with EKG changes, low bone mineral density, acute renal insufficiency, anemia, thrombocytopenia, amenorrhea, substance abuse issues, and psychiatric disorders.

REFERENCES

1. Yager JY, Andersen AE. Anorexia nervosa. N Engl J Med 2005; 353:1481–1488.

2. McIntosh V, Jordan J, Carter F, et al. Three psychotherapies for anorexia nervosa: a randomized, controlled trial. Am J Psychiatry 2005;162:741–747.

3. American Psychiatric Association (APA). Practice guidelines for the treatment of patients with eating disorders. 3rd ed. Washington (DC): American Psychiatric Association (APA), 2006 June.

4. Becker AE, Grinspoon SK, Klibanski A, et al. Eating disorders. N Engl J Med 1999;340:1092–1097.

5. Whitaker JS, Sware RD, Hards L. Anorexia nervosa. In: Merritt R, DeLegge MH, Holcombe BH, et al., eds. A.S.P.E.N. Nutrition Support Manual, 2nd ed. Silver Spring, MD, A.S.P.E.N., 2005:349–354.

6. Drug treatment for eating disorders. Pharmacist's Letter/Prescriber's Letter 2006;22:220811.

7. Walsh BT, Kaplan AS, Attia E, et al. Fluoxetine after weight restoration in anorexia nervosa: a randomized controlled trial. JAMA 2006; 295:2605–2612.

8. Woodside DB, Carter JC, Blackmore E. Predictors of premature termination on inpatient treatment for anorexia nervosa. Am J Psychiatry 2004;161:2277–2281.

69

ALZHEIMER'S DISEASE

Changing of the Guards. . . . . Level I

Cynthia P. Koh-Knox, PharmD

Robert W. Bennett, MS, RPh

LEARNING OBJECTIVES

After completing this case study, the reader should be able to:

- Recognize cognitive deficits and noncognitive/behavioral symptoms of Alzheimer's disease (AD).

- Recommend pharmacotherapy to manage the cognitive and behavioral symptoms of AD.

- Provide education and counseling to patients and caregivers about AD, the possible benefits and adverse effects of pharmacotherapy for the disorder, and the importance of adherence to therapy.

- List at least three theories of AD etiologies and agents under investigation based on those theories.

PATIENT PRESENTATION

◼ Chief Complaint

"Mom has become uninterested and apathetic in the past month. She is not always cooperative with daily functions. I am moving out of state to help take care of my own grandchildren; so my brother, Sam, is thinking about moving Mom to his house or to a nursing home. He will become her main caregiver."

◼ HPI

Norma Dale is a 74-year-old woman who presents to the geriatric care clinic for a routine visit accompanied by her daughter Ann. Norma was diagnosed with Alzheimer's disease 6 years ago. Her initial symptoms included forgetting times and dates easily, misplacing and losing items, repeating questions and current events, inability to answer questions, and increasing difficulty with managing finances. She was initially treated with tacrine, which was eventually discontinued due to complexity of QID dosing and elevated liver enzymes. Treatment with Aricept 10 mg at bedtime has been well tolerated for the past 4 years, and Norma has been participating more actively in family and social functions. Behavioral problems have been infrequent since diagnosis and have not been treated in the past. Since her last clinic visit, Norma began using Depends undergarments as extra protection for urinary incontinence.

Norma lives with her daughter, Ann, who reports that this living arrangement has been tolerable. As the principal caregiver, Ann has been able to maintain a regular routine with her mother's daily activities, nutrition, and financial responsibilities. However, Ann is moving in 1 month to live closer to her own daughter to help with grandchildren and has asked her youngest unmarried brother, Sam, to help take care of their mother. Sam has agreed to be his mother's caregiver. He lives and works across town and is not sure if he wants to move his mother into his home. There has been discussion about placing Norma in a long-term care facility. Norma displays lack of interest and apathy lately, especially when Ann and Sam are talking about her care. Ann asks about Norma's current Alzheimer's medication and her recent attitude and lack of cooperation.

◼ PMH

Osteoarthritis in both knees × 6 years
Alzheimer's disease diagnosed 6 years ago

◼ FH

Noncontributory, both parents deceased. Five children, four who live nearby

◼ SH

Lives with daughter; has been widowed for 10 years (husband died of cancer)

◼ Meds

Aricept 10 mg po at bedtime
Vitamin E 400 IU po once daily
Ensure drinks PRN
Acetaminophen PRN

◼ All

NKDA

◼ ROS

Reports occasional bladder incontinence and knee pain; no c/o heartburn, chest pain, or shortness of breath

◼ Physical Examination

Gen

WD woman who appears her stated age

VS

BP 126/76, P 76, RR 18, T 37°C; Wt 120 lb, Ht 5'6"

Skin

Normal texture and color

HEENT

WNL, TMs intact

Neck/Lymph Nodes

Neck supple without thyromegaly or lymphadenopathy

Lungs/Thorax

Clear, normal breath sounds

Breasts

No masses or tenderness

CV

RRR, no murmurs or bruits

Abd

Soft, NTND

Genit/Rect

Normal external female genitalia

MS/Ext

No CCE, normal ROM

Neuro

Motor, sensory, CNs, cerebellar, and gait normal. Folstein MMSE score 16/30, compared to a score of 17/30 and 19/30, last year and at the initial diagnosis, respectively. Disoriented to season, month, date, and day of week. Disoriented to country. Good registration but impaired attention and very poor short-term memory. Unable to remember any of three items after 3 minutes. Able to follow commands. Displayed apathy during MMSE.

◼ Labs

Na 139 mEq/L	Hgb 13.5 g/dL	T. bili 0.9 mg/dL	Ca 9.7 mg/dL
K 3.7 mEq/L	Hct 39.0%	D. bili 0.3 mg/dL	Phos 4.5 mg/dL
Cl 108 mEq/L	AST 25 IU/L	T. prot 7.5 g/dL	TSH 3.6 mIU/L
CO_2 25.5 mEq/L	ALT 24 IU/L	Alb 4.5 g/dL	T_4 5.9 ng/dL
BUN 16 mg/dL	Alk phos 81 IU/L	Chol 212 mg/dL	UA 6.8 mg/dL
SCr 1.1 mg/dL	GGT 22 IU/L	Trig 155 mg/dL	
Glu 102 mg/dL	LDH 85 IU/L		

◼ CT Scan (Head, 4 Years Ago)

Mild to moderate generalized cerebral atrophy

◼ Assessment

1. Alzheimer's disease, stage 5 on the Global Deterioration Scale (moderate AD—early dementia).

2. Behavioral problems reported by caregiver as lack of interest, apathy, and uncooperative behavior.

3. Occasional urinary incontinence.

4. Occasional knee pain secondary to osteoarthritis; generally well controlled with acetaminophen PRN.

QUESTIONS

Problem Identification

1.a. Create a list of the patient's drug therapy problems.

1.b. What information (signs, symptoms, laboratory values) indicates the presence or severity of the cognitive and noncognitive problems of this patient with Alzheimer's disease?

Desired Outcome

2. What are the goals of pharmacotherapy in this case?

Therapeutic Alternatives

3.a. What nondrug therapies might be useful for this patient?

3.b. What feasible pharmacotherapeutic alternatives are available for the treatment of the cognitive deficits of Alzheimer's disease?

3.c. What pharmacologic treatments may be useful to treat the noncognitive symptoms and behaviors of this patient?

3.d. What economic and psychosocial considerations are applicable to this patient?

Optimal Plan

4.a. What drug, dosage form, dose, schedule, and duration of therapy are best for the cognitive and noncognitive symptoms of this patient?

4.b. What alternatives would be appropriate if the initial therapy fails or cannot be used?

Outcome Evaluation

5. What clinical and laboratory parameters are necessary to evaluate the therapy for achievement of the desired therapeutic outcome and to detect or prevent adverse effects?

Patient Education

6. What information should be provided to the patient to enhance compliance, ensure successful therapy, and minimize adverse effects?

■ FOLLOW-UP QUESTION

1. For questions related to the use of ginkgo biloba for the treatment of Alzheimer's disease, please see Section 20 of the Casebook.

■ SELF-STUDY ASSIGNMENTS

1. Describe neurofibrillary tangles and neuritic plaques and their roles in AD development.

2. List at least three theories of the etiology of AD. What therapies are under investigation to support these theories?

3. Characterize the stages of cognitive decline as described by the global deterioration scale and define the stage where AD may be identified.

4. Differentiate cognitive deficits from noncognitive/psychiatric symptoms and behaviors of AD.

CLINICAL PEARL

Behavior symptoms may arise due to change in caregiver or change in living arrangements and should not be assumed to be due to cognitive decline.

REFERENCES

1. Grossberg GT, Desai AK. Management of Alzheimer's disease. J Gerontol A Biol Sci Med Sci 2003;58:331–353.
2. Doody RD, Stevens JC, Beck C, et al. Practice parameter: management of dementia (an evidence-based review). Report of the quality standards subcommittee of the American Academy of Neurology. Neurology 2001;56:1154–1166.
3. Morris MC. Diet and Alzheimer's disease: what evidence shows. MedGenMed 2004:6:48. (Published online January 16, 2004)
4. Adams LL, Gatchel RJ, Gentry C. Complementary and alternative medicine: applications and implications for cognitive functioning in elderly populations. Altern Ther Health Med 2001;7:52–61.
5. Sink KM, Covinsky KE, Barnes DE, et al. Caregiver characteristics are associated with neuropsychiatric symptoms of dementia. JAGS 2006; 54:796–803.
6. Kaduszkiewicz H, Zimmerman T, Beck-Bornholdr H-P, et al. Cholinesterase inhibitors for patients with Alzheimer's disease: systematic review of randomized clinical trials. BMJ 2005;331:321–327.
7. ADAPT Research Writing Committee. Naproxen and celecoxib do not prevent AD in early results from a randomized controlled trial. Neurology 2007;68:1800–1818.
8. Tariot PN, Farlow MR, Grossberg GT, et al. Memantine treatment in patients with moderate to severe Alzheimer disease already receiving donepezil. JAMA 2004;291:317–324.
9. Doraiswamy PM. Non-cholinergic strategies for treating and preventing Alzheimer's disease. CNS Drugs 2002;16:811–824.
10. Engelhart MJ, Geerlings MI, Ruitenberg A, et al. Dietary intake of antioxidants and risk of Alzheimer disease. JAMA 2002;287:3223–3229.
11. Boustani M, Watson L. The interface of depression and dementia. Psychiatric Times 2004;21. Available at: *http://www.psychiatrictimes.com/display/article/10168/47181.*
12. Wang PS, Schneeweiss S, Avorn J, et al. Risk of death in elderly users of conventional vs. atypical antipsychotic medications. N Engl J Med 2005;353:2335–2341.

70

ALCOHOL WITHDRAWAL

The Best Intentions Can
Have Consequences . . . . Level I

Kevin M. Tuohy, PharmD, BCPS

LEARNING OBJECTIVES

After completing this case study, the reader should be able to:

- Recognize the signs and symptoms of acute alcohol withdrawal syndrome.
- Recognize the common laboratory abnormalities seen in the alcohol-dependent patient.
- Develop a treatment plan for acute alcohol withdrawal and alcohol-related seizures.
- Recommend an appropriate regimen for electrolyte replacement in an alcohol-dependent patient.

PATIENT PRESENTATION

Chief Complaint

"My father has been confused, sweating, and shaking all day. I think he had a seizure an hour ago."

HPI

Matthew Fitzgerald is a 67-year-old man who is brought to the ED by his 38-year-old daughter. She states that her father has abused alcohol for as long as she can remember. She states that his typical weekly consumption for the past 15 years has averaged about three to four cases of beer per week. She reports that she and her younger sister staged an intervention with their father a few days earlier in an effort to curtail his alcohol abuse. He was limited to one case of beer per week with consumption only allowed between Thursday and Sunday. It is now Monday evening and he has not had a drink since Sunday afternoon.

PMH

Alcohol abuse and dependence
Alcohol withdrawal with seizure 10 years prior
Hypertension × 8 years
GERD × 5 years

SH

The patient is a retired construction worker. He retired 2 years ago. Currently unmarried, his wife died of breast cancer 4 years ago. Has been a heavy drinker for past 30 years. Drinks an average of 12 beers per day for past 15 years. (+) tobacco history—quit 6 years ago. Denies any illicit drug use.

Meds

Hydrochlorothiazide 25 mg po daily
Nifedipine XL 30 mg po daily
OTC omeprazole 20 mg po daily

All

Sulfa

ROS

The patient exhibits overall confusion and is not responsive to questions. Daughter states his mental status was normal until this afternoon when his confusion, sweating, and shakiness started.

Physical Examination

Gen

Thin, undernourished-appearing male, in mild distress who is acutely confused and tremulous

VS

BP 158/85, P 105, RR 20, T 38.3°C; Wt 60 kg, Ht 5'10"

Skin

Moist, diaphoretic

HEENT

Head—atraumatic, icteric sclera, PERRLA, EOMI, mild AV nicking seen on funduscopic exam

Neck/Lymph Nodes

Supple, no thyromegaly or lymphadenopathy

Lungs/Thorax

Symmetric, lungs CTA

CV

RRR, no MRG

Abd

Soft, nontender; (+) bowel sounds; (+) hepatomegaly

Genit/Rect

(−) occult blood in stool

MS/Ext

Confused, tremor in both hands

Neuro

A & O only to person, DTRs exaggerated

Labs

Na 137 mEq/L	Phos 2.7 mg/dL	PT 14.6 sec
K 3.2 mEq/L	Ca 9.5 mg/dL	INR 1.25
Cl 87 mEq/L	GGT 305 IU/L	ETOH (−)
CO₂ 23 mEq/L	AST 250 IU/L	
BUN 14 mg/dL	ALT 120 IU/L	
SCr 1.2 mg/dL	T. bili 1.6 mg/dL	
Glu 108 mg/dL	D. bili 0.7 mg/dL	
Mg 1.4 mEq/L	Alb 2.3 g/dL	

Assessment

Alcohol withdrawal with possible seizure

QUESTIONS

Problem Identification

1.a. Create a list of patient's drug therapy problems.

1.b. What information (signs, symptoms, laboratory values) indicates that this patient is experiencing alcohol withdrawal?

1.c. What signs, symptoms, and history are consistent with alcohol dependence in this patient?

1.d. What laboratory abnormalities may be expected in a patient with a history of alcohol abuse?

Desired Outcome

2. What are the goals of pharmacotherapy in this case?

Therapeutic Alternatives

3.a. What pharmacotherapeutic alternatives are available for the treatment of alcohol withdrawal?

3.b. How should alcohol withdrawal seizures be managed pharmacologically?

3.c. What electrolyte imbalances need to be corrected in this patient, and what vitamin deficiencies should be corrected?

Optimal Plan

4. Design an appropriate pharmacotherapy regimen for the treatment of alcohol withdrawal in this patient. Include recommendations for electrolyte replacement and correction of vitamin deficiencies, as well as for the management of the patient's other medical problems.

Outcome Evaluation

5. What clinical and laboratory parameters are necessary to evaluate your therapy for the achievement of desired therapeutic outcome and to detect or prevent adverse effects?

Patient Education

6. What information should be provided to the patient to enhance compliance, ensure successful therapy, and minimize adverse effects?

■ SELF-STUDY ASSIGNMENTS

1. Research alcohol-related treatment websites that can be recommended to patients with alcohol dependence.

2. Discuss the pharmacologic options that are currently marketed in the United States (FDA-approved drugs) for the treatment of alcohol dependence.

CLINICAL PEARL

Very high doses of benzodiazepines are often needed to control the symptoms of alcohol withdrawal. This is due to cross tolerance between alcohol and benzodiazepines.

REFERENCES

1. Mayo-Smith MF. Pharmacological management of alcohol withdrawal: a meta-analysis and evidence-based practice guideline. American Society of Addiction Medicine Working Group on Pharmacological Management of Alcohol Withdrawal. JAMA 1997;278:144–151.

2. Holbrook AM, Crowther R, Lotter A, et al. Meta-analysis of benzodiazepine use in treatment of acute alcohol withdrawal. CMAJ 1999;160:649–655.

3. Saitz R, O'Malley SS. Pharmacotherapies for alcohol abuse. Withdrawal and treatment. Med Clin North Am 1997;81:881–907.

4. Mayo-Smith MF, Beecher LH, Fischer TL, et al. Management of alcohol withdrawal delirium: an evidence-based practice guideline. Arch Intern Med 2004;164:1405–1412.

5. Rathlev NK, Ulrich AS, Delanty N, et al. Alcohol-related seizures. J Emerg Med 2006;31:157–163.

6. Hillbom M, Pieninkeroinen I, Leone M. Seizures in alcohol-dependent patients. Epidemiology, pathophysiology and management. CNS Drugs 2003;17:1013–1030.

7. Sullivan JT, Sykora K, Schniederman J, et al. Assessment of alcohol withdrawal: the revised clinical institute withdrawal assessment for alcohol scale (CIWA-Ar). Br J Addict 1989;84:1353–1357.

71

NICOTINE DEPENDENCE

Smoke Gets in Your Eyes . . . . Level I

Julie C. Kissack, PharmD, BCPP

LEARNING OBJECTIVES

After completing this case study, the reader should be able to:

- Explain the adverse effects to people exposed to second-hand smoke.

- Interpret the stage of change exhibited by a specific patient, and prepare an action plan to promote smoking cessation and nicotine abstinence based on the 5A plan.

- Design patient-specific recommendations for initiating lifestyle modifications and pharmacologic treatment to encourage reduction or elimination of cigarette smoke exposure.

- Recommend alternative treatments for nicotine dependence if an initial plan fails.

- Develop patient counseling on the use of pharmacotherapeutic agents used to treat nicotine dependence for a specific patient.

PATIENT PRESENTATION

■ Chief Complaint

"I need help!"

■ HPI

J.I. Kickit is a 59-year-old woman who presents to the community pharmacy with complaints of a biased administration at her workplace. A smoking ban at her health care facility will begin in 3 weeks. She states that "I need the income but could work part time to pay the bills. I don't want to quit smoking. What can you suggest to help me get through my shift without going though nicotine withdrawal? Oh, and don't suggest those nicotine patches. I tried those in the past and they just made me want to smoke more."

■ PMH

S/P hysterectomy 4 months prior to this visit.
Hypertension diagnosed at age 41.
Depression with anxiety diagnosed at age 35.
Chronic back pain diagnosed at age 38.
Migraine headaches diagnosed at age 23, increased frequency over the past 6 months. Headaches are so severe now that patient is calling in sick to work at least once per week.
Insomnia diagnosed at age 49.

■ FH

Mother died at age 78 of natural causes. Father died at age 61 of a heart attack. Patient is the oldest child of four siblings. All siblings have smoked cigarettes, but in the past 5 years, two of the siblings have quit smoking. Son and daughter do not smoke. Twenty-nine-year-old son has attention deficit hyperactivity disorder (ADHD). Twenty-five-year-old daughter was hospitalized with a collapsed lung 8 years ago.

■ SH

This pediatric nurse works the night shift (11 PM–7 AM) at a local hospital. She smokes 2 packs of cigarettes daily and has smoked for the past 45 years. She drinks 15 cups of coffee a day when she is working. She states that she drinks one glass of wine every 3 months. Son lives in the mother's home intermittently throughout the year. Son is a nonsmoker. Conflict arises frequently between patient and her son about her cigarette smoking.

■ Meds

Imitrex 6 mg injection PRN migraine headache, not to exceed two doses per day
Meloxicam 15 mg po daily
Amitriptyline 75 mg po at bedtime
Hydrochlorothiazide 25 mg po daily
Ambien CR 12.5 mg po at bedtime
Escitalopram 10 mg po daily

■ All

NKDA

■ ROS

No problems noted

■ Physical Examination

Gen

Disheveled, heavy-set African-American woman who looks older than her stated age, with an anxious demeanor. Strong odor of cigarette smoke.

VS

BP 118/75, P 100 obtained at the pharmacy

Skin

Pale, yellowed skin on fingers

HEENT

Yellow teeth, wrinkled facial skin
No other PE information is available

■ Labs

None available

■ Assessment

Patient's quality of life is compromised by cigarette smoking status and exposure to second-hand smoke (SHS) at work during smoke breaks, increased migraine headache frequency, and anxiety about work policy changes concerning cigarette smoking.

QUESTIONS

Problem Identification

1.a. Create a list of this patient's drug therapy problems.

1.b. What information in the patient's history can be identified as disease or symptoms directly related to the patient's smoking history (Fig. 71-1)?

1.c. Identify the stage of change that the patient is currently in at this time of her life, and describe your intervention plan using one of the A's from the 5A intervention plan for smokers (Table 71-1).

1.d. Describe aspects of the case that reveal the severity of nicotine dependence.

A Cigarette and Select Smoke Components

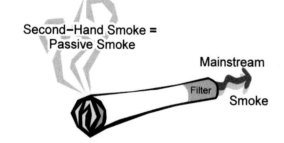

Cigarette Smoke

Gaseous Component	Particulate Component
Carbon monoxide	Nicotine
Hydrogen cyanide	Tobacco alkaloids
Toluene	Tar
Methanol	Polynuclear Aromatic
Acetone	Hydrocarbons (PAH)

FIGURE 71-1. A cigarette and select smoke components.

Desired Outcome

2. What are the goals of smoking cessation pharmacotherapy for this patient?

Therapeutic Alternatives

3.a. Describe nondrug therapies that may help this patient continue to work in her job.

3.b. What pharmacotherapeutic alternatives are available for the treatment of the nicotine dependence, and which would be an acceptable recommendation to make to this patient?

3.c. What economic, psychosocial, racial, and ethical issues need to be considered in this patient's treatment?

Optimal Plan

4. What drug, dosage form, dose, schedule, and duration of therapy are best for this patient?

Outcome Evaluation

5. What clinical and laboratory parameters are necessary to evaluate the therapy for achievement of the desired therapeutic outcome and to detect or prevent adverse effects?

Patient Education

6. What information should be provided to the patient about the medication you recommended to enhance compliance, ensure successful outcome, and minimize adverse effects?

■ SELF-STUDY ASSIGNMENTS

1. Evaluate current literature concerning the use of varenicline (Chantix). State the mechanism of action of this medication, dosing considerations, and potential adverse effects. Explain how Chantix should be used to help smokers quit when compared with other products used for smoking cessation.

2. Visit the *smokefree.gov* website and select three studies that are currently enrolling smokers to help them quit smoking. Compare and contrast the three studies. Create a flyer that could be used to recruit patients to one of the three studies.

TABLE 71-1	Stages of Change and Smoking Cessation Counseling	
Stage of Change	**Patient's Mindset**	**Response**
Precontemplation	Not interested in quitting, fails to recognize smoking as a problem.	Provide concise and relevant statement about why the smoker should think about quitting smoking.
Contemplation	Smoking is a problem and might consider quitting.	State that there is good evidence that cigarette smoke and second-hand smoke are dangerous. Encourage smoker to quit.
Preparation	Cigarette smoking is problematic and now ready to think about quitting.	Discuss options for treatment—both pharmacotherapeutic and nonpharmacotherapeutic.
Action	Motivated to quit, instituting a plan with an identified quit date and developing a plan to cope with stressors.	Encourage quit attempt, offer to be a resource during the quit attempt and praise former smokers' abstinent status.
Maintenance	Former smokers who have not smoked for a period of time.	Great job staying quit. Continued cessation is a positive move in becoming healthier.

3. Review the Surgeon General's report about second-hand smoke found at *http://www.surgeongeneral.gov/library/secondhandsmoke*. Develop a 10-item list stating how second-hand smoke acts as a toxin to cause disease. Write a two-page paper delineating how you could use this information to encourage smokers to quit smoking.

CLINICAL PEARL

No second-hand smoke exposure is safe. An intervention with a smoker must be personalized and relevant to the smoker's current stage of change status (see Table 71-1). Smoking cessation is achieved through a dynamic process involving pharmacotherapy and nonpharmacotherapy treatments.

REFERENCES

1. Okuyemi KS, Nollen NL, Ahluwalia JS. Interventions to facilitate smoking cessation. Am Fam Physician 2006;74:262–271, 276.
2. U.S. Department of Health and Human Services. The Health Consequences of Involuntary Exposure to Tobacco Smoke: A Report of the Surgeon General—Executive Summary. U.S. Department of Health and Human Services, Centers for Disease Control and Prevention, Coordinating Center for Health Promotion, National Center for Chronic Disease Prevention and Health Promotion, Office on Smoking and Health, 2006. Available at: *http://www.surgeongeneral.gov/library/secondhandsmoke*.
3. Ranney L, Melvin C, Lux L, et al. Systematic review: smoking cessation intervention strategies for adults and adults in special populations. Ann Intern Med 2006;145:845–856.
4. Feret B, Orr K. Varenicline: an oral partial nicotine agonist for smoking cessation. Formulary 2006;41:265–272.
5. Fiore MC, Jaén CR, Baker TB, et al. Treating Tobacco Use and Dependence: 2008 Update. Clinical Practice Guideline. Rockville, MD: U.S. Department of Health and Human Services. Public Health Service; 2008.

72

SCHIZOPHRENIA

A Thousand Worms Inside My Body . . . . Level I

Lawrence J. Cohen, PharmD, BCPP, FASHP, FCCP

LEARNING OBJECTIVES

After completing this case study, the reader should be able to:

- Identify the target symptoms of schizophrenia.
- Manage an acutely psychotic patient with appropriate pharmacotherapy.
- Manage adverse effects of the antipsychotics.
- Discuss the role of atypical antipsychotics in the treatment of schizophrenia.

PATIENT PRESENTATION

■ Chief Complaint

"I want to see my lawyer."

■ HPI

This is the first admission for Anita Gonzalez, a 32-year-old woman who was brought to the state hospital by the police. The patient apparently has been delusional and believes people sneak into her room at night when she is asleep and place a thousand worms inside her body. She also believes that she is being raped by passing men on the street. She is quite preoccupied about having massive wealth. She claims to have bought some gold and left it at the grocery store. She believes that her ideas have been given to a Cuban communist who has had plastic surgery to look like her and is using her ID to take possession of all of her property. She states that she is having difficulty getting her property back.

Apparently, the precipitating event causing her hospitalization was that she created a disturbance at a local fast-food restaurant, claiming that she owned it. Because of the disturbance, police were called, and she subsequently was sent here on an order of protective custody. According to the patient, she bought a hamburger and sat down to eat it, and for some reason somebody called the police and charged her with illegal trespassing. She claims that 6 years ago she was raped by a relative of a sister and broke her hip in the process. She states that her feet were cut off because she would not do what her impostors wanted her to do, and her feet were subsequently sent back to her from Central America and were reattached.

Her speech is quite rambling. She speaks of having been part of an experiment in Monterey, Mexico, in which 38 eggs were taken from her body, and children were produced from them and then killed by the government. She claims that she has worms in her that are the type that kill dogs and horses and says that they have been put there by the government. She also claims that at one time she had transmitters in her backbone and that it took 3 years to have them taken out by the government. She claims to have had surgery in the past, and the surgeon didn't know what he was doing and took out her gallbladder and put it in the intestines, where it exploded. The patient also states that on one occasion a physician was removing the snakes from her abdominal cavity, and the snakes killed the doctor and a nurse. She also claims that she worked as a surgeon herself before 1963.

■ Past Psychiatric History

The patient denies any prior hospitalization for mental problems and denies any street drugs or significant substance use. There is some history of her having frequent visits to the local hospital. She denies any drug or alcohol use. She smokes two packs of cigarettes per day.

■ PMH

The patient's past records indicate that she did have gallbladder surgery (cholecystectomy) 2 months ago.
There is no record of her ever being raped or having a broken hip.
No further medical history is known.

■ Family Psychiatric History

The patient claims that her alleged family is not really her family and that she is not sure who is her family.

■ Meds

None noted

■ All

Penicillin→rash

■ Legal/Social Status

Divorced; heterosexual; lives in an apartment alone; employment history unknown

TABLE 72-1 Lab Values

Na 140 mEq/L	Hgb 14.6 g/dL	WBC $11.0 \times 10^3/mm^3$	AST 34 IU/L	Ca 9.6 mg/dL
K 3.9 mEq/L	Hct 45.7%	Neutros 66%	ALT 22 IU/L	Phos 5.1 mg/dL
Cl 104 mEq/L	RBC $4.7 \times 10^6/mm^3$	Lymphs 24%	Alk phos 89 IU/L	TSH 4.5 μIU/mL
CO_2 22 mEq/L	MCV 90.2 μm^3	Monos 8%	GGT 38 IU/L	RPR negative
BUN 19 mg/dL	MCH 31 pg	Eos 1%	T. bili 0.9 mg/dL	Urine pregnancy (−)
SCr 1.1 mg/dL	MCHC 34.5 g/dL	Basos 1%	Alb 3.6 g/dL	
Glu 100 mg/dL		Plt $232 \times 10^3/mm^3$	T. chol 208 mg/dL	

■ Mental Status Examination

The patient is a white female of Hispanic ethnicity, modestly dressed, with some disarray. She is morbidly obese. Her hair is black and unwashed. She is alert, is oriented, and in no acute distress. Her speech is clear, constant, pressured, with many grandiose delusions and illogical thoughts. She is quite rambling, going from one subject to the other without interruption. Her affect is mood-congruent, her mood is euphoric, and there is a marked degree of grandiosity. Her thought processes are quite illogical, with marked delusional thinking. There is no evidence of auditory hallucinations, and she denies visual hallucinations. She denies any suicidal or homicidal ideation, but she is quite verbal and pressured in her thought content, verbalizing a great deal about the things that have been taken away from her illegally by people impersonating her. She has marked delusional symptoms, with paranoid ideation prominent. Her memory (immediate, recent, and remote) is fair. Her cognition and concentration are adequate. Her intellectual functioning is within the average range. Insight and judgment are markedly impaired.

■ ROS

Reports occasional GI upset; complains that worms are inside her stomach; otherwise negative

■ Physical Examination

VS

BP 140/85, P 80, RR 17, T 37.1°C; Wt 97 kg; Ht 5'3"

HEENT

PERRLA; EOMI; fundi benign; throat and ears clear; TMs intact

Skin

Scratches on both hands

Neck

Supple, no nodes; normal thyroid

Lungs

CTA & P

CV

RRR, normal S_1 and S_2

Abd

(+) BS, nontender

Ext

Full ROM, pulses 2+ bilaterally

Neuro

A & O × 3; reflexes symmetric; toes downgoing; normal gait; normal strength; sensation intact; CNs II–XII intact

■ Labs

See Table 72-1.

■ UA

Color yellow; appearance slightly cloudy; glucose (−); bili (−); ketones, trace; SG 1.025; blood (−); pH 6.0; protein (−); nitrites (−); leukocyte esterase (−)

ASSESSMENT

Axis I: schizophrenia, paranoid type, acute exacerbation
Axis II: none
Axis III: patient allergic to penicillin by history; S/P gallbladder surgery 2 months ago; obesity
Axis IV: unemployment
Axis V: Global Assessment of Functioning (GAF) Scale = 32

QUESTIONS

Problem Identification

1.a. Create a list of the patient's drug therapy problems.

1.b. Which information (signs, symptoms, laboratory values) indicates the presence or severity of an acute exacerbation of schizophrenia, paranoid type?

Desired Outcome

2. What are the goals of pharmacotherapy in this case?

Therapeutic Alternatives

3.a. What nondrug therapies might be useful for this patient?

3.b. What pharmacotherapeutic options are available for the treatment of this patient?

Optimal Plan

4.a. What drug, dosage form, dose, schedule, and duration of therapy are best for this patient?

4.b. What alternatives would be appropriate if the initial therapy fails or cannot be used?

Outcome Evaluation

5. What clinical and laboratory parameters are necessary to evaluate the therapy for achievement of the desired therapeutic outcome and to detect or prevent adverse effects?

Patient Counseling

6. What information should be provided to the patient to enhance adherence, ensure successful therapy, and minimize adverse effects?

SELF-STUDY ASSIGNMENTS

1. Perform a literature search regarding weight gain with each of the atypical antipsychotics currently marketed. Which ones are more likely to cause weight gain? Which ones are less likely to cause weight gain?

2. Perform a literature search regarding QTc changes with both typical and atypical antipsychotics. Which antipsychotics are more likely to alter the QT interval?

3. Review the pharmacoeconomic literature for the atypical antipsychotics. For your geographic area, compare costs for the average daily doses of haloperidol, aripiprazole, clozapine, olanzapine (oral, rapid-dissolving formulation and IM), risperidone (oral, rapid-dissolving formulation and long-acting injection), quetiapine, and ziprasidone (oral and IM).

CLINICAL PEARL

A benzodiazepine (lorazepam) can be scheduled routinely during the initiation of an antipsychotic to minimize aggression and allow time for the antipsychotic to take effect. The addition of lorazepam may also allow lower dosages to be used initially and during the maintenance phase of treatment.

ACKNOWLEDGMENT

Special thanks to William H. Benefield Jr., PharmD, BCPP, FASCP, for his contribution in the initial development of this case.

REFERENCES

1. Marder SR. Facilitating compliance with antipsychotic medication. J Clin Psychiatry 1998;59(Suppl 3):21–25.

2. Freedman R. Schizophrenia. N Engl J Med 2003;349:1738–1749.

3. Expert consensus panel for optimizing pharmacologic treatment of psychotic disorders. Expert consensus guideline series. Optimizing pharmacologic treatment of psychotic disorders. J Clin Psychiatry 2003;64(Suppl 12);2–97.

4. Revicki DA. Methods of pharmacoeconomic evaluation of psychopharmacologic therapies for patients with schizophrenia. J Psychiatry Neurosci 1997;22:256–266.

5. Glazer WM. Olanzapine and the new generation of antipsychotic agents: patterns of use. J Clin Psychiatry 1997;8(Suppl 10):18–21.

6. Kinon BJ, Basson BR, Gilmore JA, et al. Long-term olanzapine treatment: weight change and weight-related health factors in schizophrenia. J Clin Psychiatry 2001;62:92–100.

7. Conley RR, Kelly DL, Richardson CM, et al. The efficacy of high-dose olanzapine versus clozapine in treatment-resistant schizophrenia: a double-blind crossover study. J Clin Psychopharmacol 2003;23:668–671.

8. Nelson MW, Reynolds R, Kelly DL, et al. Safety and tolerability of high dose quetiapine in treatment refractory schizophrenia: preliminary results from an open-label trial. Schizophrenia Res 2003;60(Suppl):363. Abstract.

9. Sharma T, Mockler D. The cognitive efficacy of atypical antipsychotics in schizophrenia. J Clin Psychopharmacol 1998;18(Suppl 1):12S–19S.

10. Taylor DM, McAskill R. Atypical antipsychotics and weight gain: a systematic review. Acta Psychiatr Scand 2000;101:416–432.

ADDITIONAL RESOURCES

1. Texas Medication Algorithm Project (TMAP). Available at: *http://www.dshs.state.tx.us/mhprograms/disclaimer.shtm.*

2. Lieberman JA, Stroup TS, McEvoy JP, et al., for the Clinical Antipsychotic Trials of Intervention Effectiveness (CATIE) Investigators. Effectiveness of antipsychotic drugs in patients with chronic schizophrenia. N Engl J Med 2005;353:1209–1223.

73

MAJOR DEPRESSION

A Life Worth Living . . . . Level I

Brian L. Crabtree, PharmD, BCPP

Victor G. Dostrow, MD

LEARNING OBJECTIVES

After completing this case study, the reader should be able to:

- Identify the signs and symptoms of depression.

- Develop a pharmacotherapy plan for a patient with depression.

- Compare side effect profiles of various antidepressant drugs.

- Discuss pharmacoeconomic considerations that must be taken into account when selecting antidepressant therapy.

PATIENT PRESENTATION

Chief Complaint

"I don't know if I can handle this anymore."

HPI

Geneva Flowers is a 41-year-old woman who is referred by her family physician to an outpatient mental health clinic. She c/o feeling down and sad, with crying spells, trouble sleeping, increased eating, depression, impaired concentration, and fatigue. She has not worked in over 2 months and has used up her vacation and sick leave.

She went through treatment for alcoholism over a year ago. Things were going fairly well for her after her treatment and she remarried approximately 8 months ago. Arguments with her teenage sons about family issues and past incidents have made her increasingly depressed over the last few months. Her older son, 17, moved out to live with his father. Her younger son, 12, moved to live with his paternal grandparents.

She divorced the boys' father after approximately 10 years of marriage when she discovered he was having an affair with another woman. She left her second husband after approximately 2 years because of problems involving his children that caused increasing conflict with her then husband. Without a second income in the household, she accumulated large credit card debts. She began drinking and soon developed a pattern of using alcohol to relieve stress. Just before entering alcoholism treatment, there was a sexual fondling incident involving one of her son's friends while the friend was visiting her son at her house, but she was amnestic for the incident. Her present husband, her third, has been supportive of her, but she feels guilty about her failed previous marriages and her sons, worries about her debt, and has become more despondent. She has taken a leave of absence from her job as a school secretary.

The patient sought treatment for depression 3 months ago from her family physician, who prescribed mirtazapine. Her spirits have not improved, and she says the medication made her gain weight. Because of vague references the physician believed could possibly indicate suicidal ideas, she has been referred for psychiatric evaluation.

■ PMH

Childhood illnesses—she has had all of the usual childhood illnesses. She was hospitalized at age 3 for bacterial meningitis but knows of no residual effects.

Adult illnesses—no current nonpsychiatric adult illnesses; no previous psychiatric treatment.

Trauma—fractured arm due to bicycle accident at age 9, otherwise unremarkable.

Surgeries—Hx childbirth by C-section; tonsillectomy at age 6.

Travel—no significant travel history.

Diet—no dietary restrictions. Despite not having much of an appetite, reports eating more since taking mirtazapine.

Exercise—no regular exercise program.

Immunizations—no personal records of childhood vaccinations; had tetanus booster 9 years ago.

■ FH

Mother and father are in good health except father's well-controlled HTN. A sister has depression and anxiety, takes antidepressant medication; G.F. doesn't know its name. A second sister committed suicide.

■ SH

High school graduate; works as a school secretary but on leave of absence for approximately 2 months. Married approximately 8 months, two previous divorces. Lives with husband and sons until sons moved out in the last few weeks. Health insurance is through the school district; includes adjusted copay on prescriptions. Mental health care is covered 50%. Reports heavy credit card debt. Attended church regularly in the past (Protestant), but not recently. Attends AA weekly.

Denies drinking alcohol since treatment. Denies smoking. Drinks three to four cups of caffeinated coffee per day; usually drinks iced tea with evening meal; drinks colas as leisure beverage. Used marijuana a few times after high school, denies any use in more than 10 years; denies use of other illicit substances.

■ Meds

Mirtazapine 30 mg at bedtime (started on mirtazapine 15 mg at bedtime approximately 3 months ago)

Ortho-Novum 1/35-28, 1 po daily; hasn't taken for 2 months

St. John's wort 300 mg po TID for the last 2 weeks at suggestion of husband (purchased at health food store)

APAP 1,000–1,500 mg as needed for headaches, 2 or 3 times a week

Uses OTC antihistamines and decongestants for colds or allergies; none in recent months

■ All

NKDA

■ ROS

General appearance—pt c/o feeling tired much of the time

HEENT—wears contact lenses; no tinnitus, ear pain, or discharge; no c/o nasal congestion; Hx of dental repair for caries

Chest—no Hx of asthma or other lung disease

CV—reports occasional feelings of "pounding heart"; no Hx of heart disease

GI—reports infrequent constipation; takes MOM PRN; has gained 9 lbs in last 2 months

GU—has regular menses; LMP ended a week ago

Neuromuscular—occasional headaches, worse over the past few months; no syncope, vertigo, weakness or paralysis, numbness or tingling

Skin—no complaints

■ Physical Examination

Performed by nurse practitioner

Gen

Overweight WF, slightly unkempt

VS

BP 132/78, P 88, RR 22, T 36.9°C; Wt 187 lbs, Ht 5'8"

Skin

Normal skin, hair, and nails

HEENT

PERRLA; EOM intact, no nystagmus. Fundus—disks sharp, no retinopathy; no nasal discharge or nasal polyps; TMs gray and shiny bilaterally; minor accumulation of cerumen

Neck/Lymph Nodes

Supple without thyromegaly or lymphadenopathy

Chest/Lungs

Frequent sighing during examination, but no tachypnea or SOB; chest CTA

Breasts

No masses or tenderness

Heart

RRR without murmur

Abd

Soft, nontender; (+) BS; no organomegaly

Genit/Rect

Deferred

Ext

Unremarkable

Neuro

CN—EOM intact, no nystagmus, no weakness of facial or tongue muscles. Casual gait normal. Finger-to-nose normal. Motor—normal symmetric grip strength. DTRs 2+ and equal. Sensory—intact bilaterally.

Mental Status

When seen in the clinic, the patient is pale and appears moderately overweight, dressed in casual slacks and sweater. Grooming is fair and without makeup. She speaks slowly, often not responding to questions for approximately 30 seconds before beginning answers. She describes depressed mood and lack of energy and says she feels no pleasure in life. Her husband is good to her, but she feels everyone else she loves has left her. She has no social contacts other than occasional visits by her parents. She spends most of her time in bed. She feels worthless and blames herself for her problems. She feels particularly anguished about the incident with her son's friend even though she doesn't remember it. She is often anxious and worries about the future. She wonders if her sons love her and if they will ever return. She worries how she will repay her financial debts. Her speech is logical, coherent, and goal-oriented. She denies suicidal intent but says the future seems dim to her, and she wonders sometimes if life is worth living. She admits she sometimes wishes she could just go to sleep and not wake up. She denies hallucinations. Paranoid delusions, flight of ideas (FOI), ideas of reference (IOR), and loss of awareness (LOA) are absent. There is no dysarthria or anomia.

Labs (Collected 11:45 AM)

Na 139 mEq/L	Hgb 14.0 g/dL	AST 34 IU/L
K 4.2 mEq/L	Hct 46.2%	ALT 42 IU/L
Cl 102 mEq/L	MCV 92 μm^3	GGT 38 IU/L
CO_2 24 mEq/L	MCH 29 pg	T. bili 0.8 mg/dL
BUN 12 mg/dL	Plt 234 × 10^3/mm³	T. prot 7.0 g/dL
SCr 0.9 mg/dL	WBC 7.3 × 10^3/mm³	Alb 4.4 g/dL
Glu 98 mg/dL	Segs 49%	CK 57 IU/L
Ca 9.5 mg/dL	Bands 1%	T_4 8.6 mcg/dL
Mg 1.7 mEq/L	Lymphs 42%	T_3 uptake 29%
Uric acid 4.0 mg/dL	Monos 2%	TSH 2.8 mIU/L
	Eos 6%	

UA

Glucose (–); ketones (–); pH 5.8; SG 1.016; bilirubin (–); WBC 1/hpf; protein (–), amorphous—rare, epithelial cells 1/hpf; color yellow; blood (–), RBC 0/hpf; mucus—rare; bacteria—rare; casts 0/lpf; appearance clear

Assessment

Major depressive disorder, single episode, with melancholic features

Plan

Refer for support group, psychotherapy; begin antidepressant medication

QUESTIONS

Problem Identification

1.a. Create a list of this patient's drug therapy problems.

1.b. What signs, symptoms, and laboratory values indicate depression in this patient?

1.c. What factors in the family history support a diagnosis of depression?

1.d. Is there anything in the patient's medication history that could cause or worsen depression?

Desired Outcome

2. What are the goals of pharmacotherapy in this case?

Therapeutic Alternatives

3.a. What nonpharmacologic treatments are important in this case? Should nonpharmacologic treatments be tried before beginning medication?

3.b. What pharmacotherapeutic options are available for the treatment of depression?

Optimal Plan

4.a. What drug regimen (drug, dosage, schedule, and duration) is best for this patient?

4.b. How should the patient be advised about the herbal therapy, St. John's wort?

4.c. What alternatives would be appropriate if the patient fails to respond to initial therapy?

Outcome Evaluation

5. What clinical and laboratory parameters are necessary to evaluate the therapy for efficacy and adverse effects?

Patient Education

6. What information should be provided to the patient to enhance compliance, ensure successful therapy, and minimize adverse effects?

■ FOLLOW-UP QUESTION

For questions related to the use of St. John's wort for the treatment of depression, please see Section 20 of the Casebook.

■ SELF-STUDY ASSIGNMENTS

1. Because the SSRI antidepressants are commonly used and have the same reuptake pharmacology, contrast the agents in this class, considering relative side effects, dosing, and drug interactions.

2. Compare other antidepressants with SSRIs with regard to adverse effects and relative advantages and disadvantages.

3. Discuss pharmacoeconomic considerations in antidepressant therapy, including choice of agents for inclusion in the formulary of a hospital or health maintenance organization.

4. Review the medical literature and evaluate the scientific evidence for the efficacy of St. John's wort in the treatment of depression.

CLINICAL PEARL

Although the selective serotonin reuptake inhibitors are a pharmacologic class, they are not a chemical class. Failure to respond to one SSRI does not reliably predict failure to respond to others.

REFERENCES

1. Perry PJ. Pharmacotherapy for major depression with melancholic features: relative efficacy of tricyclic versus selective serotonin reuptake inhibitor antidepressants. J Affect Disord 1996;39:1–6.
2. Cassano P, Fava M. Tolerability issues during long-term treatment with antidepressants. Ann Clin Psychiatry 2004;16:15–25.
3. Preskorn SH, Shah R, Neff M, et al. The potential for clinically significant drug-drug interactions involving the CYP2D6 system: effects with fluoxetine and paroxetine versus sertraline. J Psychiatr Pract 2007;13:5–12.
4. Ferguson JM. SSRI antidepressant medications: adverse effects and tolerability. Primary Care Companion J Clin Psychiatry 2001;3:22–27.
5. Schmidt ME, Fava M, Robinson JM, et al. The efficacy and safety of a new enteric-coated formulation of fluoxetine given once weekly during the continuation treatment of major depressive disorder. J Clin Psychiatry 2000;61:851–857.
6. Barbui C, Percudani M, Hotopf M. Economic evaluation of antidepressive agents: a systematic critique of experimental and observational studies. J Clin Psychopharmacol 2003;3:145–154.
7. Geddes JR, Carney SM, Davies C, et al. Relapse prevention with antidepressant drug treatment in depressive disorders: a systematic review. Lancet 2003;361:653–661.
8. Linde K, Mulrow CD, Berner M, et al. St. John's wort for depression. Cochrane Database Syst Rev 2005;CD000448.
9. Nierenberg AA, Fava M, Trivedi MH, et al. A comparison of lithium and T(3) augmentation following two failed medication treatments for depression: a STAR*D report. Am J Psychiatry 2006;163:1484–1486.

74

BIPOLAR DISORDER

Don't Hate Me Because I'm Beautiful . . . . Level II

Lawrence J. Cohen, PharmD, BCPP, FASHP, FCCP

LEARNING OBJECTIVES

After completing this case study, the reader should be able to:

- Outline a mental status examination and identify target symptoms of bipolar disorder when given patient interview information.

- Recommend appropriate pharmacotherapy for patients with acute mania.

- Generate parameters for monitoring anticonvulsant therapy for bipolar disorder.

- Identify the pharmacotherapeutic options for treating the subtypes of bipolar disorder.

PATIENT PRESENTATION

■ Chief Complaint

"There are hundreds of vampires in this city, and I have the documents to prove it."

■ HPI

Michael Harrison is a 25-year-old man who was brought to the hospital by police. This is his third psychiatric admission. According to neighbors who called the police, the patient has been acting increasingly strange. The lights in the house are left on all night, and spiritual music is played at all hours. Last evening, he dug a trench around his front yard with an electric lawn edger and filled it with garlic cloves. This evening, he painted crosses on the front of the house and threw furniture into his yard and the street. When approached by neighbors, he apparently began screaming and preaching at them. When the police arrived, they found the patient standing naked on the dining room table in his front yard preaching. When the police approached, he began throwing garlic tablets at them and screaming, "Become naked in the eyes of the Lord and you will be saved." He became increasingly hostile during the arrest shouting, "Don't hate me because I'm beautiful." He then tried to bite one of the officers.

■ PMH

Manic episodes first occurred while he was in college, leading to psychiatric admissions at ages 21 and 23 for acute mania. Patient was treated with haloperidol 5 mg po once daily and lithium 600 mg po Q AM and 900 mg po at bedtime, with adequate response and discharged on both occasions after about a month.
Medical problems include migraine headaches.

■ Patient Interview

Patient is disheveled with pungent body odor. He is pacing the room, waving his hands in the air and preaching in an elated, loud, sing-songy voice. He is dressed flamboyantly in a brightly colored bathrobe and appears to be wearing a garlic necklace. He is carrying a Bible. When asked how he felt, he stated, "Playful, with intense clarity,

sharp, spiffy, and clean." He then became angry, insisting that he be discharged before sunrise or he would "face the light of the right and mighty and burn in 'demonocratic' hell." He then asked for a priest to exorcise the homosexual demons from his body. He believes that vampires live in the city. He stated he has the documents to prove it and that the vampires are pursuing him to keep him from exposing their existence to Christians everywhere. He spoke in long run-on sentences with many political, religious, and sexual references. He was very difficult to interrupt. For example, at one point he stated, "Can't you see, or are you an idiot?! I am being persecuted by the right, 100 points of light, Republicans, redeeming the public, for the republic, under which I stand because I have no one to lean on, one gay man, bitten by the Democrat, the demoncrat, doomed and miserable for loving the company I keep, and that's why misery loves company, and if you don't get that you're an idiot."

When asked about his sleep, he angrily replied, "Would you sleep at a time like this? If I sleep, America will fall, and it will all be on my shoulders. The towers in New York City have already fallen because I didn't get there in time." The patient stated that he has not been eating and has not taken his lithium in several days because, "Lithium is of the ground, the underworld. The Lord will sustain me."

Through his verbose conversation, it becomes apparent that a man he picked up in a gay bar last week bit him on the neck. He also seems to believe that he has been given a mission from God as penance for visiting this bar. Several times during the interview, he began crying and wailing loudly, begging to be saved and shouting, "I'm sorry." He said something about the trials of Job and that he would be the next to die. He sang "Swing Low Sweet Chariot" in a very loud voice. When told that he might need to stay at the hospital so we could help him with his problems, he screamed, "You can't help me! Only the Lord can help me! They have drunk from the fruit of the vine. I am that fruit."

■ Abnormal Involuntary Movement Scale (AIMS)

Excessive eye blinking and mild grimacing; unclear whether abnormal (patient states this is the "demon blood" trying to take over his body). He is bothered by it in that to him it represents "his sinful nature."

■ FH

Father has a history of depression; paternal grandmother was placed in an "asylum" for hysteria secondary to childbirth. Mother and brother have Type 2 diabetes.

■ SH

Recently fired from his job as a nurse at a local hospital. Patient is a single homosexual. Religious upbringing as a Southern Baptist. Smokes one ppd for 5 years. Patient states that he drinks "only occasionally," but he was noted to be intoxicated, with a BAC 0.14%, on a previous admission.

■ Meds

Ergotamine and ibuprofen PRN for migraines

■ All

NKDA

■ ROS

Migraine headaches about twice a month, no aura, (+) nausea and photophobia. Occasional GI upset with no clear relationship to meals or time of day; frequent loose stools.

■ Physical Examination

VS

BP 118/73, P 83, RR 16, T 37.1°C; Wt 94 kg, Ht 5'2"

TABLE 74-1 Lab Values

Na 141 mEq/L	Hgb 14.6 g/dL	WBC $12.0 \times 10^3/mm^3$	AST 32 IU/L	Ca 9.7 mg/dL
K 3.8 mEq/L	Hct 45.7%	Neutros 67%	ALT 21 IU/L	Phos 5.3 mg/dL
Cl 103 mEq/L	RBC $4.73 \times 10^6/mm^3$	Lymphs 23%	Alk Phos 87 IU/L	TSH 4.1 μIU/mL
CO_2 24 mEq/L	MCV 90.2 μm^3	Monos 7%	GGT 46 IU/L	RPR: Neg
BUN 19 mg/dL	MCH 31 pg	Eos 2%	T. bili 0.9 mg/dL	Lithium 0.1 mEq/L
SCr 1.1 mg/dL	MCHC 34.4 g/dL	Basos 1%	Alb 3.7 g/dL	
Glu 89 mg/dL	Plt $256 \times 10^3/mm^3$		T. chol 218 mg/dL	

HEENT

PERRLA; EOMI; fundi benign; throat and ears clear; TMs intact; rapid eye blinking and facial grimacing (may indicate early tardive dyskinesia)

Skin

Psoriasis evident on both elbows

Neck

Supple, bite mark, no nodes

Lungs

CTA & P

CV

RRR; S_1, S_2 normal; no MRG

Abd

(+) BS, nontender

Ext

Full ROM, pulses 2+ bilaterally

Neuro

A & O × 3; reflexes symmetric; toes downgoing; normal gait; normal strength; sensation intact; CNs II–XII intact

■ Labs

See Table 74-1.

■ UA

Color yellow; appearance slightly cloudy; glucose (–), bili (–), ketones trace; SG 1.025, blood (–), pH 6.0, protein (–), nitrites (–), leukocyte esterase (–)

■ Assessment

Axis I: bipolar disorder, current episode mixed
Axis II: deferred
Axis III: migraine headache by history

QUESTIONS

Problem Identification

1.a. From the case information and patient interview, write a mental status examination for this patient.

1.b. Create a list of this patient's drug therapy problems.

1.c. What information (target symptoms, laboratory values) indicates the presence and severity of bipolar disorder, mixed episode?

Desired Outcome

2. What are the goals of pharmacotherapy in this patient?

Therapeutic Alternatives

3.a. What nondrug therapies might be useful for this patient?

3.b. What feasible pharmacotherapeutic alternatives are available for treatment of bipolar disorder?

Optimal Plan

4.a. What drug, dosage form, dose, schedule, and duration of therapy are best for this patient?

4.b. What alternatives would be appropriate if the initial therapy fails or cannot be used?

Outcome Evaluation

5. Which clinical and laboratory parameters are necessary to evaluate response to therapy and to detect or prevent adverse effects?

Patient Education

6. What information should be provided to the patient to enhance adherence, ensure successful therapy, and minimize adverse effects?

■ SELF-STUDY ASSIGNMENTS

1. Perform a literature search and explore the role of the newer anticonvulsants (lamotrigine, gabapentin, oxcarbazepine, and topiramate) in the treatment of bipolar disorder.

2. Perform a literature search on once-daily dosing of antimanic agents. How would you go about changing a patient's dosing regimen to increase adherence? Based on the literature, which patients are most suitable for conversion to once- or twice-daily dosing with lithium, carbamazepine, or valproate? Can regular-release products be used, or must the patient be converted to extended-release products?

3. Design an algorithm for the treatment of bipolar disorder. Include treatment strategies for acute mania, rapid cycling, depression, and mixed states.

CLINICAL PEARL

When a patient admitted with acute mania is taking an antidepressant, the antidepressant should be tapered and withdrawn. In some patients, antidepressants may activate mania or increase the rate of cycling, and potentially prolong response to antimanic medication.

ACKNOWLEDGMENT

Special thanks to William H. Benefield Jr., PharmD, BCPP, FASCP, for his contribution in initial development of this case.

REFERENCES

1. Swann AC, Bowden CL, Morris D, et al. Depression during mania: treatment response to lithium or divalproex. Arch Gen Psychiatry 1997;54:37–42.
2. Freeman TW, Clothier JL, Pazzaglia P, et al. A double-blind comparison of valproate and lithium in the treatment of acute mania. Am J Psychiatry 1992;149:108–111.
3. Goldberg JF, Garno JL, Leon AC, et al. Rapid titration of mood stabilizers predicts remission from mixed or pure mania in bipolar patients. J Clin Psychiatry 1998;59:151–158.
4. Tohen M, Jacobs TG, Grundy SL, et al. Efficacy of olanzapine in acute bipolar mania: a double-blind, placebo-controlled study. The Olanzapine HGGW Study Group. Arch Gen Psychiatry 2000;57:841–849.
5. Tohen M, Sanger TM, McElroy SL, et al. Olanzapine versus placebo in the treatment of acute mania. Olanzapine HGEH Study Group Trial. Am J Psychiatry 1999;156:702–709.
6. Sachs G, Mullen JA, Devine NA. Quetiapine vs placebo as adjunct to mood stabilizer for the treatment of acute mania. Eur Neuropsychopharmacol 2002;12(Suppl 3):235–236.
7. Bowden CL, Calabrese JR, Sachs G, et al. A placebo-controlled 18-month trial of lamotrigine and lithium maintenance treatment in recently manic or hypomanic patients with bipolar disorder I. Arch Gen Psychiatry 2003;60:392–400.
8. Goldsmith DR, Wagstaff AJ, Ibbotson T, et al. Spotlight on lamotrigine in bipolar disorder. CNS Drugs 2004;18:63–67.
9. Gerner RH, Stanton A. Algorithm for patient management of acute manic states: lithium, valproate, or carbamazepine? J Clin Psychopharmacol 1992;12:57S–63S.
10. Hartong EG, Moleman P, Hoogduin CA, et al. Prophylactic efficacy of lithium versus carbamazepine in treatment-naive bipolar patients. J Clin Psychiatry 2003;64:144–151.
11. McElroy SL, Keck PE, Tugrul KC, et al. Valproate as a loading treatment in acute mania. Neuropsychobiology 1993;27:146–149.
12. Sachs GS, Printz DJ, Kahn DA, et al. The Expert Consensus Guideline Series: Medication Treatment of Bipolar Disorder 2000. Postgrad Med 2000;Spec No:1-104.
13. Ghaemi SN. New treatments for bipolar disorder: the role of atypical neuroleptic agents. J Clin Psychiatry 2000;61(Suppl 14):33–42.
14. Calabrese JR, Vieta E, Sheldon MD. Latest maintenance data on lamotrigine in bipolar disorder. Eur Neuropsychopharmacol 2003;13 (Suppl 2):S57–S66.

ADDITIONAL RESOURCES

1. Systematic Treatment Enhancement Program for Bipolar Disorder (STEP-BD). Available at: *http://www.stepbd.org/referencelist.html*.
2. Texas Medication Algorithm Project (TMAP). Available at: *http://www.dshs.state.tx.us/mhprograms/disclaimer.shtm*.

75

GENERALIZED ANXIETY DISORDER

Worried Sick . . . . Level I

Sarah T. Melton, PharmD, BCPP, CGP

Cynthia K. Kirkwood, PharmD, BCPP

LEARNING OBJECTIVES

After completing this case study, the reader should be able to:

- Identify target symptoms associated with generalized anxiety disorder (GAD).
- Construct treatment goals of pharmacotherapy for GAD.
- Recommend appropriate pharmacotherapy and duration of treatment for the acute, continuation, and maintenance phases of GAD.
- Develop a plan to counsel patients and consult with providers about the pharmacotherapy used in the treatment of GAD.
- Develop a monitoring plan for a patient treated for GAD based on the treatment regimen.

PATIENT PRESENTATION

■ Chief Complaint

"I don't think my medicine is working. I worry so much I feel sick."

■ HPI

Caroline Long is a 31-year-old woman who presents to her family physician with complaints of irritability, feelings of "being on edge," and inability to fall asleep at night. She states that she always feels tense and exhausted with constant muscle tension and body aches. She has been employed as an elementary school teacher for 3 years. Over the past school year, she has had difficulty concentrating when preparing lessons and her mind often "goes blank" in the classroom. She has frequent abdominal pain and diarrhea. She constantly worries about the children in her class, her teaching ability, finances, and her relationship with her husband. She is afraid she will receive a poor evaluation and be asked to leave the school. She states that she cannot control her worry and that her anxiety has increased in intensity over the past 6 months, despite being treated with BuSpar. She denies having obsessive-compulsive thoughts or behaviors or symptoms of panic disorder. She recently discontinued hydroxyzine 12.5 mg BID and 25 mg at bedtime PRN for anxiety, after 2 weeks secondary to excessive sedation and dry mouth. She tried kava kava from an herbal store a few months ago. It was not effective, and she discontinued it after 2 weeks because of severe abdominal pain.

■ PMH

Records from the nurse practitioner indicate frequent visits over the past year for headaches, abdominal pain, and diarrhea.
After a recent visit to the ED, she was prescribed hydroxyzine to be taken at night for sleep and during the day as needed for anxiety.
No past psychiatric history.

■ FH

Father, 62-year-old, on "nerve medication" for several years. Mother, 59-year-old, with history of major depression, now doing well. Patient has one brother who has no known psychiatric or medical problems.

■ SH

Married for 5 years; no children; master's degree in elementary education; no tobacco use; little exercise because of time constraints; drinks four to five cups of coffee per day. She drinks two alcoholic drinks every evening to help her "calm down and sleep." Has prescription drug coverage through the school system.

■ Meds

BuSpar Dividose 30 mg po BID for anxiety
Sudafed PE 10 mg po QID PRN nasal congestion
Loperamide 2 mg po Q 6 h PRN diarrhea

■ All

Penicillin (hives); iodine

■ ROS

Positive only for paresthesias and mild diaphoresis; negative for dizziness, palpitations, SOB, chest pain

■ Physical Examination

Gen

Nervous, thin woman sitting on examination table; cooperative; oriented × 3

VS

BP 100/65, P 90, RR 18, T 36.5°C; Wt 50 kg, Ht 5'5"

Skin

Clammy; no rashes, lesions, or track marks

HEENT

EOMI; PERRLA; fundi benign; ear and nose clear; dentition intact; tonsils 1+

Neck/Lymph Nodes

Supple, no lymphadenopathy; thyroid symmetric and of normal size

Lungs/Chest

Symmetric chest wall movement; BS equal bilaterally; no rub; clear to A & P

Breasts

No masses or tenderness

CV

RRR, normal S_1 and S_2, no MRG

Abd

Symmetric; NTND; normal BS; no organomegaly or masses

Genit/Rect

Deferred

MS/Ext

Small frame; normal bones, joints, and muscles

Neuro

CNs II–XII intact; motor and sensory grossly normal; coordination intact

MSE

Appearance and behavior: well-groomed, good eye contact, wringing hands and bouncing legs
Speech: well-spoken, coherent with normal rate and rhythm
Mood: anxious, worried about what is wrong with her and if she can get better
Affect: full

Thought processes: linear, logical, and goal-directed
Thought content: negative for suicidal or homicidal ideations, obsessions/compulsions, delusions, or hallucinations
Memory: 3/3 at 0 minutes, 2/3 at 5 minutes; spelled "steak" backwards
Abstractions: good
Judgment: good by testing
Insight: fair
Score on Hamilton Anxiety Scale = 28 points (see Appendix A)

■ Labs

Na 142 mEq/L	Hgb 14.0 g/dL
K 4.3 mEq/L	Hct 38%
Cl 105 mEq/L	TSH 3 mIU/L
CO$_2$ 28 mEq/L	AST 23 IU/L
BUN 15 mg/dL	ALT 20 IU/L
SCr 0.9 mg/dL	Alk Phos 23 IU/L
Glu 80 mg/dL	GGT 30 IU/L

■ ECG

NSR; rate 88 bpm

■ Urine Toxicology Screen

Negative

■ Assessment

Generalized anxiety disorder

QUESTIONS

Problem Identification

1.a. Create a list of the patient's drug therapy problems.

1.b. Is there anything in the patient's medication history that could cause or worsen anxiety?

1.c. What information (signs, symptoms, laboratory values) indicates the presence or severity of GAD?

Desired Outcome

2. What are the goals of pharmacotherapy in this case?

Therapeutic Alternatives

3.a. What nonpharmacologic therapies might be useful for this patient?

3.b. What pharmacotherapeutic alternatives are available for the treatment of GAD?

Optimal Plan

4.a. What drug, dosage form, dose, schedule, and duration of therapy are best for this patient?

4.b. What pharmacotherapeutic alternatives would be appropriate if the optimal plan fails?

Outcome Evaluation

5. What clinical and laboratory parameters are necessary to evaluate the therapy for achievement of the desired therapeutic outcome and to detect or prevent adverse effects?

Patient Education

6. What information should be provided to the patient to enhance compliance, ensure successful therapy, and minimize adverse effects?

■ FOLLOW-UP QUESTION

1. For questions related to the use of kava kava for the treatment of generalized anxiety disorder, please see Section 20 of the Casebook.

■ SELF-STUDY ASSIGNMENTS

1. Perform a literature search to obtain recent information about GAD in the elderly. Write a two-page paper detailing how the elderly present with GAD and the most appropriate pharmacotherapy for treating this special population.

2. Perform a literature search to obtain recent information about the use of pregabalin in Europe for the treatment of GAD. Write a brief critical overview of the controlled trials that support the use of pregabalin in the treatment of GAD.

3. Benzodiazepines were once prescribed on long-term basis for the treatment of GAD. Write a critical review detailing the historical basis and reasoning for the current recommendation to use benzodiazepines only in the acute management of GAD.

CLINICAL PEARL

With effective pharmacotherapy available for the acute and long-term therapy of GAD, the treatment goal for anxiety is remission. Many patients exhibit treatment response but still have anxiety symptoms and social and functional impairment. Remission is a more rigorous treatment goal that requires a HAM-A score of ≤ 7 or reduction of at least 70% in baseline levels of symptoms.

REFERENCES

1. Hamilton M. Hamilton Anxiety Scale. In: Guy W, ed. ECDEU Assessment Manual for Psychopharmacology. Rockville, MD, US Department of Health, Education, Welfare, 1976:193–198.

2. Ballenger JC, Davidson JRT, Lecrubier Y, et al. Consensus statement on generalized anxiety disorder from the International Consensus Group on Depression and Anxiety. J Clin Psychiatry 2001;62(Suppl 11):53–58.

3. National Institute for Health and Clinical Excellence. Anxiety: management of anxiety (panic disorder, with or without agoraphobia, and generalised anxiety disorder) in adults in primary, secondary and community care. London: NICE, 2004 (clinical guideline 22). *http://www.nice.org.uk/guidance/CG22/niceguidance/pdf/English.* Accessed Dec. 7, 2006.

4. Kapczinski F, Lima MS, Souza N, et al. Antidepressants for generalized anxiety disorder (Cochrane Review). Cochrane Database Syst Rev 2003;2:CD003592.

5. Baldwin DS, Anderson IM, Nutt DJ, et al. Evidence-based guidelines for the pharmacological treatment of anxiety disorders: recommendations from the British Association for Psychopharmacology. J Psychopharm 2005;19:567–596.

6. Koponen H, Allgulander C, Erickson J, et al. Efficacy of duloxetine for the treatment of generalized anxiety disorder: implications for primary care physicians. Prim Care Companion J Clin Psychiatry 2007;9:100–107.

7. Frampton JE, Foster RH. Pregabalin: in the treatment of generalized anxiety disorder. CNS Drugs 2006;20:685–693.

8. Llorca PM, Spadone C, Sol O, et al. Efficacy and safety of hydroxyzine in the treatment of generalized anxiety disorder: a 3-month double-blind study. J Clin Psychiatry 2002;63:1020–1027.

9. Connor KM, Payne V, Davidson JR. Kava in generalized anxiety disorder: three placebo-controlled trials. Int Clin Psychopharmacol 2006;21:249–253.

10. Pollack MH. Optimizing pharmacotherapy of generalized anxiety disorder to achieve remission. J Clin Psychiatry 2001;62(Suppl 19):20–25.

Appendix A

The Results of the Hamilton Anxiety (HAM-A) Scale (ECDEU Version)[1] for This Patient

Mark and score as follows: 0 = not present; 1 = mild; 2 = moderate; 3 = severe; 4 = very severe

ANXIOUS MOOD

___4___ Worries, anticipation of the worst, fearful anticipation, irritability

TENSION

___3___ Feelings of tension, fatigability, startle response, moved to tears easily, trembling, feelings of restlessness, inability to relax

FEARS

___2___ Of dark, of strangers, of being left alone, of animals, of traffic, of crowds

INSOMNIA

___3___ Difficulty in falling asleep, broken sleep, unsatisfying sleep and fatigue on waking, dreams, nightmares, night terrors

INTELLECTUAL

___3___ Difficulty in concentration, poor memory

DEPRESSED MOOD

___0___ Loss of interest, lack of pleasure in hobbies, depression, early waking, diurnal swing

SOMATIC (muscular)

___2___ Pains and aches, twitchings, stiffness, myoclonic jerks, grinding of teeth, unsteady voice, increased muscular tone

SOMATIC (sensory)

___1___ Tinnitus, blurring of vision, hot and cold flushes, feelings of weakness, pricking sensation

CARDIOVASCULAR SYMPTOMS

___1___ Tachycardia, palpitations, pain in chest, throbbing of vessels, fainting feelings, sighing, dyspnea

RESPIRATORY SYMPTOMS

___1___ Pressure or constriction in chest, choking feelings, sighing, dyspnea

GASTROINTESTINAL SYMPTOMS

___3___ Difficulty in swallowing, wind, abdominal pain, burning sensations, abdominal fullness, nausea, vomiting, borborygmi, looseness of bowels, loss of weight, constipation

GENITOURINARY SYMPTOMS

___4___ Frequency of micturition, urgency of micturition, amenorrhea, menorrhagia, development of frigidity, premature ejaculation, loss of libido, impotence

AUTONOMIC SYMPTOMS

___1___ Dry mouth, flushing, pallor, tendency to sweat, giddiness, tension, headache, raising of hair

BEHAVIOR AT INTERVIEW

___3___ Fidgeting, restlessness or pacing, tremor of hands, furrowed brow, strained face, sighing or rapid respiration, facial pallor, swallowing, etc.

TOTAL SCORE: ___28___

76

OBSESSIVE-COMPULSIVE DISORDER

Five Is the Magic Number . . . . Level I

Sarah T. Melton, PharmD, BCPP, CGP

Cynthia K. Kirkwood, PharmD, BCPP

LEARNING OBJECTIVES

After completing this case study, the reader should be able to:

- Identify target symptoms associated with obsessive-compulsive disorder (OCD).

- Discuss treatment goals of pharmacotherapy for OCD.

- Recommend nonpharmacologic therapies for OCD.

- Develop an appropriate pharmacotherapy plan and duration of therapy for the management of OCD.

- Counsel patients and consult with providers about the pharmacotherapy used for OCD.

- Develop a monitoring plan for a patient treated for OCD based on the treatment regimen.

PATIENT PRESENTATION

■ Chief Complaint

"I am afraid that I'm going to hurt my baby."

■ HPI

Kayla Mitchell is a 27-year-old woman presenting to her family physician for a 6-week postpartum check-up with complaints of anxiety and feelings of unease for the past 2 weeks. She reports that she is having intrusive thoughts of harming her baby. Because these thoughts are becoming more frequent, she feels she is a bad mother and may actually harm her baby. She has started checking all appliances in the house multiple times during the day to make sure they are turned off because she fears starting a fire that will injure the baby. At first, she incessantly checked on the baby but now is beginning to avoid the baby because of her fears. She states that she knows that these thoughts are irrational. She is concerned because the checking behavior consumes 2–3 hours each day. She has stopped going out with the baby because she has to check and recheck the car seat safety belts so often that she usually does not make it to her destination. She also reports rubbing her arm in multiples of 5 to feel some relief from the overwhelming anxiety that develops throughout the day from the intrusive thoughts. She states that she has tried to hide this behavior from her husband, but it has become so time-consuming and distressful that she asked him to accompany her on this visit to the physician.

■ PMH

G_1P_1 now at 6 weeks postpartum, normal spontaneous vaginal delivery with first-degree perineal tear

Small external hemorrhoids s/p delivery

H/O complex partial seizures in childhood and teen years (off medication and seizure-free for 7 years)

■ PPH

No hospitalizations or outpatient psychiatric treatment, but she recalls from childhood doing strange counting rituals while lying in bed or watching TV. She has always felt a need to "control things."

■ FH

Father, 68-year-old, with history of major depression. Mother, 65-year-old, with multiple sclerosis. Older brother is a "perfectionist" and has to have everything "just right."

■ SH

Married for 3 years, bachelor's degree in business, presently on maternity leave from the bank where she works part-time; undecided about returning to work, no tobacco or alcohol use. Breastfed infant for 4 weeks, now bottle-feeding. She had excessive worrying that the baby was starving because he was not getting enough breast milk. She recently lost her prescription drug insurance when her husband changed jobs.

■ Meds

Docusate sodium 100 mg po BID

■ All

Sulfa (hives), adhesive bandages

■ ROS

Unremarkable except patient reports that she feels she is "going insane" and has guilt over her obsessions. Positive for dry and red skin on right arm. Patient denies fatigue, change in appetite, sleep pattern, difficulty concentrating, and crying spells. No palpitations, dyspnea.

■ Physical Examination

Gen

Anxious, WDWN woman sitting on examination table rubbing her arm up and down, cooperative, oriented × 3

VS

BP 120/75, P 80, RR 19, T 36.5°C; Wt 60 kg, Ht 5'5"

Skin

Left arm red and slightly inflamed from elbow to wrist; no rashes, lesions, or track marks. Normal hair growth and distribution.

HEENT

EOMI; PEERLA; fundi benign; ear and nose clear; dentition intact; tonsils 1+

Neck/Lymph Nodes

Supple, no lymphadenopathy; thyroid symmetric and of normal size

Lungs/Chest

Symmetric chest wall movement, BS equal bilaterally, no rub; clear to A & P

Breasts

Slight tenderness S/P weaning from breastfeeding

CV

RRR, normal S_1 and S_2, no MRG

Abd

Symmetric; NTND; normal BS; no organomegaly or masses

Gyn

Normal hair distribution and external genitalia; normal urethra; well-healed perineum; parous cervix with no lesions or discharge; uterus normal; no adnexal masses or tenderness

MS/Ext

Small frame; normal bones, joints, muscles

Neuro

CNs II–XII intact; motor and sensory grossly normal; coordination intact; no tremor

MSE

Appearance and behavior: well-groomed, poor eye contact, rubbing arm up and down in a slow methodical manner

Speech: well-spoken, coherent with normal rate and rhythm

Mood: anxious, worried that she is a bad mother and will harm her baby

Affect: anxious, frightened

Thought processes: linear, logical, and goal-directed

Thought content: negative for suicidal or homicidal ideations; positive for obsessions about harming her child; compulsions including checking and rubbing arm in multiples of 5; denies delusions and hallucinations

Memory: 3/3 at 0 minutes, 3/3 at five minutes (ball, pencil, chair); spelled "horse" backwards

Abstractions: fair

Judgment: good by testing

Insight: good

Score on Yale-Brown Obsessive Compulsive Scale = 28 points

■ Labs

Na 140 mEq/L	Hgb 15.0 g/dL
K 3.7 mEq/L	Hct 40%
Cl 107 mEq/L	TSH 2.8 mIU/L
CO_2 28 mEq/L	AST 28 IU/L
BUN 14 mg/dL	ALT 25 IU/L
SCr 0.8 mg/dL	Alk Phos 42 IU/L
Glu 75 mg/dL	

■ ECG

NSR; rate 80 bpm

■ Urine Toxicology Screen

Negative

■ Assessment

Obsessive-compulsive disorder

■ Plan

1. Start clomipramine, 50 mg po HS
2. Refer patient to Michelle Johnston, PhD, for cognitive behavioral therapy

QUESTIONS

Problem Identification

1.a. Create a list of the patient's drug therapy problems.

1.b. Is there anything in the patient's history that could be considered a risk factor for the development of OCD?

1.c. What information (signs, symptoms, laboratory values) indicates the presence or severity of OCD?

Desired Outcome

2. What are the goals of pharmacotherapy for OCD in this case?

Therapeutic Alternatives

3.a. What nonpharmacologic therapies might be useful for this patient?

3.b. What pharmacotherapeutic alternatives are available for the treatment of OCD?

Optimal Plan

4.a. What drug, dosage form, dose, schedule, and duration of therapy are best for this patient?

4.b. What pharmacotherapeutic alternatives would be appropriate if the optimal plan fails?

4.c. When is a patient with OCD considered to be "treatment-refractory?" What other pharmacologic alternatives are available if this patient is determined to be refractory to standard pharmacotherapy?

Outcome Evaluation

5. Which clinical and laboratory parameters are necessary to evaluate the therapy for achievement of the desired therapeutic outcomes and to detect or prevent adverse effects?

Patient Education

6. What information should be provided to the patient to enhance compliance, ensure successful therapy, and minimize adverse effects?

■ FOLLOW-UP QUESTIONS

1. When is a decrease in the Y-BOCS score considered clinically significant?

2. If this patient had presented to the physician desiring to continue breastfeeding, what would your recommendations be regarding pharmacotherapy?

■ SELF-STUDY ASSIGNMENTS

1. Prepare a short paper evaluating the risks and benefits of using SSRIs in the pharmacotherapy of OCD in a woman who is pregnant or breastfeeding.

2. Perform a literature search and write a short paper describing the symptoms of body dysmorphic disorder (BDD) and the association with OCD. How is BDD treated with pharmacotherapy?

3. Discuss the pharmacotherapeutic agents used to augment antidepressant therapy in the treatment of OCD in patients who have a partial response to antidepressant monotherapy.

4. Using the Internet, find and report on several OCD or mental health foundations that provide valuable information and support for patients and families affected by OCD.

CLINICAL PEARL

Higher dosages of antidepressant medication than those typically used for depression are often required to obtain antiobsessional effects. A response to pharmacotherapy may not occur until a therapeutic dose has been maintained for at least 10–12 weeks.

REFERENCES

1. Fairbrother N, Abramowitz JS. New parenthood as a risk factor for the development of obsessional problems. Behav Res Ther 2007;45:2155–2163.
2. Ross LE, McLean LM. Anxiety disorders during pregnancy and the postpartum period: a systematic review. J Clin Psychiatry 2006;67:1285–1298.
3. Jenike MA. Obsessive-compulsive disorder. N Engl J Med 2004;350:259–265.
4. Goodman WK, Price LH, Rasmussen SA, et al. The Yale-Brown Obsessive Compulsive Scale I. Development, use, and reliability. Arch Gen Psychiatry 1989;46:1006–1011.
5. National Institute for Health and Clinical Excellence. Obsessive-compulsive disorder: core interventions in the treatment of obsessive-compulsive disorder and body dysmorphic disorder. London, NICE, 2005 (clinical guideline 31). *http://www.nice.org.uk/guidance/CG31*. Accessed Dec. 7, 2006.
6. Denys D. Pharmacotherapy of obsessive-compulsive disorder and obsessive-compulsive spectrum disorders. Psychiatr Clin North Am 2006;553–584.
7. Phelps NJ, Cates ME. The roles of venlafaxine in the treatment of obsessive-compulsive disorder. Ann Pharmacother 2005;39:136–140.
8. Hollander E, Allen A, Steiner M, et al. Acute and long-term treatment of prevention of relapse of obsessive-compulsive disorder with paroxetine. J Clin Psychiatry 2003;64:1113–1121.

77

INSOMNIA

Eating at Night. . . . . Level II

Mollie Ashe Scott, PharmD, BCPS, CPP

Amy M. Lugo, PharmD, BCPS, CDM

LEARNING OBJECTIVES

After completing this case study, the reader should be able to:

- Identify the psychosocial, disease-related, and drug-induced causes of insomnia.

- Explain the risks of sedative-hypnotics in the elderly.

- Educate a patient regarding nonpharmacologic treatments for insomnia.

- Design a therapeutic plan for treatment of insomnia.

PATIENT PRESENTATION

Chief Complaint

"My glucoses are out of control."

HPI

Mary Jane Smith is a 72-year-old woman who is referred by her primary care physician to a Pharmacotherapy Clinic for medication therapy management for diabetes. Her diabetes control has worsened over the past 2 months. She is noticeably tired and nods off during the interview. She is accompanied by her daughter who gives most of the medical history. The patient states that she has had difficulty sleeping for many years but that her sleep has improved since starting zolpidem 3 months ago. Her daughter is concerned about the patient's safety, as she recently found her wandering into the kitchen at night to prepare a sandwich on multiple occasions. The patient insists that she stays in her bed all night and is flabbergasted that her daughter would "tell such a story." The daughter recently heard that zolpidem can cause "sleep-eating" and wonders if this is why her mother is getting up at night to eat. The patient is responsible for filling her own pillbox, and the daughter has noticed that she frequently needs medication refills from the pharmacy too early.

PMH

Insomnia for many years
Osteoarthritis (right hip, right knee, and hands)
Dyslipidemia
DM Type 2 for 12 years
Peripheral neuropathy
HTN for 10 years
Depression
History of falls
Allergic rhinitis

FH

Mother died of CVA at age 65, had breast cancer; father died from myocardial infarction at age 55

SH

Divorced, lives with her daughter. Family is building a small house for her next to her daughter's house. She reports having financial stressors since her only income currently is Social Security and a small pension. She worked as a social worker in a community hospital before retiring. She has Medicare and pays for her medications with a Medicare Part D plan.

Medications

Zolpidem 10 mg po Q HS PRN sleep
Ibuprofen 600 mg po TID
Glucosamine 500 mg po TID
Amitriptyline 100 mg po Q HS
HCTZ 25 mg po Q AM
Metformin 1,000 mg po BID
Lisinopril 40 mg po once daily
Doxazosin 4 mg po Q HS
Excedrin Extra Strength 1 tablet po Q HS
Venlafaxine ER 150 mg po once daily
Aspirin 81 mg po once daily
Diphenhydramine 25 mg po TID PRN
Advil Cold and Sinus po QD PRN

All

Amlodipine—pedal edema

ROS

Patient reports that her glucoses have been elevated for the past several months. She has never attended group diabetes classes. Her recent fasting low glucose was 155 and recent fasting high glucose was 302. Patient reports difficulty going to sleep and staying asleep, and she reports having had this problem for several years. She reports that she is sleeping much better now that she is taking zolpidem. She has a long history of depression and was hospitalized for depression approximately 10 years ago. She currently denies a "blue mood" or any thoughts of suicide and her PHQ-9 score today is 5. She states she uses incontinence briefs and reports urinary frequency and urgency. She has a longstanding history of losing urine when she coughs or sneezes. Her urinary incontinence symptoms have worsened over the past several months. She has stopped going to church and to lunch with friends for fear of being incontinent. She has right knee pain and stiffness, particularly upon awakening and after sitting. Her hand and wrist pain have caused her to stop quilting, which she truly enjoys. Her verbal pain scale regarding her OA in her hip, knee and hands is 5/10. She complains of burning and tingling in her lower extremities. She feels hungry all the time, and her daughter thinks that dietary indiscretions have contributed to her worsened diabetes control. She has frequent headaches and "springtime allergies" that are causing nasal congestion. She complains of dizziness and lightheadedness if she stands up too quickly. She experienced a fall approximately 1 month ago while checking the mail.

■ Physical Examination (from the last visit with her PCP)

Gen

Elderly WDWN woman in NAD who looks her stated age

VS

BP 90/62, P 76, RR 12, T 37°C; Wt 68 kg; Ht 5'5"

Skin

Normal skin color and turgor, no lesions noted

HEENT

Normocephalic, PERRLA, EOMI, boggy turbinates

Neck/Lymph Nodes

Supple with normal size thyroid, (–) adenopathy

Lungs

CTA bilaterally

CV

Normal S_1, S_2; no MRG

Abd

NTND, no HSM

Genit/Rect

Deferred

Ext

No C/C/E; normal muscle bulk and tone; muscle strength 5/5 and equal in all extremities; 1+ popliteal and dorsalis pedis pulses; decreased lower extremity sensation to monofilament bilaterally; rotation of the right hip produced pain in her groin indicative of hip OA. Right knee demonstrates bony changes indicative of knee OA; (–) for effusions of the knee; DIP joints demonstrate bony changes associated with OA.

Neuro

Oriented to person, place, and time; CN II–XII intact; Mini Mental State Examination results: 25/30

■ Labs

			Lipid Panel:
Na 140 mEq/L	Hgb 14 g/dL	AST 34 IU/L	
K 4.2 mEq/L	Hct 43%	ALT 32 IU/L	TC 212 mg/dL
Cl 105 mEq/L	RBC 4.7 × 10⁶/mm³	LDH 112 IU/L	LDL 137 mg/dL
CO₂ 28 mEq/L	Plt 262 × 10³/mm³	GGT 47 IU/L	HDL 45 mg/dL
BUN 11 mg/dL	WBC 6.2 × 10³/mm³	T. bili 0.3 mg/dL	TG 180 mg/dL
SCr 1.6 mg/dL	TSH 1.3 mIU/L	T. prot 7.1 g/dL	
Glu 242 mg/dL	Free T₄ 4.1 ng/dL	Alb 4.0 g/dL	

A1C 9.2% (increased from 7.0% 6 months ago)

■ Assessment

1. Insomnia
2. Sleep-eating due to zolpidem
3. Diabetes Type 2, worsened control
4. Untreated urinary incontinence
5. OA
6. Untreated dyslipidemia
7. History of falls
8. Depression
9. History of HTN (current hypotension)
10. Peripheral neuropathy
11. Obesity
12. Chronic renal insufficiency
13. Allergic rhinitis
14. At risk for osteoporosis
15. At risk for GI bleed
16. Nonadherence

QUESTIONS

Problem Identification

1.a. Create a drug related problem list for the patient.

1.b. Which information (signs, symptoms, laboratory values) indicates the presence or severity of insomnia?

1.c. Could any of the patient's problems have been caused by drug therapy?

1.d. What additional information is needed to satisfactorily assess this patient's insomnia?

Desired Outcome

2. What are the goals of pharmacotherapy in this case?

Therapeutic Alternatives

3.a. What nonpharmacologic therapies might be useful for this patient's insomnia?

3.b. What feasible pharmacotherapeutic alternatives are available for treatment of insomnia?

Optimal Plan

4.a. What drug, dosage form, dose, schedule, and duration of therapy are best for this patient's insomnia?

4.b. What alternatives would be appropriate if the initial therapy fails or cannot be used?

Outcome Evaluation

5. Which clinical and laboratory parameters are necessary to evaluate the therapy for achievement of the desired therapeutic outcome and to detect or prevent adverse effects?

Patient Education

6. What information should be provided to the patient to enhance adherence, ensure successful therapy, and minimize adverse effects?

■ FOLLOW-UP QUESTION

1. What other medication adjustments should be made at this time?

2. For questions related to the use of valerian for insomnia, please see Section 20 of the Casebook.

■ SELF-STUDY ASSIGNMENTS

1. Develop a pharmacotherapy plan for the treatment of her diabetes.

2. Design a personal medication record to help the patient manage her medications at home.

3. Identify medications that the patient is taking that are on the Beers' List for medications to avoid in the elderly.

4. Summarize the published literature about hypnotic-induced sleep-eating, and discuss how this potential adverse effect impacted negatively upon this patient's health.

CLINICAL PEARL

Sedative-hypnotics should be prescribed with caution in the elderly due to the risk of potential adverse drug events.

REFERENCES

1. National Institutes of Health. National Institutes of Health state of the science conference statement: manifestations and management of chronic insomnia in adults June 13–15, 2005. Sleep 2005;28:1049–1057.

2. Morin A, Jarvis C, Lynch A. Therapeutic options for sleep-maintenance and sleep-onset insomnia. Pharmacotherapy 2007;27:89–110.

3. Morgenthaler TI, Silber MH. Amnestic sleep-eating disorder associated with zolpidem. Sleep Med 2002;3:323–327.

4. Holbrook AM, Crowther R, Lotter A, et al. Meta-analysis of benzodiazepine use in the treatment of insomnia. CMAJ 2000;162:225–233.

5. Fick DM, Cooper JW, Wade WE, et al. Updating the Beers' Criteria for potentially inappropriate medication use in older adults. Results of a US consensus panel of experts. Arch Intern Med 2003;163:2716–2724.

6. Dooley M, Plosker GL. Zaleplon. A review of its use in the treatment of insomnia. Drugs 2000;60:413–445.

7. Montplaisir J, Hawa R, Moller C, et al. Zopiclone and zaleplon vs benzodiazepines in the treatment of insomnia. Canadian consensus statement. Hum Psychopharmacol 2003;18:29–38.

8. Terzano MG, Rossi M, Palomba V, et al. New drugs for insomnia. Comparative tolerability of zopiclone, zolpidem, and zaleplon. Drug Safety 2003;26:261–282.

9. US Food and Drug Administration Center for Drug Evaluation and Research. Sleep Disorder (Sedative-Hypnotic) Drug Information. *http://www.fda.gov/cder/drug/infopage/sedative_hypnotics/default.htm.* Accessed May 10, 2007.

10. Moen M, Plosker G. Zolpidem extended-release. CNS Drugs 2006; 20:419–426.

11. Krystal AD, Walsh JK, Laska E, et al. Sustained efficacy of eszopiclone over 6 months of nightly treatment: results of a randomized, double-blind, placebo-controlled study in adults with chronic insomnia. Sleep 2003;26:793–799.

12. Johnson M, Suess P, Griffiths R. Ramelteon: a novel hypnotic lacking abuse liability and sedative adverse effects. Arch Gen Psychiatry 2006;63:1149–1157.

13. Wortelboer U, Cohrs S, Rodenbeck A, et al. Tolerability of hypnosedatives in older patients. Drugs Aging 2002;19:529–539.

14. Olde Rikkert MG, Rigaud AS. Melatonin in elderly patients with insomnia. A systematic review. Z Gerontol Geriatr 2001;34:491–497.

15. Bent S, Padula A, Moore D, et al. Valerian for sleep: a systematic review and meta-analysis. Am J Medicine 2006;119:1005–1012.

16. Holm KJ, Goa KL. Zolpidem: an update of its pharmacology, therapeutic efficacy and tolerability in the treatment of insomnia. Drugs 2000;59:865–889.

17. McEvoy GK, Snow EK, eds. AHFS Drug Information Essentials 2006–2007. American Society of Health-System Pharmacists, Bethesda MD, 2006.

78

TYPE 1 DIABETES MELLITUS AND KETOACIDOSIS

Spring Break in Key West . . . . Level II

Amy S. Nicholas, PharmD, CDE

Holly S. Divine, PharmD, CGP, CDE

LEARNING OBJECTIVES

After completing this case study, the reader should be able to:

- Identify existing and potential risk factors for diabetic ketoacidosis (DKA).

- Recognize signs and symptoms of DKA.

- Determine laboratory parameters for the diagnosis and monitoring of DKA.

- Identify anticipated electrolyte abnormalities associated with DKA and their treatment.

- Recommend appropriate insulin therapy for treating DKA.

- Identify therapeutic decision points in DKA treatment and provide parameters for altering therapy at those points.

- Propose method(s) to convert from IV to subcutaneous insulin therapy and calculate the dose of insulin that should be administered.

- Develop a plan for sick day management of patients with diabetes mellitus and prevention of future DKA.

- Provide education on lifestyle modifications to help control Type 1 diabetes and to prevent complications.

PATIENT PRESENTATION

■ Chief Complaint

Patient's roommate reports the patient stating "I feel really sick, weak, and lightheaded. I think I have an infected blister on my foot that is causing all of this" this morning just hours before she vomited and collapsed in the bathroom of their dormitory.

■ HPI

Buffy Sandoon is a 21-year-old woman with a history of Type 1 diabetes, diagnosed 5 years ago. She is a college senior at the local university. She and her mom returned 2 days ago from a 5-day vacation in Key West, and she returned to her college dormitory yesterday. It was a welcome break, as she is a 4.0 student and has been chronically tired from studying diligently this past year. She states that she has been under a "lot of stress" in the last 2 months preparing for her wedding and graduation. She wore flip-flops all week on the beach, and 5 days ago, she started to notice a blister forming between her big toe and second toe (on her left foot). She dismissed it, putting a liquid bandage on it and treating it with triple antibiotic ointment. Three days ago, it was larger and "oozing pus." She called her primary care physician, who called in a prescription that day for an oral antibiotic.

She began feeling nauseated with some stomach pains several hours after breakfast, and she began vomiting last night immediately after dinner. Her roommate suggested she call her doctor, but Buffy believed the antibiotic could be the cause of her stomach upset leading to her hyperglycemia. Her blood glucose at that time (7 PM) was 350 mg/dL. At bedtime, her blood glucose was 375 mg/dL. She tried sipping clear diet soda and eating a large popsicle, but was unable to keep any fluids down. She vomited five more times that evening before falling asleep for several hours. Since she fell asleep, she missed her evening dose of insulin glargine. Her roommate heard her fall in the bathroom around 3:30 AM. She called 911 immediately. When the paramedics arrived, she was alert but not oriented. The paramedics noted coffee ground emesis in the toilet, Kussmaul respirations (and timed it to be 30 breaths/min), and "fruity breath." Her roommate told them that she was not intoxicated but that she has Type 1 diabetes. She was very warm to the touch, and they noted the large lesion on her left foot. They immediately transported her to the ER.

Her mother arrived and provided background information to the admitting nursing staff. Buffy had a visit with her ophthalmologist over a year ago and was told there was "nothing abnormal" upon receiving a dilated eye examination. Her last screen for microalbuminuria 3 months ago was positive, although she has not had additional screenings to confirm those results. She has no paresthesias of the feet or hands and has never previously had a foot ulcer. Her last lipid panel was obtained 3 months ago and was "not good." She has had a history of DKA upon her original diagnosis of Type 1 diabetes 5 years ago and had one hospitalization with DKA 6 months ago. Her mother suspects Buffy has not been taking insulin regularly and is concerned about her recent weight loss. Her glucose control has been suboptimal, as indicated by an A1C of 10.5% from 2 months ago. She infrequently sees a dietitian and admits that she has had difficulty managing her diabetes due to the demands of college, her part-time job and planning the wedding.

■ PMH

Type 1 DM diagnosed 5 years ago; hospitalized 2 times for DKA in the past 5 years

■ PSH

Tonsillectomy 1997

■ FH

Father, age 45, has HTN and hyperlipidemia
Mother, age 43, has Type 2 diabetes and hypertension
One sister, age 15 and healthy

SH

College student; engaged to be married; no tobacco or illicit drug use; drinks two to three beers a month with friends

Meds

Insulin glargine 13 units SC at bedtime
Insulin lispro 5 units SC before breakfast, 5 units SC before lunch, and 6 units SC before dinner
Ibuprofen 200 mg PRN menstrual cramps
Glucagon injection kit

Allergies

NKDA

ROS

HEENT—Complains of blurry vision and dizziness on postural change; denies vertigo, head trauma, ear pain, tinnitus, dysphagia, odynophagia
Resp—Complains of SOB; no complaints of cough or wheezing
GI—Vomiting as noted above in HPI; complains of abdominal pain; denies constipation, diarrhea, or food intolerance
GU—Had polyuria (large volumes every hour) yesterday; incontinent when paramedics arrived
OB-GYN—G_0P_0; denies current pregnancy and has ongoing menses; menses typically flows for 5 days and is regular every 28 days; not sexually active and denies any vaginal discharge, pain, or itching
Neuro—Has never had a seizure; complains of lethargy; no complaints of headache, paresthesias, dysesthesias, or anesthesias
Derm—No history of chronic rashes or sweating abnormalities; no history of injection site reactions or problems
Endo—Denies history of goiter and has no heat or cold intolerance; she has lost 10 lb in the last year

Physical Examination

Gen

Underweight white woman with a female body habitus appearing her stated age, with deep respirations, ketones on her breath, and slurred speech; slightly confused, but responds appropriately to questions

VS

BP 110/69 supine, 105/65 sitting, P 130, RR 29, T 40.0°C; Wt 48 kg, Ht 5'6"

Skin

Unremarkable

HEENT

NCAT, PERRLA, EOM intact; mucous membranes are dry; pharynx is erythematous; tonsils have been removed; ears are unremarkable

Neck/Lymph Nodes

Thyroid is palpable but not enlarged; no masses. Cervical, axillary, and femoral lymph nodes are not palpable.

Chest

Lungs are CTA and P. There is full chest excursion.

CV

PMI is normal and non-displaced; S_1 and S_2 are normal without S_3, S_4, murmur or rub; RRR; carotid, femoral, and dorsalis pedis pulses are normal throughout; no carotid, abdominal, or femoral bruits

Abd

Soft, without organomegaly or masses; guarding noted upon palpation of suprapubic area; bowel sounds are decreased

Rect

Anus is normal; no masses or hemorrhoids are noted; stool is heme (−)

Ext

There is no pretibial edema. A 1-cm ulcer noted between big toe and 2nd toe on left foot; 0.5-cm blister noted between big toe and 2nd toe on right foot; calluses noted on heels and plantar surfaces bilaterally

Neuro

DTR's bilaterally 2+ for the biceps, brachioradialis, quadriceps, and Achilles; plantars are downgoing bilaterally; vibratory perception at the 1st MTP bilaterally is slightly depressed; muscle strength is 5/5

Labs

Na 127 mEq/L	Hgb 17 g/dL	WBC 12.5×10^3/mm³	*Fasting Lipid Panel*
K 5.9 mEq/L	Hct 44%	Neutros 55%	*(3 months prior to*
Cl 98 mEq/L	RBC 5.3×10^6/mm³	Bands 12%	*admission):*
CO_2 6.0 mEq/L	Plt 270×10^3/mm³	Lymphs 28%	T. chol 220 mg/dL
Anion gap 27	MCV 90 μm³	Monos 5%	LDL 125 mg/dL
mEq/L	MCHC 35 g/dL		HDL 44 mg/dL
BUN 23 mg/dL			Trig 244 mg/dL
SCr 1.5 mg/dL			Serum pregnancy:
Glu 775 mg/dL			Negative

ABG

On room air: pH 7.2; pCO_2 7.6; pO_2 139; HCO_3 2.0, O_2 sat 97%

UA

SG 1.0005, pH 6, glu (−), protein (−), ketones (3+), blood (−); nitrite (−); leukocyte esterase (−); 1 WBC/hpf; 0 RBC/hpf, no bacteria, 1–5 epithelial cells

Chest X-Ray

Normal

ECG

Sinus tachycardia

Assessment

1. Diabetic ketoacidosis precipitated by foot ulcer, stress, and decreased insulin adherence

2. Type 1 DM complicated by hypercholesterolemia and probable microalbuminuria

3. Underweight; possible anorexia

QUESTIONS

Problem Identification

1a. What signs, symptoms, and laboratory findings indicate the presence and severity of DKA in this patient?

1.b. What are the general risk factors for DKA, and which of those risk factors are present in this patient?

1.c. What are the diagnostic criteria for DKA?

1.d. What problems beyond hyperglycemia are encountered in DKA that may require intervention?

Desired Outcome

2. What are the goals of therapy for this patient?

Therapeutic Alternatives

3. What therapies are available to correct the metabolic derangements of DKA?

Optimal Plan

4. Outline your specific plan for providing the IV fluids and medications that should be administered to this patient.

Outcome Evaluation

5.a. What monitoring is necessary for the therapeutic plan that you developed for the patient?

5.b. What changes in the therapeutic regimen should be considered when the blood glucose drops below 200 mg/dL or the potassium drops into the range of 3.3–5.3 mEq/L? What if glucose does not fall by 50–70 mg/dL in the first hour? Provide the rationale for your answer.

5.c. At what point is the DKA considered to be resolved, and when can IV insulin therapy be converted to subcutaneous therapy?

5.d. Outline a plan for converting the patient from IV to subcutaneous insulin after resolution of the DKA.

Patient Education

6. How should this patient be counseled about self-management of her diabetes on a "sick day" (i.e., when she is anorexic, nauseated, or vomiting)?

7. What additional counseling or interventions should occur with this patient regarding prevention of future DKA?

■ FOLLOW-UP QUESTIONS

1. Are there any other medications that should be added to her regimen based on her presenting laboratory values and/or history of present illness?

2. What lifestyle recommendations, if any, would you make?

3. Describe the nonpharmacologic approaches that should be taken to prevent further complications associated with diabetes, including the prevention of future foot ulcerations.

■ SELF-STUDY ASSIGNMENTS

1. Describe the medical complications associated with DKA and DKA treatment.

2. Describe the doses and outcomes for the use of rapid acting insulin in the treatment of DKA according to recent literature.

3. What does the American Diabetes Association state about DKA and hyperosmolar hyperglycemic nonketotic syndrome (HHS) in patients with Type 2 diabetes? Compare these two disorders with respect to prevention, precipitating causes, signs and symptoms, pathophysiology, and treatment.

4. Persons with diabetes are at risk for developing cardiovascular disease and end-stage renal disease. Describe therapeutic approaches to prevent these two complications.

CLINICAL PEARL

According to the American Diabetes Association, cerebral edema is a fatal but rare complication of DKA. Cerebral edema can also occur in cases of HHS.

ACKNOWLEDGMENT

This case is based in part on the case written for the Fifth Edition by Scott Jacober, DO, CDE, and Linda A. Jaber, PharmD.

REFERENCES

1. Kitabachi AE, Umpierrez GE, Murphy MB, et al. American Diabetes Association. Hyperglycemic crises in adult patients with diabetes: a consensus statement from the American Diabetes Association. Diabetes Care 2006;29:2739–2748.

2. Trachtenberg DE. Diabetic ketoacidosis. Am Fam Physician 2005; 71:1705–1714.

3. American Diabetes Association Clinical Practice Recommendations. Diabetes Care 2007;30:S3–S103.

4. American College of Endocrinology Consensus Statement on Guidelines for Glycemic Control. Endocr Pract 2002;8(Suppl 1):Jan/Feb.

79

TYPE 2 DIABETES MELLITUS: NEW ONSET

An American Epidemic. . . . . Level III

Deanne L. Hall, PharmD, CDE

Scott R. Drab, PharmD, CDE, BC-ADM

LEARNING OBJECTIVES

After completing this case study, the reader should be able to:

• Recognize the signs, symptoms, and risk factors associated with Type 2 diabetes mellitus (DM).

• Identify the comorbidities in Type 2 DM associated with insulin resistance (metabolic syndrome).

• Compare the pharmacotherapeutic options in the management of Type 2 DM including mechanisms of action, contraindications, and side effects.

• Describe the role of self-monitoring of blood glucose (SMBG) and identify factors to enhance patient adherence.

• Develop a patient-specific pharmacotherapeutic plan for the treatment and monitoring of Type 2 DM.

PATIENT PRESENTATION

■ Chief Complaint

"My gynecologist said I should have a check-up since I am tired all the time."

HPI

Louise Jackson is a 49-year-old woman who presents to her primary care physician after her gynecologist recently diagnosed her with polycystic ovarian syndrome (PCOS) during an evaluation for amenorrhea. She complains of increasing fatigue, which she attributes to being overweight. She states her last appointment with her PCP was over 2 years ago.

PMH

PCOS × 2 months
Hyperlipidemia × 2 years (diet controlled)
HTN × 4 years

FH

Diabetes present in both mother and maternal grandmother. Father died suddenly of colon cancer at age 59, mother alive age 76 with history positive for DM Type 2, HTN, and hyperlipidemia; one younger sister with PCOS and HTN.

SH

Married × 23 years with two children. Works full-time as insurance consultant which is telephone based from home. No alcohol or tobacco use. Rarely exercises and admits to trying fad diets for weight loss with little success. She reports adherence to her medications.

Meds

Ortho-Novum 1/35 as directed
Hydrochlorothiazide 50 mg po daily

All

Codeine

ROS

Frequent fatigue. Occasional polydipsia, polyphagia, weakness, and lightheadedness upon standing. Denies blurred vision, chest pain, dyspnea, tachycardia, dizziness, or tingling or numbness in extremities, leg cramps, peripheral edema, changes in bowel movements, GI bloating or pain, nausea or vomiting, urinary incontinence, or presence of skin lesions.

Physical Examination

Gen

Patient is an African-American woman with central obesity in no apparent distress

VS

BP 152/88 sitting R arm, BP 130/70 standing R arm, P 82, RR 18, T 37.2°C; Wt 95.5 kg, Ht 5'6"

Skin

Dry with poor skin turgor; no ulcers or rash

HEENT

PERRLA; EOMI; TMs intact; no hemorrhages or exudates on funduscopic examination; mucous membranes normal; nose and throat clear w/o exudates or lesions

Neck/Lymph Nodes

Supple; without lymphadenopathy, thyromegaly, or JVD

Lungs

CTA

CV

RRR; normal S_1 and S_2; no S_3, S_4, rubs, murmurs, or bruits

Abd

Soft, NT, central obesity; normal BS; no organomegaly, or distention

GU/Rect

Deferred

Ext

Normal ROM and sensation; peripheral pulses 2+ throughout; no lesions, ulcers, or edema

Neuro

A & O × 3, CN II–XII intact; DTRs 2+ throughout; feet with normal vibratory and pinprick sensation (5.07/10 g monofilament)

Labs

Na 141 mEq/L	Ca 9.9 mg/dL
K 4.0 mEq/L	Phos 3.2 mg/dL
Cl 96 mEq/L	AST 21 IU/L
CO_2 22 mEq/L	ALT 15 IU/L
BUN 16 mg/dL	Alk phos 45 IU/L
SCr 1.2 mg/dL	T. bili 0.9 mg/dL
Random Glu 280 mg/dL	T. chol 260 mg/dL

UA

(–) ketones, (–) protein, (–) microalbuminuria

Assessment

1. Elevated random glucose; presumed newly diagnosed Type 2 diabetes mellitus; will obtain a fasting blood glucose level to confirm the diagnosis and also check A1C

2. Elevated total cholesterol; will obtain fasting lipid profile to evaluate LDL, HDL, and triglycerides

3. Hypertension with suboptimal treatment and possible side effects due to diuretic

4. Obesity

5. PCOS

Clinical Course

The patient returned to clinic 3 days later for lab work, which revealed: FBG 189 mg/dL; A1C 9.4%; FLP: T. chol 263 mg/dL, HDL 31 mg/dL, LDL 152 mg/dL, Trig 260 mg/dL.

QUESTIONS

Problem Identification

1.a. What risk factors for Type 2 DM are present in this patient?

1.b. What information (signs, symptoms, laboratory values) supports the diagnosis of Type 2 DM?

1.c. What information indicates the presence of insulin resistance?

1.d. Create a list of this patient's drug therapy problems.

Desired Outcome

2.a. What are the desired goals for the treatment of this patient's diabetes?

2.b. Considering her other medical problems, what other treatment goals should be established?

Therapeutic Alternatives

3.a. What nonpharmacologic therapies might be useful in the management of this patient?

3.b. What feasible pharmacotherapeutic alternatives are available for the treatment of this patient's DM? Identify the factors that will influence your choice of initial therapy.

Optimal Plan

4.a. Outline a complete pharmacotherapeutic plan to manage this patient's current problems, including drug, dosage form, dose, schedule, and rationale for your selections.

4.b. What changes in therapy would you recommend if your initial plan fails to achieve adequate glycemic control?

Outcome Evaluation

5.a. What clinical and laboratory parameters will you monitor to evaluate glycemic efficacy and to detect or prevent adverse effects?

5.b. The patient's physician suggested that she obtain a blood glucose meter for self-testing. What are the health care provider's responsibilities with respect to patients and self-monitoring of blood glucose (SMBG)?

5.c. Identify at least four potential situations in which the information provided by SMBG would be useful to patients and health care providers.

5.d. What factors should be considered in the selection of an appropriate blood glucose meter?

Patient Education

6.a. What information should be provided to the patient about diabetes and its treatment to enhance compliance, ensure successful therapy, minimize adverse effects, and prevent future complications?

6.b. How would you educate the patient regarding how and when to check her blood glucose?

■ FOLLOW-UP QUESTIONS

1. Which over-the-counter products could be recommended for patients to use in treating hypoglycemic episodes?

2. List several potential sources of error in SMBG.

3. When starting patients on insulin, the use of combination oral antihyperglycemic agents and insulin offers several advantages over switching entirely to insulin:

   a. What are the advantages of adding insulin to existing therapies with oral agents?

   b. List an appropriate method of starting insulin therapy to adequately control fasting hyperglycemia in patients on combination oral agents.

■ SELF-STUDY ASSIGNMENTS

1. Describe how you would evaluate and monitor this patient's quality of life.

2. Characterize the relationship between insulin resistance and the risk for atherosclerotic vascular disease.

3. Prepare a list of medications that have been associated with increasing blood glucose. Provide literature evidence on the strength of the association with each medication.

4. Review the literature and conduct a comparative review of the efficacy of inhaled insulin therapy relative to the insulin products commercially available for subcutaneous injection.

CLINICAL PEARL

PCOS affects up to 11% of women. Although the exact pathophysiology is not well understood, it is evident that women who have factors of metabolic syndrome are more likely to develop PCOS. Lowering insulin levels by improving insulin sensitivity improves ovulation, restores menstruation, and improves fertility. Therefore, insulin sensitizing agents, such as metformin, pioglitazone, and rosiglitazone, are under investigation as agents to treat PCOS and are being used clinically in some areas.

REFERENCES

1. American Diabetes Association. Standards of medical care in diabetes—2007. Diabetes Care 2007;30(1, suppl):S4–S41.

2. American Diabetes Association. Diagnosis and classification of diabetes mellitus. Diabetes Care 2007;30(1, suppl):S42–S47.

3. Bloomgarden ZT. Insulin resistance: current concepts. Clin Ther 1998; 20:216–231.

4. American College of Endocrinology and American Association of Clinical Endocrinologists. Medical guidelines for the management of diabetes mellitus: the AACE system of intensive diabetes self-management. Endocrine Practice 2002;8(Suppl. 1):40–82.

5. Grundy SM, Cleeman JI, Merz CN, et al. Implications of recent clinical trials for the National Cholesterol Education Program Adult Treatment Panel III Guidelines. Circulation 2004;110:227–239.

6. American Diabetes Association. Evidence-based nutrition principles and recommendations for the treatment and prevention of diabetes and related complications. Diabetes Care 2003;26(1, suppl):S51–S61.

7. Lanham MSM, Lebovic DI, Domino SE. Contemporary medical therapy for polycystic ovary syndrome. Int J Gynaecol Obstet 2006;95:236–241.

8. Nathan DM, Buse JB, Davidson MB, et al. Management of hyperglycemia in type 2 diabetes: a consensus algorithm for the initiation and adjustment of therapy. Diabetes Care 2006;29:1963–1972.

9. American Diabetes Association. Hypertension management in adults with diabetes. Diabetes Care 2004;27(1, suppl):S65–S67.

10. National Cholesterol Education Program (NCEP) Expert Panel: executive summary of the third report of the NCEP expert panel on detection, evaluation, and treatment of high blood cholesterol in adults (Adults Treatment Panel III). JAMA 2001;285:2486–2497.

80

TYPE 2 DIABETES MELLITUS: EXISTING DISEASE

Establishing Optimal Control . . . . .Level II

Sharon B. S. Gatewood, PharmD

Jean-Venable "Kelly" R. Goode, PharmD, BCPS, FAPhA, FCCP

LEARNING OBJECTIVES

After completing this case study, the reader should be able to:

• Identify the goals of therapy for the treatment of Type 2 diabetes mellitus (DM).

• Discuss the risk factors and comorbidities associated with Type 2 DM.

- Compare options for drug therapy management of Type 2 DM including mechanisms of action, combination therapies, co-morbidities, and patient-friendly treatment plans.

- Develop an individualized drug therapy management plan including dosage regimens, therapeutic endpoints, and monitoring parameters.

- Provide patient education regarding medications and the importance of adhering to the treatment plan, monitoring the disease state, maintaining blood glucose control, and seeking advice from health care providers when necessary.

PATIENT PRESENTATION

■ Chief Complaint

"I was recently diagnosed with possible diabetes and would like to have my blood sugar tested. I think that my blood sugar is running low because I have a terrible headache."

■ HPI

Sarah Martin is a 43-year-old woman who comes to the pharmacy for a diabetes education class taught by the pharmacist. She would like for the pharmacist to check her blood sugar before the class begins. She was diagnosed with diabetes mellitus Type 2 about 6 months ago. She has been attempting to control her disease with diet and exercise but has had no success. Her physician has recently started her on glyburide 5 mg. She has gained 15 lb over the past year. She monitors her blood sugar once a day, per her physician, with a range of 215–260 mg/dL. Her fasting blood sugars average 170 mg/dL.

■ PMH

Type 2 DM × 6 months
HTN × 15 years
Bipolar disorder × 25 years
Dyslipidemia × 10 years
Morbid obesity × 15 years

■ FH

Father has history of HTN and bipolar disorder. Mother has a history of dyslipidemia. Brother has DM secondary to alcoholism.

■ SH

Has been married for 21 years. She has two children who are teenagers. She works in a floral shop making deliveries. Denies any use of tobacco products but does drink alcohol occasionally (five beers/wine per week).

■ Meds

Glyburide 5 mg po BID
Lisinopril 20 mg po once daily
Zyprexa 5 mg po Q HS
Carbamazepine 200 mg po TID
Lorazepam 1 mg po TID PRN
Fluoxetine 20 mg po Q AM
EC ASA 81 mg po once daily
Pravastatin 40 mg po once daily

■ All

Morphine—hives

■ ROS

Complains of nocturia, polyuria, and polydipsia on a daily basis. Denies nausea, constipation, diarrhea, signs or symptoms of hypoglycemia, paresthesias, and dyspnea.

■ Physical Examination

Gen

WDWN severely obese, Caucasian woman in NAD

VS

BP 165/90, P 98, RR 18, T 38.6°C; waist circ 38 in, Wt 109 kg, Ht 5'8''

HEENT

PERRLA, EOMI, R and L fundus exam without retinopathy

Neck/Lymph Nodes

WNL

Lungs

Clear to A & P

CV

RRR, no MRG

Abd

NT/ND

Genit/Rect

Deferred

MS/Ext

Carotids, femorals, popliteals, and right dorsalis pedis pulses 2+ throughout; left dorsalis pedis 1+; feet show mild calluses on MTPs

Neuro

DTRs 2+ throughout, feet with normal sensation (5.07 monofilament) and vibration

■ Labs

Na 139 mEq/L	Ca 9.4 mg/dL	*Fasting Lipid Profile:*
K 3.6 mEq/L	Phos 3.3 mg/dL	T. chol 236 mg/dL
Cl 103 mEq/L	AST 15 IU/L	LDL 135 mg/dL
CO_2 31 mEq/L	ALT 18 IU/L	HDL 56 mg/dL
BUN 15 mg/dL	Alk Phos 62 IU/L	Trig 223 mg/dL
SCr 0.8 mg/dL	T. bili 0.4 mg/dL	TC/HDL ratio 4.2
Gluc (random) 232 mg/dL	A1C 9%	

■ UA

1+ protein, (+) microalbuminuria

■ Assessment

The patient reports that she exercises at most once a week and her diet is difficult to maintain due to the nature of her job as a delivery person. Her glycemic control has been maintained with an 8.9% A1C 6 months ago. She has had a moderate weight gain of 15 lb (6.8 kg) over the past year. Her blood pressure and cholesterol are not at goal on the current drug therapy. Her bipolar disorder is moderately controlled on the current drug therapy. When the patient is in a depression or manic phase, she tends to use food to "treat" the symptoms.

QUESTIONS

Problem Identification

1.a. What are this patient's drug therapy problems?

1.b. What findings indicate poorly controlled diabetes in this patient?

Desired Outcome

2.a. What are the goals of treatment for Type 2 diabetes in this patient?

2.b. What individual patient characteristics should be considered in determining the treatment goals?

Therapeutic Alternatives

3.a. What nonpharmacologic interventions should be recommended for this patient's drug therapy problems?

3.b. What pharmacologic interventions could be considered for this patient's drug therapy problems?

Optimal Plan

4. What pharmacotherapeutic regimen would you recommend for each of the patient's drug therapy problems?

Outcome Evaluation

5. What parameters should be monitored to evaluate the efficacy and possible adverse effects associated with the optimal regimens you selected?

Patient Education

6. What information should be given to the patient regarding diabetes mellitus, hypertension, dyslipidemia, bipolar disorder, obesity, and her treatment plan to increase adherence, minimize adverse effects, and improve outcomes? Include information on use of a glucagon emergency kit (Fig. 80-1).

■ FOLLOW-UP QUESTION

1. What alternative therapies might be appropriate if the initial plan for diabetes treatment fails?

■ SELF-STUDY ASSIGNMENTS

1. Discuss the phenomenon known as the metabolic syndrome (syndrome X) and the role that insulin resistance is postulated to play in its sequelae.

2. Explore and discuss the importance of monitoring postprandial blood glucose levels and its impact on overall glucose control, A1C levels, and progression of diabetes complications.

3. Research the various blood glucose monitors available, and compare among available monitors the features that meet the

needs of individual patients and improve adherence to testing regimens.

4. Research new therapies for diabetes and discuss their potential role in the management of patients with Type 2 DM.

CLINICAL PEARL

Although metformin is now considered the first-line therapy for a patient with Type 2 diabetes, not all patients with Type 2 diabetes are appropriate candidates for metformin. Metformin has several contraindications, and patients generally must have good renal, hepatic, cardiac, and respiratory function to be considered a candidate for metformin therapy. Thus, before prescribing metformin, a thorough assessment of the patient's comorbid conditions must be made.

REFERENCES

1. American Diabetes Association. Clinical practice recommendations 2007. Diabetes Care 2007;30(1, suppl):S3–S103.
2. Grundy SM, Cleeman JI, Merz CN, et al. Implications of recent clinical trials for the National Cholesterol Education Program Adult Treatment Panel Guidelines III. Circulation 2004;110:227–239.
3. Expert Panel on Detection, Evaluation, Treatment of High Blood Cholesterol in Adults. Executive Summary of the third report of the National Cholesterol Education Program (NCEP) Expert Panel on detection, evaluation, and treatment of high blood cholesterol in adults (Adult Treatment Panel III). JAMA 2001;285:2486–2497.
4. Joint National Committee on Prevention, Detection, Evaluation, Treatment of High Blood Pressure. The seventh report of the Joint National Committee on Prevention, Detection, Evaluation, Treatment of High Blood Pressure. Arch Intern Med 2003;42:1206–1252.
5. NHLBI Obesity Education Initiative Expert Panel on the Identification, Evaluation, and Treatment of Overweight and Obesity in Adults. National Institutes of Health. NIH Publication No. 98–4083, September 1998.
6. Haupt DW. Differential metabolic effects of antipsychotic treatments. European Neuropsychopharmacology 2006;16:S149–S155.
7. Koski RR. Practical review of oral antihyperglycemic agents for type 2 diabetes mellitus. The Diabetes EDUCATOR 2006(Nov/Dec);32:869–876.
8. Pepine CJ, Handberg EM, Cooper-DeHoff RM. A calcium antagonist vs a noncalcium antagonist hypertension treatment strategy for patients with coronary artery disease: The International Verapamil-Trandolapril Study (INVEST): a randomized control trial. JAMA 2003;290:2805–2816.
9. Colhoun HM, Betteridge DJ, Durrington PN, et al. Primary prevention of cardiovascular disease with atorvastatin in type 2 diabetes in the Collaborative Atorvastatin Diabetes Study (CARDS): multicentre randomised placebo-controlled trial. Lancet 2004;364:685–696.
10. Collins R, Armitage J. Heart Protection Study Collaborative Group: MRC/BHF heart protection study of cholesterol-lowering with simvastatin in 5963 people with diabetes: a randomised placebo-controlled trail. Lancet 2003;361:2005–2016.

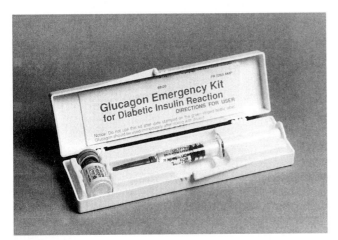

FIGURE 80-1. The Glucagon Emergency Kit for the treatment of hypoglycemia.

81

HYPERTHYROIDISM: GRAVES' DISEASE

Gland Central . . . . Level II

Kristine S. Schonder, PharmD

LEARNING OBJECTIVES

After completing this case study, the reader should be able to:

- Describe the signs, symptoms, and laboratory parameters associated with hyperthyroidism and relate them to the pathophysiology of the disease.

- Select and justify appropriate patient-specific initial and follow-up pharmacotherapy for patients with hyperthyroidism.

- Develop a plan for monitoring the pharmacotherapy for hyperthyroidism.

- Provide appropriate education to patients receiving drug therapy for hyperthyroidism.

PATIENT PRESENTATION

■ Chief Complaint

"My heart feels like it is racing and beating out of my chest."

■ HPI

Debbie James is a 32-year-old woman who returns to her PCP with complaints of worsening palpitations and continuing shortness of breath with exertion. She saw the PCP 2 weeks ago for the shortness of breath and was diagnosed with bronchitis. Despite treatment with an antibiotic and an inhaler, the symptoms have not resolved. The palpitations started a few months ago and would come and go until the past week when they began occurring more frequently, almost daily. She denies CP. She reports a 10-kg weight loss over the past 2 months, despite a good appetite. She feels hot all of the time and sweats a lot. She also reports that she has been losing her hair recently and that that she is more irritable than usual.

■ PMH

Not significant

■ FH

Father has HTN; mother has Graves' disease and a history of ovarian cysts prior to having a hysterectomy

■ SH

Lives with her husband and two daughters, ages 7 and 5 years; does not smoke and drinks alcohol socially

■ Meds

Multivitamin daily

■ All

Sulfa (rash)

■ ROS

She notes that her hair has become more fine and thinner in distribution recently. She has no visual changes, CP, or dyspnea. She has occasional N/V/D.

■ Physical Examination

Gen

Patient is a thin, tan-appearing WF in NAD

VS

BP 130/78, P 120–160 irreg, RR 20, T 38.1°C; Wt 58 kg, Ht 5'6"

Skin

Hyperpigmented on upper back and lower extremities; warm and moist. Hair is fine and sparse in the frontal area.

HEENT

PERRL, EOMI, (+) lid lag, mild proptosis (no ophthalmoplegia), mild lid retraction

Neck/Lymph Nodes

Supple, (+) smooth, symmetrically enlarged thyroid, (+) thyroid bruit, prominent pulsations in neck vessels

Lungs

CTA bilaterally, no wheezes or rales

CV

Irregularly irregular rhythm, tachycardic without murmurs; (+) carotid bruits bilaterally

Abd

Soft, NT/ND; (+) BS; no HSM or masses. Aortic pulsations palpable.

Rect

Guaiac (–) stool

Ext

2+ DP pulses bilaterally, no calf tenderness. No cyanosis. Fingernails and toenails are flaking. Thumbnails have prominent ridges.

Neuro

A & O × 3; fine tremor with outstretched hands; hyperreflexia at knees; no proximal muscle weakness

■ Labs

See Table 81-1

■ ECG

Atrial fibrillation, with ventricular response of 130 bpm

TABLE 81-1	Lab Values			
Na 138 mEq/L	Hgb 13.8 g/dL	RDW 12.4%	AST 12 IU/L	Total T$_4$ 18 mcg/dL
K 3.9 mEq/L	Hct 39.7%	WBC 6.2 × 10³/mm³	ALT 20 IU/L	TSH <0.018 mIU/L
Cl 102 mEq/L	RBC 3.24 × 10⁶/mm³	Polys 68%	T. bili 0.1 mg/dL	T$_3$ resin uptake 35%
CO$_2$ 26 mEq/L	Plt 341 × 10³/mm³	Lymphs 27%	Amylase <30 IU/L	Total T$_3$ 368 ng/dL
BUN 9 mg/dL	MCV 87.8 μm³	Monos 2%	Ca 9.7 mg/dL	Free thyroxine index 28.7
SCr 0.7 mg/dL	MCH 28.9 pg	Eos 1%	Mg 1.7 mEq/L	
Glu 101 mg/dL	MCHC 32.4 g/dL	Basos 2%	Phos 3.9 mg/dL	

■ Assessment

32-year-old white woman with goiter, probable hyperthyroidism, and new onset atrial fibrillation. Most likely cause is Graves' disease.

QUESTIONS

Problem Identification

1.a. Create a list of the patient's drug therapy problems.

1.b. What signs, symptoms, and laboratory values indicate the presence or severity of hyperthyroidism?

Desired Outcome

2. What are the goals of pharmacotherapy in this case?

Therapeutic Alternatives

3.a. What nondrug therapies and instruction might be useful for this patient?

3.b. What feasible pharmacotherapeutic alternatives are available for the treatment of hyperthyroidism in this patient?

Optimal Plan

4. What drug, dosage form, dose, schedule, and duration of therapy are best for this patient?

Outcome Evaluation

5. What clinical and laboratory parameters are necessary to evaluate the response to therapy and to detect or prevent adverse effects?

Patient Education

6. What information should be provided to the patient to enhance compliance, ensure successful therapy, and minimize adverse effects?

■ CLINICAL COURSE

The patient is started on the treatment you recommended and returns for a 1-month follow-up visit. The following information is obtained:

VS: BP 124/70, P 98 irreg, RR 16, T 37.2°C

Hgb 13.5 g/dL	WBC $5.8 \times 10^3/mm^3$	AST 14 IU/L	Total T_4 14.2 mcg/dL
Hct 38.6%	Polys 65%	ALT 22 IU/L	TSH <0.17 mIU/L
MCV 85.6 μm^3	Lymphs 30%	Alk Phos 86 IU/L	
MCH 27.5 pg	Monos 2%	T. bili 0.2 mg/dL	
MCHC 32.6 g/dL	Eos 2%	PT 21.5 sec	
RDW 13.5%	Basos 1%	INR 2.3	

■ FOLLOW-UP QUESTIONS

1. What interventions, if any, would you suggest at this point?

2. If the patient subsequently becomes hypothyroid but clinical signs indicate that the patient still has Graves' disease, what plan should be implemented?

■ SELF-STUDY ASSIGNMENTS

1. Develop a monitoring protocol for the pharmacotherapy of hyperthyroidism.

2. Design a systematic approach for a patient counseling technique for the drug therapy of hyperthyroidism.

CLINICAL PEARL

Hyperthyroidism in pregnant women must be treated to avoid fetal complications or death. Surgery and radioactive iodine are contraindicated in pregnancy. PTU is preferred because it does not cross the placental barrier as efficiently as methimazole. The lowest dose possible should be used to avoid fetal hypothyroidism and goiter. Free T_4 levels should be used to monitor therapy and should be maintained within the upper limit or slightly above normal to mimic the slightly elevated free T_4 levels seen in euthyroid pregnancies. TSH and free T_3 levels can be misleading when used to monitor therapy.

REFERENCES

1. Cooper DS. Antithyroid drugs. N Engl J Med 2005;352:905–917.
2. Bartalena L, Tanda ML, Bogazzi F, et al. An update on the pharmacological management of hyperthyroidism due to Graves' disease. Expert Opin Pharmacother 2005;6:851–861.

82

HYPOTHYROIDISM

Why Am I Always Soooo Tired?. . . . . .Level II

Michael D. Katz, PharmD

LEARNING OBJECTIVES

After completing this case study, the reader should be able to:

• Recognize the signs and symptoms of mild and overt hypothyroidism.

• Identify the goals of therapy for hypothyroidism.

• Develop an appropriate treatment and monitoring plan for thyroid replacement based on individual patient characteristics.

• Select an appropriate product for thyroid replacement therapy.

• Properly educate a patient taking thyroid replacement therapy.

PATIENT PRESENTATION

■ Chief Complaint

"I always feel so tired lately. Maybe I'm working too hard?"

■ HPI

Christina Lopez is a 45-year-old woman who presents to her new PCP complaining of feeling tired, lethargic, and "fuzzy-headed" for the last 6 months. She has seen her previous PCP several times over this period of time, and she has been told that her symptoms are probably due to anemia, depression, or perimenopause. Several months ago, she developed menorrhagia that resulted in iron deficiency anemia (hematocrit 31%, MCV 68 μm^3). However despite treatment with iron (and resultant improvement of her anemia), a hormonal contraceptive to help regulate her menstrual cycle, and an antidepressant, her symptoms have slowly worsened. She notes that

2 years ago, she attended a local health fair that provided a variety of laboratory tests. The result of her TSH at that time was 6.2 mIU/L, and her total cholesterol was 246 mg/dL. Her PCP felt that the TSH value was compatible with subclinical hypothyroidism and therefore could not explain her symptoms. She also has noticed that her skin seems more dry and itchy and that she has difficulty keeping warm and frequently wears a sweater, even in warm weather.

■ PMH

Iron deficiency anemia × 6 months
Depression × 6 months
Menorrhagia × 4 months

■ FH

Positive for CVD, CAD; father had Type 2 DM and died of CVA at age 55, mother is alive with Type 2 DM, HTN, and hypothyroidism and had an MI at 60; she has one brother with Type 2 DM and a sister with HTN.

■ SH

Married, lives with her husband of 20 years; has two children aged 16 and 12. Works as a financial advisor for a large bank. Social drinker; (–) tobacco or illicit drug use.

■ Meds

MOM 30 mL po daily PRN constipation
Fluoxetine 20 mg po daily
Ortho Tri-Cyclen-28 1 po daily
$FeSO_4$ 300 mg po daily
Calcium carbonate 500 mg po twice daily
Acetaminophen 325–650 mg po PRN headache, body aches

■ All

NKDA

■ ROS

Occasional headaches relieved with non-aspirin pain reliever; (–) tinnitus, vertigo, or infections; frequent body aches which she attributes to lack of exercise; (–) change in urinary frequency, but she has noticed an increase in the number of episodes of constipation in the past year; reports cold extremities; (–) history of seizures, syncope, or LOC, (+) dry skin

■ Physical Examination

Gen

Well-appearing, middle-aged, Hispanic woman in NAD

VS

BP 142/89, P 64, RR 18, T 36.4°C; Wt 68 kg, Ht 5'4"

Skin

Dry appearing skin and scalp; (–) rashes or lesions

HEENT

PERRLA, EOMI; trace periorbital edema; (–) sinus tenderness; TMs appear normal

Neck/Lymph Nodes

(–) thyroid nodules or goiter; (–) lymphadenopathy, (–) carotid bruits

Lungs/Thorax

CTA

Breasts

(–) lumps/masses

CV

RRR, normal S_1, S_2; (–) S_3 or S_4

Abd

NT/ND, (–) organomegaly

Neuro

A & O × 3; CN II–XII intact; DTRs 2+, symmetric

■ Labs

Na 142 mEq/L	Hgb 13.6 g/dL	Anti-TPO antibody +
K 4.1 mEq/L	Hct 40.1%	TSH 12.8 mIU/L
Cl 100 mEq/L	WBC 7.6 × 10³/mm³	Free T_4 0.71 ng/dL
CO_2 24 mEq/L	MCV 83 μm^3	T. chol 268 mg/dL
BUN 9 mg/dL	Ca 9.4 mg/dL	LDL chol 142 mg/dL
SCr 0.8 mg/dL	Mg 1.8 mEq/L	HDL chol 36 mg/dL
Glu 104 mg/dL	PO_4 3.8 mg/dL	
	Albumin 3.8 g/dL	
	AST 22 IU/L	
	ALT 19 IU/L	
	T. bili 0.4 mg/dL	
	Alk phos 54 IU/L	

■ Assessment

45-year-old woman with signs, symptoms, and laboratory tests consistent with hypothyroidism

QUESTIONS

Problem Identification

1.a. Identify this patient's drug therapy problems.

1.b. What information (signs, symptoms, laboratory values) indicates the presence of hypothyroidism?

1.c. List examples of medications that are known to cause hypothyroidism. Could any of the patient's complaints have been caused by drug therapy?

1.d. Should her previously diagnosed, mild hypothyroidism have been managed differently? Why or why not?

Desired Outcome

2. What are the goals of pharmacotherapy for this patient?

Therapeutic Alternatives

3.a. What nondrug therapies might be useful for this patient?

3.b. What feasible pharmacotherapeutic alternatives (including complementary/alternative medicine products) are available for treatment of hypothyroidism?

Optimal Plan

4. What drug, dosage form, product, dose, schedule, and duration of therapy are best for this patient?

Outcome Evaluation

5. What clinical and laboratory parameters are necessary to evaluate thyroid replacement therapy to achieve euthyroidism and prevent adverse effects?

Patient Education

6. What information should be provided to the patient to enhance adherence, ensure successful therapy, and minimize adverse effects?

■ FOLLOW-UP QUESTIONS

1. How should this patient's elevated cholesterol and BP be managed now? What if her cholesterol and BP continue to be elevated after she becomes euthyroid?

2. Evaluate this patient's continued need for ferrous sulfate therapy. Can it be discontinued? If not, what potential problems (if any) might be expected once thyroid replacement therapy is started?

3. Evaluate this patient's continued need for hormonal contraception. What potential problems (if any) might occur if the contraceptive is discontinued after her LT4 dose has been stabilized?

4. How could you determine if the patient requires continued antidepressant therapy?

■ SELF-STUDY ASSIGNMENTS

1. Research information on the U.S. bioequivalence testing of levothyroxine (LT4) products. How does U.S. bioequivalence testing of LT4 products differ from other oral products? Does LT4 bioequivalence ensure therapeutic equivalence? Is there a consensus regarding the substitution of levothyroxine products?

2. Review the therapeutic endpoints and proper methods for adjusting thyroid replacement therapy in the treatment of hypothyroidism. What are the potential effects of over- or undertreating patients with thyroid replacement therapy (i.e., TSH not in the desired target range)?

CLINICAL PEARL

In general, the TSH is the only thyroid function test that needs to be monitored on a long-term basis. However, there is controversy regarding the upper limits of the normal range for TSH, since large population studies in healthy individuals do not show a normal distribution for TSH levels. Many thyroid experts are recommending that the upper limit of the normal range be reduced to ~3 mIU/L. Routine monitoring of the total T_4 is no longer recommended due to its lack of sensitivity and specificity. The free T_4 (in addition to the TSH) may be helpful when 1) initially evaluating a patient's thyroid status; 2) the patient's thyroid status is unstable; 3) the patient is suspected to be nonadherent to the medication regimen; 4) the patient has secondary (pituitary) hypothyroidism; and 5) assessing thyroid hormone status in very young children.

REFERENCES

1. Hollowell JG, Staehling NW, Flanders WD, et al. Serum TSH, T_4 and thyroid antibodies in the United States population (1988 to 1994): National Health and Nutrition Examination Survey (NHANES III). J Clin Endocrinol Metab 2002;87:489–499.

2. Canaris GJ, Manowitz NR, Mayor G, et al. The Colorado thyroid disease prevalence study. Arch Intern Med 2000;160:526–534.

3. Wartofsky L, Dickey RA. The evidence for a narrower thyrotropin reference range is compelling. J Clin Endocrinol Metab 2005;90:5483–5488.

4. Roberts CGP, Ladenson PW. Hypothyroidism. Lancet 2004;363:793–803.

5. Blakesley V, Awni W, Locke C, et al. Are bioequivalence studies of levothyroxine sodium formulations in euthyroid volunteers reliable? Thyroid 2004;14:191–200.

6. Carr D, McLeod DT, Parry G, et al. Fine adjustment of thyroxine replacement dosage: comparison of the thyrotrophin releasing hormone test using a sensitive thyrotrophin assay with measurement of free thyroid hormones and clinical assessment. Clin Endocrinol 1988;28:325–333.

7. Dong BJ, Hauck WW, Gambertoglio JG, et al. Bioequivalence of generic and brand-name levothyroxine products in the treatment of hypothyroidism. JAMA 1997;277:1205–1213.

8. Mayor GH, Orlando T, Kurtz NM. Limitations of levothyroxine bioequivalence evaluation: an analysis of an attempted study. Am J Ther 1995;2:417–432.

9. Grozinsky-Glasberg S, Fraser A, Nahashoni E, et al. Thyroxine-triiodothyronine combination therapy versus thyroxine monotherapy for clinical hypothyroidism: a meta-analysis of randomized controlled trials. J Clin Endocrinol Metab 2006;91:2592–2599.

10. Rodondi N, Aujesky D, Vittinghoff E, et al. Subclinical hypothyroidism and the risk of coronary heart disease: a meta-analysis. Am J Med 2006;119:541–551.

83

CUSHING'S SYNDROME

When One Gland Affects Another . . . . Level II

Christopher M. Terpening, PhD, PharmD

John G. Gums, PharmD

LEARNING OBJECTIVES

After completing this case study, the reader should be able to:

- Recognize and differentiate the signs, symptoms, and laboratory changes associated with the various forms of Cushing's syndrome.

- Recognize the biochemical, anatomic, and emotional changes that can occur with Cushing's syndrome.

- Recommend appropriate treatment regimens for patients with Cushing's syndrome.

- Suggest appropriate adjunctive pharmacotherapy to other health care providers for patients with Cushing's disease.

- Provide patient counseling on proper dosing, administration, and adverse effects of treatment for Cushing's disease.

PATIENT PRESENTATION

■ Chief Complaint

"I have been tired and weak lately."

■ HPI

Susan Taylor is a 31-year-old woman who presents to her family physician complaining of fatigue and weakness. She also reports weight gain (50 lb over 2 years) and depression with insomnia.

■ PMH

Patient has been healthy with no other major medical illnesses. She had two healthy children by uncomplicated vaginal deliveries.

■ FH

Mother is alive at age 54 with Type 2 DM; father is living at age 56 with HTN. She has two sisters, one is healthy, and the other has depression.

■ SH

Patient does not smoke, and drinks occasionally. She is a photographer. Children are ages 6 and 3.

■ Meds

Triphasil-21 as directed
Unisom PRN sleep
Advil PRN headache

■ All

Sulfa—rash

■ ROS

(+) For fatigue, weakness, occasional back pain, and weight gain; also reports episodes of sadness, depressed mood, and insomnia; skin bruises easily; occasional headache, blurred vision, and heartburn; no CP, wheezing, or SOB. Normal menstruation with regular periods.

■ Physical Examination

Gen

WDWN obese, cushingoid-appearing white woman in NAD

VS

BP 154/96, HR 85, RR 14, T 37.0°C; Wt 82.1 kg, Ht 5′3″

Skin

Thin skin with some bruising and scratches; purple striae visible on abdomen

HEENT

Rounded face; moderate facial hair; PERRLA; EOMI; funduscopic exam shows normal retinal background, optic cup-to-disk ratios 0.4; visual fields appear to be grossly intact; OP moist and pink

Neck/Lymph Nodes

Supple; (−) JVD, bruits, adenopathy, or thyromegaly

Chest

CTA bilaterally

Breasts

No lumps or masses

CV

RRR, no MRG

Abd

Obese, soft, NT, (−) masses or organomegaly

Genit/Rect

Guaiac (−); normal external genitalia; no masses

MS/Ext

Appears to have decreased strength bilaterally; DTR 1–2+ and symmetric throughout all four extremities; no CCE

Neuro

Oriented × 3; flat affect; CNs II–XII intact

■ Labs

Na 138 mEq/L	Hgb 13.4 g/dL	AST 9 IU/L	TSH 2.33 mIU/L
K 3.3 mEq/L	Hct 38.5%	ALT 7 IU/L	A1C 7.1%
Cl 105 mEq/L	RBC $4.0 \times 10^6/mm^3$	Alk Phos 180 IU/L	*Fasting Lipid Profile:*
CO_2 25 mEq/L	Plt $264 \times 10^3/mm^3$	T. bili 0.5 mg/dL	T. chol 261 mg/dL
BUN 12 mg/dL	WBC $5.8 \times 10^3/mm^3$	Alb 4.5 g/dL	HDL 62 mg/dL
SCr 0.9 mg/dL		UA 5.6 mg/dL	LDL 120 mg/dL
Glu 160 mg/dL			Trig 396 mg/dL

■ Assessment

Patient appears to have Cushing's syndrome and should be evaluated by an endocrinologist.

■ Clinical Course

The patient was seen by an endocrinologist for further evaluation. Baseline 24-hour UFC was 156 and 162 mcg on separate days. A midnight salivary cortisol level was 0.54 mcg/dL. An overnight 1-mg DST showed a plasma cortisol of 9.2 mcg/dL. Plasma ACTH levels on 2 consecutive days at 1:00 PM were 103 and 110 pg/mL. A 2-day high-dose DST resulted in a UFC of 13 mcg. A CRH stimulation test revealed a baseline plasma cortisol of 10.4 mcg/dL and ACTH of 108 pg/mL, with an increase to a plasma cortisol of 13.5 mcg/dL and ACTH of 187 pg/mL following CRH administration. An MRI revealed an enlarged pituitary gland; the same finding was seen on a focused repeat MRI. There was no focal inhomogeneity that would suggest an isolated adenoma (i.e., the tumor cannot be localized).

The risks and benefits of all the treatments were explained to Ms. Taylor. She preferred to undergo radiation treatments rather than exploratory-type surgery. She indicated that she would like to have more children and would prefer to try other treatments prior to surgery.

QUESTIONS

Problem Identification

1.a. Create a list of this patient's drug therapy problems.

1.b. What information (signs, symptoms, laboratory values) indicates the presence or severity of Cushing's syndrome?

Desired Outcome

2. What are the goals of pharmacotherapy in this case?

Therapeutic Alternatives

3.a. What nondrug therapies might be useful for this patient?

3.b. What feasible pharmacotherapeutic alternatives are available for the treatment of Cushing's disease?

Optimal Plan

4. What drug, dosage form, dose, schedule, and duration of therapy are best for treating this patient's Cushing's disease?

Outcome Evaluation

5. What clinical and laboratory parameters are necessary to evaluate the therapy for achievement of the desired therapeutic outcome and to detect or prevent adverse events?

Patient Education

6. What information should be provided to the patient to enhance compliance, ensure successful therapy, and minimize adverse events?

■ FOLLOW-UP QUESTIONS

1. What advantages does measuring late-night salivary cortisol have over measuring late-night serum cortisol levels?

■ CLINICAL COURSE

The patient received radiation therapy with adjuvant pharmacotherapy to reduce cortisol levels. Given that it may take several months for therapy to normalize cortisol levels, several other interventions were initiated to ameliorate the complications of Cushing's disease. She received hydrochlorothiazide 25 mg daily for her hypertension, pioglitazone 30 mg daily for her elevated blood sugars, atorvastatin 10 mg daily for her dyslipidemia, and citalopram 20 mg daily for her depression. A DEXA scan revealed a Z-score of –2.4 standard deviations at the hip and –2.6 vertebrally. Accordingly, she received a diagnosis of steroid-induced osteoporosis. One month following initiation of the above agents, she presented to her physician for follow-up. She reported increased weakness, leg cramps, and palpitations. Lab work revealed a serum potassium of 2.7 mEq/L.

2. What pharmacologic therapy would you recommend to reduce her risk of fracture?

3. What medication changes would you suggest at this time?

■ SELF-STUDY ASSIGNMENTS

1. Many of the tests used in the differential diagnosis of Cushing's syndrome require drug therapy (e.g., DST, CRH). Create a table to assist health care providers in performing these tests correctly (include possible adverse events, timing, critical values, and evaluation of the results).

2. Compare the retail costs in your area for each of the pharmacotherapeutic alternatives for the treatment of Cushing's syndrome. Write a brief summary of your findings, and describe whether this information would cause you to change your recommendation for the initial drug therapy for this patient.

3. Describe methods that may be used to minimize drug-induced Cushing's syndrome.

CLINICAL PEARL

Most patients with Cushing's disease are treated with transsphenoidal surgery because of its high cure rate (80–90%). Pharmacotherapy is usually used as adjunctive therapy rather than primary therapy.

REFERENCES

1. Newell-Price J, Bertagna X, Grossman AB, et al. Cushing's syndrome. Lancet 2006;367:1605–1617.
2. Arnaldi G, Angeli A, Atkinson AB, et al. Diagnosis and complications of Cushing's syndrome: a consensus statement. J Clin Endocrinol Metab 2003;88:5593–5602.

84

ADDISON'S DISEASE

Tall and Tan, But Not from Ipanema . . . . Level II

Cynthia P. Koh-Knox, PharmD

Bruce C. Carlstedt, PhD, FASHP

LEARNING OBJECTIVES

After completing this case study, the reader should be able to:

- Recognize the clinical presentation, symptoms, and laboratory changes associated with Addison's disease.
- Optimize pharmacologic and nonpharmacologic therapy for patients with Addison's disease.
- Provide education and counseling to patients and family members about Addison's disease and the proper administration, side effects, and adverse effects of corticosteroids and mineralocorticoids, and the importance of adherence to therapy.
- Provide counseling and education about common side effects associated with high and low cortisol serum concentrations.
- Compare corticosteroids with respect to relative glucocorticoid and mineralocorticoid potencies.

PATIENT PRESENTATION

■ Chief Complaint

"I'm preparing for a vacation but lack the energy to plan. Besides, I look like I've been out in the sun already."

■ HPI

Carla Stanley is a 43-year-old woman who presents to the clinic for her annual visit. She has been busy at work and is excited to go on a planned and "well-deserved" vacation on a Caribbean cruise. She reports feeling continuously fatigued with bouts of nausea and anorexia for several months. She is worried she will not be well enough to prepare for the trip. Carla reports a recent craving for salty foods.

■ PMH

Hypothyroidism × 15 years

■ FH

Father had DM for 50 years; mother has HTN and osteoporosis; has three sisters with hypothyroidism and one sister with hyperthyroidism.

■ SH

Married to a professor; works as an occupational therapist; has three teenaged children; drinks wine with dinner occasionally and socially; non-smoker.

■ Meds

Levothyroxine 0.088 mg po once daily
Os-Cal 500+D daily

■ All

Penicillin—rash

■ ROS

Reports several months of nausea, profound fatigue, and a 6-lb weight loss. Claims she frequently gets dizzy when she stands up, and reports that she has had a craving for salty foods like olives and pickles for the past several months. She has significant tanning of her skin even in non–sun-exposed areas, despite her denial of recent medication changes or participation in any outdoor activities. Denies fever, night sweats, visual disturbances, or changes in menstrual cycle.

■ Physical Examination

Gen

Tired-looking, tanned woman in NAD

VS

BP 94/70 sitting, 84/60 standing; P 79 sitting, 87 standing; RR 22; T 96.8°F; Wt 60 kg, Ht 5'6"

Skin

Normal texture; slightly dry, no cracks, pigmented skin creases on palms of hand; generalized tan appearance even in unexposed areas. Darkened scar on right forearm.

HEENT

WNL except dry mucous membranes; TMs intact

Neck

Supple without thyromegaly or adenopathy

Lungs

Clear, normal breath sounds

Breasts

No masses

CV

RRR, no MRG

Abd

NTND; no HSM

GU

Normal external female genitalia

MS/Ext

No CCE; normal ROM

Neuro

A & O × 3

■ Labs (fasting, drawn at 9:00 AM)

Na 127 mEq/L	TSH 4.8 mIU/L
K 5.0 mEq/L	Free T$_4$ 1.3 ng/dL
Cl 98 mEq/L	Cortisol 1.4 mcg/dL Time drawn 0910
CO$_2$ 27 mEq/L	ACTH 2,096 pg/mL
BUN 15 mg/dL	AST 50 IU/L
SCr 1.1 mg/dL	ALT 84 IU/L
Glu 102 mg/dL	ETA-HCG Qual neg

Reference range for Cortisol: AM: 8–25 mcg/dL, PM 4–20 mcg/dL; ACTH 0–130 pg/mL

■ UA

Clear, yellow, SG 1.015, pH 7.0

■ Other

No CT scan or ECG performed

■ Assessment

1. Primary adrenal insufficiency, most likely due to an autoimmune disease

2. History of hypothyroidism, currently treated with levothyroxine

QUESTIONS

Problem Identification

1.a. Create a list of the patient's drug therapy problems.

1.b. What information (signs, symptoms, laboratory values) indicates the presence or severity of Addison's disease?

Desired Outcome

2. What are the goals of pharmacotherapy in this case?

Therapeutic Alternatives

3.a. What nondrug therapies might be useful for this patient?

3.b. What feasible pharmacotherapeutic alternatives are available for the treatment of Addison's disease?

3.c. What psychosocial considerations are applicable to this patient?

Optimal Plan

4. What drug, dosage form, dose, schedule, and duration of therapy are best for this patient?

Outcome Evaluation

5. Which clinical and laboratory parameters are necessary to evaluate the therapy for achievement of the desired therapeutic outcome and to detect or prevent adverse effects?

Patient Education

6. What information should be provided to the patient to enhance adherence, ensure successful therapy, and minimize adverse effects?

■ SELF-STUDY ASSIGNMENTS

1. Review the signs and symptoms of an acute adrenal crisis, and describe the treatment.

2. Differentiate the glucocorticoids with respect to duration of activity, glucocorticoid potency, and mineralocorticoid potency.

3. Differentiate the biologic functions of cortisol and aldosterone.

4. Explain why the skin becomes pigmented in adrenal insufficiency.

5. Identify drugs that may precipitate acute adrenal insufficiency or adrenal crisis.

CLINICAL PEARL

Salt craving is a symptom of Addison's disease. Intake of salty foods may be reported to alleviate other symptoms of the disease, such as achy joints and orthostatic hypotension.

REFERENCES

1. Wilson TA, Speiser P. Adrenal insufficiency. *http://www.emedicine.com/ped/Topic47.htm.* Accessed January 27, 2007.
2. Lovas K, Husebye E. Addison's disease. Lancet 2005;365:2058–2061.
3. Williams GH, Dluhy RG. Disorders of the adrenal cortex. In: Harrison's Principles of Internal Medicine, 16th ed. 2005. *http://online.statref.com/Document/Document.aspx?fxid=55&docid=2160.&SessionId=A564DERPNYHXRREV.* Accessed January 2, 2007.
4. Barnard C, Kanani R, Friedman JN. Her tongue tipped us off… CMAJ 2004;171:451.
5. Baker SJ, White K. Addison's disease owner manual. *http://www.addisons.org.uk/info/manual/page1.html.* Accessed January 15, 2007.
6. Chikada N, Imaki T, Hotta M, et al. An assessment of bone mineral density in patients with Addison's disease and isolated ACTH deficiency treated with glucocorticoid. Endocrine J 2004;51:355–360.
7. Thomsen AF, Kvist TK, Andersen PK, et al. The risk of affective disorders in patients with adrenocortical insufficiency. Psychoneuroendocrinology 2006;31:614–622.
8. Gebre-Medhin G, Husebye ES, Mallmin H, et al. Oral dehydroepiandrosterone (DHEA) replacement therapy in women with Addison's disease. Clin Endocrinol (Oxf) 2000;52:775–780.

85

HYPERPROLACTINEMIA

The Missing Period . . . . .Level I

Amy Heck Sheehan, PharmD

Karim Anton Calis, PharmD, MPH, FASHP, FCCP

LEARNING OBJECTIVES

After completing this case study, the reader should be able to:

- Recognize the signs and symptoms of hyperprolactinemia.
- Recommend appropriate treatment options for hyperprolactinemia.
- Outline a plan to monitor the response to the pharmacologic treatment of hyperprolactinemia.

PATIENT PRESENTATION

▦ Chief Complaint

"I haven't had my period for almost a year."

▦ HPI

Susan Oliver is a 31-year-old woman with a history of oligomenorrhea (menstrual cycle every 2–6 months) since menarche at age 14. She presents to her gynecologist after 11 months of amenorrhea and a small amount of milky discharge from her left breast, which she first noticed 1–2 months ago. The patient and her husband would like to have a baby, but she is concerned that she may be unable to have children. The patient states that she and her husband have not used birth control for more than 1 year, and she has had several negative home pregnancy tests.

▦ PMH

GERD
Migraine headaches (one to two episodes per month)
Seasonal allergies

▦ FH

Father died at age 58 from an AMI; mother (age 62) has Type 2 DM and HTN. Patient has two brothers (ages 33 and 35) who are alive and well.

▦ SH

The patient is employed as an administrative assistant. She smokes 1–2 ppd and has less than one drink of alcohol per month. She has been married for 5 years and lives with her husband and two step-daughters (ages 7 and 9).

▦ Meds

Esomeprazole 20 mg po daily
Loratadine 10 mg po daily
Sumatriptan 6 mg SC PRN migraine
Prenatal vitamins 1 tablet po daily
Acetaminophen 500 mg po PRN

▦ All

Codeine (hives)

▦ ROS

Galactorrhea of the left breast and amenorrhea for 11 months as described in HPI above. No visual defects. No active GERD or migraine symptoms.

▦ Physical Examination

Gen
The patient is a WDWN white woman in NAD

VS
BP 124/71, P 72, RR 13, T 37.1°C; Wt 72 kg, Ht 5'8"

Skin
Normal, intact, warm and dry

HEENT
PERRLA, EOMI, normal funduscopic exam, normal visual fields

Neck/Lymph Nodes
Normal thyroid, no lymphadenopathy

Lungs/Chest
Clear to A & P

Breasts
Galactorrhea of left breast, no masses

CV
RRR, S_1 and S_2 normal, no MRG

Abd
Soft, nontender, no organomegaly, (+) bowel sounds

GU
LMP 11 months ago, normal pelvic exam and Pap smear

MS/Ext
Normal range of motion, no edema, pulses 2+ throughout

Neuro

A & O × 3, bilateral reflexes intact, normal gait, CNs II–XII intact

■ Labs

Na 138 mEq/L	AST 23 IU/L	TSH 2.1 mIU/L
K 4.0 mEq/L	ALT 31 IU/L	T_3 111 ng/dL
Cl 101 mEq/L	Alk Phos 110 IU/L	Total T_4 7.5 mcg/dL
CO_2 25 mEq/L	T. bili 0.5 mg/dL	Free T_4 1.3 ng/dL
BUN 13 mg/dL		Serum β-HCG negative
SCr 0.8 mg/dL		
Glu 89 mg/dL		

Serum prolactin on three separate days: 151, 163, and 147 mcg/L

■ Other

MRI of the pituitary gland revealed an 8-mm pituitary adenoma

■ Assessment

Hyperprolactinemia due to a microprolactinoma

QUESTIONS

Problem Identification

1.a. Create a list of this patient's drug therapy problems.

1.b. What signs, symptoms, and laboratory values indicate the presence of hyperprolactinemia?

1.c. Could this patient's hyperprolactinemia be drug-induced?

Desired Outcome

2. What are the goals of treatment for a woman with hyperprolactinemia?

Therapeutic Alternatives

3.a. What nondrug therapies can be considered for the treatment of hyperprolactinemia?

3.b. What pharmacotherapeutic options are available for the treatment of hyperprolactinemia in this woman?

Optimal Plan

4. What medication regimen would you recommend for this patient?

Outcome Evaluation

5.a. What clinical and laboratory parameters are necessary to monitor the patient's response to therapy?

5.b. If the initial therapy you recommend is effective, how soon can the patient hope to become pregnant?

Patient Education

6. What information should be provided to the patient to enhance adherence, ensure successful therapy, and minimize adverse effects?

■ CLINICAL COURSE

The patient was started on the regimen that you recommended, and she returned to the clinic 4 weeks later complaining of significant nausea and abdominal pain that was temporally associated with medication administration. Serum prolactin concentrations measured 10 minutes apart were 141 mcg/L, 147 mcg/L, and 145 mcg/L. Galactorrhea and amenorrhea were unchanged.

■ FOLLOW-UP QUESTIONS

1. Identify the possible reasons for the patient's poor initial response to therapy.

2. Given the new patient information, what alternative therapies should be considered?

3. How long will this patient require drug treatment for the prolactinoma?

■ SELF-STUDY ASSIGNMENTS

1. Review the available information on the safety of bromocriptine use during pregnancy. If this patient eventually becomes pregnant, should dopamine agonist therapy be continued?

2. Research information on the use of hormone replacement therapy in patients with hyperprolactinemia. Is this patient a candidate for hormone replacement therapy? Why or why not?

3. Describe the treatment of hyperprolactinemia in the presence of a macroadenoma. How would the management of hyperprolactinemia be different if the patient were diagnosed with a macroprolactinoma instead of a microprolactinoma?

CLINICAL PEARL

Although dopamine agonists are the mainstay of therapy for hyperprolactinemia, approximately 5–10% of patients do not respond to these agents because of poor compliance, suboptimal dosing, or the presence of a treatment-resistant prolactinoma.

REFERENCES

1. Gillam MP, Molitch ME, Lombardi, et al. Advances in the treatment of prolactinomas. Endocr Rev 2006;27:485–534.

2. DiSarno A, Landi ML, Cappabianca P, et al. Resistance to cabergoline as compared with bromocriptine in hyperprolactinemia: prevalence, clinical definition, and therapeutic strategy. J Clin Endocrinol Metab 2001;86:5256–5261.

3. Schade R, Andersohn F, Suissa S, et al. Dopamine agonists and the risk of cardiac-valve regurgitation. N Engl J Med 2007;356:29–38.

4. Molitch ME. Prolactin-secreting tumors: what's new? Expert Rev Anticancer Ther 2006;6:S29–S35.

5. Molitch ME. Medical management of prolactin-secreting pituitary adenomas. Pituitary 2002;5:55–65.

6. Mah PM, Webster J. Hyperprolactinemia: etiology, diagnosis, and management. Semin Reprod Med 2002;20:365–373.

7. Schlechte JA. Prolactinoma. N Engl J Med 2003;349:2035–2041.

86

CONTRACEPTION

Babies Aren't Us Yet . . . . Level II

Julia M. Koehler, PharmD

LEARNING OBJECTIVES

After completing this case study, the reader should be able to:

- Discuss the absolute and relative contraindications to the use of hormonal contraceptives.

- Discuss the advantages and disadvantages of the various forms of hormonal contraceptives, including both oral and non-oral formulations.

- Compare and contrast the marketed oral contraceptive (OC) combinations and be able to select the best product for an individual patient.

- Develop strategies for managing the possible side effects of OCs and prepare appropriate alternative treatment plans.

- Provide specific patient education on the administration and expected side effects of selected hormonal contraceptives.

PATIENT PRESENTATION

■ Chief Complaint

"My fiancé and I are getting married soon, and we're not ready for kids just yet."

■ HPI

Madeline Macy is a 24-year-old graduate student who presents to the Family Medicine Clinic for contraceptive counseling. She and her fiancé, Fritz, are planning to be married in approximately 3 months. Madeline states that she and Fritz have been in a monogamous sexual relationship for the past 2 years, and that their primary method of contraception has been via the inconsistent use of male condoms. She is here today to be evaluated for the use of hormonal contraceptives. The patient states she began menses at age 14, with irregular cycles of 25–36 days in length. Her last menses was 2 weeks ago. The patient states she has heard about contraceptive options that "keep you from having a period," and she wants to know more about those options, and if they would be okay for her to try.

■ PMH

Migraine headaches without aura or focal neurologic symptoms; well controlled for the past 6 months on prophylactic therapy

■ FH

Mother, age 52, has HTN and osteoporosis. Grandmother died from complications of breast cancer, which was diagnosed at age 60. Father, age 53, has osteoarthritis, hypothyroidism, and hyperlipidemia. Grandfather died at age 74 of MI.

■ SH

Currently lives in a house on campus, which she rents with three other graduate students. Once she and Fritz are married, they plan to rent an apartment together until she finishes graduate school. She admits to occasional social use of tobacco and alcohol ("a few drinks and a couple of cigarettes at parties on the weekends"). Otherwise, she denies regular smoking or alcohol use during the week, and she denies illicit drug abuse.

■ Meds

Propranolol LA 160 mg po once daily for migraine prophylaxis
Naproxen 220 mg, one to two tablets po Q 8 h PRN menstrual cramps

■ All

NKDA

■ ROS

Menstrual periods are the most irregular during exam times. Migraine headaches are not accompanied by aura or focal neurologic symptoms, and have been well controlled on prophylactic medication. (Patient states she as not had a migraine for more than 6 months; however, prior to being placed on propranolol for migraine prophylaxis, she reported experiencing menstrual-related headaches in addition to frequent migraines.)

■ Physical Examination

Gen
WDWN female in NAD

VS
BP 116/74, P 66, RR 14, T 37°C; Wt 56 kg, Ht 5'6"

Skin
Mild facial acne

HEENT
PERRLA; EOMI; TMs intact; oral mucosa clear

Neck/Lymph Nodes
Supple without lymphadenopathy or thyromegaly

Lungs
CTA, no wheezing

CV
NSR; no MRG

Breasts

Equal in size without nodularity or masses, nontender

Abd

Soft, NT, no masses or organomegaly

Genit/Rect

Normal vaginal exam w/o tenderness or masses

MS/Ext

Normal ROM; normal muscle strength

Neuro

A & O × 3

■ **Labs**

Negative Pap smear and UPT

■ **Assessment**

Young, generally healthy, sexually active female with history of migraine headache disorder that has been well controlled with prophylactic medication is requesting hormonal contraceptives for birth control.

QUESTIONS

Problem Identification

1.a. Create a list of the patient's potential drug therapy problems.

1.b. What medical problems are absolute contraindications to hormonal contraceptive use, and do any of those conditions apply to this patient?

1.c. What medical problems are relative contraindications to hormonal contraceptive use, and do any of these apply to this patient?

1.d. What other information should be obtained before creating a pharmacotherapeutic plan?

Desired Outcome

2. What are the goals of pharmacotherapy in this case?

Therapeutic Alternatives

3. What pharmacotherapeutic alternatives are available for prevention of pregnancy in this patient, and what are the advantages or disadvantages of each (Fig. 86-1)?

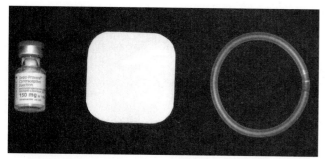

FIGURE 86-1. Three non-oral contraceptive products: Medroxyprogesterone acetate injectable suspension (Depo-Provera) for intramuscular injection *(left)*, norelgestromin/ethinyl estradiol (Ortho Evra) transdermal system for topical application *(middle)*, and etonogestrel/ethinyl estradiol (NuvaRing) ring for intravaginal use *(right)*. (Photo courtesy of R. Bowman.)

Optimal Plan

4. What contraceptive method, dose, and schedule are best for this patient?

Outcome Evaluation

5. What clinical and laboratory parameters are necessary to evaluate the therapy for efficacy and adverse effects?

Patient Education

6. What information should be provided to the patient to enhance adherence, ensure successful therapy, and minimize adverse effects?

■ **CLINICAL COURSE**

Madeline returns to the clinic in 2 months complaining of worsening acne and breakthrough bleeding.

■ **FOLLOW-UP QUESTIONS**

1. What medical conditions can be the cause of breakthrough bleeding?

2. If breakthrough bleeding is not caused by an underlying medical condition, how can it be managed?

3. What recommendations can be made to address this patient's complaint of worsening acne?

■ **SELF-STUDY ASSIGNMENTS**

1. Compare the costs of each method of birth control and prepare a report that contains your conclusions as to which method provides the best efficacy at the most reasonable cost.

2. Visit a pharmacy and review the various home pregnancy tests; determine how you would counsel a patient to use each one, and evaluate them for ease of use (Fig. 86-2).

CLINICAL PEARL

Caution patients taking oral contraceptives about the potential for drug interactions. Drugs that reduce absorption, induce metabolism, or alter gut bacterial flora can reduce oral contraceptive efficacy.

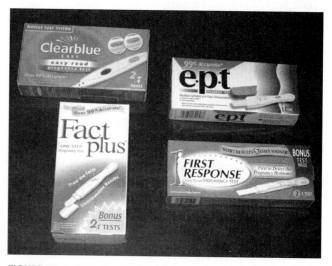

FIGURE 86-2. Several examples of home pregnancy test kits. (Photo courtesy of R. Bowman.)

REFERENCES

1. Hatcher RA, Trussell J, Stewart F, et al. Contraceptive Technology 18th revised ed. New York, Ardent Media, Inc., 2004.
2. Lewis MA, Spitzer WO, Heinemann LA, et al. Third generation oral contraceptives and risk of myocardial infarction: an international case-control study. Transitional Research Group on Oral Contraceptives and the Health of Young Women. BMJ 1996;312:88–90.
3. Joint National Committee on Prevention, Detection, Evaluation, Treatment of High Blood Pressure. The seventh report of the Joint National Committee on Prevention, Detection, Evaluation, Treatment of High Blood Pressure. JAMA 2003;289:2560–2572.
4. Schoenen J, Sándor PS. Headache with focal neurological signs or symptoms: a complicated differential diagnosis. Lancet Neurol 2004;3:237–245.
5. Knopp RH, Broyles FE, Cheung M, et al. Comparison of lipoprotein, carbohydrate, and hemostatic effects of phasic oral contraceptives containing desogestrel or levonorgestrel. Contraception 2001;63:1–11.
6. Vercellini P, Frontino G, De Giorgi O, et al. Continuous use of an oral contraceptive for endometriosis-associated recurrent dysmenorrhea that does not respond to a cyclic pill regimen. Fertil Steril 2003;80:560–563.
7. Product information for levonorgestrel 90 mcg and ethinyl estradiol 20 mc (Lybrel). Wyeth Pharmaceuticals, Inc. Philadelphia, PA. May 2007.
8. ACOG Committee on Practice Bulletins—Gynecology. ACOG practice bulletin. No. 73: use of hormonal contraception in women with co-existing medical conditions. Obstet Gynecol 2006;107:1453.
9. Audet M, Moreau M, Koltun WD, et al. Evaluation of contraceptive efficacy and cycle control of a transdermal contraceptive patch vs an oral contraceptive: a randomized controlled trial. JAMA 2001;285:2347–2354.
10. Bjarnadottir RI, Tuppurainen M, Killick SR. Comparison of cycle control with a combined contraceptive vaginal ring and oral levonorgestrel/ethinyl estradiol. Am J Obstet Gynecol 2002;186:389–395.
11. Anonymous. Treatment guidelines from the Medical Letter. Choice of contraceptives. December 2007;5:101–108.
12. Executive Summary of the Third Report of the National Cholesterol Education Program (NCEP) Expert Panel on Detection, Evaluation, Treatment of High Blood Cholesterol in Adults (Adult Treatment Panel III). JAMA 2001;285:2486–2497.

87

PREMENSTRUAL DYSPHORIC DISORDER

A Desperate Woman. Level II

Kelly R. Ragucci, PharmD, FCCP, BCPS, CDE

LEARNING OBJECTIVES

After completing this case study, the reader should be able to:

- Compare and contrast the diagnostic and clinical differences between premenstrual syndrome (PMS) and premenstrual dysphoric disorder (PMDD).

- Discuss the therapeutic goals for a patient with PMDD.

- Evaluate and/or design an appropriate treatment strategy for a patient suffering from PMDD.

- Formulate a monitoring plan for a patient with PMDD, taking into account individual patient-specific factors (Table 87-1).

- Educate patients and other health care professionals about PMDD and possible treatment options.

PATIENT PRESENTATION

Chief Complaint

"I have so many complaints that I don't know where to begin, and my husband wants to divorce me."

HPI

Jane Sullivan is a 31-year-old woman who comes into the Family Medicine clinic complaining of headaches, anxiety, depressed mood, lack of energy, insomnia, bloating, and cramping. Upon further questioning, she states that these symptoms generally occur during the week prior to menses each month. She feels like she is a different person during these days and that it is greatly affecting her relationship with her husband. In addition, she feels that she is not performing well at work and ends up calling in sick at some point during that time each month. She states that she has tried Midol Extended Relief as well as over-the-counter ibuprofen in the past, but these agents were only minimally helpful. She doesn't feel like she has any control over her emotions and what is going on physically with her body and is desperate for some help. Of additional note, she complains of increased acne/breakouts since starting her new oral contraceptive.

PMH

Hypothyroidism, asthma

FH

Sister has depression (currently well controlled). Father has hypertension and hyperlipidemia. Mother has hypothyroidism.

TABLE 87-1	Item Content of the Daily Record of Severity of Problems (DRSP)
1.a. Felt depressed, sad, "down," or "blue"	
1.b. Felt hopeless	
1.c. Felt worthless or guilty	
2. Felt anxious, tense, "keyed up," or "on edge"	
3.a. Had mood swings (e.g., suddenly felt sad or tearful)	
3.b. Was more sensitive to rejection or my feelings were easily hurt	
4.a. Felt angry, irritable	
4.b. Had conflicts or problems with people	
5. Had less interest in usual activities (e.g., work, school, friends, hobbies)	
6. Had difficulty concentrating	
7. Felt lethargic, tired, fatigued, or had a lack of energy	
8.a. Had increased appetite or overate	
8.b. Had cravings for specific foods	
9.a. Slept more, took naps, found it hard to get up when intended	
9.b. Had trouble getting to sleep or staying asleep	
10.a. Felt overwhelmed or that I could not cope	
10.b. Felt out of control	
11.a. Had breast tenderness	
11.b. Had breast swelling, felt "bloated," or had weight gain	
11.c. Had headache	
11.d. Had joint or muscle pain	
At work, at school, at home, or in daily routine, at least one of the problems noted above caused reduction of productivity or inefficiency	
At least one of the problems noted above interfered with hobbies or social activities (e.g., avoid or do less)	
At least one of the problems noted above interfered with relationships with others	

SH

Married for 5 years. No children. Denies tobacco use and only drinks alcohol on occasion, socially. She works full-time as a pharmacist at a small independent pharmacy.

Meds

Ortho-Novum 1/35
Advair 250/50 one inhalation BID
Albuterol MDI two inhalations PRN
Levothyroxine 0.137 mg po daily
Lorazepam 1 mg po PRN
Fioricet one to two tablets po Q 4 h PRN

All

NKDA

ROS

Complaints as above in HPI

Physical Examination

Gen

Tired-looking, anxious, overweight female

VS

BP 117/69, P 68, RR 16, T 97.8°F; Wt 146 lbs, Ht 5'2"

Skin

Normal, intact, warm and dry. Mixed whiteheads/blackheads on forehead and around nose.

HEENT

PERRLA, EOMI; TMs intact

Neck/Lymph Nodes

Supple without evidence of thyroid nodules/goiter or lymphadenopathy

Lungs/Thorax

CTA

Breasts

Supple; no masses; tender to touch

CV

RRR, no MRG

Abd

Soft, mildly overweight; NT/ND; + BS; no masses

Genit/Rect

Normal pelvic exam and pap smear

Ext

Normal ROM; pulses 2+; –CCE

Neuro

A & O × 3; CN II–XII intact; DTRs 2+

Labs

Na 137 mEq/L	Ca 9.5 mg/dL	TC 177 mg/dL (fasting)	WBC 7.89 × 10³/mm³
K 4.4 mEq/L	AST 20 IU/L	TG 71 mg/dL (fasting)	Hgb 13.9 g/dL
Cl 102 mEq/L	ALT 17 IU/L	LDL 111 mg/dL (fasting)	Hct 40.6%
CO₂ 27 mEq/L	Alb 3.7 g/dL	HDL 52 mg/dL (fasting)	MCV 92.8 μm³
Glu 87 mg/dL	TSH 0.74 mIU/L		MCH 31.7 pg
BUN 14 mg/dL			MCHC 34.2 g/dL
SCr 0.9 mg/dL			Plt 249 × 10³/mm³

Assessment

1. PMDD
2. Hypothyroidism, currently well controlled
3. Mild obesity
4. Asthma, currently well controlled
5. Acne

QUESTIONS

Problem Identification

1.a. What are this patient's current drug therapy and medical problems?

1.b. What signs/symptoms does this patient have that are consistent with the diagnosis of PMDD?

1.c. How do these signs/symptoms differ from those of PMS? What are the diagnostic differences between the two?

Desired Outcome

2. What are the therapeutic goals for this patient with regard to PMDD?

Therapeutic Alternatives

3.a. What nonpharmacologic treatments might be useful for a patient with PMDD?

3.b. What alternative pharmacologic treatments (e.g., vitamins, dietary supplements) might be useful for a patient with PMDD?

3.c. What pharmacotherapeutic options might be useful for a patient with PMDD?

Optimal Plan

4. Design an appropriate pharmacotherapeutic plan to treat this patient's PMDD.

Outcome Evaluation

5. What clinical parameters are necessary to evaluate and monitor the therapeutic goals listed above (see Desired Outcome)?

Patient Education

6. What information should be provided to the patient to enhance adherence, ensure successful therapy, and minimize adverse effects?

■ SELF-STUDY ASSIGNMENTS

1. Develop a patient education sheet/brochure on the diagnosis and treatment of PMDD, comparing and contrasting to PMS.

2. Explain how hypo- and/or hyperthyroidism could exacerbate the signs/symptoms of PMDD.

3. Review the various over-the-counter Midol products on the market and determine which one would be most useful, given a patient-specific situation.

CLINICAL PEARL

The etiology of PMDD is likely multifactorial, including: hormonal imbalance (specifically, low progesterone level during the luteal phase of the menstrual cycle—although treatment with progesterone is controversial at best); abnormal neurotransmitter response (specifically, changes in levels of serotonin—the reason that SSRIs have been shown to be useful); abnormal HPA-axis function; nutritional deficiency (including magnesium and calcium); and environmental factors (stress).

REFERENCES

1. American Psychiatric Association. Diagnostic and Statistical Manual of Mental Disorders, 4th ed. Washington, DC, American Psychiatric Press, 2000:771–774.
2. Futterman LA, Rapkin AJ. Diagnosis of premenstrual disorders. J Reprod Med 2006;51:349–358.
3. Endicott J, Nee J, Harrison W. Daily record of severity of problems (DRSP): reliability and validity. Arch Women Ment Health 2006;9:41–49.
4. Clinical Management Guidelines for Premenstrual Syndrome. ACOG Practice Bulletin. No. 15. Washington, D.C.: The American College of Obstetricians and Gynecologists, April 2000.
5. Kroll R, Rapkin AJ. Treatment of premenstrual disorders. J Reprod Med 2006;51:359–370.

88

MANAGING MENOPAUSAL SYMPTOMS

A Hot Topic . . . . Level II

Nicole S. Culhane, PharmD, BCPS

LEARNING OBJECTIVES

After completing this case study, the reader should be able to:

- Identify the signs and symptoms associated with menopause.
- List the risks and benefits associated with hormone replacement therapy (HRT) and identify appropriate candidates for HRT.
- Differentiate between topical and systemic forms of hormone replacement therapy.
- Recommend nonpharmacologic therapy for menopausal symptoms.
- Identify alternative, nonhormonal therapies for women unable to take HRT.
- Design a comprehensive pharmacotherapeutic plan for a patient on HRT, including treatment options and monitoring.
- Determine the desired therapeutic outcomes for a patient taking hormone replacement therapy.
- Educate patients on the treatment options, benefits, risks, and monitoring of HRT.

PATIENT PRESENTATION

Chief Complaint

"I have been having hot flashes for the past few months, and I just can't take it anymore."

HPI

Emma Peterson is a 50-year-old woman who reports experiencing two to three hot flashes per day, occasionally associated with insomnia. She also states she is awakened from sleep about two to three times per week needing to change her bed clothes and linens. Her symptoms began about 3 months ago, and over that time, they have worsened to the point where they have become very bothersome. She states that her mother was prescribed a pill for this, but she is hesitant to take the same thing because she heard on the news and from friends that the medication may not be safe. She also does not want to "get her period back," if possible. Successfully treated for depression in the past, she is currently controlled on paroxetine therapy. She currently exercises three times a week and tries to follow a low-cholesterol diet.

PMH

Depression
GERD
HTN
Hypothyroidism

FH

Mother died of stroke at age 67; father died of lung cancer at age 62. Patient has one brother, 52, and one sister, 48, who are alive and well, but both with HTN.

SH

Married, mother of two healthy daughters, ages 21 and 25. She is an RN in a neighboring physician's office. She walks on her treadmill three times a week and is trying to follow a dietitian-designed low-cholesterol diet. She does not smoke and occasionally drinks a glass of red wine with dinner.

Meds

Hydrochlorothiazide 25 mg po once daily
Omeprazole 20 mg po once daily
Paroxetine 20 mg po once daily
Synthroid 75 mcg po once daily

All

NKDA

ROS

(+) hot flashes, occasional night sweats and insomnia, vaginal dryness. (–) for weight gain, constipation. LMP 12 months ago.

Physical Examination

Gen
WDWN female in NAD

VS
BP 128/86, P 78, RR 15, T 36.4°C; Wt 76.2 kg, Ht 5'6"

Skin
Warm, dry, no lesions

HEENT
WNL

Neck/Lymph Nodes
Supple, no bruits, no adenopathy, no thyromegaly

Lungs/Thorax
CTA bilaterally

Breasts

Supple; no masses

CV

RRR, normal S_1 and S_2; no MRG

Abd

Soft, NT/ND, (+) BS; no masses

Genit/Rect

Pelvic exam normal except (+) mucosal atrophy; stool guaiac (−)

Ext

(−) CCE; pulses intact

Neuro

Normal sensory and motor levels

Labs

Na 136 mEq/L	Hgb 12.7 g/dL	Ca 9.3 mg/dL	*Fasting Lipid Profile:*
K 3.9 mEq/L	Hct 39.3%	AST 32 IU/L	T. chol 190 mg/dL
Cl 104 mEq/L	WBC $6.5 \times 10^3/mm^3$	ALT 30 IU/L	LDL 132 mg/dL
CO_2 25 mEq/L	Plt $208 \times 10^3/mm^3$	TSH 2.46 mIU/L	HDL 50 mg/dL
BUN 10 mg/dL		FSH 87.8 mIU/mL	Trig 180 mg/dL
SCr 0.7 mg/dL		UPT (−)	
Random Glu			
98 mg/dL			

Other

PAP smear and mammogram: Normal

Assessment

50-year-old, symptomatic postmenopausal woman considering HRT versus other treatment options

QUESTIONS

Problem Identification

1.a. Create a list of the patient's drug therapy problems.

1.b. What information (signs, symptoms, laboratory values) indicates the presence or severity of this patient's problems as she begins menopause?

Desired Outcome

2. What are the goals of therapy for this patient's menopausal symptoms?

Therapeutic Alternatives

3.a. What nondrug therapies might be useful for this patient?

3.b. What are the benefits and risks of HRT for this patient?

3.c. What pharmacotherapeutic **hormonal** therapies are available for the treatment of menopause?

3.d. What **nonhormonal** alternatives may be used to manage menopausal symptoms?

Optimal Plan

4. What drug, dosage form, dose, schedule, and duration are best for this patient?

Outcome Evaluation

5. What clinical and laboratory parameters are necessary to evaluate the therapy for achievement of the desired therapeutic outcome and to detect or prevent adverse effects?

Patient Education

6. What information should be provided to the patient to enhance adherence to the medication, ensure successful therapy, and minimize adverse effects?

■ CLINICAL COURSE

The patient returns to her physician after taking HRT for 1 year. She reports that her hot flashes, night sweats, and occasional insomnia have significantly decreased and would like to know if she should continue taking the HRT regimen and if so, for how long.

■ FOLLOW-UP QUESTIONS

1. What is the optimal dose and length of time for a patient to continue on HRT?

2. How should HRT be discontinued after successful treatment? Would your recommendation for HRT change if the patient had been complaining of genital symptoms only? Why or why not?

3. Would your recommendation for HRT change if this patient were to have had significant risk factors for CHD or a personal history of breast cancer? Why or why not?

4. For questions related to the use of black cohosh for managing menopausal symptoms, please see Section 20 of the Casebook.

■ SELF-STUDY ASSIGNMENTS

1. Research nonhormonal therapies that have been studied for the relief of menopausal symptoms and compare the scientific evidence of their efficacy to traditional hormonal medications.

2. Review the results of the Women's Health Initiative (WHI) study and provide a summary of the findings regarding HRT and cardiovascular risk and breast cancer risk.

CLINICAL PEARL

Women should receive a thorough history and physical exam, including assessing coronary artery disease (CAD) and breast cancer risk factors, before HRT is considered. If a woman does not have any contraindications to HRT, including CAD or significant CAD risk factors, and also does not have a personal history of breast cancer, HRT would be an appropriate therapy option as it remains the most effective treatment for vasomotor symptoms and vulvovaginal atrophy.

REFERENCES

1. Bolland MJ, Ames RW, Horne AM, et al. The effect of treatment with a thiazide diuretic for 4 years on bone density in normal postmenopausal women. Osteoporosis Int 2007;18:479–86.

2. Grady D. Management of menopausal symptoms. N Engl J Med 2006;355:2338–2347.

3. Hulley S, Grady D, Bush T, et al. Randomized trial of estrogen plus progestin for secondary prevention of coronary heart disease in postmenopausal women. Heart and Estrogen/Progestin Replacement Study (HERS) Research Group. JAMA 1998;280:605–613.

4. Rossouw JE, Anderson GL, Prentice RL, et al. Writing Group for the Women's Health Initiative Investigators. Risks and benefits of estrogen plus progestin in healthy postmenopausal women: principal results

from the Women's Health Initiative randomized controlled trial. JAMA 2002;288:321–333.

5. Anderson GL, Limacher M, Assaf AR, et al. Effects of conjugated equine estrogen in postmenopausal women with hysterectomy: the Women's Health Initiative randomized controlled trial. JAMA 2004;291:1701–1712.

6. Utian WH, Shoupe D, Backmann G, et al. Relief of vasomotor symptoms and vaginal atrophy with lower doses of conjugated equine estrogens and medroxyprogesterone acetate. Fertil Steril 2001;75: 1065–1079.

7. Fugate SE, Church CO. Nonestrogen treatment modalities for vasomotor symptoms associated with menopause. Ann Pharmacother 2004;38:1482– 1499.

8. Grady D. A 60-year-old woman trying to discontinue hormone replacement therapy. JAMA 2002;287:2130–2137.

89

ERECTILE DYSFUNCTION

Where There's a Pill, There's a Way . . . . Level III

Cara Liday, PharmD, CDE

LEARNING OBJECTIVES

After completing this case study, students should be able to:

- Identify the different etiologies of erectile dysfunction (ED).

- Recognize risk factors for the development of ED.

- Provide brief descriptions of the advantages and disadvantages of the common methods available for treating ED.

- Recommend appropriate therapy and alternative treatments for ED in a specific patient.

- Counsel patients on treatment options, proper administration of selected treatments, and possible side effects.

PATIENT PRESENTATION

▣ Chief Complaint

"I've been having some problems, you know, in the bedroom."

▣ HPI

Jack Johnson is a 65-year-old man who presents to his PCP with the above complaint. On questioning, he states that for the last year he has been able to achieve only partial erections that are insufficient for intercourse. He does not notice nocturnal penile tumescence. He feels that the problem is leading to a strained relationship with his wife.

▣ PMH

Type 1 DM × 50 years
HTN
CHF (NYHA Class I)
Dyslipidemia

▣ FH

Father deceased at age 72 of cancer; mother alive with HTN

▣ SH

Married for 32 years; no history of marital problems. He is a non-smoker and drinks two to three alcoholic beverages per week. Walks for 30 minutes 5 days/wk without significant SOB.

▣ Meds

Insulin glargine 35 units SC at bedtime
Insulin aspart 13 units SC with meals and for correction dosing
Lisinopril 40 mg po once daily
Carvedilol 25 mg po BID
Furosemide 20 mg po every morning
Simvastatin 40 mg po once daily
ASA 81 mg po once daily

▣ All

NKDA

▣ ROS

Denies significant life stressors, fatigue, nocturia, urgency, or symptoms of prostatitis. Complains of some numbness in his feet and difficulty achieving and maintaining erections. Occasionally has transient edema in his ankles, and many of his toenails are brittle and yellowing.

▣ Physical Examination

Gen

Alert, well-developed, cooperative man in NAD

VS

BP 122/76, P 60, RR 18, T 37.2°C; Wt 80 kg, Ht 5'11"

Skin

Warm, dry; no lesions

HEENT

NC/AT; EOMI; PERRLA; funduscopic examination shows no arteriolar narrowing, hemorrhages, or exudates

Neck/Lymph Nodes

Supple without JVD, lymphadenopathy, masses, or goiter

Lungs/Chest

Clear to A & P bilaterally

CV

RRR; normal S_1 and S_2; no MRG

Abd

Soft, obese; NTND; normal bowel sounds; no masses or organomegaly

Genit/Rect

Normal scrotum, testes descended; NT w/o masses; penis without discharge or curvature

MS/Ext

Muscle strength 5/5 throughout; full ROM in all extremities; pulses 2+ throughout; no edema present; multiple toenails with yellow discoloration and thickening

Neuro

CNs II–XII intact; DTRs 2+ and equal bilaterally. No sensory/motor deficits; reduced sensation in extremities bilaterally with vibratory and monofilament testing

■ Labs

Na 139 mEq/L	Hgb 16.0 g/dL	Ca 9.5 mg/dL	*Fasting Lipid Profile:*
K 3.9 mEq/L	Hct 50%	Mg 1.8 mEq/L	T. chol 153 mg/dL
Cl 102 mEq/L	BNP 79 pg/mL	A1C 7.5%	HDL 48 mg/dL
CO_2 24 mEq/L		Testosterone 700 ng/dL	LDL 86 mg/dL
BUN 12 mg/dL			TG 96 mg/dL
SCr 1.0 mg/dL			VLDL 19 mg/dL
Glu (fasting) 136 mg/dL			

■ UA

SG 1.00; pH 5.1; leukocyte esterase (–); nitrite (–); protein 100 mg/dL; ketones (–); urobilinogen normal; bilirubin (–); blood (–)

■ Assessment

1. Erectile dysfunction
2. Poor long-term control of Type 1 DM
3. Hypertension controlled on current therapy
4. Dyslipidemia controlled on current therapy
5. Probable diagnosis of onychomycosis

QUESTIONS

Problem Identification

1.a. Create a list of the patient's drug therapy problems.

1.b. What risk factors for ED are present in this patient?

1.c. What are the etiologies of ED, and what is this patient's most likely etiology?

1.d. Could any of the patient's problems have been caused by drug therapy?

Desired Outcome

2. What are the goals of therapy in this case?

Therapeutic Alternatives

3.a. What nondrug therapies are available for the treatment of ED?

3.b. What pharmacologic alternatives are available for the treatment of ED?

Optimal Plan

4. What therapy is most appropriate and effective for initial treatment of this patient? If drug therapy is indicated, list the drug, dosage form, dose, schedule, and duration of therapy.

Outcome Evaluation

5. What clinical parameters are necessary to evaluate the therapy for achievement of the desired therapeutic outcome and to detect or prevent adverse effects?

Patient Education

6. What information should be provided to the patient to enhance compliance, ensure successful therapy, and minimize adverse effects?

■ SELF-STUDY ASSIGNMENTS

1. If therapy for onychomycosis is desired, what medication would be optimal, and how would the addition of this agent change your treatment of the patient's ED?

2. Investigate the treatments for priapism, and write a two-page report that includes your conclusion about the most effective treatment.

3. Perform a literature search to identify new oral therapies and alternative routes of medication delivery for ED. Compare the potential advantages and disadvantages of each treatment.

CLINICAL PEARL

Patients with cardiovascular (CV) disease have a greater risk of developing ED. In some patients, the initial presenting symptom of CV disease is ED, which can serve as a warning signal of existing or future CV disease. Providers may use this opportunity to screen or treat CV disease appropriately.

REFERENCES

1. Schwarz ER, Rastogi S, Kapur V, et al. Erectile dysfunction in heart failure patients. J Am Coll Cardiol 2006;48:1111–1119.
2. Guay AT, Spark RF, Bansal S, AACE Male Sexual Dysfunction Task Force. American Association of Clinical Endocrinologists medical guidelines for clinical practice for the evaluation and treatment of male sexual dysfunction: a couple's problem—2003 update. Endocr Pract 2003;9:77–95.
3. Ralph D, McNicholas T, for the Erectile Dysfunction Alliance. UK management guidelines for erectile dysfunction. BMJ 2000;321:499–503.
4. De Tejada IS. Therapeutic strategies for optimizing PDE-5 inhibitor therapy in patients with erectile dysfunction considered difficult or challenging to treat. Int J Impot Res 2004;16(Suppl 1):S40–S42.
5. Gresser U, Gleiter CH. Erectile dysfunction: comparison of efficacy and side effects of the PDE-5 inhibitors sildenafil, vardenafil and tadalafil: review of the literature. Eur J Med Res 2002;7:435–446.
6. Kostis JB, Jackson C, Rosen R, et al. Sexual dysfunction and cardiac risk (the Second Princeton Consensus Conference). Am J Cardiol 2005;96:313–321.
7. Soderdahl DW, Thrasher JB, Hansberry KL. Intracavernosal drug-induced erection therapy versus external vacuum devices in the treatment of erectile dysfunction. Br J Urol 1997;79:952–957.

90

BENIGN PROSTATIC HYPERPLASIA

Size Matters . . . . Level II

Kevin W. Cleveland, PharmD, ANP

Catherine A. Heyneman, PharmD, MS, CGP, ANP, FASCP

LEARNING OBJECTIVES

After completing this case study, students should be able to:

• Recognize the clinical manifestations of benign prostatic hyperplasia (BPH).

- Differentiate between obstructive and irritative symptoms in patients with BPH.

- Recommend appropriate pharmacotherapeutic treatment for BPH.

- Identify and manage drug interactions associated with BPH pharmacotherapy.

- Recognize when surgical therapies should be considered for patients with BPH.

- Understand how some drugs can exacerbate BPH symptoms.

PATIENT PRESENTATION

Chief Complaint

"I can't sleep at night. I'm up four or five times feeling that I have to urinate, and then when I get to the bathroom all I do is dribble. Sometimes I don't even make it to the bathroom in time. I have a girlfriend now and I regularly take Cialis. Going to the bathroom all night is really impacting my love life."

HPI

Conrad McLaren is a 62-year-old man with a longstanding history of UTIs. He has been hospitalized twice in the past 3 years for urosepsis. He is being evaluated because of complaints of worsening urinary hesitancy, nocturia, and dribbling.

PMH

HTN
Laminectomy 10 years ago
BPH with urge incontinence
Chronic UTIs
Type 2 DM (well-controlled with glyburide/metformin)
Erectile dysfunction
Obesity
Hx headaches
Osteoarthritis

FH

Educated through the 8th grade. Father died of massive MI at age 72; mother died of natural causes at age 91.

SH

Worked for 35 years as a railroad diesel refrigeration mechanic; retired 7 years ago. Married once. Wife deceased 6 months ago (stroke); one daughter, two granddaughters. Lives alone but is socially active. Recently started dating a 59-year-old woman he met through his church group. Patient is emphatic about maximizing the use of natural products in his therapy. Used smokeless tobacco × 35 years; heavy ETOH in the past, occasional glass of wine now.

ROS

In conversation, he is alert, friendly, and courteous. He has no c/o dyspepsia, dysphagia, abdominal pain, hematemesis, or visible blood in the stool.

Meds

Glyburide/metformin 5/500 mg po BID
Amitriptyline 50 mg po at bedtime (H/A prophylaxis)
Lisinopril/hydrochlorothiazide 10/12.5 mg po once daily
Ibuprofen 800 mg po BID
Tadalafil 10 mg po PRN
Claritin-D 24-Hour 1 tablet po daily (allergy to cats)

All

NKDA; allergic to cat dander

Physical Examination

Gen

White male in NAD; well-kept appearance; A & O × 3

VS

BP 140/95, P 72, RR 18, T 37°C; Wt 115.2 kg, Ht 6'0"

Skin

Vertical scars on neck and lower back from laminectomies

HEENT

PERRLA; EOMI; TMs WNL; nose and throat clear w/o exudate or lesions

Neck/Lymph Nodes

Supple w/o LAD or masses; thyroid in midline

Lungs/Thorax

CTA, distant sounds

CV

RRR w/o murmurs

Abd

Soft, NTND w/o masses or scars; (+) BS

Genit/Rect

Testes ↓↓, penis circumcised w/o DC; guaiac (+) stool

MS/Ext

Neurovascular intact; distal pulses 1–2+

Neuro

DTRs 2+; CNs II–XII grossly intact

UA

Color straw; appearance clear; SG 1.010; pH 6.5; glucose (–); bilirubin (–); ketones (–); blood (–); urobilinogen 0.2 mg/dL; nitrite (–); leukocyte esterases (–); epithelial cells—occasional per hpf; WBC—occasional per hpf; RBC—none seen; bacteria—trace; amorphous—none seen; crystals—1+ calcium oxalate; mucus—none seen. Culture not indicated.

GU Consult

Patient treated for UTI 2 weeks ago with Cipro 250 mg Q 12 h × 3 days. Urine clear; negative for glucose. Bladder examination with ultrasound revealed postvoid residual estimate of 200 mL. Prostate approximately 50 g, enlarged, benign.

Assessment

BPH with urge incontinence
Erectile dysfunction
Normocytic anemia possibly secondary to UGI bleed

Labs

See Table 90-1

TABLE 90-1 Lab Values

Na 136 mEq/L	Hgb 12.6 g/dL	WBC $5.6 \times 10^3/mm^3$	AST 12 IU/L	Ca 8.5 mg/dL
K 4.1 mEq/L	Hct 37.9%	Neutros 75%	ALT 16 IU/L	Phos 3.5 mg/dL
Cl 103 mEq/L	MCV 92.5 μm^3	Lymphs 16%	Alk Phos 55 IU/L	Uric Acid 3.5 mg/dL
CO_2 41 mEq/L	MCH 30.8 pg	Monos 5%	LDH 121 U/L	T_4 7.3 mcg/dL
BUN 9 mg/dL	MCHC 33.3 g/dL	Eos 3%	T. bili 0.6 mg/dL	TSH 1.04 mIU/L
SCr 0.7 mg/dL	Plt $191 \times 10^3/mm^3$	Basos 1%	T. prot 6.1 g/dL	A1C 7.5%
Glu 120 mg/dL			T. chol 146 mg/dL	PSA 4.5 ng/mL

QUESTIONS

Problem Identification

1.a. Create a list of the patient's drug therapy problems.

1.b. Describe the natural history and epidemiologic characteristics of BPH (Fig. 90-1).

1.c. Which of this patient's complaints are consistent with obstructive symptoms of BPH? Which are consistent with irritative symptoms?

1.d. What steps are recommended in the initial evaluation of all patients presenting with BPH?

1.e. What other medical conditions should be ruled out before treating this patient for BPH?

Desired Outcome

2. What are the goals of pharmacotherapy in this case?

Therapeutic Alternatives

3. What are the treatment alternatives for BPH?

Optimal Plan

4. What drug, dosage form, dose, schedule, and duration of therapy are best for this patient?

Outcome Evaluation

5. What clinical and laboratory parameters are necessary to evaluate the therapy for achievement of the desired therapeutic outcome and to detect or prevent adverse effects?

Patient Education

6. What information should be provided to the patient to enhance compliance, ensure successful therapy, and minimize adverse effects?

■ FOLLOW-UP QUESTION

1. For questions related to the use of saw palmetto for the treatment of BPH, please see Section 20 of this Casebook.

■ CLINICAL COURSE

Mr. McLaren's blood pressure was reduced to the desired range after discontinuation of ibuprofen and a switch from Claritin-D to

Patient Name: _____ DOB: _____ ID: _____ Date of assessment: _____

Initial Assessment ( ) Monitor during: _____ Therapy ( ) after: _____ Therapy/surgery ( ) _____

AUA BPH Symptom Score

	Not at all	Less than 1 time in 5	Less than half the time	About half the time	More than half the time	Almost always	
1. Over the past month, how often have you had a sensation of not emptying your bladder completely after you finished urinating?	0	1	2	3	4	5	
2. Over the past month, how often have you had to urinate again less than two hours after you finished urinating?	0	1	2	3	4	5	
3. Over the past month, how often have you found you stopped and started again several times when you urinated?	0	1	2	3	4	5	
4. Over the past month, how often have you found it difficult to postpone urination?	0	1	2	3	4	5	
5. Over the past month, how often have you had a weak urinary stream?	0	1	2	3	4	5	
6. Over the past month, how often have you had to push or strain to begin urination?	0	1	2	3	4	5	
	None	1 time	2 times	3 times	4 times	5 or more times	
7. Over the past month, how many times did you most typically get up to urinate from the time you went to bed at night until the time you got up in the morning?	0	1	2	3	4	5	
						Total Symptom Score	

FIGURE 90-1. The American Urologic Association (AUA) symptom index for benign prostatic hyperplasia (BPH). *(Reprinted with permission from BPH, Main Report: Roehrborn CG, McConnell JD, Barry MJ, et al. AUA Guideline on the Management of Benign Prostatic Hyperplasia. American Urological Association Education and Research, Inc., © 2003.)*

Claritin. Lisinopril and tadalafil were continued; hydrochlorothiazide was discontinued due to the potential for causing or worsening ED. BPH symptoms improved within days after discontinuation of amitriptyline and pseudoephedrine and the addition of the new therapy you recommended. However, over the ensuing weeks, he continued to experience occasional urgency and hesitancy, so 6 months later he opted for laser prostatectomy. This procedure was successful in alleviating his symptoms.

■ SELF-STUDY ASSIGNMENTS

1. Compare the efficacy of saw palmetto (Serenoa repens) to finasteride and α_1-antagonists for the treatment of BPH.

2. Perform a literature search for evidence that supports the use of finasteride and α_1-antagonists as combination therapy for BPH.

3. Compare treatment options for hypertension in patients with BPH. Compare diuretic therapy to α_1-antagonists for BP control in this patient population.

4. Compare treatment options for erectile dysfunction in patients with BPH. Identify the risks and potential benefits of using α_1-antagonists and 5α-reductase inhibitors in treating comorbid ED and BPH.

CLINICAL PEARL

Physiologic measurements such as postvoid residuals, uroflowmetry, and pressure-flow studies often do not correlate well with the patient's perception of BPH symptom severity.

REFERENCES

1. Miner M, Rosenberg MT, Perelman MA. Treatment of lower urinary tract symptoms in benign prostatic hyperplasia and its impact on sexual function. Clin Ther 2006;28:13–25.
2. Kaminetsky JC. Comorbid LUTS and erectile dysfunction: optimizing their management. Curr Med Res Opin 2006;22:2497–2506.
3. AUA Practice Guidelines Committee. AUA guideline on management of benign prostatic hyperplasia (2003). Chapter 1: diagnosis and treatment recommendations. J Urol 2003;170(Pt 1):530–547.
4. Narayan P, Evans CP, Moon T. Long-term safety and efficacy of tamsulosin for the treatment of lower urinary tract symptoms associated with benign prostatic hyperplasia. J Urol 2003;170(Pt 1):498–502.
5. McConnell JD, Bruskewitz R, Walsh P, et al. The effect of finasteride on the risk of acute urinary retention and the need for surgical treatment among men with benign prostatic hyperplasia. N Engl J Med 1998;338:557–563.
6. Lowe FC, McConnell JD, Hudson PB, et al., Finasteride Study Group. Long-term 6-year experience with finasteride in patients with benign prostatic hyperplasia. Urology 2003;61:791–796.
7. Roehrborn CG, Boyle P, Nickel JC, et al. Efficacy and safety of a dual inhibitor of 5-alpha-reductase types 1 and 2 (dutasteride) in men with benign prostatic hyperplasia. Urology 2002;60:434–441.
8. McConnell JD, Roehrborn CG, Bautista OM, et al., Medical Therapy of Prostatic Symptoms (MTOPS) Research Group. The long-term effect of doxazosin, finasteride, and combination therapy on the clinical progression of benign prostatic hyperplasia. N Engl J Med 2003;349:2387–2398.
9. Bent S, Kane C, Shinohara K, et al. Saw palmetto for benign prostatic hyperplasia. N Engl J Med 2006;354:557–566.
10. Dvorkin L, Song KY. Herbs for benign prostatic hyperplasia. Ann Pharmacother 2002;36:1443–1452.

91

URINARY INCONTINENCE

Bladder Matters . . . . Level II

Mary Lee, PharmD, BCPS, FCCP

Roohollah R. Sharifi, MD, FACS

LEARNING OBJECTIVES

After completing this case study, students should be able to:

- Distinguish among four types of urinary incontinence: urge, stress, overflow, and functional incontinence.

- Define overactive bladder syndrome.

- Determine when anticholinergic drugs should be recommended for the management of overactive bladder syndrome.

- Compare and contrast the muscarinic receptor selectivity, lipophilicity, and pharmacokinetic properties of oxybutynin, tolterodine, trospium, darifenacin, and solifenacin and discuss the clinical implications of these properties.

- Compare the adverse reactions associated with oral immediate-release tablet, oral extended-release tablet, and transdermal system (patch) of oxybutynin for overactive bladder syndrome.

- Identify concomitant drug therapy that may exacerbate overactive bladder syndrome.

- Recommend appropriate nondrug therapy for the management of overactive bladder syndrome.

- Explain why anticholinergic and muscle relaxant drugs should be used cautiously in elderly patients.

PATIENT PRESENTATION

■ Chief Complaint

"I can't seem to control my urine. I feel like I have to urinate all the time. However, when I do go to the bathroom, I often pass only a small amount of urine. Sometimes I wet myself."

■ HPI

Susan Jones is a 60-year-old woman with urinary urgency and frequency. She reports soiling her underwear at least once or twice during the day and night and has resorted to wearing panty liners or changing her underwear several times a day. The patient has curtailed much of her volunteer work and social activities because of this problem. Urinary leakage is not worsened by laughing, coughing, sneezing, carrying heavy objects, or walking up and down stairs. She does not report wetting herself without warning.

■ PMH

HTN for many years, treated with medications for 10 years
Hypercholesterolemia for 5 years, controlled with a low-cholesterol diet, weight control, and weekly exercise
Menopausal; stopped ovulating at age 52; no longer has hot flashes

FH

Noncontributory

SH

Non-smoker; social drinker; married

Meds

Hydrochlorothiazide 25 mg po once daily with supper
Aspirin 325 mg po Q AM

All

NKDA

ROS

Complains that she has urinary urgency and frequency, and periodic urinary incontinence. Urinary leakage is not worsened by laughing, coughing, sneezing, or carrying heavy objects.

Physical Examination

Gen

WDWN female

VS

BP 135/84, P 90, RR 16, T 37°C; Wt 65 kg, Ht 5'2"

Skin

No rashes, wounds, or open sores

HEENT

PERRLA; EOMI; no AV nicking or hemorrhages

Neck/Lymph Nodes

No palpable thyroid masses; no lymphadenopathy

Pulm

Clear to A & P

Breasts

Normal; no lumps

CV

Regular S_1, S_2; (+) S_4; (−) S_3, murmurs, or rubs

Abd

Soft, NTND: (+) bowel sounds

Genit/Rect

Genital examination shows atrophic vaginitis consistent with menopausal status.
Pelvic examination shows no uterine prolapse and a mild degree of cystocele. Cervix is normal. No pelvic, adnexal, or uterine masses found.
External hemorrhoids; heme (−) stool.

Ext

Normal; equal motor strength in both arms and legs

Neuro

A & O × 3, CNs II–XII grossly intact; DTRs 3/5 bilaterally; negative Babinski

Labs

Na 145 mEq/L	Hgb 12 g/dL
K 4.2 mEq/L	Hct 37%
Cl 105 mEq/L	Plt 400×10^3/mm^3
CO_2 28 mEq/L	WBC 5.0×10^3/mm^3
BUN 15 mg/dL	
SCr 1.0 mg/dL	
Glu 100 mg/dL	

UA

No bacteria; no WBC

Other

The patient's bladder was catheterized. No residual urine was found. The bladder was then filled with 300 mL of saline. The patient felt an urge at 100 mL. The catheter was removed. The patient was asked to cough in different positions. No stress urinary incontinence was demonstrated. The patient voided the entire volume of saline that was instilled.

Assessment

Overactive bladder with symptoms of urinary urgency and frequency, and urinary incontinence.

QUESTIONS

Problem Identification

1.a. Create a list of the patient's drug therapy problems.

1.b. What information (signs, symptoms, medical history, laboratory values, other test results) suggests the presence or severity of urge incontinence?

1.c. Differentiate urge incontinence from stress incontinence, overflow incontinence, and functional incontinence.

1.d. Define overactive bladder syndrome.

1.e. In addition to the medications the patient is currently taking, what other drugs could exacerbate overactive bladder syndrome?

Desired Outcome

2. What are the goals of pharmacotherapy in this case?

Therapeutic Alternatives

3.a. What nondrug therapies might be useful for this patient?

3.b. What feasible pharmacotherapeutic alternatives are available for treatment of overactive bladder syndrome?

Optimal Plan

4. What drug, dosage form, dose, schedule, and duration of therapy are best for this patient?

Outcome Evaluation

5. What clinical and laboratory parameters are necessary to evaluate the therapy for achievement of the desired therapeutic outcome and to detect or prevent adverse effects?

Patient Education

6. What information should be provided to the patient to enhance compliance, ensure successful therapy, and minimize adverse effects?

◼ CLINICAL COURSE

The patient was started on oxybutynin immediate-release tablets, 10 mg two times a day. Although her voiding symptoms resolved, she experienced severe constipation and dry mouth. After 1 week of drug treatment, the patient returns to the physician complaining that she cannot tolerate the adverse effects and wants alternative drug treatment.

◼ FOLLOW-UP QUESTIONS

1. Explain why this patient is experiencing these adverse effects of oxybutynin.

2. What other dosage formulations of oxybutynin are available? Are any of these alternative formulations associated with a lower prevalence of adverse effects than oxybutynin immediate-release tablets?

3. Assume that the physician wants to switch to another anticholinergic agent. Are any of other available agents associated with a lower incidence of anticholinergic adverse effects?

4. Why should anticholinergic drugs be used cautiously in elderly patients?

◼ SELF-STUDY ASSIGNMENTS

1. Patients have been classified as extensive versus poor metabolizers of tolterodine. Describe the characteristics of these patients and the clinical implications of this patient classification.

2. Conduct a literature search to determine if anticholinergic agent–induced dry mouth is severe enough to require treatment discontinuation in all patients.

3. Oxybutynin has direct muscle relaxant effects. Is this a clinically significant action of the drug in the management of overactive bladder syndrome?

CLINICAL PEARL

A drug with pharmacologic selectivity for muscarinic receptor subtypes in the detrusor muscle produces dose-related undesired anticholinergic adverse effects outside of the urinary bladder.

REFERENCES

1. Ouslander JG. Management of overactive bladder. N Engl J Med 2004;350:786–799.

2. Andersson KE. Antimuscarinics for treatment of overactive bladder. Lancet Neurol 2004;3:46–53.

3. Stewart W, Herzog R, Wein A, et al. Prevalence and impact of overactive bladder in the US: results for the NOBLE program. Neurourol Urodyn 2001;20:406. Abstract.

4. Wein A, Rackley RR. Overactive bladder: a better understanding of pathophysiology, diagnosis and management. J Urol 2006;175:S5–S10.

5. Staskin DR, MacDiarmid SA. Using anticholinergics to treat overactive bladder: the issue of treatment tolerability. Am J Med 2006;119:9S–15S.

6. Van Kerrebroeck P, Kreder K, Jonas U, et al., on behalf of the Tolterodine Study Group. Tolterodine once daily: superior efficacy and tolerability in the treatment of overactive bladder. Urology 2001;57:414–421.

7. Hashim H, Abrams P. Drug treatment of overactive bladder. Drugs 2004;64:1643–1656.

8. Rovner ES. Trospium chloride in the management of overactive bladder. Drugs 2004;64:2433–2446.

9. Haab F, Stewart L, Dwyer P. Darifenacin, an M3 selective receptor antagonist, is an effective and well-tolerated once-daily treatment for overactive bladder. Eur Urol 2004;45:420–429.

10. Payne CK. Solifenacin in overactive bladder syndrome. Drugs 2006;66:175–190.

92

SYSTEMIC LUPUS ERYTHEMATOSUS

Tired to the Bone . . . . Level II

Nicole M. Paolini, PharmD

Holly V. Coe, PharmD

LEARNING OBJECTIVES

After completing this case study, students should be able to:

- Discuss the clinical presentation of systemic lupus erythematosus (SLE), including its complications (e.g., lupus nephritis).

- Design appropriate therapy for lupus nephritis and iron deficiency anemia associated with SLE.

- Devise a monitoring plan for SLE, including disease activity, drug efficacy, and drug toxicity.

PATIENT PRESENTATION

■ Chief Complaint

"I feel tired all the time and have abdominal pain."

■ HPI

Caroline Pentz is a 34-year-old woman who was diagnosed with SLE 2 years ago. She initially presented with a malar rash, fatigue, and arthralgias. Presently, her urinalysis and labs are significant for proteinuria, hematuria, and elevated serum creatinine. Her renal biopsy is significant for focal proliferative changes, indicative of lupus nephritis. She currently complains of increased fatigue resulting in difficulty performing her job and activities of daily living. She is currently taking ibuprofen for arthralgias. The patient also has noticed a darkening of her stools over the past few months.

■ PMH

SLE × 2 years
Asthma × 15 years
Allergic rhinitis × 20 years
Depression × 2 years

■ FH

Father alive in his 60s with hypertension and celiac disease; mother alive in her 60s with fibromyalgia

■ SH

Employed as a bank executive; married for 10 years; occasional ETOH use; no current tobacco use; previous cigarette smoker: 1 ppd × 12 years (quit 5 years ago)

■ Meds

Advair 100/50 1 inhalation BID
Albuterol 1–2 puffs Q 4–6 h PRN
Fluticasone 2 sprays in each nare once daily
Paroxetine 20 mg po once daily
Ibuprofen 800 mg po QID

■ All

NKDA

■ ROS

No fever, chills, peripheral edema, alopecia, or rashes

■ Physical Examination

Gen

Tired-looking woman in NAD

VS

BP 132/80, P 74, RR 18, T 38°C; Wt 55 kg, Ht 5'3"

Skin

Warm, moist, no rash

HEENT

PERRLA; EOMI

Neck/Lymph Nodes

Supple without adenopathy

Lungs/Thorax

CTA; no rales/rhonchi

CV

RRR; S_1 and S_2 heard

Abd

Tender, non-distended; (+) bowel sounds; stool guaiac (+)

Ext

Peripheral pulses intact; no edema

Neuro

A & O × 3; CNs II–XII intact; Babinski negative

Labs

Na 142 mEq/L	Hgb 10 g/dL	C4 10 mg/dL
K 5.0 mEq/L	Hct 30%	C3 45 mg/dL
Cl 105 mEq/L	WBC $7.2 \times 10^3/mm^3$	Anti-ds DNA antibody 550 mg/dL
CO_2 25 mEq/L	Plt $250 \times 10^3/mm^3$	ESR 66 mm/h
BUN 30 mg/dL	Fe 35 mcg/dL	
SCr 1.5 mg/dL	TIBC 450 mcg/dL	
Uric acid 9.0 mg/dL	Ferritin 8 ng/mL	
Glucose 88 mg/dL		

UA

Many RBCs; no RBC casts; 2+ proteinuria

Kidney Biopsy

Focal proliferative changes

Assessment

Mild focal proliferative lupus nephritis (class III); development of iron deficiency anemia secondary to NSAID use

QUESTIONS

Problem Identification

1.a. Create a list of the patient's drug therapy problems.

1.b. What information (signs, symptoms, laboratory values) indicates the development of iron deficiency anemia?

1.c. What information (signs, symptoms, laboratory values) indicates the development of lupus nephritis?

Desired Outcome

2.a. What are the goals of pharmacotherapy for lupus nephritis in this patient?

2.b. What are the goals of pharmacotherapy for iron deficiency anemia?

Therapeutic Alternatives

3.a. What nondrug therapies might be useful for this patient?

3.b. What feasible pharmacotherapeutic alternatives are available for the treatment of lupus nephritis?

Optimal Plan

4.a. For treatment of lupus nephritis, what drug, dosage form, dose, schedule, and duration of therapy are best for this patient?

4.b. What do you recommend for treating iron deficiency anemia in this patient?

Outcome Evaluation

5. What clinical and laboratory parameters are necessary to evaluate the therapy for achievement of the desired therapeutic outcome and to detect or prevent adverse events?

Patient Education

6. What information should be provided to the patient to enhance adherence, ensure successful therapy, and minimize adverse events?

■ FOLLOW-UP QUESTIONS

1. What other medications do you recommend for treating the non-renal manifestations of lupus in this patient (i.e., arthralgias, rash)?

2. What alternatives would be appropriate if the initial treatment fails or cannot be used?

■ SELF-STUDY ASSIGNMENTS

1. New treatment modalities such as rituximab (Rituxan) are currently under investigation for SLE. Perform a literature search regarding rituximab and its efficacy/safety in lupus.

2. It has been postulated that hormonal disturbances in estrogen and androgen metabolism may play a role in the etiology and progression of SLE. Perform a literature search on dehydroepiandrosterone (DHEA) and its efficacy in the treatment of SLE.

CLINICAL PEARL

Because UV light exacerbates SLE, drugs that induce photosensitivity should be avoided in patients with the disease.

REFERENCES

1. Fine DM. Pharmacological therapy of lupus nephritis. JAMA 2005;293:3053–3060.

2. Weening JJ, D'Agati VD, Schwartz MM, et al. The classification of glomerulonephritis in systemic lupus nephritis revisited. Kidney Int 2004;65:521–530.

3. Gourley MF, Austin HA, Scott D, et al. Methylprednisolone and cyclophosphamide, alone or in combination, in patients with lupus nephritis: a randomized, controlled trial. Ann Intern Med 1996;125:549–557.

4. Kocis P. Prasterone. Am J Health Syst Pharm 2006;63:2201–2210.

5. Yeomans ND, Tulassay Z, Juhasz L, et al. A comparison of omeprazole with ranitidine for ulcers associated with nonsteroidal antiinflammatory drugs. N Engl J Med 1998;338:719–726.

6. Austin HA III, Klippel JH, Balow JE, et al. Therapy of lupus nephritis. Controlled trial of prednisone and cytotoxic drugs. N Engl J Med 1986;314:614–619.

7. Illei GG, Austin HA, Crane M, et al. Combination therapy with pulse cyclophosphamide plus pulse methylprednisolone improves long-term renal outcomes without adding toxicity in patients with lupus nephritis. Ann Intern Med 2001;135:248–257.

8. Kapitsinou PP, Boletis JN, Skopouli FN, et al. Lupus nephritis: treatment with mycophenolate mofetil. Rheumatology 2004;43:377–380.

9. Ong LM, Hooi LS, Lim TO, et al. Randomized controlled trial of pulse intravenous cyclophosphamide versus mycophenolate mofetil in the induction therapy of proliferative lupus nephritis. Nephrology 2005; 10:504–510.

10. Ginzler EM, Dooley MA, Aranow C, et al. Mycophenolate mofetil or intravenous cyclophosphamide for lupus nephritis. N Engl J Med 2005;353:2219–2228.

11. Chan TM, Li FK, Tang CS, et al. Efficacy of mycophenolate mofetil in patients with diffuse proliferative lupus nephritis. N Engl J Med 2000;343:1156–1162.

12. Grootscholten C, Ligtenberg G, Hagen EC, et al. Azathioprine/methylprednisolone versus cyclophosphamide in proliferative lupus nephritis. A randomized controlled trial. Kidney Int 2006;70:732–742.

13. Toubi E, Kessel A, Shoenfeld Y. High-dose intravenous immunoglobulins: an option in the treatment of systemic lupus erythematosus. Hum Immunol 2005;66:395–402.

93

ALLERGIC DRUG REACTION

The Three-Day Itch . . . . Level II

Lynne M. Sylvia, PharmD

LEARNING OBJECTIVES

After completing this case study, students should be able to:

- Interpret drug allergy information (e.g., timing of the reaction, signs, and symptoms) to identify the likelihood of an IgE-mediated reaction.

- Assess the potential for cross-sensitivity between penicillins and cephalosporins.

- Identify patients who are appropriate candidates for desensitization.

- Select appropriate antibiotic therapy for a patient with multiple antibiotic allergies.

PATIENT PRESENTATION

▓ Chief Complaint

"I am more short of breath than normal and I have thick, greenish phlegm when I cough."

▓ HPI

Alan Adams is a 55-year-old man with a history of COPD who presents to the ED complaining of a 3-day history of tiredness and a cough productive of greenish sputum. He also states that he is more short of breath than usual upon ambulation. The patient has had three admissions this year for COPD and pneumonia.

▓ PMH

COPD × 17 years
Chronic empyema secondary to bronchial pleural fistulae with chest tube placement 6 months ago
Right upper lobe abscess secondary to *Candida* and *Aspergillus* S/P upper lobe lobectomy 11 years ago
Hypertension × 10 years
S/P MI 15 years ago

▓ SH

Lives with his mother; he is unemployed. He has a 40 pack-year smoking history. Admits to occasional alcohol use; denies use of recreational drugs.

▓ Meds

Albuterol MDI 2 puffs Q 6 h PRN
Ipratropium MDI 2 puffs Q 6 h
Oxycodone/APAP 5/325 mg po Q 6 h PRN pain
Aspirin 325 mg po once daily
Amlodipine 10 mg po once daily

▓ All

Ampicillin-sulbactam: facial edema, tongue swelling, periorbital edema

Ceftazidime: urticarial rash on chest and face with shortness of breath
Codeine: nausea, pruritus

▓ ROS

(+) malaise, fatigue, sore throat, shortness of breath, and cough with green sputum; (−) nausea, vomiting, diarrhea, fever, chills, or chest pain

▓ Physical Examination

Gen

55-year-old Caucasian man appearing older than his stated age in moderate respiratory distress. He is lethargic and hard of hearing.

VS

BP 100/65, P 91, RR 16, T 36.4°C; Wt 52 kg, Ht 5'5"

Skin

Dry scaly skin; no tenting

HEENT

PERRLA, EOM intact, dry mucous membranes

Neck/Lymph Nodes

(−) bruits, (−) lymphadenopathy

Lungs/Thorax

(+) diffuse crackles at the left base; wheezes throughout with poor breath sounds

CV

Normal S_1 and S_2, RRR, (−) MRG

Abd

Distended with (+) bowel sounds; (−) hepatosplenomegaly

Genit/Rect

Deferred

Ext

(+) clubbing; (−) cyanosis or edema; poor muscle tone

▓ Labs

Na 137 mEq/L	Hgb 14.8 g/dL	WBC 18.9 × 10³/mm³
K 3.7 mEq/L	Hct 44.6%	Neutros 72%
Cl 96 mEq/L	RBC 5.36 × 10⁶/mm³	Bands 9%
CO₂ 29 mEq/L	Plt 244 × 10³/mm³	Eos 0%
BUN 8 mg/dL	MCV 83.2 μm³	Lymphs 11%
SCr 0.6 mg/dL	MCHC 33.2 g/dL	Monos 8%
Glu 119 mg/dL		Basos 0%

▓ ABG

pH 7.44, pO_2 55 mm Hg, pCO_2 38 mm Hg, O_2 sat 90%

▓ Chest X-Ray

Haziness in the left lower lobe S/P right upper lobe resection. Possible fibrosis versus infiltrate.

▓ Sputum Gram Stain (available 2 hours post-admission)

2+ polys; 2+ squamous epithelial cells; 2+ Gram-positive rods; 2+ Gram-positive cocci in clusters.

▓ Sputum Cultures (available 24 hours post-admission)

3+ mixed respiratory flora; 2+ *Pseudomonas aeruginosa*; susceptibilities pending

■ Blood cultures

Pending

■ Assessment

1. Bacterial pneumonia
2. Multiple allergies to antibiotics
3. COPD
4. S/P MI

QUESTIONS

Problem Identification

1.a. Based on the patient's allergy history, how should his allergies to ampicillin-sulbactam and ceftazidime be categorized—as minor, moderate, or severe?

1.b. What additional information would be helpful to fully assess the patient's risk of hypersensitivity reactions to β-lactam antibiotics?

1.c. What additional information would be helpful to assess whether the patient experiences true hypersensitivity versus pseudoallergy to codeine?

Desired Outcome

2. What are the goals for the treatment of pneumonia in this case?

■ CLINICAL COURSE

The patient was started on moxifloxacin 400 mg po Q 24 h, albuterol 2.5 mg by nebulizer Q 2 h PRN, ipratropium 0.5 mg by nebulizer Q 2 h PRN, guaifenesin with codeine (100 mg/10 mg per 5 mL) po Q 4 h PRN, and prednisone 40 mg po once daily. On day 2, sputum cultures revealed *Pseudomonas aeruginosa*, and antibiotic therapy was changed to ciprofloxacin 400 mg IV Q 12 h. Later on day 2, the susceptibility results from the sputum cultures obtained on admission were finalized and reported (Table 93-1). Orders were written to discontinue ciprofloxacin and desensitize the patient to cefepime.

Therapeutic Alternatives

3. Based on the susceptibility test results and the patient's antibiotic allergies, what alternative treatment regimens are appropriate for this patient's pneumonia?

Optimal Plan

4. Based on the physician's order, outline a cefepime desensitization regimen for this patient. Include the initial antibiotic dose, the route of administration, the amount of each subsequent dose, the administration schedule, and any preventive measures that should be employed during the desensitization process.

TABLE 93-1	Culture Results of Sputum Sample Taken on Day 1 and Reported on Day 3	
Antibiotic	**Dilution**	**Interpretation**
Amikacin	>64	Resistant
Aztreonam	4.0	Sensitive
Cefepime	4.0	Sensitive
Ciprofloxacin	>4	Resistant
Gentamicin	>16	Resistant
Imipenem	>16	Resistant
Piperacillin/tazobactam	16	Sensitive
Tobramycin	4	Sensitive

Outcome Evaluation

5. What clinical and laboratory parameters should be evaluated during and after the desensitization procedure to detect or prevent allergic events?

Patient Education

6. What information should be provided to the patient about his drug allergies to minimize allergic events in the future?

■ SELF-STUDY ASSIGNMENTS

1. Develop a care map for patients allergic to penicillin for whom a cephalosporin is ordered. Outline the process by which the clinician would determine the most appropriate course of action for these patients. Be specific to the type of allergy to the penicillin (i.e., maculopapular rash versus Stevens-Johnson syndrome versus anaphylactic reaction).

2. Apply the concept of graded challenge dosing (see Clinical Pearl) to the issue of β-lactam hypersensitivity. Develop criteria describing those patients with history of β-lactam hypersensitivity who would be appropriate candidates for graded challenge dosing with structurally related antibiotics.

CLINICAL PEARL

A graded challenge dose (test dosing) involves the cautious administration of a medication to a patient. Graded challenge doses of a medication are often recommended for patients who have history of hypersensitivity to a structurally related medication and the risk of a cross-reaction is deemed unlikely.

REFERENCES

1. Sylvia LM. Drug allergy and pseudoallergy. In: Tisdale JE, Miller DA, eds. Drug-Induced Diseases: Prevention, Detection and Management. 1st ed. Bethesda, MD, ASHP Publications, 2005:27–55.
2. Sampson HA, Munoz-Furlong A, Campbell RL, et al. Second symposium on the definition and management of anaphylaxis: summary report—Second National Institute of Allergy and Infectious Disease/Food Allergy and Anaphylaxis Network Symposium. J Allergy Clin Immunol 2006;117:391–397.
3. Lieberman P, Kemp SF, Oppenheimer J, et al. The diagnosis and management of anaphylaxis: an updated practice parameter. J Allergy Clin Immunol 2005;115:S483–S523.
4. Solensky R. Drug hypersensitivity. Med Clin North Am 2006;90:233–260.
5. Romano A, Quaratino D, Papa G, et al. Aminopenicillin allergy. Arch Dis Child 1997;76:513–517.
6. Sastre J, Quijano LD, Novalbos A, et al. Clinical cross-reactivity between amoxicillin and cephadroxil in patients allergic to amoxicillin and with good tolerance of penicillin. Allergy 1996;51:383–386.
7. Romano A, Di Fonso M, Viola M, et al. Selective hypersensitivity to piperacillin. Allergy 2000;55:787.
8. Pichichero ME. Cephalosporins can be prescribed safely for penicillin-allergic patients. J Fam Pract 2006;55:106–112.
9. Kelkar PS, Li JT. Cephalosporin allergy. N Engl J Med 2001;345:804–809.
10. Friedman JD, Dello Buono FA. Opioid antagonists in the treatment of opioid-induced constipation and pruritus. Ann Pharmacother 2001;35:85–91.
11. Adkinson NF, Saxon A, Spence MR, et al. Cross-allergenicity and immunogenicity of aztreonam. Rev Infect Dis 1985;7(Suppl 4):S613–S621.
12. Win PH, Brown H, Zankar A, et al. Rapid intravenous cephalosporin desensitization. J Allergy Clin Immunol 2005;116:225–228.
13. Solensky R. Drug desensitization. Immunol Allergy Clin North Am 2004;24:425–443.

94

SOLID ORGAN TRANSPLANTATION

Jim's New Kidney . . . . .Level III

Kristine S. Schonder, PharmD

LEARNING OBJECTIVES

After completing this case study, students should be able to:

- Develop a patient-specific therapeutic plan for complications associated with solid organ transplantation.

- Counsel a transplant recipient on the importance of medication adherence and implement mechanisms to enhance adherence.

- Describe possible adverse effects to immunosuppressive medications and develop a plan to resolve these effects.

- Assess a transplant medication regimen for potential drug interactions and develop a plan to resolve any identified interactions.

PATIENT PRESENTATION

■ Chief Complaint

"I have had diarrhea for the past 3 days."

■ HPI

James Halper is a 58-year-old man who presents to the renal transplant clinic for evaluation of diarrhea.

■ PMH

2 months S/P cadaveric kidney transplant
ESRD secondary to DM nephropathy
Diabetes mellitus
HTN
Hypercholesterolemia

■ FH

Both parents are deceased. Mother had HTN and DM; father died from MI. Mr. Halper is married with 4 children, Michael, James, Suzanna, and Catherine, who are alive and well.

■ SH

Used to drink an occasional beer with friends, but not since his transplant. He smoked cigarettes in the past, but quit 4 years ago when he started dialysis (20 pack-years). He has no history of IVDA.

■ ROS

He has been having significant diarrhea three to four times a day and occasional N/V and nocturia.

■ Meds

Tacrolimus 7 mg po BID (last dose taken last night at 8:00 PM)
Prednisone 15 mg po once daily
Mycophenolate mofetil 1,000 mg po BID
Sulfamethoxazole 400 mg/trimethoprim 80 mg po once daily
Acyclovir 200 mg po BID
ASA 81 mg po once daily
Docusate sodium 100 mg po BID
Sodium bicarbonate 1,300 mg po TID
Ferrous sulfate 300 mg po TID
Rosiglitazone 4 mg po BID
Insulin glargine 22 units SC at bedtime
Insulin regular per sliding scale
Diltiazem CD 240 mg po once daily
Clonidine 0.1 mg po TID
Famotidine 20 mg po BID
Atorvastatin 20 mg at bedtime

■ All

Codeine (nausea)

■ Physical Examination

Gen

WDWN African-American man in NAD

VS

BP 159/85, P 76 reg, RR 16, T 37.4°C; Wt 130 kg, Ht 6'1"

Skin

Warm and dry

HEENT

PERRLA; EOMI

Chest

CTA & P

CV

Normal S_1 and S_2; no MRG

Abd

Soft, NT with palpable, nontender graft; incisional wound is healing; liver size normal

Ext

2+ pitting edema in LE; 2+ DP pulses bilaterally. No cyanosis.

Neuro

A & O × 3; CN II–XII intact; DTRs 2+ throughout

■ Labs

At 8:00 AM today (fasting):

Na 141 mEq/L	Hgb 10.2 g/dL	Ca 8.9 mg/dL	*Fasting Lipid Panel:*
K 5.7 mEq/L	Hct 31.4%	Phos 2.3 mg/dL	T. chol 182 mg/dL
Cl 104 mEq/L	RBC 2.78 × 10⁶/mm³	Mg 1.0 mEq/L	LDL-C 111 mg/dL
CO₂ 21 mEq/L	WBC 2.5 × 10³/mm³	FK 12.5 ng/mLᵃ	HDL-C 35 mg/dL
FBS 188 mg/dL	Plt 289 × 10³/mm³		Trig 180 mg/dL
BUN 40 mg/dL (last was 38 mg/dL)			CMV antigenemia test:
SCr 1.7 mg/dL (last was 2.1 mg/dL)			Positive (32/200,000 leukocytes)

ᵃTacrolimus whole blood concentration (therapeutic range, 5–20 ng/mL)

■ ECG

NSR

■ Assessment

CMV infection, hyperkalemia

QUESTIONS

Problem Identification

1.a. Create a list of the patient's drug therapy problems.

1.b. Which signs, symptoms, and laboratory values indicate the presence of CMV infection?

1.c. What are the potential causes of hyperkalemia in this patient?

1.d. What are the potential causes of the other medical problems in this patient?

Desired Outcome

2. What are the goals of pharmacotherapy in this case?

Therapeutic Alternatives

3.a. What nonpharmacologic therapies and education might be useful for this patient?

3.b. What pharmacotherapeutic alternatives are available for the treatment of CMV infection?

3.c. What pharmacotherapeutic alternatives are available for treating hyperkalemia in this patient?

Optimal Plan

4. Design a pharmacotherapeutic plan to treat this patient's CMV infection, hyperkalemia, and other medical problems.

Outcome Evaluation

5. What clinical and laboratory parameters are necessary to evaluate the response to therapy and to detect or prevent adverse effects?

Patient Education

6. What information should be provided to the patient to enhance adherence, ensure successful therapy, and minimize adverse effects?

■ CLINICAL COURSE

The patient is started on the treatment you recommended and returns for a 2-week follow-up visit. He now complains that he has been having significant swelling in his legs and his urine output has decreased. The diarrhea has still not resolved.

■ Meds

Tacrolimus 7 mg po BID (last dose taken last night at 8:00 PM)
Prednisone 15 mg po once daily
Mycophenolate mofetil 1,000 mg po BID
Sulfamethoxazole 400 mg/trimethoprim 80 mg po once daily
Ganciclovir 325 mg IV BID
ASA 81 mg po once daily
Sodium bicarbonate 650 mg po TID
Ferrous sulfate 300 mg po TID
Rosiglitazone 4 mg po BID
Insulin glargine 25 units SC at bedtime
Diltiazem CD 240 mg po once daily
Clonidine 0.2 mg po TID
Famotidine 20 mg po BID
Atorvastatin 40 mg po at bedtime

■ Physical Examination

Unremarkable, except for the following findings

Chest

Crackles at bases

Ext

4+ pitting edema bilaterally

VS

BP 165/90, P 74 reg, RR 20, T 36°C; Wt 138 kg

■ Labs

At 8:00 AM today:

Na 140 mEq/L	Ca 9.2 mg/dL	WBC $1.1 \times 10^3/mm^3$	*CMV Antigenemia*
K 5.1 mEq/L	Phos 2.5 mg/dL	Polys 68%	*Test:*
Cl 111 mEq/L	Mg 1.2 mEq/L	Lymphs 27%	Negative (CMV
CO₂ 24 mEq/L	FK 11.7 ng/mL	Monos 2%	antigenemia test
BUN 54 mg/dL	Hgb 10.2 g/dL	Eos 1%	1 week ago was
SCr 2.6 mg/dL	Hct 29.8 %	Basos 2%	12/200,000
FBS 140 mg/dL	RBC $2.97 \times 10^6/mm^3$	Plt $203 \times 10^3/mm^3$	leukocytes)

■ Renal Biopsy

Mild acute cellular rejection (Banff 2A)

■ Stool Culture

Negative

■ FOLLOW-UP QUESTIONS

1. What is the most likely cause of the patient's edema?

2. What are the potential causes of leukopenia in this patient?

3. What changes (if any) should be made in the patient's CMV treatment?

4. What are other potential causes of diarrhea in this patient?

■ SELF-STUDY ASSIGNMENTS

1. Develop a pharmacotherapeutic plan for the different strategies to prevent and manage CMV infection in solid organ transplant recipients.

2. Design a systematic approach for patient education for a new solid organ transplant recipient focusing on immunosuppressive therapies, adverse effects and drug interactions, and strategies to manage patient compliance with a complicated regimen.

CLINICAL PEARL

It is estimated that 75–90% of people are CMV-seropositive. Solid organ transplant recipients are at risk of active CMV infection due to immunosuppressive therapy. The greatest risk of CMV infection occurs in CMV-seronegative recipients who receive an allograft from a CMV-seropositive donor. Recipients who are CMV-seropositive are also at risk for reactivation of CMV.

REFERENCES

1. Sia IG, Patel R. New strategies for prevention and therapy of cytomegalovirus infection and disease in solid-organ transplant recipients. Clin Microbiol Rev 2000;13:83–121.

2. Tylicki L, Habicht A, Watschinger B, et al. Treatment of hypertension in renal transplant recipients. Curr Opin Urol 2003;13:91–98.

3. K/DOQI clinical practice guidelines for managing dyslipidemias in chronic kidney disease. *www.kidney.org/professionals/kdoqi/guidelines_lipids/index. htm.* Accessed April 19, 2008.

4. Andany MA, Kasiske BL. Dyslipidemia and its management after renal transplantation. J Nephrol 2001;14(Suppl 4):S81–S88.

95

OSTEOPOROSIS

Bone Up on Osteoporosis . . . . Level II

Emily C. Farthing-Papineau, PharmD, BCPS

Julia M. Koehler, PharmD

LEARNING OBJECTIVES

After completing this case study, students should be able to:

- Identify the risk factors for the development of osteoporosis.

- Recommend appropriate nonpharmacologic measures for the prevention and treatment of osteoporosis.

- Recommend the correct amount and form of calcium supplementation required for the prevention and treatment of osteoporosis.

- Design an appropriate pharmacologic treatment regimen for the treatment of osteoporosis in postmenopausal women.

- Provide appropriate patient education regarding osteoporosis and its therapy.

PATIENT PRESENTATION

Chief Complaint

"My back has been hurting a lot since yesterday."

HPI

Beverly Jones is a 75-year-old Caucasian woman with a history of HTN, hyperlipidemia, COPD, hypothyroidism, and osteoporosis. She presents to the family medicine clinic for a follow-up visit for her HTN and osteoporosis. She has been experiencing episodes of constipation and flatulence since she began taking Os-Cal 500 after her last clinic visit.

PMH

HTN first diagnosed at age 50.
S/P MI 12 years ago.
Hyperlipidemia × 13 years; patient modified diet and took cholestyramine for several years.
Hypothyroidism × 27 years, treated with levothyroxine.
Osteoporosis diagnosed by DXA scan 2 years ago.
COPD diagnosed several years ago. History of repeated exacerbations requiring prednisone; last exacerbation 6 months ago. Currently stable on multiple inhalers.
Breast cancer with mastectomy of left breast and radiation therapy at age 40.

Menopause at age 39.
Right carotid endarterectomy 2 years ago.
GERD.

FH

Paternal history (+) for CAD; father died at age 60 of "heart trouble." Maternal history (+) for stroke and vascular disorders; mother became menopausal at approximately age 40.

SH

Widowed; G_2P_3; $2^1/_2$ ppd smoker, quit after MI; non-drinker

ROS

Mild headaches and new onset back pain, treated with acetaminophen; vaginal dryness; has noticed that her height has decreased by 2" since she was 35 years old; denies shortness of breath or chest pain

Meds

Ramipril 10 mg po BID × 2 years
Tiotropium 18 mcg inhaled once daily × 9 months
Advair 250/50 1 puff BID × 9 months
Albuterol MDI 2 puffs Q 6 h PRN
Synthroid 100 mcg po once daily × 20 years
Atenolol 50 mg po once daily × 10 years
Aspirin 81 mg po once daily × 12 years
Omeprazole 20 mg po once daily × 1 year
Lipitor 10 mg po once daily × 3 months
Os-Cal 500 po TID × 3 months

All

NKDA

Physical Examination

Gen

WDWN Caucasian woman in NAD

VS

BP 150/94, P 64, RR 17, T 37°C; Wt 53.5 kg, Ht 5'3"

Skin

Fair complexion, color good, no lesions

HEENT

PERRLA; EOMI; eyes and throat clear; funduscopic exam reveals mild arteriolar narrowing, with AV ratio 1:3; no hemorrhages, exudates, or papilledema

Neck/Lymph Nodes

Supple, without obvious nodes; no JVD

Chest

Decreased breath sounds bilaterally; air movement decreased; no rales or rhonchi

Breasts

Mastectomy scar left breast; right breast normal

CV

RRR; no murmurs; normal S_1 and S_2, no S_3 or S_4

Abd

Soft, NT/ND, (+) BS

Genit/Rect

Deferred

MS/Ext

Good pulses bilaterally

Neuro

CN II–XII intact; DTRs 2+; sensory and motor levels intact

■ Labs

Na 141 mEq/L	TSH 3.492 mIU/L	*Current fasting lipid profile:*	*Three months ago:*
K 4.2 mEq/L	AST 32 IU/L		T. chol 250 mg/dL
Cl 104 mEq/L	ALT 27 IU/L	T. chol 177 mg/dL	Trig 265 mg/dL
CO_2 25 mEq/L		Trig 215 mg/dL	HDL 30 mg/dL
BUN 17 mg/dL		HDL 32 mg/dL	LDL 167 mg/dL
SCr 1.0 mg/dL		LDL 102 mg/dL	AST 20 IU/L
Glu 98 mg/dL			ALT 17 IU/L

■ Other

DXA scan of lumbar spine today reveals: L2–4 = 0.780 g/cm^2 (T score: –3.2 SD); right femoral neck = 0.615 g/cm^2 (T score: –3.1 SD)
X-ray of the spine today shows a new compression fracture on L3

■ Assessment

1. Back pain secondary to a vertebral compression fracture
2. Severe osteoporosis requiring further intervention
3. Hypertension not adequately controlled
4. Hyperlipidemia responding to therapy, but not at goal
5. Stage IV COPD stable on present regimen
6. Hypothyroidism well controlled on present regimen
7. Constipation

QUESTIONS

Problem Identification

1.a. Create a list of the patient's drug therapy problems.

1.b. What information (signs, symptoms, laboratory values) indicates the presence or severity of the patient's osteoporosis? What are the patient's risk factors for developing osteoporosis?

1.c. What additional information would be useful in determining the extent of the patient's osteoporosis and the need for aggressive therapy?

Desired Outcome

2. What are the goals of pharmacotherapy for osteoporosis in this case?

Therapeutic Alternatives

3.a. What nondrug therapies might be useful for this patient's osteoporosis?

3.b. What feasible pharmacotherapeutic alternatives are available for treatment of the osteoporosis?

Optimal Plan

4.a. What drug, dosage form, dose, schedule, and duration of therapy are best for treating this patient's osteoporosis?

4.b. What alternatives would be appropriate if the initial therapy fails or cannot be used?

Outcome Evaluation

5. Which clinical and laboratory parameters are necessary to evaluate the therapy for achievement of the desired therapeutic outcome and to detect or prevent adverse effects?

Patient Counseling

6. What information should be provided to the patient to enhance compliance, ensure successful therapy, and minimize adverse effects?

■ SELF-STUDY ASSIGNMENTS

1. Create a list of medications associated with an increased risk for developing osteoporosis.

2. Investigate the new drugs and drug classes under development for the treatment of osteoporosis.

3. Develop an exercise plan to prevent osteoporosis.

CLINICAL PEARL

In elderly patients or those on acid-suppressive therapy, recommend calcium citrate instead of calcium carbonate, as this salt form does not require an acidic gastric pH for dissolution.

REFERENCES

1. Yang YX, Lewis JD, Epstein S, et al. Long-term proton pump inhibitor therapy and risk of hip fracture. JAMA 2006;296:2947–2953.

2. National Institutes of Health. JNC 7 express; Seventh report of the Joint National Committee on Prevention, Detection, Evaluation and Treatment of High Blood Pressure. Bethesda, Md: National Heart, Lung, and Blood Institute. National Institutes of Health; 2003. NIH Publication No. 03-5233.

3. Feskanich D, Willett WC, Stampfer MJ, et al. A prospective study of thiazide use and fractures in women. Osteoporos Int 1997;7:79–84.

4. National Cholesterol Education Program Expert Panel. Final report of the third report of the National Cholesterol Education Program (NCEP) expert panel on detection, evaluation, and treatment of high blood cholesterol in adults (adult treatment panel III). Bethesda, MD: National Heart, Lung, and Blood Institute. National Institutes of Health; 2002. NIH Publication No. 02-5215.

5. Grundy SM, Cleeman JI, Merz CN, et al. for the Coordinating Committee of the National Cholesterol Education Program. Implications of recent clinical trials for the National Cholesterol Education Program Adult Treatment Panel III guidelines. Circulation 2004;110:227–239.

6. Global strategy for diagnosis, management, and prevention of chronic obstructive lung disease executive summary. 2006. pgs. 1–31. Available at: *www.goldcopd.org.* Accessed May 24, 2007.

7. Management of osteoporosis in postmenopausal women: 2006 position statement of The North American Menopause Society. Menopause 2006;13:340–367.

8. American Association of Clinical Endocrinologists Osteoporosis Task Force. AACE medical guidelines for clinical practice for the prevention and treatment of postmenopausal osteoporosis: 2001 edition, with selected updates for 2003. Endocr Pract 2003;9:544–564.

9. National Osteoporosis Foundation Physician's Guide to Prevention and Treatment of Osteoporosis. Available at: *http://www.nof.org/physguide/index.htm*.

10. Tucker KL, Morita K, Qiao N, et al. Colas, but not other carbonated beverages, are associated with low bone mineral density in older women: the Framingham Osteoporosis Study. Am J Clin Nutr 2006; 84:936–942.

11. Levenson DI, Bockman RS. A review of calcium preparations. Nutr Rev 1994;52:221–232.

12. American College of Rheumatology Ad Hoc Committee On Glucocorticoid-Induced Osteoporosis. Recommendations for the prevention and treatment of glucocorticoid-induced osteoporosis, 2001 update. Arthritis Rheum 2001;44:1496–1503.

13. Houghton LA, Veith R. The case against ergocalciferol (vitamin D_2) as a vitamin supplement. Am J Clin Nutr 2006;84:694–697.

14. Black DM, Schwartz AV, Ensrud KE, et al. Effects of continuing or stopping alendronate after 5 years of treatment. JAMA 2006;296:2927–2938.

15. Black DM, Delmas PD, Eastell R, et al. Once-yearly zoledronic acid for treatment of postmenopausal osteoporosis. N Engl J Med 2007;356:1809–1822.

16. Woo SB, Hellstein JW, Kalmar JR. Systematic review: bisphosphonates and osteonecrosis of the jaws. Ann Intern Med 2006;144:753–761.

17. McClung M, Recker R, Miller P, et al. Intravenous zoledronic acid 5 mg in the treatment of postmenopausal women with low bone density previously treated with alendronate. Bone 2007, DOI:10.1016/j.bone.2007.03.011

18. U.S. Preventive Services Task Force. Hormone therapy for the prevention of chronic conditions in postmenopausal women: recommendations from the U.S. Preventive Services Task Force. Ann Intern Med 2005;142:855–860.

96

RHEUMATOID ARTHRITIS

Joint Project............................ Level II

Amy L. Whitaker, PharmD

LEARNING OBJECTIVES

After completing this case study, the reader should be able to:

- Identify the signs and symptoms of rheumatoid arthritis (RA).

- Recommend appropriate drug therapy for the management of RA.

- Recognize alternative therapies for the treatment of pain and inflammation in patients with RA.

- Recommend appropriate nonpharmacologic options for managing patients with RA.

- Counsel patients about the drug therapy used to treat RA.

PATIENT PRESENTATION

▩ Chief Complaint

"I have pain in all of my joints, a swollen left knee, and stiffness every morning."

▩ HPI

Janet Hobbs is a 58-year-old woman who presents to her rheumatologist with generalized arthralgias, a swollen left knee, and morning stiffness. These symptoms have been occurring with increasing severity for the past several weeks. She presented with similar symptoms 3 months ago, at which time her drug regimen was changed from methotrexate and NSAID therapy to her current regimen below.

▩ PMH

RA × 6 years
S/P hysterectomy 4 years ago
HTN × 10 years

▩ FH

Father died from complications after a traumatic fall at age 65. Mother died of hip fracture and pneumonia at age 78. No siblings.

▩ SH

Housewife; married for 32 years; has two grown children with no known medical problems. Denies alcohol or tobacco use. Volunteers in the community extensively, but has been doing less in the past 2 months.

▩ Meds

Hydrochlorothiazide 25 mg po Q AM
Norvasc 10 mg po once daily
Nabumetone 750 mg, 2 tabs po Q HS
Prednisone 5 mg, $^1/_2$ tab po Q AM
Methotrexate 2.5 mg, 6 tabs po once a week
Hydroxychloroquine 200 mg, 1 tab po BID
Sulfasalazine EC 500 mg, 1 tab po BID
Folic acid 1 mg po once daily
Patient receives medications at a local community pharmacy. Medication profile indicates that she refills her medications on time the first of each month.

▩ All

Penicillin (rash 25 years ago)

▩ ROS

Swelling in left knee; decreased ROM in hands; morning stiffness every day for about 3 hours; fatigue experienced daily during afternoon hours; denies HA, chest pain, SOB, bleeding episodes, or syncopal attacks; denies nausea, vomiting, diarrhea, loss of appetite or weight loss; reports minor visual changes corrected with stronger prescription glasses.

▩ Physical Examination

Gen

Pleasant, middle-aged white woman in moderate distress because of pain and swelling in left knee

VS

BP 138/80, P 82, RR 14, T 37.1°C; Wt 65.3 kg, Ht 5'6"

Skin

No rashes; normal turgor; no breakdown or ulcers

HEENT

Atraumatic; moon facies; PERRLA; EOMI; AV nicking visible bilaterally; pale conjunctiva bilaterally; TMs intact; xerostomia

Neck/Lymph Nodes

Supple, no JVD or thyromegaly; no bruits; palpable lymph nodes

Chest

CTA

TABLE 96-1 Lab Values

Na 135 mEq/L	Hgb 10.0 g/dL	AST 15 IU/L	CK <20 IU/L	Fasting Lipid Profile:
K 4.1 mEq/L	Hct 31%	ALT 12 IU/L	ANA negative	T. chol 219 mg/dL
Cl 101 mEq/L	WBC 13.0×10^3/mm³	Alk phos 56 IU/L	Wes ESR 47 mm/h	LDL 106 mg/dL
CO₂ 22 mEq/L	Plt 356×10^3/mm³	T. bili 0.8 mg/dL	RF (+) 1:1,280	HDL 50 mg/dL
BUN 12 mg/dL	Ca 9.1 mg/dL	Alb 4.2 g/dL	Anti-CCP (+)	TG 150 mg/dL
SCr 0.8 mg/dL	Urate 5.1 mg/dL	HbsAg (–)	aPTT 31 sec	
Glu 103 mg/dL	TSH 0.74 mIU/L	Anti-HCV (–)	INR 1.0	

Breasts

Normal; no lumps

CV

RRR; normal S_1, S_2; no MRG

Abd

Soft, NT/ND; (+) BS

Genit/Rect

Deferred

MS/Ext

Hands: mild RA changes; swelling of the 3rd, 4th, and 5th PIP joints bilaterally; pain in the 3rd and 4th MCP joints on left; boutonnière deformity of the 3rd and 4th digits bilaterally; ulnar deviation bilaterally; decreased grip strength, L > R (patient is left-handed)

Wrists: decreased ROM

Elbows: good ROM; slight permanent contracture on right; fixed nodule at pressure point

Shoulders: decreased ROM (especially abduction) bilaterally

Hips: decreased ROM on right; atrophy of quadriceps, L > R

Knees: pain bilaterally; decreased ROM on left; effusion/edema on left

Feet: no edema; full plantar flexion and dorsiflexion; 3+ pedal pulses

■ Neuro

CN II–XII grossly intact; muscle strength 5/5 UE, 4/5 LE, DTRs 2/4 biceps and triceps, 1/4 patella

■ Labs

See Table 96-1

■ UA

Normal

■ Chest X-Ray

No fluid, masses, or infection; no cardiomegaly

■ Hand X-Ray

Erosion of MCP and PIP joints bilaterally; measurable joint space narrowing from previous x-ray 6 months ago

■ Synovial Fluid

From left knee; white cells 23.0×10^3/mm³, turbid in appearance

■ DEXA scan of hip/spine

T-score reported as –2

■ Assessment

58-year-old woman in moderate distress with acute flare of RA (functional class II). RA not adequately controlled with current therapy. Patient is adherent with current medication regimen. HTN is controlled on present therapy. DEXA scan results suggestive of osteopenia.

QUESTIONS

Problem Identification

1.a. List the patient's drug therapy problems.

1.b. What information (signs, symptoms, laboratory values) indicates the presence and severity of rheumatoid arthritis?

1.c. What additional information is needed to assess the patient?

Desired Outcome

2. What are the goals of pharmacotherapy in this case?

Therapeutic Alternatives

3.a. What nonpharmacologic modalities may be beneficial for this patient?

3.b. What pharmacologic alternatives are available for the treatment of RA?

3.c. What economic and psychosocial considerations are applicable to this patient?

Optimal Plan

4. What drug, dosage form, dose, schedule, and duration of therapy are best for this patient?

Outcome Evaluation

5. What clinical and laboratory parameters are necessary to evaluate the patient's drug therapy?

Patient Education

6. What information should be provided to the patient to enhance adherence, ensure successful therapy, and minimize adverse effects?

■ SELF-STUDY ASSIGNMENTS

1. Perform a literature search and assess the risk of cardiovascular events associated with NSAID use.

2. Create a list of the clinically significant drug interactions for NSAIDs and DMARDs, including methotrexate.

3. Compare the biologic agents used to treat rheumatoid arthritis with respect to class of agent, route of administration, efficacy, and incidence of side effects.

CLINICAL PEARL

Treat with high-dose corticosteroids to obtain short-term benefit and relieve the flare of rheumatoid arthritis. Concurrently, or shortly thereafter, begin an NSAID and a DMARD to obtain long-term benefit and prevent disease flares and progression.

REFERENCES

1. American College of Rheumatology Subcommittee on Rheumatoid Arthritis Guidelines. Guidelines for the management of rheumatoid arthritis: 2002, Update. Arthritis Rheum 2002;46:328–346.
2. Moreland LW, Schiff MH, Baumgartner SW, et al. Etanercept therapy in rheumatoid arthritis. A randomized controlled trial. Ann Intern Med 1999;130:478–486.
3. Klareskog L, van der Heijde D, De Jaager JP, et al. Therapeutic effect of the combination of etanercept and methotrexate compared with each treatment alone in patient with rheumatoid arthritis: double-blind randomised controlled trial. Lancet 2004;363:675–681.
4. St. Clair EW, van der Heijde DM, Smolen JS, et al. Combination of infliximab and methotrexate therapy for early rheumatoid arthritis: a randomized, controlled trial. Arthritis Rheum 2004;50:3432–3443.
5. Weinblatt ME, Keystone EC, Furst DE, et al. Adalimumab, a fully human antitumor necrosis factor alpha monoclonal antibody, for the treatment of rheumatoid arthritis in patients taking concomitant methotrexate: the ARMADA trial. Arthritis Rheum 2003;48:35–45.
6. Cohen SB, Moreland LW, Cush JJ, et al. A multicentre, double blind, placebo controlled trial of anakinra (Kineret), a recombinant interleukin 1 receptor antagonist, in patients with rheumatoid arthritis treated with background methotrexate. Ann Rheum Dis 2004;63:1062–1068.
7. Nogid A, Pham DQ. Role of abatacept in the management of rheumatoid arthritis. Clin Ther 2006;28:1764–1778.
8. Summers KM, Kockler DR. Rituximab treatment of refractory rheumatoid arthritis. Ann Pharmacother 2005;39:2091–2095.
9. Pucino F, Harbus PT, Goldback-Mansky R. Use of biologics in rheumatoid arthritis: where are we going? Am J Health-Syst Pharm 2006;63(Suppl 4):S19–S41.

97

OSTEOARTHRITIS

Wear and Tear . . . . Level II

Christopher M. Degenkolb, PharmD, BCPS

LEARNING OBJECTIVES

After completing this case study, the reader should be able to:

- Recognize the most common signs and symptoms of osteoarthritis.

- Design an appropriate pharmacotherapeutic regimen for treating osteoarthritis, taking into account a patient's other medical problems and drug therapy.

- Incorporate potential adjunctive therapies (pharmacologic, nonpharmacologic, and alternative) into the regimen of a patient with osteoarthritis.

- Assess and evaluate the efficacy of an analgesic regimen for a patient with osteoarthritis, and formulate an alternative plan if the regimen is inadequate or causes unacceptable toxicity.

PATIENT PRESENTATION

■ Chief Complaint

"My joints are killing me; I need something else for this pain."

■ HPI

Donald Abernathy is a 73-year-old man who presents to the Ambulatory Care Clinic for his regular follow-up appointment complaining of increasing pain in his lower back, hips, and right knee. Six months ago, the patient was started on acetaminophen 500 mg tablets, two tablets four times daily, and has been taking more than prescribed over the last few weeks. (He admits to taking three 500 mg tablets four times daily.) The patient is in clinic today complaining that this increased dose has not been working, and that he has been in moderate to severe pain for the last 3–4 weeks. He has been adherent to all other drug therapies.

The patient is a veteran who served in the Korean conflict and worked in a factory for 35 years after his time in the military. His factory job often puts strain on his back and legs due to heavy lifting. Since retiring 15 years ago, the patient states that he has put on excess weight and developed many medical problems that are frustrating him.

■ PMH

OA × 18 years
Obesity × 15 years
Type 2 DM × 5 years
Hyperlipidemia × 5 years
HTN × 10 years
BPH × 4 years

■ PSH

Appendectomy 27 years ago

■ FH

Mother died at 81 of CVA; father died at age 75 secondary to pancreatic cancer; no siblings

■ SH

Retired; receives all medications from the VA; occasional alcohol, no tobacco or illicit drug use
Married; lives with wife at home; has one daughter who is a registered nurse

■ Meds

Lisinopril 10 mg po Q AM
Metformin 500 mg po BID
Acetaminophen 500 mg po 2 tablets four times daily
Amitriptyline 25 mg po at bedtime for sleep
Loratadine 10 mg po PRN
Terazosin 2 mg po at bedtime

■ All

Sulfa—hives
Egg products

■ ROS

Positive for pain and stiffness in right knee; low back pain with "shooting pains" radiating to the buttocks and groin area; "deep, boring" pain originating in the right pretibial area and extending distally to the right ankle and toes. Negative for headache, neck stiffness, joint swelling, or erythema; no SOB or palpitations; has been experiencing urinary hesitancy and occasional constipation; no diarrhea, no tarry stools. Fingerstick blood glucose concentrations have been running in the low 140s (he checks them once to twice per week). No blurred vision.

■ Physical Examination

Gen

Well-developed, obese, Caucasian male slightly uncomfortable, but otherwise in NAD

VS

BP 148/88, P 84, RR 16, T 37.1°C; Wt 225 lb, Ht 5'11". No orthostatic changes.

Skin

Warm, dry; LE—shiny, somewhat discolored areas on the pretibial area bilaterally, consistent with venous stasis dermatitis

HEENT

NC/AT; PERRLA; funduscopic exam reveals sharp disks; mild AV nicking, but no hemorrhages or exudates; no scleral icterus; TMs intact; mucous membranes moist; poor dentition with gingival erythema; no lateral deviation of tongue; no pharyngeal edema or erythema.

Neck/Lymph Nodes

Supple; no thyromegaly or lymphadenopathy; no carotid bruits

Lungs

CTA

CV

Distant heart sounds, Normal S_1 and S_2; PMI at 5th ICS/MCL; RRR; no MRG; no JVD or HJR

Abd

Obese, soft, nontender; no guarding; (+) BS; unable to assess liver size upon palpation

Genit/Rect

Prostate gland slightly enlarged; normal sphincter tone; guaiac (–) stool in rectal vault

MS/Ext

Back pain radiating to right buttock with straight leg raising at 60°; right hip pain with flexion >90° and with internal and external rotation >45°; both hips tender to palpation; right knee (+) crepitus; right ankle with full ROM, no swelling or edema.

Neuro

Oriented × 3; normal affect; appears at times to alternate between apathy and anger/frustration; CN II–XII intact; DTRs equal bilaterally except for slightly diminished Achilles reflexes bilaterally; no focal deficits; gait impaired secondary to hip and knee pain. Slightly decreased sensation to pinprick and vibration on the distal half of right foot. Babinski's downgoing.

■ Labs

Na 135 mEq/L	Hgb 12.8 g/dL	AST 38 IU/L	Ca 11.2 mg/dL
K 4.7 mEq/L	Hct 36.7%	Alk Phos 96 IU/L	Phos 4.5 mg/dL
Cl 98 mEq/L	WBC $4.5 \times 10^3/mm^3$	T. prot 7.4 g/dL	T. chol 206 mg/dL
CO_2 26 mEq/L	Plt $286 \times 10^3/mm^3$	Alb 4.4 g/dL	HDL chol 33 mg/dL
BUN 15 mg/dL	MCV 85.3 μm^3	Uric acid 7.2 mg/dL	LDL chol 137 mg/dL
SCr 1.6 mg/dL	MCH 28.4 pg	ESR 18 mm/h	TG 184 mg/dL
Glu 248 mg/dL	MCHC 34.5 g/dL	CRP 0.2 mg/dL	A1C 8.1%

■ UA

SG 1.011; pH 6.5; WBC (–), RBC (–), leukocyte esterase (–), nitrite (–), 1+ protein. Microscopic examination reveals 2 to 5 epithelial cells/hpf and no bacteria.

■ X-Rays

Lumbar spine: advanced degenerative changes at L3-4 and at L4-5.
Right hip: moderate degenerative changes with some spurring of the femoral head and slight decrease in joint space.
Right knee: moderate degenerative changes. No effusion.

■ Assessment

1. Pain secondary to moderate to severe OA of the lumbar spine, hips, and right knee
2. Obesity (127% of IBW, BMI = 31 kg/m²)
3. Hyperlipidemia
4. DM
5. HTN
6. BPH

QUESTIONS

Problem Identification

1.a. Create a list of the patient's drug therapy problems.

1.b. What information (symptoms, signs, laboratory values) indicates the presence or severity of the primary problem (osteoarthritis)?

1.c. What additional information is needed to satisfactorily assess this patient's major medical problems?

Desired Outcome

2. What are the goals of pharmacotherapy for each of this patient's drug related problems?

Therapeutic Alternatives

3.a. What nondrug therapies might be useful for this patient?

3.b. What feasible pharmacotherapeutic alternatives are available for treatment of this patient's osteoarthritis?

Optimal Plan

4.a. What drug, dosage form, schedule, and duration of therapy are best for treating this patient's osteoarthritis?

4.b. What alternatives would be appropriate if the initial therapy fails or cannot be used?

Outcome Evaluation

5. What clinical and laboratory parameters are necessary to evaluate the therapy for achievement of the desired therapeutic outcome and to detect or prevent adverse effects?

Patient Education

6. What information should be provided to the patient to enhance adherence, ensure successful therapy, and minimize adverse effects?

■ FOLLOW-UP QUESTIONS

1. Evaluate this patient's continued need for amitriptyline therapy, taking into account benefit versus risk, potential drug interactions, and any other important considerations.

2. Evaluate this patient's therapy for diabetes mellitus. What additional information do you need to determine the adequacy of therapy? What modifications to the diabetes treatment should be considered?

3. Evaluate this patient's regimen for hypertension. Is blood pressure controlled according to recommended guidelines? If not, what is an appropriate next step of treatment?

4. Is the combination of glucosamine and chondroitin more effective than monotherapy with glucosamine? Which form of glucosamine is best to suggest to patients?

5. The patient tells you that one time his friend received an injection into his knee that really helped his arthritis. When should intra-articular injections be considered, and what are some of their limitations?

6. For additional questions related to the use of glucosamine for OA, please see Setion 20 of this Casebook.

■ SELF-STUDY ASSIGNMENTS

1. Patients whose arthritis is poorly or inadequately controlled often turn to alternative, homeopathic, or herbal remedies for relief. Develop a list of nontraditional therapies that have been used for treating arthritis.

2. Identify an Internet website that provides useful information to patients about osteoarthritis. Identify one site that you think provides misleading or potentially dangerous information to patients.

CLINICAL PEARL

Pain relief is the top priority when treating osteoarthritis. Use a systematic approach to assessing and treating pain in order to achieve total (or near-total) pain relief, avoid wasting resources, and prevent drug misuse/addiction.

REFERENCES

1. Recommendations for the medical management of osteoarthritis of the hip and knee: 2000 update. American College of Rheumatology Subcommittee on Osteoarthritis Guidelines. Arthritis Rheum 2000;43:1905–1915.

2. Felson DT. Osteoarthritis of the knee. N Engl J Med 2006;354:841–848.

3. Simon LS, Lipman AG, Jacox AK, et al. Pain in Osteoarthritis, Rheumatoid Arthritis and Juvenile Chronic Arthritis. 2nd ed. Glenview IL, American Pain Society, 2002:1–179. (Clinical practice guideline; no. 2). Available at: www.guideline.gov. Accessed July 16, 2007.

4. Neustadt DH. Intra-articular injections for osteoarthritis of the knee. Cleve Clin J Med 2006;73:897–911.

5. Lozada CJ. Glucosamine in osteoarthritis: questions remain. Cleve Clin J Med 2007;74:65–71.

6. Clegg DO, Reda DJ, Harris CL, et al. Glucosamine, chondroitin sulfate, and the two in combination for painful knee osteoarthritis. N Engl J Med 2006;354:795–808.

98

GOUT AND HYPERURICEMIA

The Disease of Kings . . . . Level II

Geoffrey C. Wall, PharmD, BCPS, CGP

LEARNING OBJECTIVES

After completing this case study, the reader should be able to:

- Recognize major risk factors for developing gout in a given patient, including drugs that may contribute to or cause this disorder.

- Develop a pharmacotherapeutic plan for a patient with acute gouty arthritis that includes individualized drug selection and assessment of the treatment for efficacy or toxicity.

- Identify patients in whom maintenance therapy for gout and hyperuricemia is warranted.

- Select medications that treat hypertension or dyslipidemia that may have a beneficial effect on serum uric acid levels in patients with gout.

PATIENT PRESENTATION

■ Chief Complaint

"I can't walk because my ankle is killing me."

■ HPI

Nathan Vance is a 66-year-old man with a history of dyslipidemia who presents to the emergency department of his local hospital. He is suffering from sudden onset of excruciating pain in his left ankle that woke him up at 5:00 AM this morning. Over the last 2 hours, his left ankle has become red and swollen, and the pain from the joint is so bad that he cannot walk. He relates no trauma or injury to the ankle and has not exerted himself more than usual in the recent past. He also denies having experienced these symptoms previously.

■ PMH

Dyslipidemia, peptic ulcer disease (duodenal ulcer discovered 6 months ago), and obesity

■ SH

The patient drinks "a can of beer or two" daily. He does not smoke or use illicit drugs.

■ Meds

Extended-release niacin (Niaspan) 1,000 mg po at bedtime, started 2 months ago
Omeprazole 20 mg po daily

■ All

Simvastatin and atorvastatin (both caused severe muscle aches, and the patient was forced to discontinue them)

■ ROS

The patient has no major complaints prior to this emergency room visit. He relates feeling "hot and flushed" occasionally after taking his niacin, but this has not been a major problem for him. No chest pain, nausea/vomiting or respiratory symptoms. Bowel habits are normal. He has no prior history of arthritic symptoms or joint problems.

■ Physical Examination

Gen

A healthy appearing, obese, white male in acute distress

VS

BP 135/88, P 100, RR 18, T 37.5°C; Wt 97 kg, Ht 5'11"

Skin

No rashes or other dermatologic abnormalities. Has a "skull" tattoo on his left arm.

HEENT

PERRLA, throat/ears clear of redness or inflammation

Neck/Lymph Nodes

Negative for lymph node swelling or masses

Lungs/Thorax

Clear to auscultation bilaterally, symmetric movement with inspiration

CV

RRR, normal S_1 and S_2

Abd

Obese, but soft, nontender. Positive bowel sounds in all quadrants.

Genit/Rect

Deferred

MS/Ext

Left ankle with 3+ edema around joint, contrasted erythema present, and very warm to touch. Joint is exquisitely painful with patient relating the pain as currently a 10/10 (on a 1–10 scale with "1" being no pain and "10" being the worse pain the patient has ever suffered). No swelling of any other joints including great toe. No signs of tophi present.

Neuro

A & O × 3. CN II–XII grossly intact, no focal neurologic deficits.

■ Labs

Na 138 mEq/L	Hgb 15.1 g/dL	WBC $12.8 \times 10^3/mm^3$	Lipid panel (fasting):
K 3.9 mEq/L	Hct 45%	Neutros 88%	HDL-C 25 mg/dL
Cl 101 mEq/L	RBC $4.9 \times 10^6/mm^3$	Bands 0%	Trig 280 mg/dL
CO_2 23 mEq/L	Plt $210 \times 10^3/mm^3$	Eos 1%	LDL-C 99 mg/dL
BUN 9 mg/dL	MCV 81 μm^3	Lymphs 10%	T. chol 180 mg/dL
SCr 1.0 mg/dL	MCHC 35 g/dL	Monos 1%	
Glu 105 mg/dL	ESR 45 mm/h	RF negative	
Uric acid 11.6 mg/dL			

Ankle radiograph: negative for break or damage
Aspirated fluid from ankle joint tap: >50 WBC/HPF, containing negatively birefringent monosodium urate crystals

■ Assessment

1. Primary presentation of acute gouty arthritis
2. Type V dyslipidemia uncontrolled on medical therapy
3. Probable adverse drug reaction: drug-induced gout
4. History of duodenal ulcer on maintenance antisecretory therapy

QUESTIONS

Problem Identification

1.a. Create a list of the patient's drug therapy problems.

1.b. What patient information (symptoms, signs, laboratory values) indicates the presence or severity of acute gouty arthritis?

1.c. What medication is the patient taking that could contribute to or cause gouty arthritis?

Desired Outcome

2. What are the goals of pharmacotherapy in this case?

Therapeutic Alternatives

3.a. What nondrug therapies may be useful for this patient?

3.b. What pharmacotherapeutic modalities are available for the treatment of acute gouty arthritis?

3.c. Should chronic treatment to decrease the patient's serum uric acid level be initiated at this time? Why or why not?

Optimal Plan

4.a. Considering the patient's information, what drug, dosage form, schedule, and duration of therapy are best in this case?

4.b. What agent would be best to treat the patient's hyperlipidemia?

Outcome Evaluation

5. Which clinical and laboratory parameters should be monitored to assess the efficacy of the pharmacotherapeutic plan and to prevent adverse effects?

Patient Education

6. What information should be provided to the patient to enhance adherence, ensure successful therapy, and to avoid adverse effects?

■ CLINICAL COURSE

The patient responded to the therapy you recommended, and within 96 hours his pain has subsided significantly. Ankle redness and swelling have decreased to near normal. After consultation with you, the patient's physician decides against maintenance therapy to decrease serum uric acid levels. The patient, remembering the severe pain this episode caused, follows your recommended lifestyle changes and is adherent to the new medication you recommend for his dyslipidemia. At his 6-month follow-up appointment, he reports no more attacks of gout. He has lost 20 lb and no longer drinks ethanol. His serum uric acid level has decreased to 6.9 mg/dL and a fasting lipid profile demonstrates a triglyceride level of 168 mg/dL and HDL-C of 41 mg/dL.

■ FOLLOW-UP QUESTIONS

1. At what point should maintenance therapy to decrease serum uric acid levels be considered?

2. If this patient developed hypertension, which antihypertensive may be most appropriate, because it has been shown to significantly decrease serum uric acid levels?

■ SELF-STUDY ASSIGNMENTS

1. List antihyperuricemic agents that are available in the United States and their relative advantages and disadvantages. Describe new agents that are being studied for this indication and what clinical data support their use.

2. Describe the concept "relative COX-2 selectivity" in relation to the nonsteroidal anti-inflammatory drugs (NSAIDs). Based on this concept, outline your selection of an NSAID approved for acute gout.

CLINICAL PEARL

Although it is less likely to cause the GI toxicity seen with the oral form of the drug, IV colchicine should be avoided for the treatment of gout. Colchicine-associated GI side effects are employed as a clinical endpoint for discontinuing the drug, as these side effects tend to occur prior to the more severe adverse effects of colchicine-induced myopathy and myelosuppression.

REFERENCES

1. Eastmond CJ, Garton M, Robins S, et al. The effects of alcoholic beverages on urate metabolism in gout sufferers. Br J Rheumatol 1995;34:756–769.
2. Rott KT, Agudelo CA. Gout. JAMA 2003;289:2857–2860.
3. Conaghan PG, Day RO. Risks and benefits of drugs used in the management and prevention of gout. Drug Safety 1994;11:252–258.
4. Schlesinger N. Management of acute and chronic gouty arthritis. Drugs 2004;64:2399–2416.
5. Feher MD, Hepburn AL, Hogarth MB, et al. Fenofibrate enhances urate reduction in men treated with allopurinol for hyperuricaemia and gout. Rheumatology (Oxford) 2003;42:321–325.
6. Mikuls TR, MacLean CH, Olivieri J, et al. Quality of care indicators for gout management. Arthritis Rheum 2004;50:937–943.
7. Wurzner G, Gerster JC, Chiolero A, et al. Comparative effects of losartan and irbesartan on serum uric acid in hypertensive patients with hyperuricaemia and gout. J Hypertens 2001;19:1855–1860.
8. Hunter DJ, York M, Chaisson CE, et al. Recent diuretic use and the risk of recurrent gout attacks: the online case-crossover gout study. J Rheumatol 2006;33:1341–1345.

99

GLAUCOMA

Another Silent Disease . . . . .Level III

Tien T. Kiat-Winarko, PharmD, BSc

LEARNING OBJECTIVES

After completing this case study, students should be able to:

- Recognize the importance of regular eye examinations and the difference between glaucoma and ocular hypertension.

- List the risk factors for developing open-angle glaucoma.

- Select and recommend agents from different pharmacologic classes when indicated and provide the rationale for drug selection.

- Recommend conventional glaucoma therapy as well as other options in glaucoma management when indicated.

- Implement the basic ophthalmologic monitoring parameters used in glaucoma therapy.

- Counsel patients on their medication regimen and proper ophthalmic administration technique.

- Explain and discuss possible adverse drug reactions with patients to increase therapy adherence.

PATIENT PRESENTATION

Chief Complaint

"My left eye is foggy, and I get blurred vision and headaches."

HPI

Lee Angeles is a pleasant 44-year-old man with a history of advanced open-angle glaucoma who presents to his ophthalmologist with complaints of fogging and distortion of vision in the left eye lasting 6–12 hours. This occasionally progresses to tunnel vision, with chronic sensitivity to fluorescent lights and throbbing band-like squeezing headaches lasting for hours. He also complains of periodic distortion in the left eye for the past 3 months, sometimes associated with central area visual blurring. Despite his condition, he continues to maintain self-independence. He often drives from Los Angeles to his weekend home in Palm Springs.

He was in his usual state of health until he had a skydiving accident 19 years ago and fractured his thoracic spine at the level of T9-10. During that hospitalization, he complained of blurred vision. Ophthalmology consult was sought, and he was ultimately diagnosed with advanced open-angle glaucoma (Fig. 99-1). He was managed by a general ophthalmologist for several years, who prescribed Timoptic 0.5% in both eyes BID, Propine 0.1% in both eyes BID, and Ocusert Pilo-40 in right eye and Ocusert Pilo-20 in left eye once every week. He was subsequently referred to a glaucoma specialist because of worsening of his condition. He had undergone laser trabeculoplasty in both eyes prior to his referral. The glaucoma specialist examined the patient, and a complete work-up was done on the initial visit.

Bilateral laser trabeculoplasty was performed 18 years ago with an initial decrease in IOP; however, IOP subsequently increased several months later. Filtering surgery was performed in Boston on both eyes 17 years ago. Multiple prior brain MRIs revealed no abnormal findings. Other ocular history includes severe myopia since childhood, history of dry eyes, and history of contact lens wear.

PMH

Childhood asthma that resolved at puberty
Depression as a consequence of chronic open-angle glaucoma and worsening of vision after completion of his PhD program
S/P ultrasonic renal lithotripsy secondary to nephrolithiasis associated with acetazolamide use
S/P tonsillectomy as a child

FH

Father, mother, and sister have glaucoma. Father has HTN.

SH

PhD in molecular biology from Harvard. Single. No history of smoking. Drank four cans of beer per day for 3 years during postgraduate study. Currently drinks two to three cans of beer/wk.

ROS

Negative except for occasional episodes of erectile dysfunction

Meds

Betoptic 0.5% in both eyes BID
Iopidine 0.5% in left eye TID
Trusopt 2% in left eye TID
FML 0.1% in both eyes TID
Bion Tears in both eyes BID
Nifedipine 10 mg po TID
Trental 400 mg po TID
Paxil 20 mg po once daily
Also performs eye massage on both eyes QID
Past medications include pilocarpine 4%, Timoptic 0.5%, Propine, Diamox sequels 500 mg, and Pred-Forte 1%

All

NKDA

Physical Examination

VS

BP 120/82, P 70, R 18, T 36.8°C

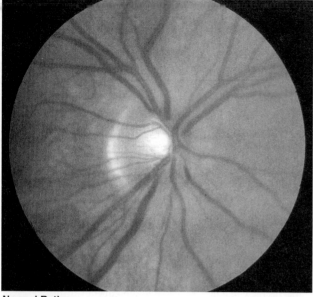
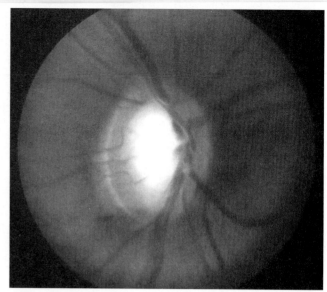

Normal Retina

Retina with Glaucoma

FIGURE 99-1. Comparison of the retina in a patient with a healthy optic nerve *(left)* and in a patient with glaucoma and a large cup with a disc hemorrhage, typical of chronic open-angle glaucoma *(right)*. *(Photo courtesy of Dr. Donald Minckler, University of California-Irvine.)*

Eyes

Visual acuity: OD—hand motion at 3 inches with correction spectacles; OS—20/30.

Slit-lamp exam: Lid margins were without inflammation in both eyes; conjunctiva without injection; normal tear break-up, did not stain with fluorescein; cornea clear and smooth; anterior chamber deep and quiet; lenses—clear in both eyes; iris round without neovascularization or abnormality; no mass/nodules; filtering bleb is visible at 11 o'clock meridian.

Intraocular pressure: OD—14 mm Hg; OS—20 mm Hg.

Vitreous examination: Clear in both eyes.

Disks: OD—the disc appeared whitish, fully cupped and showed marked pallor; cup-to-disk (C/D) ratio = 1.0; OS—C/D ratio = 0.99 with only a narrow rim present (normal C/D ratio = < 0.33).

Color vision: OD—unable to see; OS—WNL.

Visual fields: OD—unable to see the Amsler grid; can only see hand motion at 3 inches away; OS—several paracentral scotomata with the Amsler grid; 20/30. Diurnal curve of IOP revealed pressures between 10 mm Hg and 21 mm Hg.

CV

RRR without MRG; carotid pulses are brisk and equal bilaterally without bruits

Neuro

Smell and corneal sensation are intact bilaterally. Facial symmetry, tone, and sensation are intact bilaterally. Cranial nerves VIII through XII were intact. Gait was intact. Finger-to-nose and rapid alternating movement tests were normal. Reflexes were symmetric and normal. Sensation was intact and symmetric to pinprick, proprioception, and light touch. Motor strength of all extremities was 5/5.

▓ Labs

Na 138 mEq/L	BUN 10 mg/dL
K 3.7 mEq/L	SCr 0.9 mg/dL
Cl 99 mEq/L	FBG 105 mg/dL
CO_2 25 mEq/L	

▓ Assessment

1. High myopia with advanced chronic juvenile open-angle glaucoma

2. No evidence of macular edema

3. No cataracts

4. S/P filtering procedure in both eyes

5. Depression associated with chronic open-angle glaucoma

▓ Plan

Increase eye massage to 8 times/day

Follow-up in 6 weeks

Repeat filtering surgery/trabeculectomy with mitomycin C to further lower IOP

Switch nifedipine to nimodipine for better CNS/ophthalmic absorption to increase blood flow

Counsel with neuro-ophthalmologist, retina ophthalmologist, and neurologist

QUESTIONS

Problem Identification

1.a. Identify this patient's drug therapy problems.

1.b. What risk factors for primary open-angle glaucoma (POAG) are present in this patient?

1.c. What information (signs, symptoms) indicates the presence or severity of this patient's glaucoma?

1.d. The patient reports occasional episodes of erectile dysfunction. Are phosphodiesterase-5 inhibitors such as sildenafil safe for patients with high intraocular pressure?

Desired Outcome

2. What are the goals of pharmacotherapy in this case?

Therapeutic Alternatives

3.a. What nondrug therapies might be useful for this patient?

3.b. What feasible pharmacotherapeutic alternatives are available for treating this patient's glaucoma?

3.c. Is antioxidant supplementation beneficial in maintaining eye health?

3.d. Discuss the possible benefit of neuroprotective agents such as memantine in patients with glaucoma.

Optimal Plan

4.a. Devise an optimal pharmacotherapeutic regimen for treating this patient's glaucoma.

4.b. What alternatives would be appropriate if the initial therapy fails or cannot be used?

Outcome Evaluation

5. What clinical and laboratory parameters are necessary to evaluate the therapy for achievement of the desired therapeutic outcome and to detect or prevent adverse effects?

Patient Education

6. What information should the patient receive about the disease of glaucoma, proper medication administration technique, and possible side effects of treatment?

■ SELF-STUDY ASSIGNMENTS

1. Perform a literature search on the reason why antimetabolites such as mitomycin C and 5-FU are used in glaucoma surgery. What is the mechanism of action of these antimetabolites in trabeculectomy pressure-lowering surgery?

2. Perform a literature search and explain the rationale for using nimodipine and pentoxifylline in advanced open-angle glaucoma. How do these agents work to increase blood flow to the eye and retard the progression of nerve damage?

3. Under what circumstances should the product Ocusert-pilo be used? Compare the advantages and disadvantages of using this long-acting ocular insert.

REFERENCES

1. Schwartz,GF. Compliance and persistency in glaucoma follow-up treatment. Curr Opin Ophthalmol 2005;16:114–121.
2. US Food and Drug Administration. Medwatch 2005 safety alerts for drugs, biologics, medical devices, and dietary supplements. *www.fda.gov/ medwatch/safety/2005/safety05.htm#ED*.
3. Kane H, Gaasterland DE, Monsour M. Response of filtered eyes to digital ocular pressure. Ophthalmology 1997;104:202–206.
4. Liu JH. Circadian rhythm of intraocular pressure. J Glaucoma 1998; 7:141–147.
5. Brandt JD, VanDenburgh AM, Chen K, et al. Comparison of once- or twice-daily bimatoprost with twice-daily timolol in patients with elevated IOP: a 3-month clinical trial. Ophthalmology 2001;108:1023–1031.
6. Aung T, Chew PT, Yip CC, et al. A randomized double-masked crossover study comparing latanoprost 0.005% with unoprostone 0.12% in patients with primary open-angle glaucoma and ocular hypertension. Am J Ophthalmol 2001;131:636–642.
7. Mundorf T, Williams R, Whitcup S, et al. A 3-month comparison of efficacy and safety of brimonidine-purite 0.15% and brimonidine 0.2% in patients with glaucoma or ocular hypertension. J Ocul Pharmacol Ther 2003;19:37–44.
8. Glaucoma Research Foundation. Alternative medicine. *www.glaucoma. org/treating/alternative_med.html*.
9. Doshi M, Edward DP, Osmanovic S. Clinical course of bimatoprost-induced periocular skin changes in Caucasians. Ophthalmology 2006; 113:1961–1967.

100

ALLERGIC RHINITIS

College Congestion . . . . .Level II

W. Greg Leader, PharmD

LEARNING OBJECTIVES

After completing this case study, students should be able to:

• Classify a patient's allergic rhinitis based on the signs and symptoms of the disease.

• Educate patients on appropriate measures to limit or avoid exposure to specific antigens.

• Compare and contrast available agents used to treat allergic rhinitis with respect to efficacy and safety.

• Develop a safe and effective therapeutic regimen for the management of allergic rhinitis based on disease severity.

• Educate patients with allergic rhinitis on appropriate medication use.

PATIENT PRESENTATION

■ Chief Complaint

"My nose is stopped up and I can't sleep at night. I wake up with a dry mouth, and it stays dry all day. Sometimes I start sneezing and can't stop. When I do stop sneezing, my nose starts running and then plugs up again. I am having trouble in school because I am always tired, and now my eyes are itchy and watery all the time."

■ HPI

Angele Boudreaux is a 19-year-old woman who presents to her physician with complaints of upper respiratory symptoms. The symptoms have occurred off and on since she was a child, worsening in the fall and lessening in the spring; however, they have been continuous for the last 7 months. Additionally, she has developed itchy, watery eyes that did not occur with rhinitis symptoms she had in the past. She has not run a fever and does not have throat pain, but she does have an occasional nonproductive cough that gets worse at night.

■ PMH

Allergic rhinitis × 14 years
Tonsillectomy and adenoidectomy at age 8
Anterior cruciate ligament reconstruction at age 16
Sinusitis 5 months ago

■ FH

Father age 43, with a history of HTN and hyperlipidemia. Mother age 39, with a history of major depressive disorder. Brother age 17, with moderate persistent asthma, and sister age 14, with allergic rhinitis.

■ SH

Lives in a 3-bedroom house built on a concrete slab with two roommates. She has been living there for approximately 9 months.

One roommate smokes cigarettes, but not in the house. Angele smokes occasionally when she drinks alcohol. She drinks 5 or 6 drinks once or twice a week when she goes out. One of her roommates has a cat that lives indoors. Last August (about 8 months ago) Angele started attending the State University where she is a nursing major. Angele plays intramural flag football and basketball at the University and competes locally and regionally in triathlons. Angele claims she is not sexually active but is considering having intercourse with her boyfriend of 7 months.

▓ Meds

Tavist 1 tablet po BID
Oxymetazoline nasal spray PRN at night (once or twice a week)
Butterbur Extract 1 capsule po BID

▓ All

Codeine (itching)

▓ ROS

Admits to occasional headaches but denies shortness of breath, wheezing, chest pain, or abdominal discomfort

▓ Physical Examination

Gen

The patient is a young woman who looks her stated age. She appears tired with darkened areas under her eyes. She sounds congested and is continually rubbing her nose and eyes.

VS

BP 102/62, P 64, RR 14, T 36.9°C; Wt 114 lb, Ht 5'4"

HEENT

NC/AT; PERRLA; EOMI. Chemosis and conjunctival injection. Periorbital edema and discoloration. TMs are intact. Nasal mucous membranes and turbinates are swollen and pale with no epistaxis. There is no tenderness over frontal and maxillary sinuses. There are no oropharyngeal lesions, and the throat is non-erythematous.

Neck

No lymphadenopathy or thyromegaly

Chest

CTA bilaterally; no wheezes

Breast

Deferred

Heart

RRR without murmur or rub

Abdomen

Soft, nontender, (+) BS

Genit/Rect

Deferred

Extremities

No CCE, pulses 2+ throughout

Neuro

A & O × 3; DTRs 2+ throughout; 5/5 strength; CN I–XII intact

▓ Assessment

This is a 19-year-old woman with nasal congestion, chemosis, and conjunctival injection most likely due to seasonal and perennial allergies.

▓ Plan

Perennial rhinitis with seasonal exacerbations: Discontinue butterbur. Continue Tavist; start Singulair 10 mg 1 tablet po at bedtime.

QUESTIONS

Problem Identification

1.a. Create a list of the patient's drug therapy problems.

1.b. What information (signs, symptoms, laboratory values) indicates the presence or severity of allergic rhinitis?

1.c. Could any of the patient's problems have been caused by drug therapy?

1.d. What additional information from the patient history is needed to satisfactorily assess this patient?

Desired Outcome

2. What are the goals of pharmacotherapy in this case?

Therapeutic Alternatives

3.a. What nondrug therapies might be useful for this patient?

3.b. What feasible pharmacotherapeutic alternatives are available for treatment of allergic rhinitis?

Optimal Plan

4.a. What drug, dosage form, dose, schedule, and duration of therapy are best for this patient?

4.b. What alternatives would be appropriate if the initial therapy fails?

Outcome Evaluation

5. What clinical and laboratory parameters are necessary to evaluate the therapy for achievement of the desired therapeutic outcome and to detect or prevent adverse effects?

Patient Education

6.a. What information should be provided to a patient receiving an intranasal corticosteroid to enhance compliance, ensure successful therapy, and minimize adverse effects?

6.b. What information should be provided to a patient receiving an ophthalmic antihistamine?

▓ SELF-STUDY ASSIGNMENTS

1. If the patient tries out for and makes the university track or swim team, what issues concerning her therapy would have to be evaluated, and how would her therapy be impacted?

2. Make recommendations for a single first-generation antihistamine, second-generation antihistamine, and intranasal corticosteroid to include on a hospital or HMO formulary. Support your recommendations with efficacy, safety, and economic data.

3. Search the literature on the use of complementary or alternative therapies for treatment of allergic rhinitis and prepare a table summarizing the results of controlled clinical trials.

4. Outline a treatment plan for a pregnant patient with allergic rhinitis. Justify your selection of pharmacologic agents based on their efficacy and safety profiles.

CLINICAL PEARL

Immunotherapy is the only treatment for allergic rhinitis that has been demonstrated to alter the natural course of the disease.

REFERENCES

1. Bosquet J, Van Cauwenberge P, Khaltaev N. Aria Workshop Group; World Health Organization. Allergic rhinitis and its impact on asthma. J Allergy Clin Immunol 2001;108(5, Suppl):S147–S334.
2. Fornadley JA, Corey JP, Osguthorpe JD, et al. Allergic rhinitis: clinical practice guideline. Committee on Practice Standards, American Academy of Otolaryngic Allergy. Otolaryngol Head Neck Surg 1996;115:115–122.
3. Hendeles L, Hatton RC. Oral phenylephrine: an ineffective replacement for pseudoephedrine? J Allergy Clin Immunol 2006;118:279–280.
4. Casale TB, Blaiss MS, Gelfard E, et al. First do no harm: managing antihistamine impairment in patients with allergic rhinitis. J Allergy Clin Immunol 2003;111:S835–S842.
5. Weiner JM, Abramson MJ, Puy RM. Intranasal corticosteroids versus oral H_1-receptor antagonists in allergic rhinitis: systematic review of randomised controlled trials. BMJ 1998;317:1624–1629.
6. Scadding GK. Corticosteroids in the treatment of pediatric allergic rhinitis. J Allergy Clin Immunol 2001;108(1, Suppl):S59–S64.
7. Pedersen S. Assessing the effect of intranasal steroids on growth. J Allergy Clin Immunol 2001;108(1, Suppl):S40–S44.
8. Nathan RA. Pharmacotherapy for allergic rhinitis: a critical review of leukotriene receptor antagonists compared with other treatments. Ann Allergy Asthma Immunol 2003;90:182–190.
9. Rodrigo GJ, Yanez A. The role of antileukotriene therapy in seasonal allergic rhinitis: a systematic review of randomized trials. Ann Allergy Asthma Immunol 2006;96:779–786.
10. Bielory L. Ocular allergy guidelines: a practical treatment algorithm. Drugs 2002;62:1611–1634.
11. Schapowal A. Petasites Study Group. Butterbur Ze339 for the treatment of intermittent allergic rhinitis: dose-dependent efficacy in a prospective, randomized, double-blind, placebo-controlled study. Arch Otolaryngol Head Neck Surg 2004;130:1381–1386.
12. Schapowal A. Petasites Study Group. Randomised controlled trial of butterbur and cetirizine for treating seasonal allergic rhinitis. BMJ 2002;324:144–146.
13. Plaut M, Valentine MD. Allergic rhinitis. N Engl J Med 2005;353:1934–1944.

101

CUTANEOUS REACTION TO DRUGS

TEN . . . . .Level III

Rebecca M. T. Law, BS Pharm, PharmD

LEARNING OBJECTIVES

After completing this case study, students should be able to:

- Understand the approach to identifying or ruling out a suspected drug-induced skin reaction.

- Recognize the signs and symptoms of drug-induced Stevens-Johnson syndrome (SJS) and toxic epidermal necrolysis (TEN).

- Name the drugs most commonly implicated in causing SJS and TEN.

- Determine an appropriate course of action for a patient with a suspected drug-induced skin reaction.

- Counsel patients with suspected drug-induced SJS or TEN about the nature of the reaction and necessary precautions, including which medications to avoid in the future.

- Identify patients with potentially serious skin reactions who should be referred for further medical evaluation and treatment.

PATIENT PRESENTATION

Chief Complaint

"My child has a blistering rash all over her body and is really sick!"

HPI

April Rayne is a 14-year-old Caucasian girl who presented to the ED with a high fever, vomiting, diarrhea, and a 3-day history of a skin rash. The rash is maculopapular with blisters and has spread to involve 75% of her body surface area. She had a UTI about $1^1/_2$ weeks ago and was prescribed a 7-day course of trimethoprim-sulfamethoxazole (TMP/SMX). She adhered to the regimen; her urinary tract symptoms of dysuria and frequency and her abdominal discomfort resolved within 2–3 days. This was her first UTI. She continued to take the TMP/SMX as directed. Seven days after starting therapy, she noticed red spots on her arms and legs that began to spread over the whole body. The rash began to blister. She became febrile, and last night she began vomiting and had two bouts of diarrhea. This morning her mother brought her to the ED and she was admitted to the ICU, where she was immediately intubated to protect her airway patency.

PMH

Unremarkable

FH

Parents A & W, no siblings

SH

April is a student who just began taking jazz classes about 2 months ago, which she really enjoys. She is not sexually active, does not smoke, and does not use alcohol. There have been no recent changes in diet or in her living environment.

Meds

Just completed a 7-day course of TMP/SMX. No additional drugs taken including OTCs, vitamins, herbals, or drugs of abuse. Not on oral contraceptives.

Meds in Hospital

For intubation: Ketamine 40 mg IV × 1, midazolam 1 mg IV × 1, propofol 120 mg IV × 1
For BP Support: Dopamine IV infusion at 12 mcg/kg/min

All

NKDA

ROS

Skin is tender to the touch, with rash and blisters. Continues to have loose BM. Vomited × 1 in ED. Otherwise negative except for complaints noted above.

Physical Examination

Gen

Fairly anxious 14-year-old Caucasian girl looking acutely ill

VS

BP 90/50, HR 90, RR 25, T 40.1°C

Skin

Extensive maculopapular rash over 75% of BSA. Blisters involve over 30% of BSA and appear to still be spreading. Small blisters on discrete dark-red purpuric macules symmetrically over face, hands, feet, limbs, and trunk with widespread erythema. Blisters and intensely red oozing erosions over lips (especially vermilion border), oral mucosa, and vaginal area. Some ruptured blisters on skin and some with necrotic centers. Positive Nikolsky's sign. Skin is tender to the touch.

HEENT

PERRLA, EOMI, fundi benign, TMs intact. Corneal abrasions but no blisters. Conjunctivitis with some debris collecting under eyelids. External nares clear. Blisters in oral cavity and ulceration on lower lip. Pharynx erythematous and blistering.

Chest

Upper airway congestion; debris and ulceration in mouth, throat, and epiglottis. (She was immediately intubated to protect airway patency.)

Cor

RRR without murmurs, rubs or gallops; S_1 and S_2 normal

Abd

(+) BS, soft, nontender, no masses

Genitourinary

Blistering in vaginal area. Foley catheter inserted—urine output approx. 40–50 mL/h.

Rectal

Deferred

MS/Ext

Maculopapular rash and some blisters on arms and legs. Bilateral arthralgias and myalgias. Peripheral pulses present.

Neuro

Oriented × 3. No signs of confusion.

Labs

Na 140 mEq/L	Glucose 95 mg/dL	WBC 11×10^3/mm³	Hgb 12 g/dL
K 4.0 mEq/L	BUN 9 mg/dL	PMNs 65%	Hct 31%
Cl 101 mEq/L	SCr 0.7 mg/dL	Bands 5%	Plt 239×10^3/mm³
CO_2 32 mEq/L	AST 15 IU/L	Eos 8%	INR 1.24
PO_4 2.2 mg/dL	ALT 22 IU/L	Monos 1%	aPTT 32.4 sec
T. protein 6.5 g/dL	LDH 120 IU/L	Basos 1%	ESR 35 mm/h
Albumin 3.1 g/dL		Lymphs 20%	RF negative

Urinalysis: No protein, ketones, blood, WBC, or bacteria

Chest X-Ray

WNL

Clinical Course

Day 2 of Admission:

Urine output still approx. 40–50 mL/h; 1,050 mL/previous 24 hours.

Day 3 of Admission:

Histopathology of biopsy specimen from lesion on lip: Epidermal degeneration with intra-epidermal vesiculation and subepidermal bullae. Mild perivascular lymphocytic infiltrate.

Direct immunofluorescence of biopsy specimen from lip lesion: Negative.

Swab from blisters on arm: Coagulase-negative *Staphylococcus*, *Pseudomonas aeruginosa*.

Blood cultures: Coagulase-negative *Staphylococcus*, sensitive to vancomycin.

Urine culture (mid-stream urine): No growth.

Assessment

This is a 14-year-old girl with toxic epidermal necrolysis, likely drug-induced, who has probably developed secondary *Staphylococcus epidermidis* bacteremia.

QUESTIONS

Problem Identification

1.a. Create a drug therapy problem list for this patient.

1.b. What signs and symptoms of toxic epidermal necrolysis (TEN) does this patient demonstrate?

1.c. Could the patient's signs and symptoms be caused by a drug?

Desired Outcome

2. What are the treatment goals for this patient?

Therapeutic Alternatives

3.a. What nonpharmacologic alternatives are available for managing TEN in this patient?

3.b. What pharmacotherapeutic alternatives are available for managing this patient's TEN?

Optimal Plan

4. Design an optimal pharmacotherapeutic plan for TEN in this patient.

Outcome Evaluation

5. What efficacy and adverse effects monitoring is needed for the management strategies you recommended?

Patient Education

6. How would you inform this patient (and her caregivers) about her drug therapies?

■ SELF-STUDY ASSIGNMENTS

1. Differentiate among the various manifestations of cutaneous drug reactions, including fixed drug reactions, photoallergic and phototoxic reactions, bullous reactions, morbilliform and urticarial reactions, pigmentation, lichenoid eruptions, Stevens-Johnson syndrome, toxic epidermal necrolysis, hypersensitivity syndrome, and vasculitis.

2. If this patient had Stevens-Johnson syndrome, how would the clinical presentation, disease course, and treatment differ from that of toxic epidermal necrolysis?

3. Obtain information on the nonsteroidal anti-inflammatory drugs and anticonvulsants that have been most commonly implicated in causing TEN.

CLINICAL PEARL

Aggressive and vigilant nondrug supportive therapies are vital to the effective management of toxic epidermal necrolysis.

REFERENCES

1. Cohen V, Jellinek SP, Schwartz RA. Toxic epidermal necrolysis. eMedicine May 16, 2006, available at *www.emedicine.com/med/topic2291.htm*. Accessed April 21, 2008.

2. Garra GP, Viccellio P. Toxic epidermal necrolysis. eMedicine Sep. 26, 2007, available at *www.emedicine.com/EMERG/topic599.htm*. Accessed April 21, 2008.

3. Klein PA. Stevens-Johnson syndrome and toxic epidermal necrolysis. eMedicine Sep. 4, 2006. Available at: *www.emedicine.com/DERM/topic405.htm.* Accessed April 21, 2008.

4. Playe S, Murphy G. Recognizing adverse reactions to antibiotics. Emerg Med 2006;38:11–20. Available at: *www.emedmag.com/html/pre/fea/features/061506.asp.* Accessed April 21, 2008.

5. Roujeau JC, Kelly JP, Naldi L, et al. Medication use and the risk of Stevens-Johnson syndrome or toxic epidermal necrolysis. N Engl J Med 1995;333:1600–1607.

6. Mittmann N, Chan BC, Knowles S, et al. IVIG for the treatment of toxic epidermal necrolysis. Skin Therapy Lett 2007;12:7–9. ©2007 SkinCareGuide.com. Posted by Medscape April 10, 2007. Available at: *www.medscape.com/viewarticle/554693.* Accessed April 21, 2008.

7. Tilles SA. Practical issues in the management of hypersensitivity reactions: sulfonamides. South Med J 2001;94:817–824.

8. Johnson KK, Green DL, Rife JP, et al. Sulfonamide cross-reactivity: fact or fiction? Ann Pharmacother 2005;39:290–301.

9. Strom BL, Schinnar R, Apter AJ, et al. Absence of cross-reactivity between sulfonamide antibiotics and sulfonamide nonantibiotics. N Engl J Med 2003;349:1628–1635.

10. deShazo RD, Kemp SF. Allergic reactions to drugs and biologic agents. JAMA 1997;278:1895–1906.

102

ACNE VULGARIS

The Graduate . . . . Level II

Rebecca M. T. Law, BS Pharm, PharmD

Wayne P. Gulliver, MD, FRCPC

LEARNING OBJECTIVES

After completing this case study, students should be able to:

- Understand risk factors and aggravating factors in the pathogenesis of acne vulgaris.

- Understand the treatment strategies for acne, including appropriate situations for using nonprescription and prescription medications and use of topical and systemic therapies.

- Educate patients with acne on systemic therapies.

- Monitor the safety and efficacy of selected systemic therapies.

PATIENT PRESENTATION

Chief Complaint

"I can't stand this acne!"

HPI

Elaine Morgan is an 18-year-old woman with a history of facial acne since age 15. One month ago, she completed a 3-month course of minocycline in combination with Differin (adapalene). Her acne has flared up again, and she has again presented to her family physician for treatment.

PMH

Has irregular menses as a result of polycystic ovary syndrome diagnosed 3 years ago, which has not required medical treatment.

However, it has resulted in an acne condition that was initially quite mild; she responded well to nonprescription topical products. In the past 2 years, the number of facial lesions has increased despite OTC, and, later, prescription drug treatments. Initially, Benzamycin Gel was beneficial, but this had to be discontinued because of excessive drying. Differin was used next, and it controlled her condition for about 6 months, then the acne worsened and oral antibiotics were added. Most recently, she has received two 3-month courses of minocycline over the past year. She has also noted some scarring and cysts in the past few months.

FH

Parents alive and well; two older brothers (ages 21 and 25). Father had acne with residual scarring.

SH

The patient is under some stress because she is graduating in a few weeks. She wants to do well in school so she will qualify for the best colleges. Both of her brothers graduated with honors. She is sexually active, and her boyfriend uses condoms.

Meds

None currently

All

NKDA

ROS

In addition to the complaints noted above, the patient has irregular menstrual periods and mild hirsutism.

Physical Examination

Gen

Alert, moderately anxious teenager in NAD

VS

BP 110/70, RR 15, T 37°C; Wt 45 kg, Ht 5'2"

Skin

Comedones on forehead, nose, and chin. Papules and pustules on the nose and malar area. A few cysts on the chin. Scars on malar area. Increased facial hair.

HEENT

PERRLA, EOMI, fundi benign, TMs intact

Chest

CTA bilaterally

Cor

RRR without MRG, S_1 and S_2 normal

Abd

(+) BS, soft, non-tender, no masses

MS/Ext

No joint aches or pains; peripheral pulses present

Neuro

CN II–XII intact

■ Labs

Na 140 mEq/L	Hgb 13.0 g/dL	AST 21 IU/L	T. chol 170 mg/dL
K 3.7 mEq/L	Hct 38%	ALT 39 IU/L	LDL-C 90 mg/dL
Cl 100 mEq/L	Plt 300 × 10³/mm³	LDH 105 IU/L	Trig 90 mg/dL
CO₂ 25 mEq/L	WBC 7.0 × 10³/mm³	Alk phos 89 IU/L	HDL 45 mg/dL
BUN 12 mg/dL		T. bili 1.0 mg/dL	DHEAS 221 mcg/dL
SCr 1.0 mg/dL		Alb 3.9 g/dL	Testosterone (free)
Glu 100 mg/dL		FSH 30 mIU/mL	2.3 ng/mL
		LH 150 mIU/mL	Prolactin 15 ng/mL

QUESTIONS

Problem Identification

1.a. Create a drug therapy problem list for this patient.

1.b. What signs and symptoms consistent with acne does this patient have?

1.c. How does polycystic ovary syndrome contribute to this patient's acne and other physical findings?

Desired Outcome

2. What are the treatment goals for this patient?

Therapeutic Alternatives

3. What feasible therapeutic alternatives are available for management of this patient's acne and hyperandrogenism?

Optimal Plan

4. What treatment regimen is best suited for this patient?

Outcome Evaluation

5. How would you monitor the therapy you recommended for efficacy and adverse effects?

Patient Education

6. How would you educate the patient about this treatment regimen to enhance compliance and ensure successful therapy?

■ CLINICAL COURSE

Two months later, the patient has developed bloating, weight gain, and increased appetite, likely related to the therapy prescribed. She also reveals that her maternal grandmother and aunt both died of melanoma, and a friend told her that she should not be using her new therapy.

■ FOLLOW-UP QUESTION

1. What is the most appropriate course of action?

■ SELF-STUDY ASSIGNMENTS

1. Review the dysmorphic syndrome associated with acne.

2. Review the nonpharmacologic management of acne, including stress reduction and dietary changes.

CLINICAL PEARL

In females with acne, scarring + cysts + two courses of oral antibiotics means hormonal therapy and "consider isotretinoin."

REFERENCES

1. Costello M, Shrestha B, Eden J, et al. Insulin-sensitising drugs versus the combined oral contraceptive pill for hirsutism, acne and risk of diabetes, cardiovascular disease, and endometrial cancer in polycystic ovary syndrome. Cochrane Database Syst Rev 2007 Jan 24:CD005552.

2. Cheung AP, Chang RJ. Polycystic ovary syndrome. Clin Obstet Gynecol 1990;33:655–667.

3. Gollnick H, Cunliffe W, Berson D, et al. Management of acne: a report from a Global Alliance to Improve Outcomes in Acne. J Am Acad Dermatol 2003;49(1 Suppl):S1–S37.

4. Zaenglein AL, Thiboutot DM. Expert committee recommendations for acne management. Pediatrics 2006;118:1188–1199.

5. Law RM. The pharmacist's role in the treatment of acne. America's Pharmacist 2003;125:35–42.

6. Lehmann HP, Robinson KA, Andrews JS, et al. Acne therapy: a methodologic review. J Am Acad Dermatol 2002;47:231–240.

7. Agency for Healthcare Research and Quality, September 2001. Evidence report/technology assessment number 17: management of acne. www.ahcpr.gov/clinic/epcsums/acnesum.htm. Accessed July 28, 2007.

8. Goldsmith LA, Bolognia JL, Callen JP, et al. American Academy of Dermatology Consensus Conference on the safe and optimal use of isotretinoin: summary and recommendations. J Am Acad Dermatol 2004;50:900–906.

9. Wooltorton E. Diane-35 (cyproterone acetate): safety concerns. CMAJ 2003;168:455–456.

10. Karagas MR, Stukel TA, Dykes J, et al. A pooled analysis of 10 case-control studies of melanoma and oral contraceptive use. Br J Cancer 2002;86:1085–1092.

103

PSORIASIS

The Harried School Teacher . . . . Level II

Rebecca M. T. Law, BS Pharm, PharmD

Wayne P. Gulliver, MD, FRCPC

LEARNING OBJECTIVES

After completing this case study, students should be able to:

• Understand the pathophysiology of plaque psoriasis, including clinical presentation and skin changes.

• Understand the sequence of using topical, photochemical, and systemic treatment modalities for psoriasis.

• Compare the efficacy and adverse effects of systemic therapies for psoriasis, including standard therapies (methotrexate, acitretin, cyclosporine, azathioprine, hydroxyurea, and sulfasalazine), newer agents (efalizumab and alefacept), and investigational agents (infliximab and etanercept).

• Select appropriate therapeutic regimens for patients with plaque psoriasis.

• Educate patients with psoriasis about proper use of pharmacotherapeutic treatments, potential adverse effects, and necessary precautions.

PATIENT PRESENTATION

Chief Complaint

"Nothing is helping my psoriasis."

HPI

Gerald Kent is a 50-year-old man with a 25+ year history of psoriasis who presented to the outpatient dermatology clinic 2 days ago with another flare-up of his psoriasis. He was admitted to the inpatient dermatology service for a severe flare-up of plaque psoriasis involving his arms, legs, elbows, knees, palms, abdomen, back, and scalp (Fig. 103-1).

He was diagnosed with plaque psoriasis at age 23. He initially responded to topical therapy with medium-potency topical corticosteroids, later to calcipotriol. He subsequently required photochemotherapy using psoralens with UVA phototherapy (PUVA) to control his condition. PUVA eventually became ineffective, and 10 years ago, he was started on oral methotrexate 5 mg once weekly. Dosage escalations kept his condition under fairly good control for about 5 years. Flare-ups during that period were initially managed with SCAT (short-contact anthralin therapy), but they eventually became more frequent and lesions were more widespread despite increasing the methotrexate dose. A liver biopsy performed about 5 years ago showed no evidence of fibrosis, hepatitis, or cirrhosis.

After requiring two SCAT treatments in a 4-month period, along with methotrexate 25 mg once weekly po (given as two doses of 12.5 mg 12 hours apart), a change in therapy was considered necessary at that time. Because he was receiving maximum recommended methotrexate doses and had already reached a lifetime cumulative methotrexate dose of 2.2 grams, he was changed to his current cyclic regimen of cyclosporine microemulsion (Neoral) 75 mg twice daily for 3 months, followed by acitretin (Soriatane) 25 mg once daily with dinner for 3 months, and repeat. Flare-ups became infrequent and were again successfully managed by SCAT. However, in the last 6 months, he has already required two SCAT treatments for flare-ups. This is his third flare-up this year.

PMH

One episode of major depressive illness triggered by the death of his first wife, which occurred 16 years ago (age 34). He was treated by his family physician who prescribed fluoxetine for 6 months. He has had no recurrences. He has no other chronic medical conditions and no other acute or recent illnesses.

FH

Parents alive and well. Father has HTN and Type 2 diabetes. Two older sisters and a younger brother. Younger brother was diagnosed with psoriasis about 5 years ago. No history of other immune disorders or malignancy.

SH

Patient is an elementary school teacher; non-smoker; social use of alcohol (glass of wine with dinner). He is married and has two children ages 10 and 12 with his second wife. There has been an increased workload for the past year because of layoffs at his school board.

Meds

Neoral 75 mg twice daily po; in 1 month, he is scheduled to change to acitretin 25 mg once daily for the following 3 months (cyclic therapy)
Acetaminophen for occasional headaches

All

NKDA

ROS

Skin feels very itchy despite using a nonmedicated moisturizer TID. No joint aches or pains. No complaints of shortness of breath. Occasional nausea associated with a cyclosporine dose. Has been feeling jumpy and stressed because of tensions at work but does not feel depressed.

Physical Examination

Gen

Alert, mildly anxious 50-year-old white man in NAD

VS

BP 139/86, P 88, T 37°C; Wt 75 kg, Ht 5'9"

Skin

Confluent plaque psoriasis with extensive lesions on abdomen, arms, legs, back, and scalp. Thick crusted lesions on elbows, knees, palms, and soles. Lesions are red to violet in color, with sharply demarcated borders except where confluent, and are loosely covered with silvery-white scales. There are no pustules or vesicles. There are excoriations on trunk and extremities consistent with scratching.

HEENT

PERRLA, EOMI, fundi benign, TMs intact; extensive scaly lesions on scalp as noted

Neck/Lymph Nodes

No lymphadenopathy; thyroid non-palpable

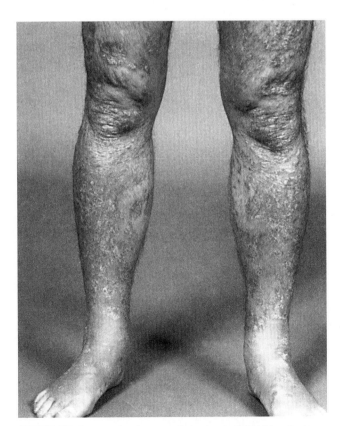

FIGURE 103-1. Example of severe plaque psoriasis involving the lower extremities in a male patient. (*Photo courtesy of Wayne P. Gulliver, MD.*)

Chest

CTA bilaterally

CV

RRR without MRG; S$_1$ and S$_2$ normal

Abd

(+) BS, soft, nontender, no masses; extensive scaly lesions and excoriations on skin as noted above in the Skin section

Genit

WNL

Rect

Deferred

MS/Ext

No joint swelling, increased warmth, or tenderness; skin lesions as noted above in Skin section; no nail involvement; peripheral pulses 2+ throughout

Neuro

A & O × 3; CN II–XII intact; DTRs 2+ toes downgoing

■ Labs

Na 139 mEq/L	Hgb 13.5 g/dL	AST 22 IU/L
K 4.0 mEq/L	Hct 35.0%	ALT 38 IU/L
Cl 102 mEq/L	Plt 255 × 10^3/mm^3	LDH 107 IU/L
CO$_2$ 25 mEq/L	WBC 6.0 × 10^3/mm^3	Alk phos 98 IU/L
BUN 14 mg/dL		T. bili 1.0 mg/dL
SCr 1.0 mg/dL		Alb 3.7 g/dL
Glu 98 mg/dL		Uric acid 4 mg/dL
		T. chol 180 mg/dL

QUESTIONS

Problem Identification

1.a. Create a list of this patient's drug therapy problems.

1.b. What signs and symptoms consistent with psoriasis does this patient demonstrate?

1.c. What risk factors for developing psoriasis or experiencing a disease flare-up are present in this patient?

1.d. Could the signs and symptoms be caused by any drug therapy he is receiving?

Desired Outcome

2. What are the goals of pharmacotherapy for psoriasis in this patient?

Therapeutic Alternatives

3.a. What nonpharmacologic alternatives are available for managing the patient's psoriasis and its related symptoms?

3.b. What feasible pharmacotherapeutic alternatives are available for controlling the patient's disease and its related symptoms at this point?

Optimal Plan

4. What drug regimen is best suited for treating this flare-up of the patient's psoriasis and its related symptoms?

Outcome Evaluation

5. How should you monitor the therapy you recommended for efficacy and adverse effects?

Patient Education

6. What information should be provided to the patient to enhance compliance and ensure successful therapy?

■ SELF-STUDY ASSIGNMENTS

1. Perform a literature search to identify potential future therapies for psoriasis: topical therapies such as NSAIDs, protein kinase C inhibitors, methotrexate gel, an implantable 5-fluorouracil formulation; systemic therapies such as glucosamine, monoclonal antibodies, and cytokines.

2. Perform a literature search to review the current guidelines, opinions, and evidence regarding liver biopsies and long-term methotrexate use for patients with psoriasis.

CLINICAL PEARL

The "3 Rs" of systemic therapy for psoriasis are Rotate Regimens Regularly.

REFERENCES

1. Law RMT. Psoriasis. In: Chisholm MA, Wells BG, Schwinghammer TL, et al., eds. Pharmacotherapy Principles and Practice. New York, McGraw-Hill, 2007:949–958.
2. Schon MP, Boehncke WH. Psoriasis. N Engl J Med 2005;352:1899–1912.
3. Rahman P, Elder JT. Genetic epidemiology of psoriasis and psoriatic arthritis. Ann Rheum Dis 2005;64(Suppl 2):ii37–ii39.
4. Krueger JG, Bowcock A. Psoriasis pathophysiology: current concepts of pathogenesis. Ann Rheum Dis 2005;64(Suppl 2):ii30–ii36.
5. Callen JP, Krueger GG, Lebwohl M, et al. AAD consensus statement on psoriasis therapies. J Am Acad Dermatol 2003;49:897–899.
6. Guenther L, Langley RG, Shear NJ, et al. Integrating biologic agents into management of moderate-to-severe psoriasis: a consensus of the Canadian Psoriasis Expert Panel. J Cutan Med Surg 2004;8:321–337.
7. Lebwohl M, Menter A, Koo J, et al. Combination therapy to treat moderate to severe psoriasis. J Am Acad Dermatol 2004;50:416–430.
8. Hengge UR, Ruzicka T, Schwartz RA, et al. Adverse effects of topical glucocorticosteroids. J Am Acad Dermatol 2006;54:1–15.
9. Henning JS, Gruson LM, Strober BE, et al. Reconsidering liver biopsies during methotrexate therapy. J Am Acad Dermatol 2007;56:893–894.
10. Pariser DM, Gordon KB, Papp KA, et al. Clinical efficacy of efalizumab in patients with chronic plaque psoriasis: results from three randomized placebo-controlled Phase III trials: Part l. J Cutan Med Surg 2005;9:303–312.
11. Papp KA, Camisa C, Stone SP, et al. Safety of efalizumab in patients with moderate to severe chronic plaque psoriasis: review of clinical data. Part 2. J Cutan Med Surg 2005;9:313–323.

104

ATOPIC DERMATITIS

The Itch That Erupts When Scratched. . . . . Level I

Rebecca M. T. Law, BS Pharm, PharmD

Poh Gin Kwa, MD, FRCPC

LEARNING OBJECTIVES

After completing this case study, students should be able to:

- Understand risk factors and aggravating factors in the pathophysiology of atopic dermatitis.

- Understand the treatment strategies for atopic dermatitis, including nonpharmacologic management.

- Educate patients and/or their caregivers about management of atopic dermatitis.

- Monitor the safety and efficacy of selected pharmacologic therapies.

PATIENT PRESENTATION

▨ Chief Complaint

As stated by the patient's mother, "My child constantly wants to scratch her skin, and she can't sleep well during the night."

▨ HPI

Julia Chan is a $3^1/_2$-year-old girl who just started attending daycare about 1 month ago. She did not want to go and still exhibits a lot of clinging behavior when her mother tries to leave; she still cries when her mother eventually does manage to leave. Her mother says that Julia's atopic dermatitis has flared up again. Julia has had atopic dermatitis since she was about 6 months old. It had been well controlled by topical corticosteroids and liberal use of moisturizers. Her recent flare-up began about 2–3 weeks ago. She has not been sleeping well and is constantly trying to scratch her skin at night. Her mother has been using 100% cotton sheets for her bed since she was an infant. She has sewn mittens on Julia's 100% cotton pajamas to prevent her from scratching, because she had previously caused excoriations from scratching, which then became infected. During the day, Julia constantly wants to scratch her skin but has been told to just "pat" the itchy area. The caregivers at the daycare center keep an eye on her scratching behavior as well but aren't always able to prevent her from scratching herself. They also inform her mother that Julia likes to eat food shared by other children.

▨ PMH

Julia was breastfed from birth for a total of 8 weeks, when her mother decided to return to work. Julia was then cared for at home by a babysitter and fed cow's milk, with oatmeal cereal being introduced as the first solid food. She was fed some lemon meringue pie (made with egg white) once, and developed generalized hives, which led to the recognition that Julia has an egg allergy. This was confirmed by allergic skin testing. Julia's atopic dermatitis presented at 6 months of age. The parents have recently become aware that the babysitter left Julia alone a lot (sitting on the floor/carpet to play by herself). That was the major reason for sending Julia to a daycare center.

▨ SH

Julia is the only child of a professional couple. Her father is an engineer and her mother is a litigation lawyer who often works long hours. The couple has a stressful lifestyle, and it appears that the stress is reflected in Julia's care. Sometimes Julia would be driven to one or another babysitter's homes at the last minute, when something urgent arises that the couple must attend to. There is very little family time. Unfortunately, their relatives do not live in the same city, and there is little social support for Julia on a day-to-day basis. The parents were hoping that the daycare center would be helpful, but so far that has proven to be another issue for Julia. She doesn't

want to participate in activities there and has lots of temper tantrums. She doesn't play well with other children. Julia had been toilet trained but has now lost her toilet training and is using diapers again. Julia's mother started smoking again due to the recent stress; Julia keeps her up at night, and she's having difficulty dealing with Julia's multiple issues at home and at the daycare center.

▨ FH

There is a strong family history of atopy. Julia's father has a severe allergy to shellfish, and her mother has a history of hay fever. Her father's sister has multiple food allergies. Her maternal grandmother had asthma. Her paternal first cousin had infantile eczema. Her maternal first cousin has a severe peanut allergy (generalized hives).

▨ Meds

Hydrocortisone 1% cream applied to affected areas two to four times a day; although twice daily is her usual maintenance dose, she is currently using it three to four times a day
Vaseline ad lib
Diphenhydramine $^1/_2$ teaspoonful at bedtime as needed (when skin is excessively itchy, to allow Julia to sleep)

▨ Allergies

NKDA. Multiple food allergies: egg (hives, developed allergy as an infant), strawberries, raspberries, tomatoes.

▨ ROS

Not obtained

▨ Physical Examination

Gen

Unhappy, cranky, thin, clinging girl who keeps sucking her thumb

VS

BP 98/50, HR 96, RR 18, T 37°C; Wt 12.2 kg (10th percentile), Ht 98 cm (38.6"; 50th percentile), head circumference 49.5 cm (19.5"; 50th percentile)

Skin

Generally dry. Eczematous skin lesions in flexure areas (behind ears, wrist joints, elbows, knees). Likely pruritic papules in flexure areas. Excoriations from scratching. Some bleeding seen but does not appear infected. Some cracking skin lesions seen behind the ears and knees. There are no lesions on the extensor parts of her body, no lesions on top of her nose, and no lesions in the diaper area.
The remainder of the physical exam was normal.

▨ Labs

Na 135 mEq/L	Hgb 12.0 g/dL	WBC differential	AST 20 IU/L
K 4.0 mEq/L	Hct 35%	Neutros 50%	ALT 7 IU/L
Cl 102 mEq/L	Plt 230 × 10³/mm³	Bands 3%	IgE 300 IU/mL
CO₂ 26 mEq/L	WBC 5.0 × 10³/mm³	Eosinophils 18%	D-dimer—90 ng/mL
BUN 8 mg/dL		Lymphs 27%	RAST elevated
SCr 0.2 mg/dL		Basophils 1%	INR 1.1
		Monos 1%	aPTT 30 sec

Note: References ranges at age $3^1/_2$: BUN 8–20 mg/dL, SCr 0.2–0.8 mg/dL, AST 20–60 IU/L, ALT 0–37 IU/L, IgE 0–25 IU/mL; WBC differential: Neutros 20–65%, Eos 0–15%, Basos 0–2%, Lymphs 20–60%, Monos 0–10%
Swab of skin lesion where there is bleeding: No growth

▨ Assessment

This is a $3^1/_2$-year-old child with an exacerbation of atopic dermatitis, likely stress-induced.

QUESTIONS

Problem Identification

1.a. Create a drug therapy problem list for this patient.

1.b. What signs and symptoms of atopic dermatitis does this patient demonstrate?

1.c. What risk factors or aggravating factors may have contributed to the patient's atopic dermatitis flare?

1.d. Could the patient's signs and symptoms be caused by a drug?

Desired Outcome

2. What are the treatment goals for this patient?

Therapeutic Alternatives

3. What feasible nonpharmacologic and pharmacologic alternatives are available to manage this patient's pruritus and atopic dermatitis?

Optimal Plan

4. What treatment regimen is best suited for this patient?

Outcome Evaluation

5. What efficacy and adverse effects monitoring is needed for the management strategies you recommended?

Patient Education

6. How would you inform the patient's caregiver about the treatment regimen to enhance compliance and ensure successful therapy?

■ SELF-STUDY ASSIGNMENTS

1. Review the use of phototherapy for atopic dermatitis.

2. Discuss how an 8-month-old infant with atopic dermatitis might differ from a $3^1/_2$-year-old child (with respect to clinical presentation and treatment strategies).

CLINICAL PEARL

In atopic dermatitis, minimizing preventable risk factors such as stress, eliminating triggers, providing appropriate skin care, and controlling the itch are as important as pharmacologic treatment.

REFERENCES

1. Eichenfield LFF, Hanifin JM, Luger TA, et al. Consensus conference on pediatric atopic dermatitis. J Am Acad Dermatol 2003;49:1088–1095.

2. Beltrani VS, Boguneiwicz M. Atopic dermatitis. Dermatol Online J 2003;9:1. http://dermatology.cdlib.org/92/reviews/atopy/beltrani.html. Accessed May 10, 2007.

3. National Institute of Arthritis and Musculoskeletal and Skin Diseases. Handout on health: atopic dermatitis. US Department of Health and Human Services, revised April 2003. www.niams.nih.gov/hi/topics/dermatitis. Accessed April 22, 2008.

4. Koblenzer CS. Itching and the atopic skin. J Allergy Clin Immunol 1999;104(3, Pt 2):S109–S113.

5. Reitamo S, Ansel JC, Luger TA. Itch in atopic dermatitis. J Am Acad Dermatol 2001;45(1, Suppl):S55–S56.

6. Hanifin JM, Cooper KD, Ho VC, et al. Guidelines of care for atopic dermatitis. J Am Acad Dermatol 2004;50:391–404. National Guideline Clearinghouse: www.guideline.gov/summary/summary.aspx?ss=15&doc_id=4361&nbr=3286. Accessed May 10, 2007.

7. Lynde C, Barber K, Claveau J, et al. Canadian practical guide for the treatment and management of atopic dermatitis. J Cutan Med Surg 2005, June 30 (epub). www.springerlink.com/content/104877/?k=++Lynde++atopic+dermatitis+. Accessed May 10, 2007.

8. Lewis E. Atopic dermatitis: disease overview and the development of topical immunomodulators. Formulary 2002;37(Suppl 2):3–15.

9. Lever R. The role of food in atopic eczema. J Am Acad Dermatol 2001;45(1, Suppl):S57–S60.

10. Murch SH. Probiotics as mainstream allergy therapy? Arch Dis Child 2005;90:881–882.

11. Hengge UR, Ruzicka T, Schwartz RA, et al. Adverse effects of topical glucocorticosteroids. J Am Acad Dermatol 2006;54:1–15.

105

IRON DEFICIENCY ANEMIA

Walter Is "Sick and Tired" . . . . .Level I

William J. Spruill, PharmD, FASHP, FCCP

William E. Wade, PharmD, FASHP, FCCP

LEARNING OBJECTIVES

After completing this case study, the student should be able to:

- Recognize that NSAID use is a common cause of chronic blood loss and iron deficiency anemia.

- Identify the signs, symptoms, and laboratory manifestations of iron deficiency anemia.

- Select appropriate iron therapy for the treatment of iron deficiency anemia.

- Understand the monitoring parameters for both short- and long-term treatment of iron deficiency anemia.

- Inform patients of the potential adverse effects of iron therapy.

- Educate patients about the importance of adherence to their iron therapy regimen.

PATIENT PRESENTATION

▓ Chief Complaint

"I feel weak and tired and think I have low blood."

▓ HPI

Walter Adams is a 71-year-old man who presents to the hospital complaining of being fatigued, particularly over the past week. Five days ago, he noted dark and black stool that has continued. He went to a local health clinic and was told that he was very anemic and needed to go to a hospital for a blood transfusion. He states that he takes ibuprofen, 600-mg tablets 3 or 4 times a day, for "old-age" arthritis, which is especially bad in his knees. He denies hematemesis but has been nauseated, dizzy, and lightheaded. He was evaluated 7 years ago for GI bleeding but has no recollection of a diagnosis being made.

▓ PMH

Gastrointestinal bleeding 7 years ago
CAD with 98% blockage of right coronary artery; angioplasty done 3 years ago
von Recklinghausen disease (neurofibromatosis)
Chronic headaches

▓ PSH

Inguinal hernia repair last year

▓ FH

Mother died in childbirth in 1937; father died of cancer at age 93

▓ SH

No smoking; quit in 1982. No alcohol; quit in 1990. He is married.

▓ ROS

No fever or chills; (+) burning pain in stomach after meals; denies heartburn or melena; good appetite, has one daily BM; no significant weight changes over past 5 years; (+) fatigue, tires easily; (−) paralysis, fainting, numbness, paresthesia, or tremor; headache only occasionally; has myopic vision; (−) tinnitus or vertigo; has hay fever in spring; (−) cough, sputum production, or wheezing; denies chest pain, edema, dyspnea, or orthopnea; denies nocturia, hematuria, dysuria, or Hx of stones; (+) unilateral joint pain in right knee for over 5 years

▓ Meds

Ibuprofen 600 mg 3 or 4 times a day for knee pain
Antacids PRN for stomach pain

▓ All

Codeine (upset stomach)
Aspirin (upset stomach)

▓ Physical Examination

Gen

WM in NAD who appears his stated age

VS

BP 168/71, P 79, RR 22, T 36.2°C, pulse oximetry 99% on room air; Wt 61 kg, Ht 5'11"

Skin

Multiple neurofibromatosis-related nodules over entire face and body

HEENT

PERRL; EOMI; conjunctivae are pale; upper and lower dentures in place; membranes moist; normal funduscopic examination with no retinopathy noted; deviated nasal septum; no sinus tenderness; oropharynx clear

Neck/Lymph Nodes

Neck supple without masses; trachea midline; no thyromegaly, (−) JVD

Thorax

Lungs clear to A & P; breath sounds equal bilaterally

CV

Regular rhythm with a soft systolic murmur; PMI at 5th ICS, MCL; (−) bruits

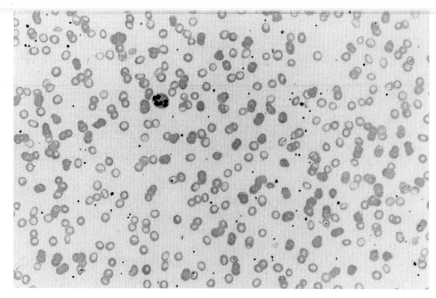

FIGURE 105-1. Blood smear with hypochromic, microcytic red blood cells (Wright-Giemsa × 330). *(Photo courtesy of Lydia C. Contis, MD.)*

Abd

Soft, tender to palpation; no masses or organomegaly; normal peristalsis

Genit/Rect

Normal external male genitalia; rectal examination (+) stool guaiac

MS/Ext

Slight joint enlargement, with pain and tenderness noted, and limited ROM of right knee; crepitation noted on dorsiflexion of joint; changes consistent with OA; strong pedal pulses bilaterally; no peripheral edema; spooning of fingernails

Neuro

A & O × 3; DTR 2+; normal gait

Other

Peripheral blood smear: hypochromic, microcytic red blood cells (Fig. 105-1)

■ **Labs**

See Table 105-1

■ **Assessment**

1. Chronic, severe iron deficiency anemia with melena, probably of GI origin; possibly secondary to NSAID-induced gastropathy

2. OA of right knee

3. Neurofibromatosis

4. FULL CODE status but patient does not wish to be left on a machine if there is no hope of recovery

■ **Plan**

Infuse 4 units PRBCs
Ferrous sulfate 325 mg TID
Begin esomeprazole (Nexium) 40 mg IV daily
Refer to gastroenterologist

■ CLINICAL COURSE

The next day, the patient was seen by a gastroenterologist and underwent both EGD and colonoscopy. Findings included severe gastritis, with multiple small bleeds noted with small hiatal hernia and normal duodenum. Colonoscopy results were normal.

Final assessment: chronic, severe IDA secondary to unspecified GI blood loss. Gastroenterology consult concluded that the bleeding was likely related to either NSAID-induced gastritis and/or small bowel arteriovenous malformations (AVMs) perhaps associated with neurofibromatosis.

QUESTIONS

Problem Identification

1.a. What potential drug therapy problems does this patient have?

1.b. What signs, symptoms, and laboratory findings are consistent with the finding of iron deficiency anemia secondary to blood loss?

TABLE 105-1	**Lab Values**			
Na 138 mEq/L	Hgb 7.2 g/dL	WBC 10.7 × 10³/mm³	AST 10 IU/L	Ca 8.7 mg/dL
K 3.7 mEq/L	Hct 25%	Segs 61%	ALT 23 IU/L	Iron 4 mcg/dL
Cl 104 mEq/L	RBC 3.77 × 10⁶/mm³	Bands 2%	T. bili 0.3 mg/dL	TIBC 465 mcg/dL
CO₂ 27 mEq/L	MCV 66.2 μm³	Lymphs 23%	LDH 85 IU/L	Transferrin sat 1%
BUN 12 mg/dL	MCH 19 pg	Monos 10%	T. prot 6.3 g/dL	Ferritin 5 ng/mL
SCr 0.8 mg/dL	MCHC 28.7 g/dL	Eos 3%	Alb 3.7 g/dL	B₁₂ 680 pg/mL
Glucose 90 mg/dL	RDW 20.9%	Basos 1%		Folic acid 8.2 ng/mL
	MPV 8.1 fl			
	Microcytosis 2 +			
	Anisocytosis 1 +			

Desired Outcome

2. What are the goals of pharmacotherapy for this patient's anemia?

Therapeutic Alternatives

3.a. What nondrug therapy may be effective for managing this anemia?

3.b. What pharmacotherapeutic alternatives could be used to treat this patient's anemia?

Optimal Plan

4. Outline an optimal pharmacotherapy plan for this patient.

Outcome Evaluation

5. What clinical and laboratory parameters are necessary to evaluate the therapy for achievement of the desired therapeutic outcome and to detect and prevent adverse effects?

Patient Education

6. What information should be provided to the patient to enhance compliance, ensure successful therapy, and minimize adverse effects?

■ CLINICAL COURSE

Mr. Adams' hemoglobin and hematocrit slowly increased as a result of the PRBCs to 12.6 g/dL and 40.8% by the fourth day of hospitalization. At that time, he was discharged and referred for outpatient management of his chronic iron deficiency anemia. In addition to the recommended anemia therapy, Walter is given a prescription for omeprazole 20 mg po once daily.

On his return to the clinic 1 month later for evaluation, he has no complaints of adverse effects from his medications. He indicates that he is fairly compliant with his iron therapy and is not experiencing any dose-limiting side effects. At that time, he is instructed to return in 3 months. Laboratory values continue to improve and his next follow-up visit is in 6 months. Laboratory values at 1, 3, and 6 months into therapy are shown in Table 105-2.

■ SELF-STUDY ASSIGNMENTS

1. Assume that on the patient's initial presentation the physician wanted to correct the anemia using parenteral iron dextran. Calculate the correct total dose iron dextran for this patient, and write a comprehensive order for its administration.

2. Make a list of oral medications that should not be taken close to the time of iron administration; note the medications for which ferrous salts may interfere with their absorption.

3. Perform a literature search to determine the evidence supporting use of various sustained-release iron preparations, and determine the incremental cost of such products.

4. What monitoring steps should be incorporated into your pharmaceutical care plan to:

a. Check for recurrence of signs/symptoms of iron deficiency due to his chronic GI bleed?

b. Educate the patient concerning his risk of GI bleed associated with NSAID therapy and how he can minimize this risk?

c. Monitor for recurrence of signs and symptoms of gastropathy?

d. Monitor for efficacy of new treatments (such as acetaminophen or glucosamine) for his osteoarthritis?

CLINICAL PEARL

In otherwise healthy patients, a transient increase in the reticulocyte count 3–10 days after beginning therapy can be used to confirm the correct diagnosis and treatment and to rule out other causes of anemia.

Therapeutic doses of iron must be given for 3–6 months to ensure repletion of all iron stores; the serum ferritin is the best parameter for monitoring iron stores after correction of the hemoglobin and hematocrit.

REFERENCES

1. Akarsu S, Taskin E, Yilmaz E, et al. Treatment of iron deficiency anemia with intravenous iron preparations. Acta Haematol 2006;116:51–57.
2. Gotloib L, Silverberg D, Fudin R, et al. Iron deficiency is a common cause of anemia in chronic kidney disease and can often be corrected with intravenous iron. J Nephrol 2006;19:161–167.
3. Marignani M, Angeletti S, Filippi L, et al. Occult and obscure bleeding, iron deficiency anemia and other gastrointestinal stories (review). Int J Mol Med 2005;15:129–135.

106

VITAMIN B$_{12}$ DEFICIENCY

Not a Minor Problem . . . . Level I

Elaine M. Ladd, PharmD

Joseph R. Ineck, PharmD

Barbara J. Mason, PharmD, FASHP

LEARNING OBJECTIVES

After completing this case study, students should be able to:

- Recognize the signs, symptoms, and laboratory abnormalities associated with vitamin B$_{12}$ deficiency anemia.

- Select an appropriate dosage regimen for treatment of anemia resulting from vitamin B$_{12}$ deficiency.

TABLE 105-2 Laboratory Test Values at 1, 3, and 6 Months			
Test (Units)	1 Mo	3 Mo	6 Mo
RBC count (× 10^6/mm^3)	4.1	4.2	4.8
Hgb (g/dL)	11.1	13.0	14.9
Hct (%)	36	40	47
MCV (μm^3)	86	90	92
MCH (pg)	25	30	33
MCHC (g/dL)	31	34	36
RDW (%)	15.8	13.2	11.3
Serum iron (mcg/dL)	45	80	105
TIBC (mcg/dL)	489	491	500
Transferrin sat (%)	9.0	19.0	21.0
Ferritin (ng/mL)	69	120	163
Stool guaiac	Negative	Negative	Negative

- Describe monitoring parameters for the initial and subsequent evaluations of patients with anemia caused by vitamin B_{12} deficiency.

- Educate patients about appropriate vitamin B_{12} therapy.

PATIENT PRESENTATION

Chief Complaint

"I've been feeling really tired for the last couple of months and I've noticed my hands and feet feel like they are buzzing, tingly, and numb."

HPI

Ann Minor is a 71-year-old woman who presents to the Veterans Affairs Medical Center (VAMC) emergency department accompanied by her daughter. On questioning, she states that she has been experiencing fatigue, lethargy, and generalized weakness for 2–3 months. She also has been experiencing tingling and numbness in her feet and hands, especially while knitting or manipulating small objects. Patient denies weight loss, fever, night sweats, or vision changes.

PMH

Allergic rhinitis
HTN
Hyperlipidemia
Type 2 DM
Insomnia
Menopause
History of DVT (November 1971)
PTSD (Military related; 1965)

FH

Father deceased at age 64 of MI
Mother deceased at age 86; had Alzheimer's disease

SH

Widowed × 4 years, lives alone approximately 45 miles from VAMC; family lives on the same farm $1/4$ mile away. (+) tobacco, 1 ppd since age 19; (+) alcohol, 1 glass of wine occasionally. She lives on limited income and social security benefits.

ROS

(+) fatigue, paresthesias, tongue soreness; (–) SOB, headache, chest pain, joint pain, hot flashes, polyuria, or polydipsia

Meds

Docusate sodium 100 mg po BID
Aspirin 81 mg po daily
Chlorpheniramine maleate 8 mg po BID
Omeprazole 20 mg po once daily before breakfast
Multivitamin 1 tab po daily
Metformin 500 mg po BID
Pravastatin 20 mg po at bedtime
Lisinopril 10 mg po daily
Amitriptyline 50 mg po daily

All

NKDA

Physical Examination

Gen

Elderly, thin Caucasian woman in NAD, with normal affect and speech, who is pleasant and cooperative and appears tired

VS

BP 146/88, P 89, RR 18, T 36.9°C; Wt 50.9 kg, Ht 5'6", BMI 18.1

Skin

Pale, turgor normal

HEENT

PERRLA; EOMI; fundi showed no cotton-wool exudates; (–) photophobia; (+) glossitis; poor dentition

Neck

Supple without LAD; normal carotid upstrokes; no masses; no lymphadenopathy or thyromegaly

Lungs

Bilateral breath sounds; no rales, rhonchi, or wheezes

CV

RRR by auscultation; no murmurs or gallops

Abd

Soft, nontender; no organomegaly; no masses; normal bowel sounds present; no abdominal bruits

Ext

No lower extremity erythema, pain, or edema; normal pulses; (+) paresthesias

Rect

Good sphincter tone; guaiac (–) stool

Neuro

A & O × 3; CN: visual field intact, hearing intact; sensory: proprioception intact bilaterally; coordination intact; decreased pinprick on both UE and LE; decreased vibratory sensation LE; (–) ataxia

Labs (All Fasting)

Na 139 mEq/L	Hgb 11.8 g/dL	AST 89 IU/L	Iron 94 mcg/dL
K 4.3 mEq/L	Hct 37.6%	ALT 21 IU/L	Ferritin 48 ng/mL
Cl 108 mEq/L	RBC 4.47×10^6/mm³	Alk phos 62 IU/L	Transferrin 259 mg/dL
CO_2 28 mEq/L	Plt 261×10^3/mm³	T. bili 1.2 mg/dL	Direct Coombs' (–)
BUN 13 mg/dL	WBC 7.6×10^3/mm³	D. bili 0.2 mg/dL	EPO 26 IU/L
SCr 0.9 mg/dL	MCV 110 μm³	T. chol 178 mg/dL	B_{12} 162 pg/mL
Glu 94 mg/dL	MCH 32.2 pg	LDL-C 113 mg/dL	Folate 8.7 ng/mL
A1C 6.1%	MCHC 34.1 g/dL	HDL 45 mg/dL	
TSH 2.34 mIU/L	Retic (corr) 0.4%	Trig 100 mg/dL	

Peripheral Blood Smear Morphology

Anisocytosis +1, basophilic stippling, poikilocytosis, hypersegmented neutrophils, large platelets 2+, and macrocytic red blood cells with megaloblastic changes (Fig. 106-1).

Assessment

1. Macrocytic anemia consistent with vitamin B_{12} deficiency

2. Peripheral sensory neuropathy possibly associated with vitamin B_{12} deficiency

QUESTIONS

Problem Identification

1.a. Create a drug therapy problem list for this patient.

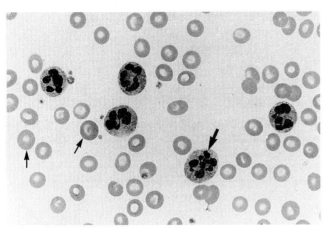

FIGURE 106-1. Blood smear with enlarged hypersegmented neutrophils, one with eight nuclear lobes *(large arrow)*, and macrocytes *(small arrows)* (Wright-Giemsa × 1,650). *(Photo courtesy of Lydia C. Contis, MD.)*

1.b. What information indicates the presence or severity of the vitamin B_{12} deficiency?

1.c. Could the vitamin B_{12} deficiency have been caused by drug therapy?

1.d. What additional information is needed to assess this patient's vitamin B_{12} deficiency?

Desired Outcome

2. What are the goals of pharmacotherapy in this case?

Therapeutic Alternatives

3.a. What nondrug therapies might be useful for this patient?

3.b. What pharmacotherapeutic alternatives are available for treatment of the vitamin B_{12} deficiency?

Optimal Plan

4. What drug, dosage form, dose, schedule, and duration of therapy are best for this patient?

Outcome Evaluation

5. What clinical and laboratory parameters are necessary to evaluate the therapy for achievement of the desired therapeutic outcome and to detect or prevent adverse effects?

Patient Education

6. What information should be provided to the patient to enhance compliance, ensure successful therapy, and minimize adverse effects?

■ FOLLOW-UP QUESTION

1. What is the role of screening for vitamin B_{12} deficiency in the absence of symptoms?

■ SELF-STUDY ASSIGNMENTS

1. How would antibiotic treatment of a patient with *Helicobacter pylori* affect concurrent cobalamin deficiency?

2. Describe the potential relationship among vitamin B_{12} deficiency, cardiovascular disease, and plasma homocysteine levels.

3. What is the rationale for screening for iron deficiency in patients with pernicious anemia?

REFERENCES

1. Wulffele M, Kooy A, Lehert P, et al. Effects of short-term treatment with metformin on serum concentrations of homocysteine, folate, and vitamin B_{12} in type 2 diabetes mellitus: a randomized, placebo-controlled trial. J Intern Med 2003;254:455–463.

2. Force RW, Meeker AD, Cady PS, et al. Increased vitamin B_{12} requirement associated with chronic acid suppression therapy. Ann Pharmacother 2003;37:490–493.

3. Andres E, Loukili NH, Noel E, et al. Vitamin B_{12} (cobalamin) deficiency in elderly patients. CMAJ 2004;171:251–259.

4. Dharmarajan TS, Adiga GU, Norkus EP. Vitamin B_{12} deficiency. Recognizing subtle symptoms in older adults. Geriatrics 2003;58:30–38.

5. Tefferi A. Anemia in adults: a contemporary approach to diagnosis. Mayo Clin Proc 2003;78:1275–1284.

6. Bain B. Diagnosis from the blood smear. N Engl J Med 2005;353:498–507.

7. Ting RZ, Szeto CC, Chan MH, et al. Risk factors of vitamin B_{12} deficiency in patients receiving metformin. Arch Intern Med 2006;166:1975–1979.

8. Hvas AM, Nexo E. Diagnosis and treatment of vitamin B_{12} deficiency—an update. Haematologica 2006;91:1506–1512.

9. Vidal-Alaball J, Butler CC, Cannings-John R, et al. Oral vitamin B_{12} versus intramuscular vitamin B_{12} for vitamin B_{12} deficiency. Cochrane Database Syst Rev 2005 Jul 20:CD004655.

10. Lindren A, Lindstedt G, Kilander AF. Advantages of serum pepsinogen A combined with gastrin or pepsinogen C as first-line analytes in the evaluation of suspected cobalamin deficiency: a study in patients previously not subjected to gastrointestinal surgery. J Intern Med 1998;244:341–349.

11. Lynch RJ, Eisenberg D, Bell RL. Metabolic consequences of bariatric surgery. J Clin Gastroenterol 2006;40:659–668.

12. Aronow WS. Homocysteine: the association with atherosclerotic vascular disease in older persons. Geriatrics 2003;58:22–28.

13. Clarke R. Vitamin B_{12}, folic acid, and the prevention of dementia. N Engl J Med 2006;354:2817–2819.

14. Murphy MF, Wallington TB, Kelsey P, et al. British Committee for Standards in Haematology, Blood Transfusion Task Force. Guidelines for the clinical use of red cell transfusions. Br J Haematol 2001;113:24–31.

15. Smellie WS, Wilson D, McNulty CA, et al. Best practice in primary care pathology: review 1. J Clin Pathol 2005;58:1016–1024.

16. Carmel R, Sarrai M. Diagnosis and management of clinical and subclinical cobalamin deficiency: advances and controversies. Curr Hematol Rep 2006;5:23–33.

107

FOLIC ACID DEFICIENCY

Scotch on the Rocks . . . . Level I

Joseph R. Ineck, PharmD

Elaine M. Ladd, PharmD

Barbara J. Mason, PharmD, FASHP

LEARNING OBJECTIVES

After completing this case study, students should be able to:

- Recognize the signs, symptoms, and laboratory abnormalities associated with folic acid deficiency.

- Identify the confounding factors that may contribute to the development of folic acid deficiency (e.g., medications, concurrent disease states, dietary habits).

- Recommend an appropriate treatment regimen to correct anemia resulting from folic acid deficiency.

- Educate patients with folic acid deficiency regarding pharmacologic and nonpharmacologic interventions used to correct folic acid deficiency.

- Describe appropriate monitoring parameters for initial and subsequent monitoring of folic acid deficiency.

PATIENT PRESENTATION

Chief Complaint

"I have been feeling really tired, and I just don't have much energy to do anything lately."

HPI

Jeffrey Wayne is a 59-year-old man with a history of multiple medical conditions and continued chronic alcohol use who presents to the medicine clinic for his annual comprehensive exam with the above complaints. He reports feeling tired and sluggish and that these symptoms have been progressively worsening for the past several months. He now feels that he is fatigued to the point of being unable to do any activities other than routine ADLs.

PMH

History of chronic alcohol use
History of depression
HTN
Hyperlipidemia
Osteoarthritis
Chronic low back pain
Lumbosacral radiculopathy
GERD
Umbilical hernia
Questionable compliance with medications in the past

FH

Negative for DM, CAD, CVA, CA

SH

Divorced, lives with significant other; (+) alcohol—three to four glasses of "scotch on the rocks" per day; (+) smoking tobacco 1.5 ppd × 30 years, (–) recreational drug use; unemployed

Meds

Docusate sodium 100 mg po BID
Aspirin 81 mg po daily
Omeprazole 20 mg po once daily before breakfast
Pravastatin 20 mg po at bedtime
Morphine sulfate 15 mg SA po Q 12 h for pain
Hydrocodone/APAP 5/500 mg 1 tablet po Q 8 h PRN pain
Gabapentin 600 mg po TID
Methocarbamol 500 mg po QID PRN back spasms
Lisinopril 20 mg po daily

All

NKDA

ROS

(+) generalized malaise and becomes easily fatigued; (+) low back pain well controlled with current medications; (+) occasional back spasms and stiffness; (+) BLE paresthesias, consistent with radiculopathy; (–) weight gain or loss; (–) fever; (–) vision or hearing changes; (–) cough, chest pain, palpitations, shortness of breath; (–) nausea/vomiting, abdominal pain, constipation, loose stools, rectal bleeding; (–) nocturia or dysuria; (–) edema; (–) symptoms of depression or anxiety

Physical Examination

Gen

Caucasian male in NAD, smells like cigarette smoke, appears older than stated age of 59, cooperative, oriented × 3, somewhat of a poor historian

VS

BP 146/82, P 74, RR 20, T 35.7°C

Skin

Faint spider angiomata noted on chest; pale skin tone with no apparent jaundice; normal turgor

HEENT

Atraumatic/normocephalic; nonicteric sclera, PERRLA, EOMI; normal funduscopic examination; TMs intact and reactive; (–) glossitis

Neck/Lymph Nodes

Normal ROM; trachea midline; submandibular, supraclavicular, axillary, and inguinal nodes not enlarged

Lung/Thorax

Lungs CTA; (+) gynecomastia

CV

RRR, no MRG

Abd

NTND, (+) bowel sounds

Genit/Rect

Deferred

MS/Ext

Decreased spinal ROM; (+) straight leg test bilaterally; lower extremities warm with bipedal pulses weak bilaterally; decreased hair on lower extremities; no clubbing, edema, or cyanosis; tobacco stains on index and middle fingers

Neuro

CN II–XII grossly intact; decreased muscle strength 2/5 bilaterally in upper and lower extremities; DTRs throughout; vibratory sense intact; Babinski ↓

■ Labs

Na 138 mEq/L	Hgb 12.6 g/dL	RDW 13.5%	*Fasting Lipid Profile:*
K 4.4 mEq/L	Hct 38.1%	AST 58 IU/L	T. chol 227 mg/dL
Cl 97 mEq/L	RBC $3.97 \times 10^6/mm^3$	ALT 62 IU/L	LDL 123 mg/dL
CO_2 25 mEq/L	Plt $181 \times 10^3/mm^3$	Alk phos 78 IU/L	HDL 37 mg/dL
BUN 12 mg/dL	WBC $6.3 \times 10^3/mm^3$	T. bili 1.1 mg/dL	Trig 272 mg/dL
SCr 0.8 mg/dL	MCV 110.4 μm^3	Alb 3.4 g/dL	Iron 67 mcg/dL
Glu 82 mg/dL	MCH 38.0 pg	TSH 1.76 mIU/L	Folate 0.8 ng/mL
PSA 0.4 ng/dL	MCHC 34.4 g/dL	T_4, free 0.99 ng/dL	B_{12} 365 pg/mL
		MMA 0.29 $\mu mol/L$	Homocysteine 52.4 $\mu mol/L$

■ Assessment

Macrocytic anemia secondary to folate deficiency

QUESTIONS

Problem Identification

1.a. Create a drug therapy problem list for this patient.

1.b. What signs, symptoms, and laboratory values indicate that this patient has anemia secondary to folate deficiency?

1.c. Could the patient's folate deficiency have been caused by drug therapy?

1.d. What additional information is needed to satisfactorily assess this patient's folate deficiency?

1.e. Why is it important to differentiate folate deficiency from vitamin B_{12} deficiency, and how is this accomplished?

Desired Outcome

2. What are the goals of pharmacotherapy for this patient's anemia?

Therapeutic Alternatives

3.a. What nondrug therapies may be used to correct this patient's folic acid deficiency?

3.b. What pharmacotherapeutic alternatives are available for treating this patient's anemia?

Optimal Plan

4. What is the most appropriate drug, dosage form, dose, schedule, and duration of therapy for resolving this patient's anemia?

Outcome Evaluation

5. What parameters should be used to evaluate the efficacy and adverse effects of folic acid replacement therapy in this patient?

Patient Education

6. What information would you provide to this patient about his folic acid replacement therapy?

■ SELF-STUDY ASSIGNMENTS

1. Why is periconceptional folic acid supplementation necessary? What might the consequences be if the folic acid requirements are not met?

2. What is the dual interaction between phenytoin and folic acid, and how should this interaction be managed?

3. How does folate deficiency relate to plasma homocysteine levels, and what role does this relationship have in the development of cardiovascular disease?

CLINICAL PEARL

The strongest determinant of plasma homocysteine is the plasma folate level. However, homocysteine levels may be elevated due to causes other than low folate levels. Impaired renal function is associated with higher plasma homocysteine levels, and patients with end-stage renal disease often have homocysteine levels three times higher than the upper limit of normal.

REFERENCES

1. Coppen A, Bolander-Gouaille C. Treatment of depression: time to consider folic acid and vitamin B_{12}. J Psychopharmacol 2005;19:59–65.
2. Bottiglieri T. Homocysteine and folate metabolism in depression. Prog Neuropsychopharmacol Biol Psychiatry 2005;29:1103–1112.
3. Klee GG. Cobalamin and folate evaluation: measurement of methylmalonic acid and homocysteine vs vitamin B_{12} and folate. Clin Chem 2000;46(Pt 2):177–1283.
4. Snow CF. Laboratory diagnosis of vitamin B_{12} and folate deficiency: a guide for the primary care physician. Arch Intern Med 1999;159:1289–1298.
5. Mason JB, Choi SW. Effects of alcohol on folate metabolism: implications for carcinogenesis. Alcohol 2005;35:235–241.
6. Galloway M, Rushworth L. Red cell or serum folate? Results from the National Pathology Alliance benchmarking review. J Clin Pathol 2003;56:924–926.
7. Bazzano LA, Reynolds K, Holder KN, et al. Effect of folic acid supplementation on risk of cardiovascular diseases: a meta-analysis of randomized controlled trials. JAMA 2006;296:2720–2726.
8. Rampersaud GC, Kauwell GP, Bailey LB. Folate: a key to optimizing health and reducing disease risk in the elderly. J Am Coll Nutr 2003;22:1–8.
9. Herrmann W. Significance of hyperhomocysteinemia. Clin Lab 2006;52:367–374.
10. Swain RA, St. Clair L. The role of folic acid in deficiency states and prevention of disease. J Fam Pract 1997;44:138–144.
11. Rader JI. Folic acid fortification, folate status and plasma homocysteine. J Nutr 2002;132(8 Suppl):2466S–2470S.
12. Mills JL. Fortification of foods with folic acid—how much is enough? N Engl J Med 2000;342:1442–1445.
13. Morris MS, Fava, M, Jacques PR. Depression and folate status in the US population. Psychother Psychosom 2003;72:80–87.
14. Smellie WS, Wilson D, McNulty CA, et al. Best practice in primary care pathology: review 1. J Clin Pathol 2005;58:1016–1024.

108

SICKLE CELL ANEMIA

A Crisis Situation . . . . Level I

Christine M. Walko, PharmD, BCOP

LEARNING OBJECTIVES

After completing this case study, students should be able to:

- Recognize the clinical characteristics associated with an acute sickle cell crisis.

- Discuss the presentation of acute chest syndrome and treatment options.
- Recommend optimal analgesic therapy based on patient-specific information.
- Identify optimal endpoints of pharmacotherapy in sickle cell anemia patients.
- Recommend treatment that may reduce the frequency of sickle cell crises.

PATIENT PRESENTATION

Chief Complaint

"My hip and leg pain is keeping me from sleeping, and now it's so bad I can't even walk."

HPI

Kimberly Johnson is a 23-year-old African-American woman with a history of sickle cell anemia who woke up 4 nights ago with pain in her left hip. Over the last four days, it has spread to both hips and down the legs and is not controlled by her home pain medication of oxycodone 5 mg/acetaminophen 325 mg. She has been taking 2 tablets every 4 hours for 2 days now. She currently rates her pain as 9 out of 10. She states she has had a cough for the last week, with some productive green to yellow sputum. Within in the last day, she has also noticed some mild sweats and chills and thinks she may have a fever.

PMH

Sickle cell anemia (SS disease) diagnosed before the age of 1, with approximately five to eight crises per year requiring hospitalization
Bilateral hip replacement at age 15
One previous episode of acute chest syndrome 5 years ago

FH

Mother and father alive and well, both with sickle cell trait. Patient is an only child.

SH

Currently starting dental school in the fall; lives with two female roommates

ROS

Denies nausea, vomiting, diarrhea, or constipation. No evidence of heart failure, but mild cardiomegaly is noted. Has had productive cough with yellowish-green sputum for approximately 1 week and some sweats and chills.

Meds

Folic acid 1 mg po daily
Multivitamin (Women's One-a-Day) 1 tablet daily
Oxycodone 5 mg/acetaminophen 325 mg 1–2 tablets po Q 4–6 h PRN

All

Penicillin (shortness of breath when very young)
Sulfa (reported rash when very young)

Physical Examination

Gen

Thin, well-developed African-American female in moderately high distress

VS

BP 136/74, P 115, RR 24, T 39.0°C; 51 kg; O_2 sat is 85% on room air and 96% on 4 L O_2

HEENT

PERRL; EOMI; oral mucosa soft and moist; normal sclerae and funduscopic examination; no sinus tenderness

Skin

Normal turgor; no rashes or lesions

Neck

Supple; no lymphadenopathy or thyromegaly

CV

RRR; II/VI SEM; no rubs or gallops

Lungs

Crackles in both bases on auscultation; dullness to percussion

Abd

Soft and nontender with normoactive bowel sounds; no rebound or guarding; mild splenomegaly; no hepatomegaly or masses

Ext

Pulses 2+ bilaterally, no edema; local bilateral lower extremity tenderness, erythema and inflammation are present

Neuro

A & O × 3; normal strength, reflexes intact

Labs

Na 139 mEq/L	Hgb 8.5 g/dL	MCV 85 μm^3	Ca 8.8 mg/dL
K 4.2 mEq/L	Hct 24.3%	Retic 18.2%	Mg 1.9 mEq/L
Cl 99 mEq/L	Plt 544 × 10³/mm³	AST 48 IU/L	Phos 3.9 mg/dL
CO₂ 30 mEq/L	WBC 24.8 × 10³/mm³	ALT 39 IU/L	(+) anti-E red cell
BUN 28 mg/dL	Neutros 89%	Alk phos 77 IU/L	antibody
SCr 0.8 mg/dL	Bands 2%	LDH 957 IU/L	
Glu 81 mg/dL	Eos 1%	T. bili 6.8 mg/dL	
	Lymphs 3%	D. bili 0.8 mg/dL	
	Monos 5%	I. bili 6.0 mg/dL	
		Alb 3.8 g/dL	

Other

Arterial blood gas: pH 7.49; pCO_2 38; O_2 72; bicarb 30; O_2 sat 96% on oxygen
Hgb electrophoresis: Hgb A_2 2%; Hgb F 6%; Hgb S 92%
Peripheral blood smear: Sickle forms and target cells present (Fig. 108-1).

Chest X-Ray (Fig. 108-2)

This is a portable chest x-ray remarkable for diffuse interstitial infiltrates in both lung fields consistent with acute chest syndrome. Cardiomegaly is also notable.

ECG

Normal sinus rhythm
Echocardiogram
Normal LV function

Assessment

A 23-year-old African-American woman in sickle cell crisis with probable acute chest syndrome

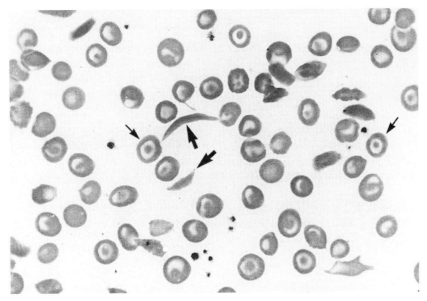

FIGURE 108-1. Peripheral blood with sickle cells *(large arrows)* and target cells *(small arrows)* (Wright-Giemsa × 1,650). *(Photo courtesy of Lydia C. Contis, MD.)*

QUESTIONS

Problem Identification

1.a. Create a list of the patient's drug therapy problems.

1.b. What signs, symptoms, and laboratory values are consistent with an acute sickle cell crisis in this patient?

1.c. What signs, symptoms, and laboratory values support a diagnosis of acute chest syndrome in this patient?

1.d. What additional information is needed to satisfactorily assess this patient?

Desired Outcome

2. What are the goals of pharmacotherapy in this case?

Therapeutic Alternatives

3.a. What nondrug therapies might be useful for this patient?

3.b. What feasible pharmacotherapeutic alternatives are available for treatment of the patient's pain?

3.c. What feasible pharmacotherapeutic alternatives are available for preventing opioid-induced constipation?

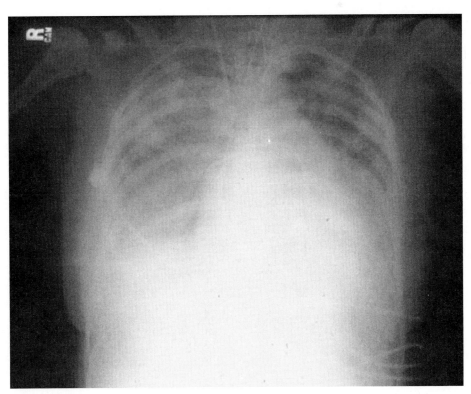

FIGURE 108-2. Lung radiograph of patient with acute chest syndrome secondary to sickle cell anemia. *(Photo courtesy of Kenneth I. Ataga, MD.)*

Optimal Plan

4. Outline a detailed therapeutic plan to treat all facets of this patient's acute sickle cell crisis and acute chest syndrome. For all drug therapies, include the dosage form, dose, schedule, and duration of therapy.

Outcome Evaluation

5.a. What clinical and laboratory parameters are necessary to evaluate therapy for achievement of the desired therapeutic outcome and to detect or prevent adverse effects?

Clinical Course

The plans you recommended have been initiated, and on the third day of hospitalization the patient's pain is markedly improved, oxygen saturation is improved to 97% on room air, and she is afebrile. She is only using two to three demands on her PCA per day and is asking to switch back to oral medication.

5.b. Considering this information, what changes (if any) in the pharmacotherapeutic plan are warranted while the patient is hospitalized?

5.c. What changes (if any) could be made to the patient's home medication regimen to decrease the number of hospitalizations for pain crisis?

5.d. If you recommended any new medications in the answer to the previous question, what laboratory parameters should be followed to evaluate adherence and hematologic response while minimizing toxicity?

Patient Education

6. What information should be provided to the patient to enhance compliance, ensure successful therapy, and minimize adverse effects?

■ SELF-STUDY ASSIGNMENTS

1. Determine the likelihood of the patient's offspring having sickle cell trait and/or disease if the father has:

   a. Normal hemoglobin
   b. Sickle cell trait
   c. Sickle cell disease

2. Describe the complications associated with frequent crises in each organ system.

3. Discuss the differences between sickle cell anemia and β-thalassemia in terms of etiologies, laboratory abnormalities, and disease complications.

CLINICAL PEARL

Allogeneic bone marrow transplantation has proved curative in pediatric sickle cell anemia patients. Approximately 20% of patients have a matched sibling donor, and matches may also be found through the National Marrow Donor Program.

REFERENCES

1. Vichinsky EP, Neumayr LD, Earles AN, et al. Causes and outcomes of the acute chest syndrome in sickle cell disease. National Acute Chest Syndrome Study Group. N Engl J Med 2000;342:1855–1865.
2. Vichinsky EP, Styles LA, Colangelo LH, et al. Acute chest syndrome in sickle cell disease: clinical presentation and course. Cooperative Study of Sickle Cell Disease. Blood 1997;89:1787–1792.
3. Steinberg MH. Management of sickle cell disease. N Engl J Med 1999;340:1021–1030.
4. Morris CR, Singer ST, Walters MC. Clinical hemoglobinopathies: iron, lungs and new blood. Curr Opin Hematol 2006;13:407–418.
5. Bellet PS, Kalinyak KA, Shukla R, et al. Incentive spirometry to prevent acute pulmonary complications in sickle cell diseases. N Engl J Med 1995;333:699–703.
6. Herndon CM, Jackson KC, Hallin PA. Management of opioid-induced gastrointestinal effects in patients receiving palliative care. Pharmacotherapy 2002;22:240–250.
7. Steinberg MH, Barton F, Castro O, et al. Effect of hydroxyurea on mortality and morbidity in adult sickle cell anemia: risks and benefits up to 9 years of treatment. JAMA 2003;289:1645–1651.

109

USING LABORATORY TESTS IN INFECTIOUS DISEASES

Health Care–Associated Pneumonia . . . . Level III

Steven J. Martin, PharmD, BCPS, FCCP, FCCM

Eric G. Sahloff, PharmD

LEARNING OBJECTIVES

After completing this case study, the reader should be able to:

- Describe the various methods for collection of respiratory secretions and outline the qualitative evaluation of the Gram stain.

- Discuss the value of culture data collected through different techniques of accessing respiratory secretions.

- Discuss the use of urine antigen testing in the diagnosis of pneumonia.

- Describe the value of blood culture in health care–associated pneumonia and outline the proper method for blood collection for culture.

- Discuss the proper means for identifying extended-spectrum β-lactamase production in clinical bacterial specimens.

- Describe the appropriate serum sampling times for antibiotic concentration determination to individualize drug dosing.

- Discuss the interpretation of antibiotic concentrations in the therapeutic plan for pneumonia management.

PATIENT PRESENTATION

Chief Complaint

Confusion and change in mental state; obtained through the patient's daughter

HPI

Evelyn Johnson is a 76-year-old woman who lives in an assisted-living community, and she has been brought to the ED of the University Medical Center by her daughter who was concerned about a change in her mother's mental status. Over the past 24 hours, she became confused and uncommunicative and developed a fever (39.8°F). Her breathing has become coarse and labored. Mrs. Johnson has a history of cigarette use and has chronic bronchitis, which limits her mobility and independent living.

PMH

Coronary artery disease
Hypercholesterolemia
Hypertension
Chronic bronchitis
Chronic obstructive pulmonary disease
Osteoarthritis
Epilepsy

FH

Both parents are deceased (mother, aged 66, of CHF; father, aged 72, of stroke). She is widowed, with two adult children (54-year-old daughter and 52-year-old son).

SH

Retired secretary and homemaker; has lived in the assisted-living facility for 2 years; no alcohol; 1 pack per day of cigarette use × 35 years; no illicit drug use

Meds

Amlodipine 5 mg po once daily
Hydrochlorothiazide 25 mg po daily
Pravastatin 30 mg po at bedtime
Valproic acid 1,000 mg po sustained-release at bedtime
Lamotrigine 25 mg po every other day
Naproxen 500 mg po BID
Albuterol/ipratropium (Combivent) inhaler 2 inhalations QID
Fluticasone propionate inhaler 2 inhalations BID

All

Sulfa (produces rash)

ROS

Unable to obtain due to patient's condition

Physical Examination

Gen

The patient is an obese elderly woman in respiratory distress

VS

BP 144/98, P 100, RR 29, T 41°C; Wt 154 lb, Ht 5'5"

Skin

Warm and diaphoretic

HEENT

NC/AT; PERRLA; conjunctivae pink; sclerae clear; EOMI; disk margins sharp; no arteriolar narrowing, AV nicking, hemorrhages, or exudates; ear canals clear and drums negative; nares normal; teeth intact, tonsils intact and normal; pharynx negative

Neck/Lymph Nodes

Trachea midline; thyroid palpable; no nodes

Chest

Rhonchi bilaterally; dullness to percussion and diminished breath sounds in RLL

CV

Tachycardic; normal S_1 and S_2; no heaves, thrills, or bruits

Abd

Soft, non-distended; no masses or tenderness; liver, spleen, and kidneys not felt; no CVA tenderness

Genit/Rect

Not performed

MS/Ext

Deferred

Neuro

Does not respond to voice; responds to pain with withdrawal

▓ Labs

Na 142 mEq/L	Hgb 13.1 g/dL	WBC 21.1×10^3/mm³
K 4.3 mEq/L	Hct 39.5%	Neutros 78%
Cl 106 mEq/L	RBC 4.7×10^6/mm³	Bands 9%
CO₂ 23 mEq/L	Plt 155×10^3/mm³	Lymphs 12%
BUN 26 mg/dL	MCV 81.8 μm³	Monos 1%
SCr 1.8 mg/dL	MCH 27.1 pg	PT 12.6 sec
Glu 97 mg/dL	MCHC 33.1 g/dL	aPTT 29.1 sec
	RDW 15%	

ABG: pH 7.50; pO_2 69 mm Hg; pCO_2 29 mm Hg; HCO_3 22 mEq/L O_2 saturation 89% on FiO_2 1 L via non-rebreather mask

▓ Chest X-Ray

Infiltrate in right lower lobe; bilateral pleural effusions

▓ Assessment

1. RLL pneumonia with increased work of breathing
2. Respiratory alkalosis secondary to pneumonia and tachypnea

▓ Plan

1. Induced sputum for respiratory secretion collection, Gram stain, culture, and sensitivity.
2. Collect two sets of blood cultures (anaerobic and aerobic) from two separate sites.

QUESTIONS

Problem Identification

1.a. Create a list of this patient's drug therapy problems.

1.b. What subjective and objective data indicate the presence of infection?

Desired Outcome

2.a. What are the desired treatment goals for this patient's current medical problems?

2.b. Why are two sets of blood culture obtained?

Clinical Course

Induced sputum was collected and sent to the microbiology laboratory for C/S. In the ED, the patient's respiratory rate increased to >40 breaths/min, requiring emergent endotracheal intubation. The patient was placed on mechanical ventilation with 100% O_2. Gram stain results from the laboratory were received, revealing many WBCs, few epithelial cells, many Gram-negative rods, and moderate Gram-positive cocci in clusters. The patient was started on ceftazidime, 1 g IV Q 12 h; gentamicin, 180 mg IV Q 24 h; and vancomycin 1 g IV Q 24 h.

2.c. The microbiology laboratory performed a Gram stain on the pulmonary secretion sample. How should the microbiologist evaluate the sample quality, and how is the semi-quantitative analysis helpful in directing initial empiric therapy?

2.d. In addition to the pulmonary secretion sample, describe how urinary antigen tests can assist in the identification of the pathogen responsible for this patient's pneumonia.

Therapeutic Alternatives

3.a. When should serum gentamicin and vancomycin concentrations be collected for individualization of drug dosing?

Clinical Course

Two days after admission the patient has not shown signs of improvement clinically and continues to have fevers of >40°C. A diagnostic fiberoptic bronchoscopy with protective specimen brush lavage for evaluation of the lung fields and collection of distal pulmonary secretion samples for Gram stain, culture, and sensitivity is performed. A sample of alveolar washing is sent to the microbiology laboratory for direct examination and culture. Later that afternoon, results of the first induced sputum C/S are reported by the laboratory, identifying *Enterobacter cloacae* and methicillin-resistant *Staphylococcus aureus* as the predominant pathogens in the respiratory culture. The susceptibility profile for the Gram-negative bacillus is shown in Table 109-1.

3.b. The microbiology lab does not routinely test cefepime using automated methods. Because of its stability to many β-lactamases, cefepime may be a viable therapeutic option. What other testing methods are available to determine the activity of cefepime against this isolate?

3.c. Given the unusual resistance profile for this organism, what additional testing should be performed on this isolate to identify specific resistance mechanisms?

Clinical Course

The Gram stain from the BAL is reported with many WBCs, no epithelial cells, and many Gram-negative rods.

Optimal Plan

4.a. The Gram stain from the BAL differs from the Gram stain performed on induced sputum. How should the difference be interpreted?

TABLE 109-1 Preliminary Susceptibility Report	
Antibiotic	**Interpretation**
Aztreonam	Resistant
Amikacin	Resistant
Ampicillin/sulbactam	Resistant
Ceftazidime	Resistant
Ceftriaxone	Resistant
Cefotaxime	Resistant
Ciprofloxacin	Resistant
Imipenem	Sensitive
Gentamicin	Resistant
Piperacillin/tazobactam	Resistant
Tobramycin	Resistant

4.b. The microbiology laboratory provided both a minimum inhibitory concentration (MIC) and an interpretation of that MIC for each antimicrobial agent tested. How are the MIC and the interpretation correlated?

Clinical Course

The patient's antibiotic regimen was switched to imipenem 500 mg IV Q 12 h, but the intensivist is concerned about the use of this drug in a patient with epilepsy and renal dysfunction. She has requested the laboratory test cefepime against the *Enterobacter* isolate. The cefepime MIC for this organism was 8 mcg/mL. The patient's antibiotic was again switched to cefepime 2 g IV Q 12 h. The patient's fever abated, and her WBC count (day 3 of hospitalization) was $13.0 \times 10^3/mm^3$, with 77% neutros, 2% bands, 18% lymphs, 2% monos, 1% eosin.

Outcome Evaluation

5.a. Would the determination of the minimum bactericidal concentration (MBC) for this organism against cefepime or the evaluation of the serum bactericidal titer (SBT) be helpful in the management of this infection?

5.b. Outline a follow-up plan for monitoring the efficacy of this therapeutic regimen.

■ SELF-STUDY ASSIGNMENTS

1. What is the expected turnaround time for the microbiology laboratory to provide a full organism identification and susceptibility profile for a sputum specimen?

2. What difference does the method of obtaining respiratory secretions for culture and sensitivity play in mortality?

3. What diagnostic significance do quantitative cultures provide?

CLINICAL PEARL

When patients with pneumonia are receiving antimicrobial agents at the time respiratory tract secretions are obtained through induced sputum or blind bronchial suctioning, cultures may be negative, and concentrations of bacteria may be below the diagnostic threshold. Several studies suggest that the sensitivity of protected specimen brush (PSB) and BAL for the diagnosis of pneumonia is unchanged in patients who acquire pneumonia while on antibiotics for >72 hours. This suggests that BAL with PSB along with quantitative culture is a preferred method for diagnosis of pneumonia.

REFERENCES

1. Al Balooshi N, Jamsheer A, Botta GA. Impact of introducing quality control/quality assurance (QC/QA) guidelines in respiratory specimen processing. Clin Microbiol Infect 2003;9:810–815.
2. Tan MJ, Tan JS, File TM. Legionnaires' disease with bacteremic coinfection. Clin Infect Dis 2002;35:533–539.
3. Roson B, Fernandez-Sabe N, Carratala J, et al. Contribution of a urinary antigen assay (Binax NOW) to the early diagnosis of pneumococcal pneumonia. Clin Infect Dis 2004;38:222–226.
4. Clinical and Laboratory Standards Institute. Methods for Dilution Antimicrobial Susceptibility Tests for Bacteria that Grow Aerobically: Approved Standard, 7th ed. NCCLS document M07-A7. Clinical and Laboratory Standards Institute, 940 West Valley Road, Suite 1400, Wayne, PA 19087–1898, 2006.
5. Sahloff EG, Martin SJ. Extended-spectrum beta-lactamase resistance in the ICU. J Pharm Pract 2002;15:96–105.
6. Chastre J, Fagon J-Y, Bornet-Lecso M, et al. Evaluation of bronchoscopic techniques for the diagnosis of nosocomial pneumonia. Am J Respir Crit Care Med 1995;152:231–240.

110

BACTERIAL MENINGITIS

Space Invaders: The Cerebral Kind . . . . Level II

Sherry A. Luedtke, PharmD

LEARNING OBJECTIVES

After completing this case study, the reader should be able to:

- Identify risk factors and common presenting signs and symptoms of bacterial meningitis in infants and children.
- Differentiate common bacterial pathogens associated with meningitis in children of different ages.
- Recommend appropriate empiric and definitive antimicrobial therapy for bacterial meningitis.
- Identify appropriate parameters for monitoring antimicrobial therapy for treatment of bacterial meningitis.

PATIENT PRESENTATION

■ Chief Complaint

From mom: "My son has a fever and is not acting right!"

■ HPI

Jonathan Cruz is a 9-month-old, 8.4 kg, male infant who presents to the emergency department in the arms of his mother. She reports that he developed a fever (T_{max} 103°F/39.4°C) 1 day prior to presentation with some mild rhinorrhea and decreased appetite. She indicates that he had a restless night, waking up numerous times with irritability and was inconsolable. This morning, she had difficulty arousing him. She immediately called her pediatrician, who instructed her to take him to the emergency department for evaluation.

■ PMH

Jonathan was born at 34 weeks' gestation and spent 3 weeks in the neonatal intensive care unit. He underwent an uncomplicated vaginal delivery. He has been relatively healthy to date, except for an ear infection at 6 months of age, which was treated with amoxicillin.

■ FH

Paternal grandparent with diabetes mellitus, father with hypertension

■ SH

Lives with mother and father, one sibling (4 years old). Both children attend daycare.

■ Meds

None; immunizations up to date

■ All

NKDA

■ Physical Examination

Gen

Lethargic, ill-appearing infant

VS

BP 85/50, HR 148, RR 52, T 39.7°C; Wt 8.4 kg

HEENT

PERRL, left tympanic membrane slightly erythematous

Chest

Lungs clear bilaterally

CV

Sinus tachycardia, regular rhythm, no murmurs

Abd

Soft, distended, (+) BS

Extremities

Capillary refill 3–4 seconds, extremities are somewhat mottled in appearance and cool to touch.

Neuro

Lethargic but arousable, (–) Kernig's and Brudzinski's sign

■ Labs

Na 133 mEq/L	Hgb 15.4 g/dL	*CBG*
K 3.9 mEq/L	Hct 46.2%	pH 7.32
Cl 105 mEq/L	Plt 297 × 10³/mm³	pO_2 47 mm Hg
CO_2 18 mEq/L	WBC 16.0 × 10³/mm³	pCO_2 53 mm Hg
SCr 1.1 mg/dL	Neutros 45%	HCO_3 13 mEq/L
Glu 153 mg/dL	Bands 19%	BE –10 mEq/L
Ca 8.1 mg/dL	Lymphs 34%	CRP 12.5 mg/L
Mg 1.6 mEq/L	Eos 1%	
PO_4 3.5 mg/dL	Basos 1%	
TP 6.2 g/dL		
Alb 3.8 g/dL		
Bili 1.0 mg/dL		
AST 79 IU/L		
ALT 19 IU/L		
ALP 365 IU/L		

Urine and CSF serology: *Haemophilus influenzae* Type B (–), *Streptococcus pneumoniae* (+), Group B Streptococcus (–), *Neisseria meningitidis* (–), *N. meningitidis* B/*Escherichia coli* (–)

CSF chemistry/cell count: color/appearance hazy, glucose 40 mg/dL, protein 281 mg/dL, WBC 300/mm³ (5% lymphs, 62% monos, 33% neutros), RBC 16/mm³

Gram stain (CSF): Gram-positive cocci in pairs

Cultures: Blood, urine, CSF pending

■ Chest X-Ray

Unremarkable

■ Assessment

1. Suspected pneumococcal meningitis
2. Hypotension

QUESTIONS

Problem Identification

1.a. What drug therapy problems does this infant have?

1.b. What risk factors does this patient have for bacterial meningitis?

1.c. What clinical and laboratory findings indicate the presence of meningitis and its severity?

Desired Outcome

2. What are the goals of drug therapy in this situation?

Therapeutic Alternatives

3.a. What nondrug therapies might be useful for managing this patient?

3.b. Describe the empiric antimicrobial regimen that should be used in this patient.

3.c. Discuss adjuvant drug therapy options for the management of infants and children with meningitis.

3.d. What supportive therapies may be used to manage the patient's hypotension and resulting metabolic acidosis?

■ CLINICAL COURSE

Blood cultures returned positive for *S. pneumoniae*. CSF cultures (drawn after antibiotics were initiated) and urine cultures were negative. Sensitivity studies revealed intermediate sensitivity to penicillin (MIC >0.01 mcg/mL) and cefotaxime/ceftriaxone (MIC >2.0 mcg/mL).

Repeat CRP in 24 hours was 3.5 mg/L and the repeat CBC at that time revealed: Hgb 14.5 g/dL, Hct 43.5%, Plt 230 × 10³/mm³, WBC 8.6 × 10³/mm³ (32% segs, 12% bands, 55% lymphs, 1% basos).

Optimal Plan

4. Given this new information, are there any changes in drug therapy that you would recommend? What duration of therapy do you recommend?

Outcome Evaluation

5. Describe the monitoring parameters necessary to evaluate the efficacy and safety of the therapy.

■ CLINICAL COURSE

The infant was treated with the regimen you recommended and blood pressure and neurologic status improved within the first 24 hours of treatment. Seventy-two hours after initiation of antibiotic therapy, a repeat lumbar puncture was performed and was clear. The patient was discharged on day 10 of therapy. Audiometry testing performed after completion of antibiotic therapy was normal. The child had no evidence of neurologic impairment as a consequence of the infection at follow-up evaluations.

■ SELF-STUDY ASSIGNMENTS

1. Discuss the impact of universal pneumococcal immunization of infants with the conjugated pneumococcal polysaccharide vaccine on invasive pneumococcal infections in children.

2. Describe the penetration of antimicrobials into the CNS and the properties that influence their penetration.

3. List the definitive therapies for the management of confirmed bacterial meningitis caused by common organisms.

4. Discuss the use of alternative agents (i.e., meropenem and/or quinolones) in the management of resistant pneumococcal meningitis.

CLINICAL PEARL

Empiric therapy and management of children should NOT be altered regardless of the immunization status or number of doses received of the conjugated pneumococcal vaccine (Prevnar).

REFERENCES

1. Chavez-Bueno S, McCracken GH. Bacterial meningitis in children. Pediatr Clin N Am 2005;52:795–810.
2. Tunkel AR, Hartman BJ, Kaplan SL, et al. Practice guidelines for the management of bacterial meningitis. Clin Infect Dis 2004;39:1267–1284.
3. Hengst JM. The role of C-reactive protein in the evaluation and management of infants with suspected sepsis. Adv Neonatal Care 2003;3:3–13.
4. Saez-Llorens X, McCracken GH. Bacterial meningitis in children. Lancet 2003;361:2139–2148.
5. Kaplan SL. Management of pneumococcal meningitis. Pediatr Infect Dis J 2002;21:589–591.

111

ACUTE BRONCHITIS

Mr. Comeaux's Cough. . . . . Level II

Justin J. Sherman, MCS, PharmD

W. Greg Leader, PharmD

LEARNING OBJECTIVES

After completing this case study, the reader should be able to:

- Identify signs and symptoms of acute bronchitis and their duration, and evaluate relevant laboratory values in order to rule out more serious illness such as pneumonia for elderly patients.

- Discuss why obtaining sputum cultures and Gram stains is not relevant in evaluation and treatment of patients with uncomplicated acute bronchitis.

- Discuss why antibiotic treatment is not indicated for uncomplicated acute bronchitis.

- Identify clinical cases when an elderly patient should be reevaluated for another ongoing illness that has been previously undetected.

- Select nonpharmacologic and pharmacologic treatment alternatives for supportive care, incorporating new data regarding efficacy.

PATIENT PRESENTATION

Chief Complaint

"My father has been coughing and wheezing for several days. He has been staying with my brother for the past month, but he didn't even take my father to the doctor, let alone start him on antibiotics."

HPI

Kathryn Comeaux appears distraught and hurried as she brings her father, Cole Comeaux, into the primary care clinic. She states that her father, a 63-year-old widower, has been complaining of a productive, purulent cough, wheezing, and rhinorrhea for the past 5 days. Upon questioning the patient, Mr. Comeaux denies that he has had any fever, chills, or myalgia. He also insists that the only problem he has now is the cough, and the wheezing and rhinorrhea have almost stopped. He states that, besides having "children who constantly bicker with each other," he is almost completely free of problems and is "feeling much better than before, thank you very much."

PMH

Hypertension × 10 years
Diabetes × 5 years
Hyperlipidemia × 2 years

FH

The patient's wife passed away at age 60 (6 months ago) due to a stroke, and his father and mother both lived to be in their 90s and died of "natural causes." He was vaccinated for pneumonia last year.

SH

Mr. Comeaux's children, both divorced, have taken turns letting him live with them after the death of their mother, since he has no gainful employment and could not keep up with his house mortgage. He used to write children's books, including the Boudreaux's Bayou Adventures series, but his last meaningful project was over a decade ago. He spends most of his time reading and smoking Barrington cigarettes (1 ppd × 30 years). Also, he admits that he would like to quit before he starts having any chronic lung problems. He tried quitting 1 year ago and was smoke-free for 2 days, but he could not tolerate the itchiness that the nicotine patches caused. Once he stopped using the patches, he started smoking again. He denies any alcohol use.

This month is his daughter's turn to serve as caretaker, but she is distressed that she will have to send him to a senior daycare center during the day while she starts her new job as a waitress at a local restaurant that serves Cajun cuisine. She is also upset because she thinks that her brother has not been taking care of their father well, since he did not take Mr. Comeaux to the doctor, let alone start him on antibiotics.

Meds

Lisinopril 40 mg daily
Metformin 1,000 mg BID
Simvastatin 20 mg daily
Note: This is patient's current list over the past 6 months. He is unsure what he took in the past because his wife used to take care of his medication responsibilities.

All

NKDA

ROS

No fever, chills, myalgia, chest pain, or shortness of breath; no nausea, vomiting, or diarrhea

Physical Examination

Gen

Well-developed, overweight male in NAD; overall demeanor seems slightly disheartened, but he is communicative and clean and well-shaven in appearance

VS

BP 142/92 mm Hg, P 84, RR 17, T 37°C; Wt 78 kg, Ht 5'6"

HEENT

PERRLA, conjunctivae clear, TMs intact. No epistaxis or nasal discharge. No sinus swelling or tenderness, and mucous membranes are moist. There are no oropharyngeal lesions. Wears dentures.

Neck

Supple without adenopathy or thyromegaly

Chest

(–) rhonchi, rales, increased fremitus, wheezing, or egophony

Heart

RRR without MRG

Abd

Soft, nontender, (+) BS

Ext

Pulses 2+ throughout

Neuro

A & O × 3; 2+ reflexes throughout, 5/5 strength; CN II–XII intact

■ Labs

Na 140 mEq/L	FPG 104 mg/dL	WBC $4.9 \times 10^3/mm^3$	*Fasting Lipid Profile*
K 4.5 mEq/L	A1C 6.4%	Segs 55%	*(from outpatient visit*
Cl 102 mEq/L	Hgb 14 g/dL	Bands 3%	*1 month ago):*
HCO_3 24 mEq/L	Hct 45%	Lymphs 33%	T. chol 150 mg/dL
BUN 14 mg/dL	RBC $5.0 \times 10^6/mm^3$	Monos 6%	TG 145 mg/dL
SCr 0.9 mg/dL	Plt $250 \times 10^3/mm^3$	Eos 2%	LDL 69 mg/dL
		Basos 1%	HDL 52 mg/dL

■ Sputum culture

No pathogens isolated

■ Assessment

A 63-year-old man with presumed acute bronchitis that is likely viral in origin

(+) smoking history; patient currently expressing desire to quit

Diabetes and dyslipidemia—well controlled on current medication regimen

Family/caregiver issues that should be further explored and addressed

QUESTIONS

Problem Identification

1.a. Create a list of the patient's drug therapy problems.

1.b. What information (signs, symptoms, laboratory values) indicates the presence or severity of acute bronchitis?

1.c. Could any of the patient's symptoms have been caused by drug therapy?

1.d. What additional information must be considered before deciding whether antimicrobial therapy is indicated?

Desired Outcome

2. What are the goals of pharmacotherapy in this case?

Therapeutic Alternatives

3.a. What nondrug therapies might be useful for this patient?

3.b. What feasible pharmacotherapeutic alternatives are available for treatment of uncomplicated acute bronchitis?

3.c. What are the most likely alternatives for the uncontrolled hypertension and smoking cessation attempt?

3.d. What psychosocial considerations are applicable to this patient?

Optimal Plan

4.a. What drugs, dosage form, dose, schedule, and duration of therapy are best to alleviate this patient's symptoms of acute bronchitis?

4.b. What medication and dosage should be recommended for this patient's elevated blood pressure and smoking cessation plan?

Outcome Evaluation

5. What clinical and laboratory parameters are necessary to evaluate the therapy for achievement of the desired outcome and to detect or prevent adverse effects?

Patient Education

6. What information should be provided to the patient to enhance compliance, ensure successful therapy, and to minimize adverse effects?

■ FOLLOW-UP QUESTION

1. What vaccinations should this patient receive?

■ SELF-STUDY ASSIGNMENTS

1. Outline a treatment plan for a patient with chronic bronchitis presenting with an acute exacerbation, and contrast how this treatment would differ from treatment for a patient with a new diagnosis of acute bronchitis.

2. Prepare a patient education pamphlet on acute bronchitis. Be sure to address why antibiotics are not usually first-line therapy for uncomplicated acute bronchitis.

3. Discuss the differences in presentation and treatment, if any, of uncomplicated acute bronchitis for a child versus an elderly patient.

CLINICAL PEARL

Many patients who present with symptoms of acute bronchitis expect to receive an antibiotic. Therefore, time should be spent with the patient to explain what goes into the decision to not prescribe an antibiotic, and why excessive use of unnecessary antibiotics could harm the community at large.

REFERENCES

1. Braman SS. Chronic cough due to acute bronchitis: ACCP evidence-based clinical practice guidelines. Chest 2006;129:95S–103S.

2. Wenzel RP, Fowler AA. Acute bronchitis. N Engl J Med 2006;355:2125–2130.

3. Steinman M, Sauaia A, Masseli J, et al. Office evaluation and treatment of elderly patients with acute bronchitis. J Am Geriatr Soc 2004;52:875–879.

4. Linder JA, Sim I. Antibiotic treatment of acute bronchitis in smokers. J Gen Intern Med 2002;17:230–234.

5. Smucny J, Flynn C, Becker L, et al. Beta2-agonists for acute bronchitis. Cochrane Database Syst Rev (database online), Issue 1, 2004.

6. Gonzales R, Bartlett JG, Besser RE, et al. Principles of appropriate antibiotic use for treatment of uncomplicated acute bronchitis: background. Ann Intern Med 2001;134:521–529.

7. Irwin RS, Baumann MH, Boulet L, et al. Diagnosis and management of cough executive summary: ACCP evidence-based clinical practice guidelines. Chest 2006;129:1S–23S.

8. Mandell LA, Bartlett JG, Dowell SF, et al. Update of practice guidelines for the management of community-acquired pneumonia in immuno-competent adults. Clin Infect Dis 2003;37:1405–1433.

9. Expert Panel on Detection, Evaluation, and Treatment of High Blood Cholesterol in Adults. Executive Summary of the Third Report of the National Cholesterol Education Program (NCEP) Expert Panel on Detection, Evaluation, and Treatment of High Blood Cholesterol in Adults (Adult Treatment Panel III). JAMA 2001;285:2486–2497.

10. Phillips TG, Hickner J. Calling acute bronchitis a chest cold may improve patient satisfaction with appropriate antibiotic use. J Am Board Fam Pract 2005;18:459–463.

11. Brunton S, Carmichael BP, Colgan R, et al. Acute exacerbation of chronic bronchitis: a primary care consensus guideline. Am J Manag Care 2004;10:689–696.

112

INFLUENZA: PREVENTION AND TREATMENT

Run Over by the Flu . . . . Level II

Margarita V. DiVall, PharmD, BCPS

LEARNING OBJECTIVES

After completing this case study, the reader should be able to:

- Recognize the clinical presentation of influenza.

- Discuss influenza-related complications.

- Develop a patient-specific treatment plan for influenza.

- Identify appropriate target populations for vaccination against influenza.

- Compare and contrast available options for preventing influenza.

- Discuss strategies to control influenza outbreaks.

PATIENT PRESENTATION

Chief Complaint

"I feel like a truck ran over me. Every muscle and bone hurts, and I am burning up."

HPI

Vladimir Kharitonov is a 57-year-old Russian man who presents in mid-December to an Urgent Care clinic with complaints of 1 day history of fever, up to 39°C (102.2°F), muscle and bone aches, feeling tired, and headache. He has not had anything to eat in the past 12 hours due to loss of appetite and has not taken his glyburide this morning. He has been in his usual state of health previously and reports that some of his coworkers have been sick with the "flu." He decided to come to the clinic in hopes that an antibiotic can allow him to recover sooner since his son is getting married next weekend. He missed his regular physical appointment 1 month ago because he was "too busy."

PMH

Type 2 DM for 14 years
Hyperlipidemia
HTN

SH

Lives at home with his wife; works full time; quit smoking 10 years ago, but smokes occasionally when really stressed or in a social setting; drinks alcohol in social a setting—mostly vodka.

Meds

Aspirin 81 mg po daily
HCTZ 25 mg po daily
Glyburide 5 mg po every morning
Metformin 1 g po twice daily
Lantus 35 units SC at bedtime
Lipitor 10 mg po daily
Centrum Silver 1 tab po daily

All

NKDA

ROS

Patient complains of severe fatigue, body aches, alternating between being too cold or sweating, sore throat, non-productive cough, and a headache. He denies nasal congestion, nausea, vomiting or diarrhea.

Physical Examination

Gen

WDWN overweight man in NAD

VS

BP 145/85, P 95, RR 18, T 38.5°C; Wt 95.5 kg, Ht 5'10"

Skin

Warm and moist secondary to diaphoresis, no lesions

HEENT

PERRLA; EOMI; TMs intact; wears dentures; mild pharyngeal erythema with no exudates

Neck/Lymph Nodes

Neck is supple and without adenopathy; no JVD

Lungs/Thorax

CTA; no crackles or wheezing

CV

RRR; Normal S_1, S_2; no murmurs

Abd

Soft, slightly obese; NT/ND; normal BS

Genit/Rect

Not performed

MS/Ext

Muscle strength and tone 4–5/5; no CCE

Neuro

A & O × 3; CN II–XII intact; decreased sensation to light touch of the lower extremities (both feet)

■ Labs

Na 138 mEq/L	Hgb 13.2 g/dL	WBC 10 × 10³/mm³	*Fasting Lipid Profile:*
K 3.8 mEq/L	Hct 41%	Neutros 50%	T. chol 177 mg/dL
Cl 98 mEq/L	Plt 275 × 10³/mm³	Bands 4%	LDL 110 mg/dL
CO₂ 24 mEq/L		Eos 0%	HDL 35 mg/dL
BUN 26 mg/dL		Lymphs 39%	Trig 160 mg/dL
SCr 1.3 mg/dL		Monos 7%	
Glu 185 mg/dL			
A1C 8.5%			

■ Diagnostic Tests

QuickVue Influenza test—positive

■ Assessment

57-year-old man with diabetes, hypertension, and hyperlipidemia presents with influenza

QUESTIONS

Problem Identification

1.a. Create a list of patient's drug therapy problems.

1.b. What information (signs, symptoms, laboratory values) indicates the presence of influenza?

1.c. What influenza-related complications is this patient at risk for developing?

Desired Outcome

2. What are the goals of pharmacotherapy in this case?

Therapeutic Alternatives

3.a. List available options for treating influenza in this patient. Include the drug name, dose, dosage form, route, frequency, and treatment duration.

3.b. What other therapies are available to help this patient with his symptoms?

Optimal Plan

4.a. Provide your individualized treatment recommendations for treating this patient's influenza, including symptom management.

4.b. Outline your plans for managing each of the patient's other drug therapy problems.

Outcome Evaluation

5. What clinical and laboratory parameters are necessary to evaluate the therapy for achievement of the desired therapeutic outcome and detect or prevent adverse effects?

Patient Education

6. What information should be provided to the patient to enhance compliance, ensure successful therapy, and minimize adverse effects?

■ CLINICAL COURSE

In October of the following year, Mr. Kharitonov presents for his routine physical exam. He has been doing very well. His diabetes, hypertension, and hyperlipidemia are well controlled.

■ FOLLOW-UP QUESTIONS

1. What indications does this patient have for administration of the influenza vaccine?

2. If the vaccine is desirable, what is the optimal time frame for this patient to receive the influenza vaccine?

3. List available options for vaccination against influenza.

4. Provide your individualized recommendations for protecting this patient against influenza virus infection.

■ SELF-STUDY ASSIGNMENTS

1. Prepare an educational pamphlet on influenza prevention and treatment directed at both patients and general practice physicians. Be sure to include recommendations for controlling influenza outbreaks.

2. Investigate the expanded role of pharmacists as immunization providers.

3. Investigate the threat of human infection with avian influenza viruses. Are currently available influenza prevention strategies effective against avian flu?

CLINICAL PEARL

Development of antibodies takes approximately 2 weeks after influenza vaccination in adults, during which time they remain at high risk for influenza infection. If the immunization occurs during an influenza outbreak, chemoprophylaxis with antiviral agents can be administered for 2 weeks immediately after vaccination to minimize the risk of infection.

REFERENCES

1. Centers for Disease Control and Prevention. Prevention and control of influenza: Recommendations of the Advisory Committee on Immunization Practices (ACIP). MMWR 2007;56:1–54.

2. Cooper NJ, Sutton AJ, Abrams KR, et al. Effectiveness of neuraminidase inhibitors in treatment and prevention of influenza A and B: systematic review and meta-analyses of randomised controlled trials. BMJ 2003;326:1235.

3. Jefferson T, Demicheli V, Deeks J, et al. Neuraminidase inhibitors for preventing and treating influenza in healthy adults. Cochrane Database Syst Rev 2000;3:CD001265.

4. Bright RA, Shay DK, Shu B, et al. Adamantane resistance among influenza A viruses isolated early during the 2005–2006 influenza season in the United States. JAMA 2006;295:891–894.

5. Centers for Disease Control and Prevention. Prevention and control of influenza: recommendations of the Advisory Committee on Immunization Practices (ACIP). MMWR 2006;55(RR-10):1–42.

6. American Diabetes Association. Standards for medical care in diabetes—2007. Diabetes Care 2007;30(Suppl 1):S4–S41.

7. Chobanian AV, Bakris GL, Black HR, et al. The seventh report of the Joint National Committee on Prevention, Detection, and Treatment of High Blood Pressure. JAMA 2003;289:2560–2572.

8. Jones P, Kafonek S, Laurora I, et al. Comparative dose efficacy study of atorvastatin versus simvastatin, pravastatin, lovastatin, and fluvastatin in patients with hypercholesterolemia (the CURVES study). Am J Cardiol 1998;81:582–587.

9. Relenza. [Patient Information Leaflet] Research Triangle Park, NC: GlaxoSmithKline, NC; 2007.

10. FluMist. [Package Insert] Gaithersburg, MD: Medimmune Vaccines, Inc; 2007.

113

COMMUNITY-ACQUIRED PNEUMONIA

Fever with a Cough . . . . Level II

Trent G. Towne, PharmD

Sharon M. Erdman, PharmD

LEARNING OBJECTIVES

After completing this case study, the reader should be able to:

- Recognize the typical signs, symptoms, physical examination, and laboratory/radiographic findings in a patient with community-acquired pneumonia (CAP).

- Describe the most common causative pathogens of CAP, including their frequency of occurrence and susceptibility to commonly used antimicrobials.

- Discuss the risk stratification strategies that can be employed to determine whether a patient with CAP should be treated as an inpatient or outpatient.

- Provide recommendations for initial empiric antibiotic therapy for an inpatient or outpatient with CAP based on clinical presentation, age, presence of comorbidities, and presence of allergies.

- Define the goals of antimicrobial therapy for a patient with CAP, including monitoring parameters that should be used to assess the response to therapy as well as the occurrence of adverse effects.

- Describe the clinical parameters that should be considered when changing a patient from IV to oral antimicrobial therapy in the treatment of CAP.

PATIENT PRESENTATION

■ Chief Complaint

"I have been short of breath and have been coughing up brown mucus for the past 3 days."

■ HPI

James Thompson is a 55-year-old man with a 3-day history of worsening shortness of breath, subjective fevers, chills, right-sided chest pain, and a productive cough. The patient states that his initial symptom of shortness of breath began approximately 1 week ago after delivering mail on an extremely cold winter day. After several days of not feeling well, he went to an immediate care clinic and received a prescription for levofloxacin 750 mg po for 5 days, which he never filled due to financial reasons. He has been taking acetaminophen and an over-the-counter cough and cold preparation, but feels that his symptoms are getting "much worse." The patient

began experiencing pleuritic chest pain and a productive cough over the past 3 days, and feels that he has been feverish with chills, although he did not take his temperature. Upon presentation to the ED, he is febrile and appears to be visibly short of breath.

■ PMH

HTN × 15 years
COPD × 10 years

■ SH

Lives with wife and four children.
Employed as a mail carrier for the U.S. Postal Service
Smokes 2 ppd for the past 30 years
Denies alcohol use or IV drug use

■ Meds

Patient states that he has only been sporadically taking his medications due to financial issues.
Lisinopril 10 mg po once daily
Hydrochlorothiazide 12.5 mg po once daily
Ipratropium/albuterol MDI two inhalations four times daily
Albuterol MDI two inhalations PRN shortness of breath
Acetaminophen 650 mg po Q 6 h PRN pain
Guaifenesin/dextromethorphan (100 mg/10 mg/5 mL) 2 teaspoonfuls Q 4 h PRN cough

■ All

NKDA

■ ROS

Patient is a good historian. Patient has been experiencing shortness of breath, a productive cough, subjective fevers, chills, and pleuritic chest pain that is "right in the middle of my chest." He denies any nausea, vomiting, constipation, or problems urinating.

■ Physical Examination

Gen

Patient is a well-developed, well-nourished, African-American man in moderate respiratory distress appearing somewhat anxious and uncomfortable.

VS

BP 156/90, P 127, RR 31, T 39.1°C; Wt 88 kg, Ht 6'1"

Skin

Warm to the touch; poor skin turgor

HEENT

PERRLA; EOMI; moist mucous membranes

Neck/Lymph Nodes

No JVD; full range of motion; no neck stiffness; no masses or thyromegaly; no cervical lymphadenopathy

Lungs/Thorax

Tachypneic, labored breathing; coarse rhonchi diffusely throughout right lung fields; decreased breath sounds in right middle and lower lung fields

CV

Audible S_1 and S_2; tachycardic with regular rhythm; no MRG

Abd

NTND; (+) bowel sounds

Genit/Rect

Deferred

Extremities

No CCE; 5/5 grip strength; 2+ pulses bilaterally

Neuro

A & O × 3; CN II–XII intact

▓ Labs on Admission

Na 140 mEq/L	Hgb 12.1 g/dL	WBC $17.2 \times 10^3/mm^3$
K 4.3 mEq/L	Hct 35%	Neutros 67%
Cl 102 mEq/L	RBC $3.8 \times 10^6/mm^3$	Bands 5%
CO_2 22 mEq/L	Plt $220 \times 10^3/mm^3$	Lymphs 16%
BUN 31 mg/dL	MCV 91 μm^3	Monos 12%
SCr 1.4 mg/dL	MCHC 35 g/dL	
Glu 101 mg/dL		

▓ ABG

pH 7.410; pCO_2 29; pO_2 65 with 85% O_2 saturation on room air

▓ Chest X-Ray

Right middle and lower lobe airspace disease, likely pneumonia. Left lung is clear. Heart size is normal.

▓ Chest CT Scan without Contrast

No axillary, mediastinal, or hilar lymphadenopathy. The heart size is normal. There is consolidation of the right lower lobe and lateral segment of the middle lobe, with air bronchograms. No significant pleural effusions. The left lung is clear.

▓ Sputum Gram Stain

>25 WBC/hpf, <10 epithelial cells/hpf, many Gram (+) cocci in pairs

▓ Sputum Culture

Pending

▓ Blood Cultures × Two Sets

Pending

▓ Assessment

Probable multilobar community-acquired pneumonia involving the RML and RLL

Hypoxemia

QUESTIONS

Problem Identification

1.a. Create a list of the patient's drug therapy problems.

1.b. What clinical, laboratory, and radiographic findings are consistent with the diagnosis of CAP in this patient?

1.c. What are the common causative bacteria of CAP?

1.d. What clinical, laboratory, and physical examination findings should be considered when deciding on the site of care for a patient with CAP (inpatient or outpatient)?

Desired Outcome

2. What are the goals of pharmacotherapy in the treatment of CAP?

Therapeutic Alternatives

3. What feasible pharmacotherapeutic alternatives are available for treatment of CAP?

Optimal Plan

4.a. What drug, dose, route of therapy, dosing schedule, and duration of treatment should be used in this patient?

■ CLINICAL COURSE

While in the ED, the patient was placed on 4L NC of O_2, and his oxygen saturation improved to 98%. The patient was initiated on ceftriaxone 1 g IV daily and azithromycin 500 mg IV daily and admitted to the hospital. Over the next 48 hours, the patient's clinical status improved with resolving fever, tachypnea, tachycardia, and shortness of breath. On hospital day 2, the blood cultures were reported positive with growth of *Streptococcus pneumoniae*, resistant to penicillin (MIC ≥2) and erythromycin (MIC ≥1), but susceptible to ceftriaxone (MIC ≤0.06), levofloxacin (MIC ≤0.5), and vancomycin (MIC ≤1). The sputum culture demonstrated only the presence of normal respiratory flora.

4.b. Given this new information, what changes in the antimicrobial therapy would you recommend?

■ CLINICAL COURSE

Gradually over the course of the next 7 days, the patient's clinical symptoms resolved, and blood cultures performed on hospital day 7 were negative. On hospital day 10, the patient was discharged home on oral antibiotics to complete a 14-day course of treatment.

4.c. What oral antibiotic would be suitable to complete the course of therapy for CAP?

Outcome Evaluation

5.a. What clinical and laboratory parameters should be monitored to ensure the desired therapeutic outcome and to detect or prevent adverse effects?

5.b. When is it appropriate to convert a patient from IV to oral therapy for the treatment of CAP?

Patient Education

6. What information should be provided to the patient about his oral outpatient antibiotic therapy to enhance compliance, ensure successful therapy, and minimize adverse effects?

■ SELF-STUDY ASSIGNMENTS

1. Review the most recent practice guidelines for the treatment of community-acquired pneumonia from the Infectious Diseases Society of America (IDSA)/American Thoracic Society, and evaluate changes from the last published guidelines.

2. Review national, regional, and local patterns of *S. pneumoniae* susceptibility and compare the data to what is seen at your institution or clinic setting.

3. Describe the role of short-course antibiotic therapy in the management of CAP.

CLINICAL PEARL

Influenza and pneumococcal vaccines for appropriate patient types are important components in reducing the morbidity and mortality associated with CAP.

REFERENCES

1. Mandell LA, Wunderink RG, Anzueto A, et al. Infectious Diseases Society of America/American Thoracic Society Consensus Guidelines

on the Management of Community-Acquired Pneumonia in Adults. Clin Infect Dis 2007;44 (Suppl 2).

2. Infections of the lower respiratory tract. In: Forbes BA, Sahm DF, Weissfeld AS, eds. Diagnostic Microbiology, 11th ed. St. Louis, Mosby, 2002:884–898.

3. Segreti J, House HR, Siegel RE. Principles of antibiotic treatment of community-acquired pneumonia in the outpatient setting. Am J Med 2005;118:21S–28S.

4. Bochus PY, Moser F, Erard P, et al. Community-acquired pneumonia: a prospective outpatient study. Medicine 2001;80:75–87.

5. File TM. Community-acquired pneumonia. Lancet 2003;362:1991–2001.

6. Aujesky D, Auble TE, Yealy DM. Prospective comparison of three validated prediction rules for prognosis in community-acquired pneumonia. Am J Med 2005;118:384–392.

7. Fine MJ, Auble TE, Yealy DM, et al. A prediction rule to identify low-risk patients with community-acquired pneumonia. N Engl J Med 1997;336:243–250.

8. Lim WS, van der Eerden MM, Laing R, et al. Defining community-acquired pneumonia severity on presentation to hospital: an international derivation and validation study. Thorax 2003;58:377–382.

9. Mandell LA, File TM. Short-course treatment of community-acquired pneumonia. Clin Infect Dis 2003;37:761–763.

10. Fine MJ, Stone RA, Singer DE, et al. Process and outcomes of care for patients with community-acquired pneumonia: results from the Pneumonia Patients Outcomes Research Team (PORT) cohort study. Arch Intern Med 1999;159:970–980.

114

OTITIS MEDIA

Tug-of-War . . . . Level I

Rochelle Farb, PharmD

Nicole S. Culhane, PharmD, BCPS

LEARNING OBJECTIVES

After completing this case study, the reader should be able to:

- Identify the signs and symptoms of acute otitis media (AOM).

- Identify risk factors associated with an increased incidence of AOM.

- Identify the pathogens most commonly causing AOM.

- Recommend an effective and economical treatment regimen including specific agent(s), route of administration, and dose(s) of antibiotics and analgesic medications.

- Recognize the role of delaying antibiotic therapy for AOM.

- Educate parents about recommended drug therapy using appropriate non-technical terminology.

PATIENT PRESENTATION

■ Chief Complaint

"My ear hurts."

■ HPI

Jacob Rodriguez is a 26-month-old boy who is brought to his pediatrician by his mother on a Monday morning in late January. Mom describes a 1-day history of tugging at his right ear and crying, and a 2-day history of decreased appetite, decreased playfulness, and difficulty sleeping. Mom states that his temperature last night was normal by electronic axial thermometer (37.0°C). Jacob has not been given any analgesics, as his mom states she wanted to wait to hear what the pediatrician had to say. When Jacob is asked if anything hurts, he points to his right ear and says "boo-boo."

■ PMH

Former 38-week, 3.5-kg healthy infant at birth, breast-fed for 3 months.

Immunizations are up-to-date, including 7-valent pneumococcal vaccination (Prevnar).

First and only episode of AOM at age 11 months treated successfully with amoxicillin and no adverse effects.

Jacob was seen approximately 3 months ago for wound treatment after he fell and cut his cheek on the fireplace. The wound has healed completely with no scar.

■ FH

Parents both in good health. One sibling, 4 years old, in good health.

■ SH

Jacob lives at home with his parents and sister. His father is employed, and his mother takes care of both children. Both parents are smokers. There is a pet dog in the home. Jacob uses a pacifier to fall asleep, but he does not use one during the day.

■ Meds

None

■ All

NKDA

■ Physical Examination

Gen

WDWN Hispanic male, now crying

VS

BP 110/60, HR 126, RR 32, T 37.8°C; Wt 11.6 kg, Ht 28"

HEENT

Both TMs erythematous (with R > L); right TM non-bulging and mobile with copious cerumen and questionable purulent fluid behind TM; both TMs landmarks appear normal including the pars flaccida, the malleus, and the light reflex below the umbo. However, the left TM landmarks are more clear than the right landmarks. Throat is erythematous; nares patent.

Neck

Supple

Chest

Clear, no crackles, wheezes, or rhonchi

CV

RRR

Abd

Soft, nontender

Genit

Tanner stage I

Ext

No CCE; moves all extremities well; warm, pink, no rashes

Neuro

Responsive to stimulation, DTR 2+ no clonus, CN intact

■ Assessment

Possible right ear AOM

QUESTIONS

Problem Identification

1.a. Create a drug therapy problem list for this patient.

1.b. What subjective and objective data support the diagnosis of AOM, and is the diagnosis certain or uncertain in this case?

1.c. How would you distinguish AOM from otitis media with effusion (OME)?

1.d. How is the severity of otitis media determined?

1.e. What risk factors for AOM are present in this child?

Desired Outcome

2. What are the goals of pharmacotherapy for AOM in this child?

Therapeutic Alternatives

3.a. What organisms typically cause AOM?

3.b. What pharmacotherapeutic alternatives are available for treatment of AOM in this patient?

3.c. Should this patient receive antibiotic therapy at this time, or should watchful waiting (observation) be the course of action? Defend your answer.

Optimal Plan

4.a. If antibiotics are indicated, which of the alternatives would you recommend to treat this child's AOM? Include the dose, duration of therapy, and rationale for your selection.

4.b. What other therapies could you recommend to treat this child's symptoms?

Outcome Evaluation

5. How should the therapy you recommended be monitored for efficacy and adverse effects?

Patient Education

6. How would you provide important information about this therapy to the child's mother?

■ SELF-STUDY ASSIGNMENTS

1. Describe a scenario in which it would be appropriate to use azithromycin to treat AOM.

2. Review the literature for evidence supporting antibiotic prophylaxis therapy in children with frequent ear infections.

CLINICAL PEARL

The rate of spontaneous AOM resolution is 81% without any antibiotic therapy, while the use of routine antibiotic treatment only proves beneficial in another 13.7% of patients.

REFERENCES

1. American Academy of Pediatrics Subcommittee on Management of Acute Otitis Media. Diagnosis and management of acute otitis media. Pediatrics 2004;113:1451–1465.
2. American Academy of Pediatrics, American Academy of Otolaryngology–Head and Neck Surgery, and American Academy of Pediatrics Subcommittee on Otitis Media with Effusion. Otitis media with effusion. Pediatrics 2004;113:1412–1429.
3. Hendley JO. Otitis media. N Engl J Med 2002;347:1169–1174.
4. Spiro DM, Tay KY, Arnold DH, et al. Wait-and-see prescription for the treatment of acute otitis media. JAMA 2006;196:1235–1241.
5. Bertin L, Pons G, d'Athis P, et al. A randomized, double-blind, multicentre controlled trial of ibuprofen versus acetaminophen and placebo for symptoms of acute otitis media in children. Fundam Clin Pharmacol 1996;10:387–392.
6. Neto JFL, Hemb L, Silva DB. Systematic literature review of modifiable risk factors for recurrent otitis media in childhood. J Pediatr 2006; 82:87–96.

115

RHINOSINUSITIS

Sick Sinus . . . . .Level II

Michael B. Kays, PharmD, FCCP

LEARNING OBJECTIVES

After completing this case study, the reader should be able to:

• Compare and contrast the clinical signs and symptoms of acute viral and bacterial rhinosinusitis in a given patient.

• Differentiate viral versus bacterial etiology in rhinosinusitis based on a patient's symptoms.

• Identify the most common pathogens that cause acute bacterial rhinosinusitis.

• Formulate a treatment plan for a patient with acute bacterial rhinosinusitis based on severity of symptoms and history of previous antibiotic use.

• Revise the treatment plan for a patient who fails the initially prescribed therapy.

PATIENT PRESENTATION

■ Chief Complaint

"I feel awful and congested, and my head hurts. I think my sinus infection is back."

◼ HPI

Maurice Simmons is a 51-year-old man who presents to his primary care physician with fever, purulent nasal discharge from the left naris, facial pain (L > R), nasal congestion, headache, and fatigue. He states that his symptoms began 5 days ago and have progressively worsened over the last few days. He also complains of intense facial pressure when he bends forward to tie his shoes or to pick up something. He has noticed a decreased ability to smell and occasional episodes of dizziness, tremors, and palpitations over this time period. He has been taking ibuprofen as needed and Claritin-D every 12 hours but has received little relief from his symptoms. Mr. Simmons states that he was treated for a sinus infection about 2 weeks ago with an antibiotic that he only had to take one time but he does not remember the drug name (later determined to be azithromycin extended-release oral suspension 2 g). When questioned further, he states that he presented to an urgent care clinic complaining of a runny nose, congestion, sneezing, cough, and a sore throat of 3-days' duration. He was leaving the next day for a business trip and asked the physician for an antibiotic prescription. His symptoms slowly improved over several days, and he was symptom-free for 1 day before his current symptoms began 5 days ago. He states that he rarely gets sick and hasn't had an infection in at least the last 10 years prior to these episodes.

◼ PMH

Sinus infection 2 weeks ago
Hypertension (well controlled with medication)
Hypercholesterolemia

◼ FH

Father died of MI at 76 years of age
Mother with hypertension and diabetes mellitus

◼ SH

Smokes cigars on occasion (one to two per week). Denies cigarette smoking and illicit drug use. Drinks socially (three to four beers and one bottle of red wine per week). He is divorced with 2 children (26-year-old son, 23-year-old daughter).

◼ Meds

Lisinopril 20 mg po daily
Hydrochlorothiazide 25 mg po daily
Simvastatin 20 mg po daily
Ibuprofen 200 mg po as needed
Claritin-D 12 hour (desloratadine 2.5 mg/pseudoephedrine 120 mg) po Q 12 h

◼ All

None

◼ ROS

Patient with a 5-day history of fever, purulent nasal drainage, congestion, facial pain, headache, fatigue, hyposmia, and occasional dizziness and palpitations. In addition, the patient complains of insomnia, which may be contributing to the fatigue. He denies nausea, vomiting, diarrhea, chills, diaphoresis, dyspnea, productive cough, or allergies.

◼ Physical Examination

Gen

Tired-looking, overweight white man in mild distress; appears uncomfortable

VS

BP 158/102, P 90, RR 16, T 38.4°C; Wt 103 kg, Ht 6'1"

Skin

Warm to touch; good skin turgor; no other abnormalities

HEENT

NC/AT; PERRLA; EOMI; funduscopic exam normal; injected conjunctivae; anicteric sclerae. Thick, purulent, yellow-green nasal discharge; mucosal hypertrophy (L > R) without evidence of nasal polyps. Facial pain over L maxillary and frontal sinuses. No oral lesions; no periorbital swelling. Tympanic membranes intact, non-erythematous, non-bulging. Throat erythematous.

Neck/Lymph Nodes

Supple, no JVD, mild lymphadenopathy

Lungs/Thorax

CTA; no crackles or wheezing

CV

Slightly tachycardic; normal S_1 and S_2, no MRG

Abd

Soft, nontender; bowel sounds present; no masses

Genit/Rect

Deferred

MS/Ext

No CCE

Neuro

A & O × 3; CN II–XII intact

◼ Labs

None drawn

◼ Assessment

Recurrent sinusitis
Hypertension
Dizziness, tremors, palpitations

QUESTIONS

Problem Identification

1.a. Create a drug therapy problem list for this patient.

1.b. What subjective and objective data support the diagnosis of acute bacterial rhinosinusitis versus viral rhinosinusitis?

1.c. What other diagnostic studies (cultures, radiographs, sinus CT, etc.), if any, would you suggest before recommending therapy?

1.d. Should the patient have been treated with an antibiotic for his initial presentation 2 weeks ago? Why or why not? If yes, what antibiotic should the patient have received?

Desired Outcome

2. What are the goals of pharmacotherapy for this patient?

Therapeutic Alternatives

3.a. What are the most likely causative pathogens in this patient?

3.b. What antibiotics and dosage regimens are appropriate treatment options for the patient at this time?

3.c. What are the most likely reasons why this patient has an infection despite receiving previous antibiotic therapy?

Optimal Plan

4.a. Based on the patient's clinical presentation, what antibiotic would you recommend for therapy? Include drug name, dosage form, schedule, and duration of therapy.

4.b. What adjunctive measures can be employed to optimize the patient's medical therapy?

4.c. What alternatives, if any, would be appropriate if the patient fails to respond to the initial regimen?

Outcome Evaluation

5. How should the therapy you recommend be monitored for efficacy and adverse effects?

Patient Education

6. What information should be provided to the patient to ensure successful therapy, enhance compliance, and minimize adverse effects?

■ SELF-STUDY ASSIGNMENTS

1. Determine if a change in mucus color from clear to yellow or green is an indication of a bacterial infection or if it is the natural course of a viral infection.

2. If the patient had a penicillin allergy, review the likelihood of an allergic reaction if he had received a cephalosporin.

3. Review the pharmacokinetic and pharmacodynamic properties of antibacterial agents commonly used in the treatment of acute bacterial rhinosinusitis.

4. Review the most common mechanisms of bacterial resistance in pathogens frequently encountered in acute bacterial rhinosinusitis.

CLINICAL PEARL

The etiology of most cases of acute sinusitis is viral; however, an antibiotic is prescribed in 85–98% of cases. In patients with a clinical diagnosis of acute bacterial rhinosinusitis, the spontaneous resolution rate is 50–60%. This information is important to consider when evaluating antimicrobial efficacy from comparative clinical studies.

REFERENCES

1. Sinus and Allergy Health Partnership. Antimicrobial treatment guidelines for acute bacterial rhinosinusitis. Otolaryngol Head Neck Surg 2004;130:1–45.

2. Scheid DC, Hamm RM. Acute bacterial rhinosinusitis in adults: part I. Evaluation. Am Fam Physician 2004;70:1685–1692.

3. Garau J, Dagan R. Accurate diagnosis and appropriate treatment of acute bacterial rhinosinusitis: minimizing bacterial resistance. Clin Ther 2003;25:1936–1951.

4. Benninger MS, Payne SC, Ferguson BJ, et al. Endoscopically directed middle meatal cultures versus maxillary sinus taps in acute bacterial maxillary rhinosinusitis: a meta-analysis. Otolaryngol Head Neck Surg 2006;134:3–9.

5. Marple BF, Brunton S, Ferguson BJ. Acute bacterial rhinosinusitis: a review of U.S. treatment guidelines. Otolaryngol Head Neck Surg 2006;135:341–348.

6. Martin CL, Njike VY, Katz DL. Back up antibiotic prescriptions could reduce unnecessary antibiotic use in rhinosinusitis. J Clin Epidemiol 2004; 57:429–434.

7. Benninger M, Brook I, Farrell DJ. Disease severity in acute bacterial rhinosinusitis is greater in patients infected with Streptococcus pneumoniae than in those infected with Haemophilus influenzae. Otolaryngol Head Neck Surg 2006;135:523–528.

8. Scheid DC, Hamm RM. Acute bacterial rhinosinusitis in adults: part II. Treatment. Am Fam Physician 2004;70:1697–1704.

9. Anon JB. Current management of acute bacterial rhinosinusitis and the role of moxifloxacin. Clin Infect Dis 2005;41:S167–S176.

10. Sharp HJ, Denman D, Puumala S, Leopold DA. Treatment of acute and chronic rhinosinusitis in the United States, 1999–2002. Arch Otolaryngol Head Neck Surg 2007;133:260–265.

116

ACUTE PHARYNGITIS

A Case That Is Difficult to Swallow . . . . Level I

John L. Lock, PharmD

Jarrett R. Amsden, PharmD

LEARNING OBJECTIVES

After completing this case study, the reader should be able to:

• Evaluate the need for antibiotic therapy in a patient with pharyngitis based on signs and symptoms as well as microbiological and immunological diagnostic studies.

• Identify the most common organisms responsible for causing pharyngitis.

• Select an appropriate pharmacologic regimen for a patient with acute pharyngitis, including route, frequency, and duration.

• List the suppurative and nonsuppurative complications of acute pharyngitis, as well as the prevalence of these complications, and the measures to prevent occurrence.

PATIENT PRESENTATION

■ Chief Complaint

"My throat hurts, and I just don't want to get out of bed."

■ HPI

James Hershey is a 14-year-old previously healthy boy who presents to the emergency department complaining of sore throat, headache, fever, and malaise. Since the symptoms developed, about 24 hours prior, he has declined to eat anything solid because he complains it is too painful. Additionally, he has been unwilling to leave his bed except to use the restroom. He does not complain of a cough, shortness of breath, or difficulty breathing. Patient denies nausea, vomiting, and abdominal pain. Mother states that nobody in the family has been ill, but the neighbor that James spends most afternoons with has been sick lately.

PMH

The patient is an otherwise healthy teenager. His mother states that he is up-to-date on all vaccines. Mother states that he has seasonal allergies relieved with over-the-counter antihistamines.

FH

Noncontributory

SH

James is an only child and lives with his parents. He is in the 8th grade at a local public school.

Meds

Loratadine 10 mg daily as needed (patient not currently taking)

All

NKDA

ROS

Negative except for complaints noted in the HPI

Physical Examination

Gen

WDWN 14-year-old male, clearly fatigued

VS

BP 118/74, P 84, RR 15, T 38.5°C; Wt 71 kg, Ht 5'8"

Skin

Pale, warm, no sign of rash

HEENT

PERRLA

Tonsils erythematous, with associated white exudate. Uvula edematous. Soft palate petechiae.

Neck/Lymph Nodes

Supple, no lymphadenopathy

Lungs/Thorax

CTA bilaterally, (–) shortness of breath, (–) cough

CV

RRR, no MRG, normal S_1 and S_2

Abd

Soft, nontender, nondistended, (+) BS

Genit/Rect

Deferred

Neuro

CN II–XII intact

Labs

RADT: positive

Assessment

14-year-old male presents to the emergency department with Group A β-hemolytic streptococcus (GABHS) pharyngitis.

QUESTIONS

Problem Identification

1.a. List the patient's drug therapy problem(s).

1.b. What signs and symptoms in this patient are indicative of GABHS infection?

1.c. What diagnostic tool(s) may be used to facilitate a diagnosis?

Desired Outcome

2. List the goals of therapy.

Therapeutic Alternatives

3.a. What nonpharmacologic therapies are available for treatment of GABHS acute pharyngitis?

3.b. What are the pharmacologic options for GABHS acute pharyngitis?

Optimal Plan

4.a. What is the preferred treatment for this patient's acute pharyngitis? Include dose, route, frequency, and duration.

4.b. Which option would be most appropriate if he reported a penicillin allergy?

Outcome Evaluation

5.a. What should be monitored to evaluate successful therapy and/or development of adverse effects?

5.b. What would be the appropriate treatment if this infection did not resolve?

Patient Education

6. What information should be shared with James and his parents regarding his drug therapy?

■ SELF-STUDY ASSIGNMENTS

1. Create a table that lists the suppurative and nonsuppurative complications of GABHS acute pharyngitis.

2. Prepare a one-page paper which describes the signs and symptoms of scarlet and rheumatic fever.

CLINICAL PEARL

Immediate administration of antibiotics is not necessary to treat pharyngitis, because:

- Even untreated, most signs and symptoms of pharyngitis are absent within 3–4 days,

- Treatment with antibiotics decreases length of illness only by approximately 24 hours, and

- Antibiotic therapy can be withheld for over 1 week without significantly increasing risk of rheumatic fever.

REFERENCES

1. Bisno AL, Gerber MA, Gwaltney, Jr JM, et al. Practice guidelines for the diagnosis and management of group A streptococcal pharyngitis. Clin Infect Dis 2002;35:113–125.

2. Bisno AL. Acute pharyngitis. N Engl J Med 2001;344:205–211.

3. Vincent MT, Celestin N, Hussein AN. Pharyngitis. Am Fam Physician 2004;69:1465–1470.
4. Snow V, Mottur-Pilson C, Cooper RJ, et al. Principles of appropriate antibiotic use of acute pharyngitis in adults. Ann Intern Med 2001;134:506–508.
5. McIsaac WJ, Goel V, To T, et al. The validity of a sore throat score in family practice. CMAJ 2000;163:811–815.
6. Thomas M, Del Mar C, Glasziou P. How effective are treatments other than antibiotics for acute sore throat? Br J Gen Pract 2000;50: 817–820.

117

CELLULITIS

A Case of "Gripping" Pain. . . . . Level II

Jarrett R. Amsden, PharmD

LEARNING OBJECTIVES

After completing this case study, the reader should be able to:

- Evaluate the signs and symptoms of cellulitis.

- Recommend appropriate empiric pharmacologic and nonpharmacologic treatment options for patients presenting with cellulitis.

- Develop a list of alternative therapeutic options for the treatment of uncomplicated cellulitis and refractory (complicated) cellulitis.

- Design an antimicrobial treatment regimen for a methicillin-resistant *Staphylococcus aureus* (MRSA) cellulitis.

PATIENT PRESENTATION

Chief Complaint

"My left forearm is swollen and painful, especially when I grip or flex."

HPI

Christoph Kottingheimer is a 45-year-old man who presents to the ED with increasing pain and swelling in his left forearm and some decreased range of motion and tenderness in his right shoulder. At his last visit to the ED 5 days ago, he was diagnosed with left upper extremity cellulitis and given a prescription for cephalexin 500 mg po TID for 7 days. Since that time, the patient's car was stolen, and inside the car were his antibiotics. As a result, the patient reports today that he has not taken any of his cephalexin doses. In addition to the increased pain and swelling in his left arm, he now also presents with new-onset pain in his right shoulder and fever.

PMH

Left-arm cellulitis, diagnosed 5 days ago (Rx for cephalexin given but patient reports nonadherence).
Type 2 diabetes mellitus (DM) (recently diagnosed; patient reports nonadherence to prescribed oral hypoglycemic agent).

Surgical History

1980—Involved in MVA; acquired a large bump on forehead
1982—Sustained a facial electrical burn that required a skin graft
2002—Had a benign cyst removed from neck

SH

Smokes two ppd × 20 years; drinks alcohol occasionally; denies any illicit drug use

Meds

Cephalexin 500 mg po TID (prescribed at ED visit 5 days ago; patient did not take)
Metformin 500 mg po BID (patient states that he filled prescription but has only taken "a couple of doses")

All

NKA

Immunizations

Only reports childhood vaccinations

ROS

Negative except for complaints noted in HPI

Physical Examination

Gen

WDWN Caucasian male in no acute distress, but with noticeable pain in his left upper extremity

VS

BP 129/74, P 96, RR 16, T 38.3°C; Wt 117 kg, Ht 6'0"

Skin

Left forearm is red, warm, and tender to touch; increased swelling and pitting edema

HEENT

PEERLA; EOMI, oropharynx clear
3 cm × 3 cm bump on over his forehead, which is not red or tender to touch

Neck/Lymph Nodes

Supple, no lymphadenopathy
4 mm × 4 mm deep hole on his right dorsal neck with no discharge, redness, or tenderness

Lungs/Thorax

CTA, no rales or wheezing

CV

RRR, no MRG

Abd

Soft, NT/ND; (+) BS

Genit/Rect

Deferred

MS/Ext

RUE: shoulder with decreased range of motion and tenderness

LUE: forearm that is red, warm, and tender to touch; increased swelling and pitting edema

Lower extremities: WNL and 2+ pulses bilaterally

Neuro

A & O × 3

▨ Labs

Na 129 mEq/L	Hgb 15.5 g/dL	WBC 26.3 × 10³/mm³
K 3.6 mEq/L	Hct 44%	Neutros 81%
Cl 87 mEq/L	Plt 329 × 10³/mm³	Bands 10%
CO_2 21 mEq/L		Lymphs 7%
BUN 23 mg/dL		Monos 2%
SCr 0.9 mg/dL		
Glu 400 mg/dL		
Ca 8.4 mg/dL		

▨ Imaging Studies

Doppler: Left forearm (–) for DVT

▨ Urine Drug Screen

(+) marijuana, (–) cocaine and other substances

▨ Assessment

Progressive left arm cellulitis. Negative for left upper extremity DVT.

New onset pain and tenderness in the right shoulder—questionable right shoulder bursitis versus septic joint versus progressing cellulitis.

Hyponatremia secondary to hyperglycemia.

Uncontrolled Type 2 DM—likely secondary to medication nonadherence.

QUESTIONS

Problem Identification

1.a. Create a list of the patient's drug-related problems.

1.b. What subjective and objective clinical data are consistent with the diagnosis of cellulitis?

1.c. What are the most common causative organisms of cellulitis?

Desired Outcome

2. What are the goals of pharmacotherapy for the treatment of this patient's cellulitis and diabetes?

Therapeutic Alternatives

3.a. What nondrug therapies might be useful in the treatment of cellulitis?

3.b. What feasible antimicrobial options are available for the treatment of cellulitis?

Optimal Plan

4.a. What antimicrobial agent, dosage form, dose, schedule, and duration of therapy are best for this patient?

4.b. What antimicrobial alternatives would be appropriate if your initial antimicrobial regimen fails or is not tolerated?

▪ CLINICAL COURSE

After 5 days of cephalexin therapy, the patient again returns to the ED with progressing left arm cellulitis with continued pain, redness, tenderness, and increased edema; continued right shoulder pain and tenderness with new-onset right axilla pain and swelling; and left lower extremity pain radiating from the lower back. Upon physical exam, the patient is found to have increased pitting edema of the left arm, a right scapular fluid collection, and a swollen right axilla and adjacent lymphadenopathy. An MRI of the left arm was done to rule out compartment syndrome. Two sets of blood cultures were drawn, and orthopedics was consulted for potential incision and drainage (I & D) of the left arm cellulitis. Cefazolin 1 g IV × one dose was started in the ED and the patient was admitted for progressive cellulitis versus necrotizing fasciitis.

4.c. Based upon the above information, the patient has failed oral cephalexin therapy. What antimicrobial regimen would you now recommend for this patient? (Please specify dose, schedule, and duration of therapy.)

4.d. What antimicrobial alternatives would be appropriate if the antimicrobial regimen you recommended in 4.c. fails or is not tolerated?

Outcome Evaluation

5. What clinical and laboratory parameters are necessary to evaluate the therapy for its effectiveness in treating this patient's cellulitis?

Patient Education

6. What information should be provided to the patient to ensure successful therapy?

▪ SELF-STUDY ASSIGNMENTS

1. In addition to vancomycin, compare and contrast the therapeutic alternatives for the treatment of MRSA infections including cellulitis.

2. Prepare a table that differentiates the presentation, signs, and symptoms of the patient in this case with that of a patient presenting with erysipelas as well as necrotizing fasciitis.

CLINICAL PEARL

In progressive multifocal cases of cellulitis/pyomyositis where there are frank fluid collections and pus, surgical debridement is essential, followed by antimicrobial agents directed towards *S. aureus* (including MRSA) and *Streptococcus* species.

REFERENCES

1. Stevens DL, Bisno AL, Chambers HF, et al. Practice guidelines for the diagnosis and management of skin and soft-tissue infections. Clin Infect Dis 2005;41:1373–1406.

2. Bisno AL, Stevens DL. *Streptococcus pyogenes*: In: Mandell GL, Bennett JE, Dolin R, eds. Mandell, Douglas, and Bennett's Principles and Practices of Infectious Diseases, 6th ed. Philadelphia, Elsevier, Churchill and Livingstone, 2005:2362–2379.

3. Pendland SL, Fish DN, Danziger LH. Skin and soft tissue infections: In: DiPiro JT, Talbert RL, Yee GC, et al., eds. Pharmacotherapy: A Pathophysiologic Approach, 6th ed. New York, McGraw-Hill, 2005:1977–1995.

4. Moran GJ, Krishnadasan A, Gorwitz RJ, et al. Methicillin-resistant *S. aureus* infections among patients in the emergency department. N Engl J Med 2006;55:666–674.

5. Rube JJ, Smith N, Bradsher RW, et al. Community onset methicillin resistant *Staphylococcus aureus* skin and soft-tissue infections: impact of antimicrobial therapy on outcome. Clin Infect Dis 2007;44:777–784.

6. Rybak MJ, LaPlante KL. Community-associated methicillin-resistant *Staphylococcus aureus*: a review. Pharmacotherapy 2005;25:74–85.

118

DIABETIC FOOT INFECTION

Watch Your Step . . . . Level II

A. Christie Graham, PharmD

Renee-Claude Mercier, PharmD, BCPS, PhC

LEARNING OBJECTIVES

After completing this case study, the reader should be able to:

- Recognize the signs and symptoms of diabetic foot infections and identify the risk factors and the most likely pathogens associated with these infections.

- Recommend appropriate antimicrobial regimens for diabetic foot infections, including for patients with drug allergies or renal insufficiency.

- Recommend appropriate home IV therapy and proper counseling to patients.

- Outline monitoring parameters for achievement of the desired pharmacotherapeutic outcomes and prevention of adverse effects.

- Counsel diabetic patients about adequate blood glucose control as part of an overall plan for good foot health.

PATIENT PRESENTATION

Chief Complaint

As per the patient's daughter: "She stepped on a piece of metal and now her foot is swollen."

HPI

Mary Littlehorse is a 67-year-old Native-American woman, Navajo-speaking only, who presents to the ED complaining of a sore and swollen foot. Five days ago, she stepped on a piece of metal and later noticed redness and soreness in the area, which increased over the next several days. History is per translation by patient's daughter.

Primary care physician is Dr. Kinder, Shiprock Indian Health Service.

PMH

Type 2 DM × 18 years

Hospitalized 2 months ago for hyperosmolar hyperglycemic syndrome (HHS)

Hospitalized 9 months ago with MI, received PCI with bare metal stents placed in the RCA and LAD

Left second toe amputation 1 year ago secondary to diabetic foot infection

Hyperlipidemia

Hypertension

Obesity

Chronic renal insufficiency

Depression

FH

Father is deceased (56 yo) secondary to MI, DM Type 2, HTN

Mother is deceased secondary to breast cancer (41 yo)

One daughter, alive and well, 42 yo

SH

The patient lives with her 42-year-old daughter in Shiprock, NM. She has been widowed × 2 years and has been significantly depressed since her husband's death. She denies tobacco, alcohol, and illicit drug use. She admits to nonadherence with her medications and glucometer.

Meds

Novolin 70/30 60 units Q AM and Q PM

Metformin 1,000 mg po twice daily

Aspirin 81 mg po once daily

Lisinopril 20 mg po once daily

Simvastatin 40 mg po once daily

Citalopram 20 mg po once daily

Trazodone 50 mg po at bedtime

All

Sulfa—severe rash

ROS

Negative except as noted above in HPI

Physical Examination

Gen

Patient is an obese Native-American woman with a dull affect but in NAD

VS

BP 122/76, P 92, RR 20, T 37.4°C; Wt 95 kg, Ht 5'1"

Skin

Warm, coarse, and very dry

HEENT

PERRLA; EOMI; funduscopic exam is normal with absence of hemorrhages or exudates. TMs are clouded bilaterally but with no erythema or bulging. Oropharynx shows poor dentition but is otherwise unremarkable.

Neck/Lymph Nodes

Neck is supple; normal thyroid; no JVD; no lymphadenopathy

Chest

CTA

Heart

RRR, normal S_1 and S_2

Abd

Distended, (+) BS, no guarding, no hepatosplenomegaly or masses felt

Ext

2+ edema with markedly diminished sensation of the right foot. Area of redness and induration 4–5 cm from portal of entry. Pedal pulses present but diminished. Normal range of motion. Poor nail care with some fungus and overgrown toenails.

Neuro

A & O × 3; CN II–XII intact. Motor system intact (overall muscle strength 4–5/5). Sensory system exam showed a decreased sensation to light touch of the lower extremities (both feet); intact upper body sensation.

■ Labs

Na 136 mEq/L	Hgb 12.6 g/dL
K 3.6 mEq/L	Hct 37.8%
Cl 98 mEq/L	Plt 390 × 10³/mm³
CO_2 24 mEq/L	WBC 16.4 × 10³/mm³
BUN 30 mg/dL	PMNs 71%
SCr 1.7 mg/dL	Bands 8%
Glu 181 mg/dL	Lymphs 15%
A1C 11.8%	Monos 6%
ESR 32 mm/h	

■ X-Ray

Right foot: There is a metallic foreign body approximately 2 cm in length in the soft tissue inferior to the third metatarsal. No evidence of adjacent periosteal reactions or erosions to suggest radiographic evidence of osteomyelitis. No definite subcutaneous air is evident. Presence of vascular calcifications.

■ Assessment

Diabetic foot infection in a patient with poorly controlled diabetes mellitus.

■ Clinical Course

On the day of admission, the patient went to surgery for an I & D and removal of the foreign body. Blood and tissue specimens were sent for culture and sensitivity testing.

QUESTIONS

Problem Identification

1.a. Create a list of the patient's drug therapy problems.

1.b. What signs, symptoms, or laboratory values indicate the presence of an infection?

1.c. What risk factors for infection does the patient have?

1.d. What organisms are most likely involved in this infection?

Desired Outcome

2. What are the therapeutic goals for this patient?

Therapeutic Alternatives

3.a. What nondrug therapies might be useful for this patient?

3.b. What feasible pharmacotherapeutic alternatives are available for the empiric treatment of diabetic foot infection?

3.c. What economic and social considerations are applicable to this patient?

Optimal Plan

4. Outline a drug regimen that would provide optimal initial empiric therapy for the infection.

Outcome Evaluation

5.a. What clinical and laboratory parameters are necessary to evaluate your therapy for achievement of the desired therapeutic outcomes and monitoring for adverse effects?

■ CLINICAL COURSE

Ms. Littlehorse received the empiric therapy you recommended until the tissue cultures were reported positive for *Staphylococcus aureus*, reported sensitive to vancomycin, linezolid, quinupristin/dalfopristin, and daptomycin and resistant to oxacillin (and other β-lactams), tetracycline, erythromycin, clindamycin, and sulfamethoxazole/trimethoprim. The blood cultures were all found to have no growth. The patient remained hospitalized for an additional 10 days and received a more directed antimicrobial regimen and multiple surgical debridements of the wound. The cellulitis slowly improved over this time and multiple x-rays did not suggest osteomyelitis. She was then discharged to complete her antimicrobial regimen on an outpatient basis. Over the next 2 weeks, she received wound care at home and showed significant but slow progress in healing of the wound.

5.b. What therapeutic alternatives are available for treating this patient after results of cultures are known to contain methicillin-resistant *S. aureus* (MRSA)?

5.c. Design an optimal drug treatment plan for treating the MRSA infection while she remains hospitalized.

5.d. Design an optimal pharmacotherapeutic plan for completion of her treatment after she is discharged from the hospital.

Patient Education

6. What information should be provided to the patient to enhance compliance, ensure successful therapy, and minimize adverse effects with IV vancomycin?

■ SELF-STUDY ASSIGNMENTS

1. Review in more detail different therapeutic options available for home IV therapy, including the antimicrobial agents suitable for use, types of IV lines available, and contraindications to home IV therapy.

2. Outline the patient counseling you would provide for successful home IV therapy.

3. Describe how you would educate this diabetic patient about proper foot care to prevent further skin or tissue breakdown.

CLINICAL PEARL

Treatment of diabetic foot infections with antimicrobial agents alone is often inadequate; local wound care (incision, drainage, debridement, and amputation), good glycemic control, and immobilization of the limb are often required.

REFERENCES

1. Lipsky BA, Berendt AR, Deery G, et al. Diagnosis and treatment of diabetic foot infections. Clin Infect Dis 2004;39:885–910.
2. Levin ME. Management of the diabetic foot: preventing amputation. South Med J 2002;95:10–20.
3. Rybak JM, LaPlante KL. Community-associated methicillin-resistant *Staphylococcus aureus*: a review. Pharmacotherapy 2005;25:74–85.
4. Boyce JM. Methicillin-resistant *Staphylococcus aureus*. Detection, epidemiology, and control measures. Infect Dis Clin North Am 1989;3:901–913.

5. Herwaldt LA. Control of methicillin resistant *Staphylococcus aureus* in the hospital setting. Am J Med 1999;106:11S–18S; discussion 48S–52S.

6. Asensio A, Guerrero A, Quereda C, et al. Colonization and infection with methicillin-resistant *Staphylococcus aureus*: associated factors and eradication. Infect Control Hosp Epidemiol 1996;17:20–28.

7. Wieman TJ, Smiell JM, Su Y. Efficacy and safety of a topical gel formulation of recombinant human platelet-derived growth factor-B (becaplermin) in patients with chronic neuropathic diabetic ulcers. A phase III randomized, placebo-controlled, double-blind study. Diabetes Care 1998;21:822–827.

8. Weigelt J, Itani K, Stevens D, et al. Linezolid versus vancomycin in the treatment of complicated skin and soft tissue infections. Antimicrob Agents Chemother 2005;46:2260–2266.

119

INFECTIVE ENDOCARDITIS

Weight on Your Heart . . . . Level II

Manjunath P. Pai, PharmD, BCPS

Keith A. Rodvold, PharmD, FCCP

LEARNING OBJECTIVES

After completing this case study, the reader should be able to:

- Differentiate the signs and symptoms of infective endocarditis compared to bacteremia.

- Select appropriate antimicrobial therapy based on a particular organism and the patient's drug allergies.

- Recognize common adverse reactions of the chosen drug therapy and establish monitoring parameters in the treatment of a patient with infective endocarditis.

- Identify candidates for outpatient antimicrobial therapy (OPAT) for the treatment of infective endocarditis.

- Educate inpatients who are being discharged on OPAT for completion of infective endocarditis therapy.

PATIENT PRESENTATION

■ Chief Complaint

"I have been feeling feverish and short of breath all week long."

■ HPI

Jill Cuore is a 53-year-old woman who presents to the ED with complaints of fever, chills, and worsening shortness of breath. These symptoms developed approximately 2 weeks ago. The patient was seen in the ED 3 months earlier for incision and drainage of a skin abscess.

■ PMH

Type 2 diabetes mellitus diagnosed 10 years ago
Hypertension diagnosed 15 years ago
Valvular abnormalities secondary to fenfluramine use

■ FH

Noncontributory

■ SH

No H/O IDU; denies ETOH use, smokes one pack/day and has a 10 pack-year tobacco history.

■ Meds

Tylenol 650 mg po Q 4–6 h PRN headaches
Metformin 500 mg po Q 12 h
Lisinopril 20 mg po Q 24 h

■ All

Penicillin (hives)

■ ROS

Noncontributory except for complaints noted in HPI

■ Physical Examination

Gen

Patient is a morbidly obese Caucasian woman in mild distress

VS

BP 136/84, P 118, RR 24, T 38.9°C; Wt 128 kg, Ht 5'4"

Skin/Nails

Splinter hemorrhages noted on right thumb nail, 4–6 mm painful nodular lesions noted on left and right foot pads

HEENT

Anicteric sclerae, PERRLA, pink conjunctivae, dry oral mucosa, no Roth spots; poor dentition

Neck/Lymph Nodes

No lymphadenopathy, JVD, or thyromegaly

Lungs

Crackles in RLL; no wheezing

CV

RRR, normal S_1 and S_2, S_3 present, III/VI holosystolic murmur

Abd

Soft with mild diffuse tenderness, liver and spleen margins difficult to assess secondary to obesity

Genit/Rect

Normal; guaiac negative stool

Ext

Reflexes bilaterally 4/5 UE, 3/5 LE, Babinski decreased; no edema

Neuro

Non-focal; A & O × 3, (−) asterixis

■ Labs

Na 133 mEq/L	Hgb 8.1 g/dL	WBC $15.4 \times 10^3/mm^3$
K 5.6 mEq/L	Hct 23.6%	Neutros 78%
Cl 91 mEq/L	Plt $180 \times 10^3/mm^3$	Bands 8%
CO_2 17 mEq/L	RDW 17.3%	Lymphs 12%
BUN 15 mg/dL	MCV 81.1 μm^3	Monos 2%
SCr 1.9 mg/dL	MCH 26.3 pg/cell	Alb 2.6 g/dL
Glu 185 mg/dL	MCHC 34 g/dL	INR 1.0
		ESR 93 mm/h

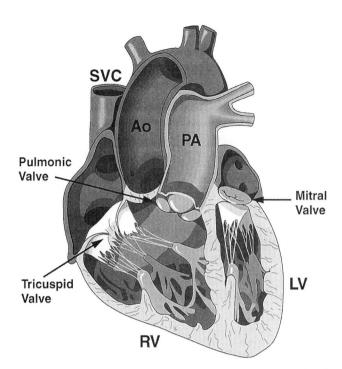

FIGURE 119-1. Diagram illustrating the location of the tricuspid, pulmonic, and mitral valves. Ao, aorta; LV, left ventricle; PA, pulmonary artery; RV, right ventricle; SVC, superior vena cava.

ECG

Nonspecific T-wave changes; increased QTc interval

Two-Dimensional Echocardiogram (Transthoracic)

Unable to accurately visualize heart valves

Transesophageal Echocardiogram

8 mm vegetation on the mitral valve with severe mitral regurgitation, and no perivalvular abscess noted. Moderate left ventricular hypertrophy (see Fig. 119-1 for location of heart valves and other cardiac structures).

Blood Cultures

3 of 3 sets (+) for *Staphylococcus aureus* (collection times: 13:40, 15:20, 16:15).

Assessment

53-year-old female with history of diabetes, recent I & D of a skin abscess, valvular abnormalities secondary to fenfluramine presents with *S. aureus* endocarditis (vegetation on mitral valve).

Additional problems include hyperkalemia, renal insufficiency and possible acidosis (on metformin), and hypertension.

QUESTIONS

Problem Identification

1.a. Identify all of the drug therapy problems of this patient.

1.b. What signs, symptoms, and other information indicate the presence of endocarditis in this patient?

1.c. What risk factors does this patient have for developing endocarditis?

1.d. Based on this patient's risk factors and location of the vegetation, does this patient have right-sided or left-sided endocarditis, and what is the prognostic relevance of left- versus right-sided endocarditis?

1.e. What additional information (laboratory tests or patient information) is needed to satisfactorily assess this patient?

Desired Outcome

2. What are the goals of pharmacotherapy for infective endocarditis?

■ CLINICAL COURSE

The patient was started on empiric vancomycin with doses adjusted for her decreased renal function until susceptibilities for the *S. aureus* isolate became available. Susceptibility testing subsequently showed the organism to be resistant to oxacillin, but sensitive to vancomycin, linezolid, quinupristin/dalfopristin, tigecycline, daptomycin, and minocycline.

Therapeutic Alternatives

3.a. What nondrug therapies might be used to treat this patient's endocarditis?

3.b. Identify the therapeutic alternatives for the treatment of *S. aureus* endocarditis based on the organism's susceptibilities. Include the drug names, doses, dosage forms, schedules, and durations of therapy in your answer.

Optimal Plan

4.a. What is the most appropriate treatment plan for this patient (give drug name, dose, dosage form, schedule, and duration of therapy).

■ CLINICAL COURSE

After 8 days of IV vancomycin therapy, the patient's blood cultures are still positive despite vancomycin trough concentrations of 15–20 mcg/mL. The organism continues to be noted as susceptible, and the MIC is reported to be 2 mcg/mL.

4.b. What information supported the possibility of therapeutic failure in this clinical scenario?

4.c. Given this new information, what is an appropriate, nonsurgical, therapeutic alternative for this patient?

Outcome Evaluation

5.a. What clinical and laboratory parameters should be monitored to evaluate the efficacy of therapy and to prevent adverse reactions?

■ CLINICAL COURSE

The patient was treated for 8 days with vancomycin followed by 3 weeks of the therapy chosen in question 4.c. Blood cultures became negative 4 days after the new regimen was instituted. She is now afebrile (T_{max} 36.3°C [97.3°F]), her white count is normalizing (WBC $10.4 \times 10^3/mm^3$ with no bands), her ESR is now 33 mm/h, she is feeling much better, and she wishes to leave the hospital now.

5.b. Based on your assessment of this patient's response and her past history, what alternatives are available for completing her course of therapy?

Patient Education

6. If this patient is discharged home after 4 weeks of IV antibiotic therapy to complete her regimen on oral antibiotics, what information should be provided to her to enhance adherence and ensure successful therapy?

■ SELF-STUDY ASSIGNMENTS

1. Compare the clinical data supporting the role of daptomycin and linezolid versus vancomycin for the management of methicillin-resistant *S. aureus* bacteremia including infective endocarditis.

2. Identify equations used to estimate glomerular filtration rate and creatinine clearance and critique the inherent bias of these equations when assessing renal function in morbidly obese patients.

CLINICAL PEARL

The probability of treatment failure remains high in patients with left-sided endocarditis. Daptomycin has received an FDA-approved indication for *S. aureus* bacteremia, including right-sided endocarditis, caused by methicillin-resistant *S. aureus* and methicillin-sensitive *S. aureus*. Only a limited number of patients with left-sided endocarditis have been treated with daptomycin during clinical trials.

REFERENCES

1. Bonnow RO, Carabello BA, Kanu C, et al. ACC/AHA 2006 guidelines for the management of patients with valvular heart disease: a report of the American College of Cardiology/American Heart Association Task Force on Practice Guidelines. Circulation 2006;114:e84–231.

2. Fowler VG, Boucher HW, Corey GR, et al. Daptomycin versus standard therapy for bacteremia and endocarditis caused by *Staphylococcus aureus*. N Engl J Med 2006;355:653–665.

3. Bauer LA, Black DJ, Lill JS. Vancomycin dosing in morbidly obese patients. Eur J Clin Pharmacol 1998;54:621–625.

4. Green B, Duffull SB. What is the best size descriptor to use for pharmacokinetic studies in the obese? Br J Clin Pharmacol 2004;58:119–133.

5. Levey AS, Coresh J, Greene T, et al. Using standardized serum creatinine values in the modification of diet in renal disease study equation for estimating glomerular filtration rate. Ann Intern Med 2006;145:247–254.

6. Hidayat LK, Hsu DI, Quist R, et al. High-dose vancomycin therapy for methicillin-resistant *Staphylococcus aureus* infections. Arch Intern Med 2006;166:2138–2144.

7. Andrews MM, von Reyn CF. Patient selection criteria and management guidelines for outpatient parenteral antibiotic therapy for native valve infective endocarditis. Clin Infect Dis 2001;33:203–209.

120

TUBERCULOSIS

Close Encounters . . . . Level II

Sharon M. Erdman, PharmD

LEARNING OBJECTIVES

After completing this case study, the reader should be able to:

- Recognize the typical signs and symptoms of pulmonary tuberculosis.

- Design a therapeutic regimen for the treatment of a patient with newly-diagnosed pulmonary tuberculosis based on the presenting signs and symptoms of infection, history of present illness, subjective and objective clinical findings, and desired clinical response.

- Develop a monitoring plan that should be used during the treatment of pulmonary tuberculosis to ensure efficacy and prevent toxicity.

- Provide patient education on the proper administration of drug therapy for pulmonary tuberculosis, including directions for use, the administration of therapy in relation to meals, the importance of adherence, and potential side effects of the medications.

- Describe the appropriate diagnostic work-up that should be performed on close contacts of patients with active pulmonary tuberculosis.

PATIENT PRESENTATION

■ Chief Complaint

"I have been coughing up blood for the past 3 days."

■ HPI

Jose Rodriguez is a 35-year-old Hispanic man who presents to the Emergency Department at the county hospital in Chicago, Illinois, with a 3–4 week history of a productive cough, which was originally productive of yellow sputum but is now accompanied by the presence of blood in the sputum for the past 3 days. Along with the cough, the patient also complains of subjective fevers, chills, night sweats, dyspnea, pleuritic chest pain, fatigue, and an unintentional 10-lb weight loss over the past several weeks. The patient moved to the United States from Mexico 4 years ago and has not recently traveled.

■ PMH

None

■ FH

Mother has DM and HTN
Father died of MI 6 months ago

■ SH

Patient has a 10 pack-year history of smoking but quit several weeks ago when the current illness started. The patient denies illicit drug use, but does report drinking alcohol on weekends.

Patient is a laborer and is currently working for cash on a new home construction project in close contact with other workers. Several of his coworkers have recently moved to the United States from Mexico and have similar respiratory symptoms. The patient does not have any medical insurance.

Patient is married and lives with his wife and young child (2 years old), who are not currently experiencing the same symptoms.

■ Meds

OTC antitussives, which did not provide any relief

■ All

No known drug allergies

■ ROS

Patient complains of a productive cough with hemoptysis for the past few days. He also complains of shortness of breath that worsens with exertion, pleuritic chest pain, subjective fevers, chills, night sweats, fatigue, and a 10-lb weight loss over the past several weeks.

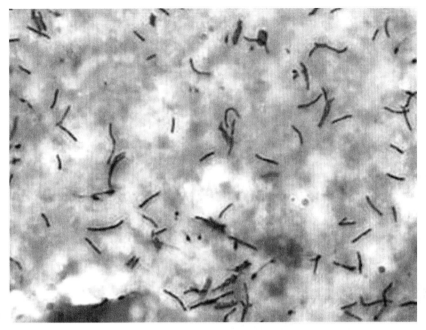

FIGURE 120-1. Acid-fast bacilli (AFB) smear. AFB (*shown as thin rods*) are tubercle bacilli.

▓ Physical Examination

Gen

Somewhat thin-appearing Hispanic male in mild respiratory distress

VS

BP 131/70, P 94, R 24, T 38.8°C; Wt 68 kg, Ht 5'9"

Skin

No lesions

HEENT

PERRLA, EOMI, no scleral icterus

Neck

Supple

Chest

Bronchial breath sounds in RUL

CV

Slightly tachycardic, no MRG

Abd

Soft NTND; (+) bowel sounds; no hepatosplenomegaly or tenderness

Ext

No CCE, pulses 2+ throughout; full ROM

Neuro

A & O × 3; CN II–XII intact; reflexes 2+, sensory and motor levels intact

▓ Labs

Na 143 mEq/L	Hgb 11.6 g/dL	WBC 11.3 × 10³/mm³	Bili 0.6 mg/dL
K 3.7 mEq/L	Hct 34.8%	Neutros 74%	Alk phos 120 U/L
Cl 106 mEq/L	RBC 3.8 × 10⁶/mm³	Bands 8%	ALT 45 IU/L
CO₂ 22 mEq/L	Plt 269 × 10³/mm³	Lymphs 10%	AST 34 IU/L
BUN 21 mg/dL	MCV 92 μm³	Monos 8%	
SCr 0.9 mg/dL	MCHC 33 g/dL		
Glu 101 mg/dL			

PPD Skin Test Result: Pending
Sputum AFB stain: Numerous AFB (Fig. 120-1)
Sputum AFB Culture: Pending
HIV Antibody Test (ELISA and Western Blot): Pending

▓ Radiology

CXR: RUL consolidation and cavitary lesion (Fig. 120-2)
Chest CT: Focal airspace disease in the RUL, including a cavitary lesion measuring 3.5 × 3.5 cm. Right hilar lymphadenopathy, with scattered mediastinal lymphadenopathy. There is no pleural effusion or pneumothorax. Findings are consistent with tuberculosis infection.

▓ Assessment

Active pulmonary tuberculosis

QUESTIONS

Problem Identification

1.a. What clinical, laboratory, and radiographic findings are consistent with the diagnosis of active pulmonary tuberculosis in this patient?

1.b. What factors place this patient at increased risk for acquiring TB?

Desired Outcome

2. What are the therapeutic goals in the treatment of active pulmonary tuberculosis?

Therapeutic Alternatives

3.a. What nonpharmacologic therapies should be considered in the management of a patient with active pulmonary tuberculosis?

3.b. What are the general principles of therapy in the management of active pulmonary tuberculosis?

3.c. What pharmacologic therapies and dosing strategies are available for the treatment of active pulmonary tuberculosis?

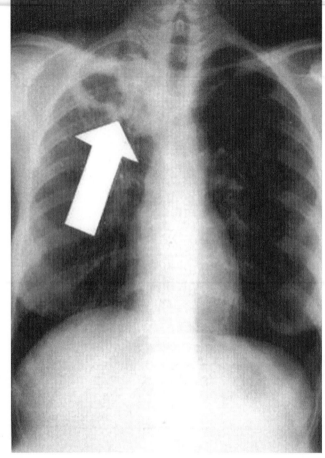

FIGURE 120-2. Chest radiograph. *Arrow* points to cavitation in patient's upper right lobe.

Optimal Plan

4.a. What drugs, dosage forms, doses, schedules, and duration of therapy are best for the treatment of this patient's active pulmonary tuberculosis? Include regimens that employ twice- or thrice-weekly administration of antituberculosis medications.

4.b. What economic and social considerations are applicable to this patient?

4.c. How should other close contacts of the patient, including his wife and child, be evaluated and treated?

Outcome Evaluation

5. What clinical and laboratory parameters should be monitored to evaluate the efficacy of therapy and to detect or prevent adverse effects?

Patient Education

6. What information should be provided to the patient to ensure successful therapy, enhance adherence, and minimize adverse effects?

■ CLINICAL COURSE

The patient was admitted to the hospital for appropriate management, including placement in a negative pressure hospital room to provide respiratory isolation. Because the initial sputum sample demonstrated the presence of numerous acid-fast bacilli (AFB), the patient was started on the therapy you recommended while waiting for the results of culture and susceptibility tests. On hospital day 2, his PPD skin test was positive (measuring 20 mm) and his HIV test was negative. The patient tolerated the four-drug antituberculosis regimen during the initial weeks of therapy, and subsequent sputum AFB smears became negative 2 weeks after the initiation of therapy. The sputum AFB culture eventually grew *Mycobacterium tuberculosis*, which was found to be susceptible to isoniazid, rifampin, pyrazinamide, ethambutol, and streptomycin. During the third week of antituberculosis therapy, an increase in the patient's AST and ALT were noted, although the patient appeared asymptomatic. The AST increased to 140 IU/L, while the ALT increased to 120 IU/L. The total bilirubin and alkaline phosphatase remained within normal limits. Follow-up mycobacterial sputum cultures obtained after 2 months of antituberculosis therapy were negative.

■ FOLLOW-UP QUESTIONS

1. How should the results of the susceptibility report of this patient's *Mycobacterium tuberculosis* isolate influence his drug therapy?

2. How should the increase in AST and ALT in this patient be managed? What changes should be made to the current antituberculosis regimen and/or monitoring plan?

3. How should a patient with AST and ALT elevations greater than five times the upper limit of normal be managed?

■ SELF-STUDY ASSIGNMENTS

1. Review the safety and efficacy of rifapentine in the management of active pulmonary tuberculosis.

2. Perform a literature search to determine the national and regional rates of isoniazid resistance in clinical isolates of *Mycobacterium tuberculosis*. How do these rates compare to those reported in other areas of the world where tuberculosis is endemic?

3. Review the management strategies of active pulmonary tuberculosis in an HIV-infected patient on antiretroviral therapy, with special attention to potential drug interactions between first-line antituberculosis agents and the non-nucleoside reverse transcriptase inhibitors or protease inhibitors.

CLINICAL PEARL

The treatment of tuberculosis in patients with HIV infection must take into consideration the many drug interactions that can occur among the antiretroviral agents and the rifamycins.

REFERENCES

1. Quast TM, Browning RF. Pathogenesis and clinical manifestations of pulmonary tuberculosis. Dis Mon 2006;52:413–419.
2. American Thoracic Society, Centers for Disease Control and Prevention, Infectious Diseases Society of America. Controlling tuberculosis in the United States. Am J Respir Crit Care Med 2005;172:1169–1227.
3. American Thoracic Society. Targeted tuberculin testing and treatment of latent tuberculosis infection. Am J Respir Crit Care Med 2000;161:S221–S247.
4. American Thoracic Society, Centers for Disease Control and Prevention, and Infectious Diseases Society of America. Treatment of tuberculosis. Am J Resp Crit Care Med 2003;167:603–662.
5. Gleeson TD, Decker CF. Treatment of tuberculosis. Dis Mon 2006;52:428–434.

6. Palomino JC. Newer diagnostics for tuberculosis and multi-drug resistant tuberculosis. Curr Opin Pulm Med 2006;12:172–178.

7. Munsiff SS, Kambili C, Ahuja SD. Rifapentine for the treatment of pulmonary tuberculosis. Clin Infect Dis 2006;43:1468–1475.

8. Chang KC, Leung CC, Yew WW, et al. Dosing schedules of 6-month regimens and relapse for pulmonary tuberculosis. Am J Respir Crit Care Med 2006;174:1153–1158.

9. Saukkonen JJ, Cohn DL, Jasmer RM, et al. An official ATS statement: hepatotoxicity of antituberculosis therapy. Am J Respir Crit Care Med 2006;174:935–952.

121

CLOSTRIDIUM DIFFICILE–ASSOCIATED DISEASE

The Real Poop on *Clostridium difficile* . . . . Level II

Michael J. Gonyeau, BS, PharmD, BCPS

LEARNING OBJECTIVES

After completing this case study, the reader should be able to:

- Recognize the clinical presentation of *Clostridium difficile*–associated disease (CDAD).

- Discuss CDAD complications.

- Develop an optimal patient-specific treatment plan for initial and recurrent CDAD including drug, dose, frequency, route of administration, and duration of therapy.

- Develop a pertinent monitoring plan for a CDAD regimen from a therapeutic and toxic standpoint.

- Discuss strategies to prevent and/or control CDAD outbreaks.

PATIENT PRESENTATION

Chief Complaint

"I have to go frequently, and when I have to go, I have to go NOW."

HPI

Helen Pratt, a 71-year-old woman, is transferred to your medical team from the MICU after requiring intubation. Over the past 2 days, she has been complaining of frequent foul-smelling stools that began after completing a 14-day course of antibiotic therapy for peritonitis.

Three weeks prior to being transferred to your team, the patient was admitted to the hospital with a history of severe abdominal pain quantified in intensity as 10/10 by the patient. She also described the pain as diffuse, associated with nausea, two episodes of vomiting of food and bilious material, and loose stools for 2–3 days. She denied any fever or chills upon admission but subsequently developed fevers during her hospital stay. Peritoneal fluid was sent for microbiology upon admission and showed growth of *Klebsiella pneumoniae* with more than 100,000 colonies. The patient was started on broad-spectrum antibiotics with cefepime and ciprofloxacin. After sensitivities were available, the cefepime was discontinued and the patient remained on ciprofloxacin for a total course of 14 days. She subsequently required admission to the MICU for intubation due to

a severe COPD exacerbation. Upon transfer to your medical team, the patient was noticed to have foul-smelling stools.

PMH

ESRD on peritoneal dialysis for 13 years
COPD
HTN
Hyperlipidemia
S/P CABG × 2 in 1999

SH

Lives at home with her son, lifetime smoker (half pack per day for 54 years), drinks alcohol socially. At baseline, patient is not very physically active because of SOB related to COPD.

Meds on Admission

Aspirin 81 mg po once daily
Calcium acetate 667 mg po twice daily
Irbesartan 150 mg po once daily
Cinacalcet 30 mg po once daily
Epogen 10,000 units IV once per week
Amlodipine 5 mg po once daily
Atorvastatin 10 mg po once daily
Fluticasone/salmeterol 250/50 Diskus 1 inhalation twice daily
Tiotropium 18 mcg inhaler 1 capsule inhaled once daily
Esomeprazole 40 mg po once daily

All

NKDA

Physical Examination

Gen

Patient is very thin and frail looking, but in no acute distress

VS

BP 139/85, P 98, RR 20, T 38.2°C; Wt 47.2 kg, Ht 5'2"

Skin

Warm and moist secondary to diaphoresis, no lesions

HEENT

PERRLA; EOMI; TMs intact; clear oropharynx, moist oral mucosa

Neck/Lymph Nodes

Neck is supple and without adenopathy; no JVD

Lungs/Thorax

Diffuse bilateral rhonchi and wheezing

CV

RRR; Normal S_1, S_2; no murmurs

Abd

Peritonial dialysis port left upper quadrant. Abdomen is soft and non-distended, diffusely tender to palpation. Slight rebound and guarding. Positive bowel sounds.

Genit/Rect

Not performed

MS/Ext

Muscle strength and tone 5/5 in upper and lower; no CCE

Neuro

A & O × 3; CN II–XII intact

■ Labs

Na 138 mEq/L	Hgb 11.8 g/dL	WBC 13.9 × 10³/mm³	*Fasting Lipid Profile:*
K 3.5 mEq/L	Hct 34.8%	Neutros 50%	T. chol 205 mg/dL
Cl 102 mEq/L	Plt 375 × 10³/mm³	Bands 9%	LDL 139 mg/dL
CO₂ 22 mEq/L	Alb 1.5 g/dL	Eos 0%	HDL 29 mg/dL
BUN 36 mg/dL		Lymphs 35%	Trig 183 mg/dL
SCr 7.3 mg/dL		Monos 6%	
Glu 81 mg/dL			
Ca 7.8 mg/dL			
Phos 6.9 mg/dL			
Mg 1.7 mg/dL			

CXR: Clear

EKG: NSR, unchanged from previous

C. difficile toxin enzyme immunoassay (EIA) test: A/B toxin assay positive

Fecal leukocytes: Not performed

■ Assessment

71-year-old woman presents with frequent foul-smelling stools for 2 days after completing a 14-day course of antibiotic therapy for peritonitis; *C. difficile* toxin positive.

QUESTIONS

Problem Identification

1.a. Create a list of the patient's drug therapy problems.

1.b. How common is CDAD in hospitalized patients?

1.c. What risk factors for CDAD are present in this patient?

1.d. What information (signs, symptoms, laboratory values) indicates the presence of CDAD?

1.e. Which antibiotics are most likely to cause CDAD?

Desired Outcome

2. What are the goals of pharmacotherapy in this case?

Therapeutic Alternatives

3.a. What nonpharmacologic strategies would be prudent to implement in this patient?

3.b. List available options for treating CDAD in this patient. Include the drug name, dose, dosage form, route, frequency, and treatment duration.

Optimal Plan

4.a. Provide your individualized treatment recommendations for treating this patient's CDAD.

■ CLINICAL COURSE

Metronidazole 500 mg po every 8 hours was initiated. Two days after starting metronidazole, the patient continued to have frequent foul-smelling stools, diffuse cramping and abdominal pain, and mild fever. A subsequent *C. difficile* toxin EIA test remained positive. At this time, vancomycin 125 mg po four times daily was added to the regimen.

4.b. Your medical team wants to start the patient on loperamide 2 mg po after each bowel movement. Do you agree with this course of action? Why or why not?

4.c. Was the addition of vancomycin therapy to metronidazole appropriate in this case? Why or why not?

4.d. Outline your plans for managing each of the patient's other drug therapy problems.

Outcome Evaluation

5. What clinical and laboratory parameters are necessary to evaluate the therapy for achievement of the desired therapeutic outcome and detect or prevent adverse effects?

Patient Education

6. What information should be provided to the patient to enhance compliance, ensure successful therapy, and minimize adverse effects?

■ FOLLOW-UP QUESTIONS

1. How can CDAD development be prevented?

2. If your patient develops similar signs and symptoms 3 weeks after successful CDAD treatment, what would be your recommendation for management?

■ SELF STUDY ASSIGNMENTS

1. Develop a plan for assessing need for rehydration therapy in patients presenting with CDAD, and discuss the pros and cons of available drug and nondrug options.

2. Conduct a literature search and develop a policy regarding infection control procedures to reduce the risk of CDAD.

3. Conduct a literature search and outline treatment options for a patient who develops fulminant *C. difficile* colitis.

4. Conduct a literature search to assess the potential role of tolevamer in the treatment of CDAD.

CLINICAL PEARL

A recent increase in CDAD infections and hospital outbreaks has been reported. Subsequently, a highly toxigenic *C. difficile* strain was identified, with increased toxin production. This "difficult clostridium" variant strain appears to have developed increasing resistance to antibiotic treatment, which again highlights the importance of infection control procedures in health care institutions. The CDC recommends metronidazole as the primary treatment for this variant strain in most cases, with careful patient monitoring for adequate clinical response. In addition, health care facilities are encouraged to monitor the number of CDAD cases and continuously reassess compliance with infection control practices.

REFERENCES

1. McDonald LD, Owings M, Jernigan DB. *Clostridium difficile* infection in patients discharged from US short-stay hospitals, 1996–2003. Emerg Infect Dis 2006;12:409–415.

2. Loo VG, Poirier L, Miller MA, et al. A predominantly clonal multi-institutional outbreak of *Clostridium difficile*-associated diarrhea with high morbidity and mortality. N Engl J Med 2005;353:2442–2449.

3. McDonald LC, Killgore GE, Thompson A, et al. An epidemic, toxin gene–variant strain of *Clostridium difficile*. N Engl J Med 2005;353:2433–2441.

4. Eggertson L, Sibbald B. Hospitals battling outbreaks of *C. difficile*. CMAJ 2004;171:19–21.

5. Simor AE, Bradley SF, Strausbaugh LJ, et al. *Clostridium difficile* in long-term-care facilities for the elderly. Infect Control Hosp Epidemiol 2002;23:696–703.

6. Barbut F, Petit JC. Epidemiology of *Clostridium difficile*-associated infections. Clin Microbiol Infect 2001;7:405–410.

7. Pepin J, Saheb N, Coulombe MA, et al. Emergence of fluoroquinolones as the predominant risk factor for *Clostridium difficile*-associated diarrhea: a cohort study during an epidemic in Quebec. Clin Infect Dis 2005;41:1254–1260.

8. McCusker ME, Harris AD, Perecevich E, et al. Fluoroquinolone use and *Clostridium difficile* associated diarrhea. Emerg Infect Dis 2003;9:730–733.

9. Yassin SF, Young-Fadok TM, Zein NN, et al. *Clostridium difficile*-associated diarrhea and colitis. Mayo Clin Proc 2001;76:725–730.

10. Malnick SD, Zimhony O. Treatment of *Clostridium difficile*-associated diarrhea. Ann Pharmacother 2002;36:1767–1775.

11. Centers for Disease Control and Prevention. Recommendations for preventing the spread of vancomycin resistance: recommendations of the Hospital Infection Control Practices Advisory Committee. MMWR 1995;44:1–13.

12. Musher DM, Aslam S, Logan N, et al. Relatively poor outcome after treatment of *Clostridium difficile* colitis with metronidazole. Clin Infect Dis 2005;40:1586–1590.

13. Cone LA, Lopez C, Tarleton HL, et al. A durable response to relapsing *Clostridium difficile* colitis may require combined therapy with high dose oral vancomycin and intravenous immune globulin. Infect Dis Clin Pract 2006;14:217–220.

14. Musher DM, Logan N, Hamill RJ, et al. Nitazoxanide for the treatment of *Clostridium difficile* colitis. Clin Infect Dis 2006;43:421–427.

15. McFarland LV. Meta-analysis of probiotics for the prevention of antibiotic associated diarrhea and the treatment of *Clostridium difficile* disease. Am J Gastroenterol 2006;101:812–822.

16. Cone JB, Wetzel W. Toxic megacolon secondary to pseudomembranous colitis. Dis Colon Rectum 1982;25:478–482.

17. National Kidney Foundation. K/DOQI clinical practice guidelines for chronic kidney disease: evaluation, classification, and stratification. Am J Kidney Dis 2002,39;S1–S266.

18. Johnson S, Homann SR, Bettin KM, et al. Treatment of asymptomatic *Clostridium difficile* carriers (fecal excretors) with vancomycin or metronidazole. A randomized, placebo-controlled trial. Ann Intern Med 1992;117:297–302.

122

INTRA-ABDOMINAL INFECTION

Like Mother, Like Son . . . . Level II

Renee-Claude Mercier, PharmD, BCPS, PhC

A. Christie Graham, PharmD

LEARNING OBJECTIVES

After completing this case study, the reader should be able to:

- Recognize the clinical manifestations of bacterial peritonitis.
- Identify the normal microflora found in the various segments of the GI tract.
- List the goals of antimicrobial therapy for bacterial peritonitis.
- Recommend appropriate empiric and definitive antibiotic therapy for primary bacterial peritonitis (also known as spontaneous bacterial peritonitis).
- Monitor antibiotic therapy for safety and efficacy.

- Recommend secondary prophylaxis for primary bacterial peritonitis.
- Establish a long-term plan for the patient regarding alcohol abuse and hepatitis C, including monitoring parameters and counseling.

PATIENT PRESENTATION

Chief Complaint

"My belly hurts so bad I can barely move."

HPI

John Chavez is a 67-year-old Hispanic man who was brought to the ED by his wife. She stated that he has been suffering from nausea, vomiting, severe abdominal pain, and has been acting "goofy" for the last 2–3 days. His intake of food and fluids has been minimal over the past several days. He is a well-known patient of the ED who often presents with alcohol intoxication and severe hepatic encephalopathy.

PMH

Cirrhosis with ascites for the last 4 years
Hepatic encephalopathy
GERD
HTN
Cholecystectomy 15 years ago
Hepatitis C+ × 4 years
Spontaneous bacterial peritonitis—one episode 9 months ago

FH

Mother was alcoholic; died 10 years ago in car accident. Father's history unknown.

SH

Retired construction worker; ETOH abuse with 10–12 cans of beer per day × 25 years; denies use of tobacco or illicit drugs; poor compliance with medications and dietary restrictions.

Meds

Lactulose 30 mL po QID PRN
Amlodipine 10 mg po once daily
Inderal LA 80 mg po once daily
Spironolactone 100 mg po once daily
Famotidine 20 mg po BID
Maalox 30 mL po QID PRN

All

NKDA

ROS

As noted above in HPI

Physical Examination

Gen

Elderly man who appears older than his stated age and is in severe pain

VS

BP 154/82, P 102, RR 32, T 38.2°C; current Wt 92 kg, IBW 68 kg

Skin

Jaundiced, warm, coarse, and very dry. Facial spider angiomata present.

HEENT

Yellow sclerae; PERRLA; EOMI; funduscopic exam is normal. Tympanic membranes are clouded bilaterally, but with no erythema or bulging. Oropharynx show poor dentition but are otherwise unremarkable.

Neck/Lymph Nodes

Supple; normal size thyroid; no JVD or palpable lymph nodes

Chest

Lungs are CTA; shallow and frequent breathing

Heart

Tachycardia, normal S_1 and S_2 with no S_3 or S_4

Abd

Distended; pain upon pressure or movements; pain is sharp and diffuse throughout abdomen; (+) guarding. (+) HSM. Decreased bowel sounds.

Genit/Rect

Prostate normal size; guaiac (–) stool

Ext

Unremarkable

Neuro

Oriented × 2 (time and person); lethargic and apathetic, slumped posture, slowed movements. CN II–XII intact. Motor system intact; overall muscle strength equal to 4–5/5; poor coordination and gait. Sensory system intact. Reflexes 3+.

■ Labs

Na 142 mEq/L	Hgb 13.1 g/dL	AST 290 IU/L
K 3.9 mEq/L	Hct 40.6%	ALT 320 IU/L
Cl 96 mEq/L	Plt 101 × 10³/mm³	Alk phos 350 IU/L
CO_2 20 mEq/L	WBC 12.25 × 10³/mm³	T. bili 3.2 mg/dL
BUN 44 mg/dL	Neutros 73%	D. bili 1.4 mg/dL
SCr 1.1 mg/dL	Bands 9%	Albumin 2.8 g/dL
Glu 101 mg/dL	Lymphs 13%	NH_3 104 mcg/dL
	Monos 5%	INR 1.34

■ Abdominal X-Ray

No evidence of free air

■ Chest X-Ray

No infiltrates; heart normal size and shape

■ Blood Cultures

Pending × 2

■ Paracentesis

Ascitic fluid: leukocytes 720/mm³, protein 2.8 g/dL, albumin 1.6 g/dL, pH 7.28, lactate 30 mg/dL. Gram-stain: numerous PMNs, no organisms

■ Assessment

Primary bacterial peritonitis

■ Clinical Course

Because of the recent low intake of food and fluids and the high BUN-to-creatinine ratio, the patient was thought to be dehydrated and was given 1 L/h of 0.9% NaCl IV in the ED. His breathing became progressively worse, and he had to be intubated and transferred to the intensive care unit.

QUESTIONS

Problem Identification

1.a. Create a list of the patient's drug therapy problems.

1.b. What signs, symptoms, and laboratory values indicate the presence of primary bacterial peritonitis?

1.c. What risk factors for infection are present in this patient?

1.d. Which organisms are the most likely cause of this infection?

Desired Outcome

2. What are the therapeutic goals for this patient?

Therapeutic Alternatives

3.a. What nondrug therapies might be useful for this patient?

3.b. What feasible pharmacotherapeutic alternatives are available for the treatment of primary bacterial peritonitis?

Optimal Plan

4.a. Given this patient's condition, which drug regimens would provide optimal therapy for the infection?

4.b. In addition to antimicrobial therapy, what other drug-related interventions are required for this patient?

Outcome Evaluation

5. What clinical and laboratory parameters are necessary to evaluate the therapy for achievement of the desired therapeutic outcome and to detect or prevent adverse effects?

Patient Education

6. What information should be provided to the patient to enhance compliance, ensure successful therapy, and minimize adverse effects?

■ CLINICAL COURSE

After 48 hours of IV antibiotics, Mr. Chavez was extubated. The blood cultures were reported positive for *Klebsiella pneumoniae*, resistant to ampicillin and ampicillin/sulbactam, and sensitive to aztreonam, ceftriaxone, levofloxacin, and piperacillin/tazobactam. The ascitic fluid culture grew *K. pneumoniae* as well. He received cefotaxime 2 g IV Q 8 h for a total of 10 days. After 3 days of antimicrobial treatment, repeat blood cultures were negative. He rapidly improved, and upon discharge his mental status had returned to baseline.

■ SELF-STUDY ASSIGNMENTS

1. Develop a table that illustrates the primary differences (clinical manifestations, pathogens involved, diagnosis methods, and treatment) between primary and secondary bacterial peritonitis.

2. Describe risk factors, clinical signs and symptoms, modes of transmission, diagnostic methods, prognosis, and therapeutic options associated with hepatitis C.

CLINICAL PEARL

Bacteremia is present in up to 75% of patients with primary peritonitis caused by aerobic bacteria but is rarely found in those with peritonitis caused by anaerobes.

REFERENCES

1. Runyon BA, McHutchison JG, Antillon MR, et al. Short-course versus long-course antibiotic treatment of spontaneous bacterial peritonitis: a randomized controlled study of 108 patients. Gastroenterology 1991;100:1737–1742.

2. Runyon BA. American Association for the Study of Liver Diseases (AASLD) Practice Guidelines: management of adult patients with ascites caused by cirrhosis. Hepatology 2004;39:841–856.

3. Parsi MA, Atreja A, Zein NN. Spontaneous bacterial peritonitis: recent data on incidence and treatment. Clev Clin J Med 2004;71:569–576.

4. Felisart J, Rimona A, Arroyo V, et al. Cefotaxime is more effective than is ampicillin-tobramycin in cirrhotics with severe infections. Hepatology 1985;5:457–462.

5. Such, J, Runyon BA. Spontaneous bacterial peritonitis. Clin Infect Dis 1998;27:669–676.

6. Sort P, Navasa M, Arroyo V, et al. Effect of intravenous albumin on renal impairment and mortality in patients with cirrhosis and spontaneous bacterial peritonitis. N Engl J Med 1999;341:403–409.

123

LOWER URINARY TRACT INFECTION

Where Is the Bathroom?.................Level I

Sharon M. Erdman, PharmD

Keith A. Rodvold, PharmD, FCCP

LEARNING OBJECTIVES

After completing this case study, the reader should be able to:

- Recognize the typical signs and symptoms of an uncomplicated urinary tract infection (UTI) in females.

- Design a therapeutic regimen for the treatment of acute cystitis after consideration of patient symptoms, history, objective findings, and desired clinical response.

- Describe parameters that should be monitored during the treatment of acute uncomplicated cystitis to ensure efficacy and prevent toxicity.

- Provide patient education on the proper administration of drug therapy for acute uncomplicated cystitis, including directions for use, the administration of therapy in relation to meals, proper storage, and potential side effects of the medication.

PATIENT PRESENTATION

▓ Chief Complaint

"It burns when I urinate, and I am urinating all the time."

▓ HPI

Sarah Ramsey is a 26-year-old woman who presents to a family practice clinic in Seattle, with continuing complaints of dysuria, frequency of urination, and urgency to urinate. She was seen in the clinic 3 days prior with the same complaints and was started on trimethoprim-sulfamethoxazole DS, 1 tablet twice daily.

▓ PMH

Diagnosed with three UTIs over the past 8 months, each treated with TMP-SMX

▓ FH

Mother has DM; remainder of FH is noncontributory

▓ SH

Denies smoking but admits to occasional marijuana use and social ETOH use. Patient has been sexually active with one partner for the past 9 months and typically uses spermicide-coated condoms for contraception.

▓ Meds

None

▓ All

No known allergies

▓ ROS

Patient reports urethral pain and burning during urination, as well as mild suprapubic tenderness. Patient denies systemic symptoms such as fever, chills, vomiting, or back pain and does not report any urethral or vaginal discharge.

▓ Physical Examination

Gen

Cooperative woman in no acute distress

VS

BP 110/60, P 68, R 18, T 36.8°C; Wt 57 kg, Ht 5'5"

Skin

No skin lesions

HEENT

PERRLA; EOMI; fundi benign; TMs intact

Neck/Lymph Nodes

Supple without lymphadenopathy

Chest

CTA

CV

RRR

Back

No CVA tenderness

Abd

Soft; (+) bowel sounds; no organomegaly or tenderness

Pelvic

No vaginal discharge or lesions; LMP 2 weeks ago; mild suprapubic tenderness

Ext

Pulses 2+ throughout; full ROM

Neuro

A & O × 3; CN II–XII intact; reflexes 2+; sensory and motor levels intact

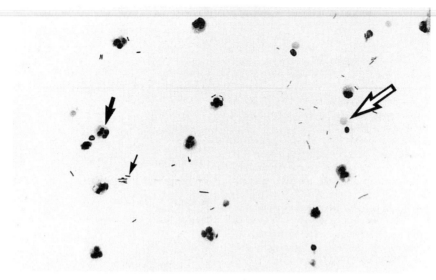

FIGURE 123-1. Urine sediment with neutrophils *(solid arrow)*, bacteria *(small arrow)*, and occasional red blood cells *(open arrow)* (Wright-Giemsa × 1,650). *(Photo courtesy of Lydia C. Contis, MD.)*

▪ Labs

Urinalysis (from clinic visit 3 days ago)

Yellow, cloudy; pH 5.0; WBC 10–15 cells/hpf; RBC 1–5 cells/hpf; protein 10 mg/dL; trace blood; glucose (–); leukocyte esterase (+); nitrite positive; many bacteria (Fig. 123-1)

Urine Culture

Not performed

▪ Assessment

Acute uncomplicated cystitis, not responding to empiric antibiotic therapy (Fig. 123-2)

QUESTIONS

Problem Identification

1.a. What clinical and laboratory findings are consistent with the diagnosis of an acute uncomplicated lower UTI (cystitis) in this patient?

1.b. How is the diagnosis of cystitis differentiated from that of urethritis (caused by *Chlamydia trachomatis*, *Neisseria gonorrhoeae*, or herpes simplex virus) or vaginitis (caused by *Candida* or *Trichomonas* species)?

1.c. How should a patient with acute uncomplicated cystitis who is not responding to empiric antibiotic therapy be managed? Should a urine culture and sensitivity test be performed? Is this patient a candidate for prophylactic antibiotics to prevent further episodes of acute uncomplicated cystitis?

1.d. What are the most likely pathogens causing this patient's acute uncomplicated cystitis, and how often are these pathogens implicated in the etiology of acute uncomplicated cystitis?

1.e. What factors can increase the risk of developing a UTI?

1.f. List potential reasons why this patient may not be responding to treatment.

Desired Outcome

2. What are the therapeutic goals in the treatment of acute uncomplicated cystitis?

Therapeutic Alternatives

3.a. What are the desirable characteristics of an antibiotic in the treatment of acute uncomplicated cystitis?

3.b. What feasible pharmacotherapeutic alternatives are available for empiric first-line and second-line treatment of an uncomplicated UTI?

3.c. What nonpharmacologic therapies may be useful in preventing uncomplicated UTIs?

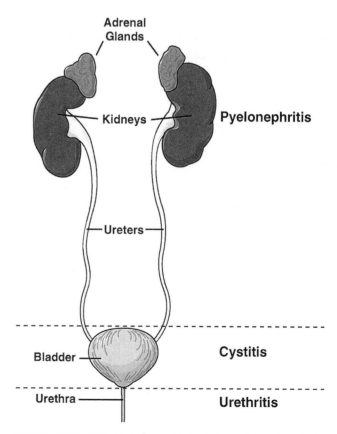

FIGURE 123-2. Anatomy and associated infections of the urinary tract.

Optimal Plan

4. What drug, dosage form, dose, schedule, and duration of therapy are best for the treatment of this patient's acute uncomplicated cystitis?

Outcome Evaluation

5. What clinical and laboratory parameters should be monitored to evaluate the efficacy of therapy and to detect or prevent adverse effects?

Patient Education

6. What information should be provided to the patient to ensure successful therapy, enhance compliance, and minimize adverse effects?

■ SELF-STUDY ASSIGNMENTS

1. Review the safety and efficacy of single-dose, 3-day, and 7-day antimicrobial therapy for the treatment of acute uncomplicated bacterial cystitis.

2. Perform a literature search to obtain information on the national and regional rates of resistance of outpatient urinary isolates of *Escherichia coli* to TMP-SMX and fluoroquinolone antibiotics. How do these rates compare to those reported at your institution, your clinic, or your geographic area?

3. Provide an assessment and recommendation on the role of phenazopyridine in treatment of UTIs.

CLINICAL PEARL

UTIs occur rarely in young males, unless there is an underlying structural abnormality or instrumentation of the urinary tract.

REFERENCES

1. Hooton TM. The current management strategies for community-acquired urinary tract infection. Infect Dis Clin North Am 2003;17:303–332.
2. Fihn SD. Acute uncomplicated urinary tract infection in women. N Engl J Med 2003;349:259–266.
3. Hooton TM. Recurrent urinary tract infection in women. Int J Antimicrob Agents 2001;17:259–268.
4. Gupta K, Sahm DF, Mayfield D, et al. Antimicrobial resistance among uropathogens that cause community-acquired urinary tract infections in women: a nationwide analysis. Clin Infect Dis 2001;33:89–94.
5. Zhanel GG, Hisanaga TL, Laing NM, et al. Antibiotic resistance in *Escherichia coli* outpatient urinary tract isolates: final results from the North American Urinary Tract Infection Collaborative Alliance (NAUTICA). Int J Antimicrob Agents 2006;27:468–475.
6. Karlowsky JA, Kelly LJ, Thornsberry C, et al. Trends in antimicrobial resistance among urinary tract infection isolates of *Escherichia coli* from female outpatients in the United States. Antimicrob Agents Chemother 2002;46:2540–2545.
7. Warren JW, Abrutyn E, Hebel JR, et al. Guidelines for antimicrobial treatment of uncomplicated acute bacterial cystitis and acute pyelonephritis in women. Infectious Diseases Society of America (IDSA). Clin Infect Dis 1999;29:745–758.
8. Wright SW, Wrenn KD, Haynes ML. Trimethoprim-sulfamethoxazole resistance among urinary coliform isolates. J Gen Intern Med 1999;14:606–609.
9. Gupta K. Emerging antibiotic resistance in urinary tract pathogens. Infect Dis Clin North Am 2003;17:243–259.
10. Stapleton A. Novel approaches to prevention of urinary infections. Infect Dis Clin North Am 2003;17:457–471.

124

ACUTE PYELONEPHRITIS

Outflanked . . . . .Level II

Brian A. Potoski, PharmD

LEARNING OBJECTIVES

After completing this case study, the reader should be able to:

- Differentiate the signs, symptoms, and laboratory findings associated with pyelonephritis from those seen in lower urinary tract infections.
- Recognize patient risk factors that predispose to development of pyelonephritis.
- Recommend appropriate empiric antimicrobial and symptomatic pharmacotherapy for a patient with suspected pyelonephritis.
- Make appropriate adjustments in pharmacotherapy based on patient response and culture results.
- Design a monitoring plan for a patient with pyelonephritis that allows objective assessment of the response to therapy.

PATIENT PRESENTATION

■ Chief Complaint

"There's pain in my stomach and back."

■ HPI

Theresa Mitch is a 53-year-old woman with a history of asthma, GERD, HTN, and CVA. She reports that she has had pain in her left flank region over the last 3 days, as well as pain in her abdomen. She complains of some nausea and reports four episodes of vomiting over the past 3 days. She has recently skipped several meals as a result. The patient reports urinary burning and frequency. She states that often she feels feverish and at times has chills. She reports no substernal chest pain, shortness of breath, cough, or sputum production. She denies any diarrhea. There is no new paresthesia, but she claims that she feels weak and worn down.

■ PMH

Hypertension (duration unknown); BP averages 142/84 mm Hg on medication
GERD (duration unknown)
Asthma (duration unknown)
S/P stroke with right hemiparesis approximately 2 years ago

■ FH

Father died at age 72 with lung cancer; mother is 75 years old and alive with CAD and CHF; one sister with diabetes; no other siblings

■ SH

Non-smoker, no IVDA, occasional alcohol use. Divorced. Currently lives with her two sons from the previous marriage. She is employed at the local post office.

■ Meds

Warfarin 5 mg po once daily
Hydrochlorothiazide 25 mg po once daily
Ranitidine 150 mg po once daily
Captopril 12.5 mg po TID
Naproxen sodium 220 mg po TID

■ All

Penicillin (develops an itchy rash)

■ ROS

Reports recently taking naproxen sodium OTC PRN for her back and abdominal pain, which doesn't seem to help. She has had one UTI in the past year but cannot remember others since.

■ Physical Examination

Gen

Conscious, alert, and oriented middle-aged, African-American woman in mild distress

VS

BP 142/84, P 77, RR 21, T 38.2°C, O_2 sat 97% room air; Wt 59.6 kg (IBW 52.4 kg), Ht 5'3"

Skin

No tenting; dry

HEENT

NCAT; EOMI; funduscopic examination with no evidence of exudates or cotton wool spots; pharynx clear and dry

Neck

Supple, flat JVP

Chest

CTA

CV

RRR, normal S_1 and S_2; no S_3 or S_4

Abd

Mildly obese; active bowel sounds; soft with suprapubic tenderness to deep palpation; no rebound or guarding. There is no hepatosplenomegaly or masses.

Back

(+) CVAT; no paraspinal or spinal tenderness; complains of pain

Genit/Rect

Normal female genitalia; no abnormal vaginal discharge; normal sphincter tone; last menstrual period 3 months ago

Ext

No CCE; dry flaky skin on lower legs bilaterally; pulses 2+ bilaterally

Neuro

A & O × 3; CN II–XII intact; sensory and perception intact; old weakness noted on right side from previous CVA

■ Labs and UA on Admission

See Table 124-1 and Fig. 124-1

■ Chest X-Ray

No infiltrates, no consolidation seen

■ CT Abdomen with Contrast

Findings: Liver, gallbladder, pancreas, spleen, and adrenals are unremarkable. No evidence of pneumoperitoneum or hemoperi-

TABLE 124-1 Laboratory Tests and Urinalyses on Days 1 through 3 of Hospitalization

Parameter (units)	Day 1	Day 2	Day 3
Serum chemistry			
Na (mEq/L)	134	136	138
K (mEq/L)	3.1	3.2	3.6
Cl (mEq/L)	99	101	105
CO_2 (mEq/L)	27	28	28
BUN (mg/dL)	45	32	17
SCr (mg/dL)	1.5	1.2	1.0
Glucose (mg/dL)	181	119	110
Hematology			
Hgb (g/dL)	10.3	9.5	8.8
Hct (%)	34.8	29.2	25.9
Plt ($\times 10^3$/mm³)	119	76	46
WBC ($\times 10^3$/mm³)	20.2	18.5	15.6
PMN/B/L/M (%)	82/10/8/0	85/9/3/3	80/5/13/2
Urinalysis			
Appearance	Hazy		
Color	Amber		
pH	5.0		
Specific gravity	1.017		
Blood	2+		
Ketones	Negative		
Leukocyte esterase	3+		
Nitrites	2+		
Urine protein, qualitative	Trace		
Urine glucose, qualitative	Trace		
WBC/hpf	487		
RBC/hpf	102		
Bacteria	Many		
WBC casts	2+		

B, bands; L, lymphocytes; M, monocytes; PMN, polymorphonuclear leukocytes.

toneum. No evidence of ascites or focal areas of fluid collection. The right kidney is unremarkable. A hypoattenuating lesion is seen involving the left kidney from mid-pole to lower-pole.

Impression: Hypoattenuating lesion in left kidney consistent with pyelonephritis, correlate with clinical picture.

■ Abdominal Ultrasound

Findings: No hydrocephalus of the kidneys bilaterally. Within the lateral cortex of the left kidney, there is a hypoechoic region, which does not display through transmission.

Impression: Focal cortical thickening with decreased echogenicity involving the mid left renal cortex, similar to the recent CT scan, most likely representing focal pyelonephritis. No renal abscess identified. No hydronephrosis.

■ Urine Gram Stain

Many Gram-negative rods

■ Assessment

Pyelonephritis
Volume depletion
Hypertension

QUESTIONS

Problem Identification

1.a. Create a list of the patient's drug therapy problems.

1.b. What information (signs, symptoms, laboratory tests) indicates the presence and severity of pyelonephritis in this patient?

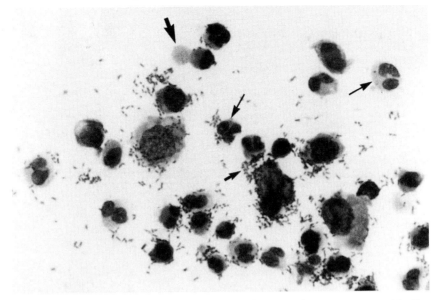

FIGURE 124-1. Urine sediment with red blood cells *(large arrow)*, numerous neutrophils *(line arrows)*, and bacteria *(small arrow)* (Wright × 1,650). *(Photo courtesy of Lydia C. Contis, MD.)*

1.c. List any potential contributing factors, including drug therapy, that may have predisposed this patient to developing pyelonephritis (Fig. 124-2).

1.d. What additional information is needed to fully assess the patient?

Desired Outcome

2. What are the goals of pharmacotherapy in this patient?

Therapeutic Alternatives

3.a. What nondrug therapies might be useful for this patient?

3.b. What organisms are commonly associated with pyelonephritis?

3.c. What feasible pharmacotherapeutic alternatives are available for the empiric treatment of pyelonephritis?

Optimal Plan

4. Outline an antimicrobial regimen that will provide appropriate empiric therapy for pyelonephritis in this patient.

Outcome Evaluation

5.a. What clinical and laboratory parameters are necessary to evaluate the antibiotic therapy for achievement of the desired therapeutic outcomes and to detect or prevent adverse effects?

■ CLINICAL COURSE

The patient was started on the empiric antimicrobial regimen you recommended. She required acetaminophen Q 6 h for back and abdominal pain, as well as occasional oxycodone 5 mg po Q 8 h PRN. Her fevers subsided with the initiation of acetaminophen. On day 3 of hospitalization, she was much improved and had begun to eat a normal diet. Laboratory tests for days 2 and 3 are included in Table 124-1. Culture results from admission were finalized on day 3 (late in the day) and are shown in Table 124-2.

5.b. What recommendations, if any, do you have for changes in the initial drug regimen?

Patient Education

6. What information should be provided to the patient on discharge to enhance adherence, ensure successful therapy, and minimize adverse effects?

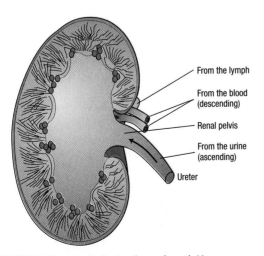

FIGURE 124-2. Routes of infection for pyelonephritis.

From the lymph

From the blood (descending)

Renal pelvis

From the urine (ascending)

Ureter

TABLE 124-2	Culture Results of Urine and Blood Samples Taken on Day 1 and Reported on Day 3
Urine Culture	
Result: >100,000 cfu/mL *Escherichia coli*	
Antibiotic	**Kirby-Bauer Interpretation**
Ampicillin/sulbactam	Intermediate
Ampicillin	Resistant
Cefazolin	Intermediate
Cefuroxime	Sensitive
Ceftriaxone	Sensitive
Levofloxacin	Sensitive
Piperacillin/tazobactam	Sensitive
Tobramycin	Sensitive
TMP/SMX	Sensitive
Blood culture × 2 sets	
Result: no growth × 5 days—report final	

■ **SELF-STUDY ASSIGNMENTS**

1. Develop a protocol for switching patients from IV to oral therapy when treating pyelonephritis.

2. Perform a literature search to find clinical trials comparing drug therapy in pyelonephritis, and compare inclusion criteria, drug regimens, outcomes, and costs of therapy.

3. Develop a clinical pathway that could be used for the management of suspected pyelonephritis.

CLINICAL PEARL

Pyelonephritis can be managed with many different drugs; choose drugs that are bactericidal and cleared in the active form by the kidney. Drugs suitable for once-daily therapy help to reduce treatment costs.

REFERENCES

1. Jinnah F, Islam MS, Rumi MA, et al. Drug sensitivity pattern of *E. coli* causing urinary tract infection in diabetic and nondiabetic patients. J Int Med Res 1996;24:296–301.

2. Warren JW, Abrutyn E, Hebel JR, et al. Guidelines for antimicrobial treatment of uncomplicated acute bacterial cystitis and acute pyelonephritis in women. Infectious Diseases Society of America (IDSA). Clin Infect Dis 1999;29:745–758.

3. Hooton TM, Stamm WE. Diagnosis and treatment of uncomplicated urinary tract infection. Infect Dis Clin North Am 1997;11:551–581.

4. Bailey RR, Begg EJ, Smith AH, et al. Prospective, randomized controlled study comparing two dosing regimens of gentamicin/oral ciprofloxacin switch therapy for acute pyelonephritis. Clin Nephrol 1996;46:183–186.

5. Talan DA, Stamm WE, Hooton TM, et al. Comparison of ciprofloxacin (7 days) and trimethoprim-sulfamethoxazole (14 days) for acute uncomplicated pyelonephritis in women. A randomized trial. JAMA 2000;283:1583–1590.

6. Klausner HA, Brown P, Peterson J, et al. A trial of levofloxacin 750mg once daily for 5 days versus ciprofloxacin 400mg and/or 500mg twice daily for 10 days in the treatment of acute pyelonephritis. Curr Med Res Opin 2007;23:2627–2628.

7. Pinson AG, Philbrick JT, Lindbeck GH, et al. ED management of acute pyelonephritis in women: a cohort study. Am J Emerg Med 1994;12:271–278.

125

PELVIC INFLAMMATORY DISEASE AND OTHER SEXUALLY TRANSMITTED DISEASES

Frankie and Jenny Were Lovers . . . . Level II

Denise L. Howrie, PharmD

Pamela J. Murray, MD, MHP

LEARNING OBJECTIVES

After completing this case study, the reader should be able to:

- Identify relevant information from patient history, physical examination, and laboratory data suggestive of the diagnosis of a sexually transmitted disease (STD).

- List major complications of STDs and appropriate strategies for prevention and/or treatment.

- Discuss other health issues that may be present in patients referred for treatment of STDs.

- Provide appropriate treatment plans for patients with STDs, including drug(s), doses, and monitoring.

- Develop patient counseling strategies regarding drug treatment and possible adverse effects.

PATIENT PRESENTATION

■ **Chief Complaint**

"My lady and I don't feel good."

■ **HPI**

Frankie Mason is a 28-year-old man who presents to a health clinic with complaints of 5 days of painful urination and increasing amounts of discolored urethral discharge. Today, he noted four painful blisters on the penis. He is single, is sexually active with two to three concurrent partners, and admits to unprotected sex "at least once" in the past 2 weeks. He does not know the sexual histories of his current or past sexual partners or their sexual partners. He denies IV drug use, is heterosexual, and has no active medical problems. He denies oral or rectal intercourse. He admits to over 15 lifetime sexual partners.

■ **PMH**

History of genital herpes 2 years ago, otherwise negative. He has not undergone testing for HIV and has not been immunized against hepatitis B. He is unaware of hepatitis A or C as infectious diseases, asking "Do you get that from sex or restaurant food?"

■ **FH**

Noncontributory

■ **SH**

Denies cigarette use; has two to four beers "on weekends"; may be unreliable in keeping follow-up appointments because he states, "I don't like doctors."

■ **Meds**

None

■ **All**

Cipro ("makes me dizzy")

■ **ROS**

Occasional headaches; denies stomach pain, constipation, vision problems, night sweats, weight loss, or fatigue

■ **Physical Examination**
Gen

Patient is a well-developed male in NAD, very talkative

VS

BP 104/80, HR 72, RR 12, T 37.6°C; Wt 78 kg

Skin

No rashes or other lesions seen

HEENT

No erythema of pharynx or oral ulcers

Neck/Lymph Nodes

No lymphadenopathy; neck supple

Chest

Normal breath sounds; good air entry

CV

RRR; no murmurs

Abd

No tenderness or rebound; no HSM

Genit/Rect

Tanner stage V; testes descended, nontender, without erythema. Thick gray-white urethral discharge; four small erupting vesicles on penile tip and glans; negative rectal examination; no scrotal tenderness or swelling. No genital growths visualized.

MS/Ext

No inguinal or other lymphadenopathy; no lesions or rashes; muscle strength and tone normal

Neuro

CN II–XII intact; DTRs 2+ bilaterally and symmetric

■ Urethral Smear

15 WBC/hpf; Gram stain (+) for intracellular Gram-negative diplococci (Fig. 125-1); rare flagellated organisms by saline prep microscopy

■ Assessment

1. Urethritis caused by gonococcal and *Trichomonas* infections

2. Recurrent genital herpes

PATIENT PRESENTATION

■ Chief Complaint

"I feel sick to my stomach."

■ HPI

Jenny Klein is a 22-year-old female sexual partner of Frankie who reports a 1-day history of increasingly severe dysuria, lower abdominal pain, fever, nausea, emesis × 2, and vaginal discharge. She is sexually active with "only Frankie," has no previous history of urinary or genital infection, and denies IV drug use. She is unaware of Frankie's multiple sexual partners. Her last menses ended 10 days ago and last intercourse was 7 days ago without use of a condom. She noted the vaginal discharge yesterday, which she describes as thick and yellow. She denies oral or rectal intercourse. She admits to three lifetime sexual partners.

■ PMH

Negative with no pregnancies. She has not been immunized against hepatitis B or A and has not received the human papillomavirus vaccine (Gardasil), because she believes she is "low risk."

■ FH

HTN in maternal grandmother; history of depression

■ SH

Denies nicotine or recreational drug use; occasional one to two glasses of wine; does not use hormonal or other contraception, reports occasional use of condoms; no routine medical care

■ Meds

None

■ All

NKDA

■ ROS

Occasional painful menses self-treated with acetaminophen

■ Physical Examination

Gen

Well-developed woman in moderate-to-severe abdominal discomfort

VS

BP 110/76, HR 120, RR 16, T 39.2°C; Wt 52 kg

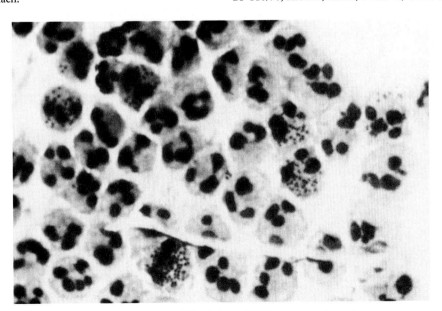

FIGURE 125-1. Gram-negative intracellular diplococci *(Neisseria gonorrhoeae).*

Skin

No rashes seen

HEENT

No erythema of pharynx or oral ulcers

Neck/Lymph Nodes

No lymphadenopathy; neck supple

Chest

Normal breath sounds; good air entry; breasts Tanner stage V

CV

RRR; no murmurs

Abd

Guarding of right and mid-lower quadrants with palpation

Genit/Rect

Pubic hair Tanner stage V; vulva with no ulcers visible; moderate erythema with mild excoriations. Vagina with large amount of thick yellow-white discharge and mild erythema. Cervix shows erythema and extensive yellow-white discharge from the os; no masses on bimanual examination; cervical motion tenderness; adnexal tenderness and fullness. No genital growths visualized.

MS/Ext

No adenopathy, lesions or rashes; no arthritis or tenosynovitis

Neuro

CN II–XII Intact, DTRs 2+ and symmetric bilaterally

◾ Labs

Na 138 mEq/L	Hgb 12.2 g/dL	WBC $12.75 \times 10^3/mm^3$
K 4.2 mEq/L	Hct 37%	Neutros 66%
Cl 102 mEq/L	Plt $250 \times 10^3/mm^3$	Bands 12%
BUN 22 mg/dL		Lymphs 10%
SCr 0.9 mg/dL		Monos 12%
Glu 106 mg/dL		

◾ Other

Examination of vaginal discharge: pH 6.0, no yeast or hyphae seen; KOH prep negative, "whiff" test negative; flagellated organisms and increased WBC seen by saline prepared microscopy; negative for clue cells

◾ UA

Rare WBC/hpf; protein 100 mg/dL; Gram stain (–)

◾ Assessment

PID
Infection of the genital tract: cervicitis, vaginitis, and urethritis

QUESTIONS

Problem Identification

1.a. For each patient, create a list of drug therapy problems.

1.b. What information indicates the presence or severity of each STD in each patient?

1.c. Should any additional tests be performed in these patients?

1.d. What complications of infection can be reduced or avoided with appropriate therapy for each patient?

Desired Outcome

2. State the goals of treatment for each patient.

Therapeutic Alternatives

3. What therapeutic options are available for treatment of each patient?

Optimal Plan

4.a. What treatment regimen (drug, dosage form, dose, schedule, and duration) is appropriate for these patients?

4.b. What alternatives would be appropriate if the initial therapy cannot be used?

Outcome Evaluation

5.a. What clinical and laboratory parameters are necessary to evaluate the therapy for achievement of the desired outcome and to detect or prevent adverse effects?

◾ CLINICAL COURSE

Eight hours later, *Chlamydia* PCR positive test results received on samples from both patients.

Two days later, bacterial cultures of urethral discharge (Frankie) and vaginal secretions (Jenny) are reported positive for *Neisseria gonorrhoeae*.

5.b. What changes, if any, in antibacterial therapy are required?

Patient Education

6. What information should be provided to Frankie to enhance compliance, ensure success of therapy, and minimize adverse effects?

◾ SELF-STUDY ASSIGNMENTS

1. Because fluoroquinolones are no longer recommended for gonococcal infections, research alternative options to fluroquinolones for treatment in patients with severe drug hypersensitivity to cephalosporins.

2. Sexually active adolescents are a high risk group for development of STDs. Identify biologic, social, and psychological factors that affect this risk, and discuss how clinicians can assist in addressing some adolescent risk behaviors.

3. Review the definitions and legal status of expedited partner therapy (EPT) in your areas of practice. Identify and discuss legal, ethical, and public health implications of this practice (see *www.cdc.gov/std/ept*).

CLINICAL PEARLS

Quinolones such as ciprofloxacin are no longer recommended for infections in which gonococcus may be present because of increasing rates of drug resistance.

Partner notification and treatment may be enhanced through "expedited partner therapy" strategies in which a sexual partner receives medication(s) or prescription(s) from a patient with a documented STD, in addition to information and referral for evaluation.

REFERENCES

1. Centers for Disease Control and Prevention. Sexually transmitted diseases treatment guidelines, 2006. MMWR Morb Mortal Wkly Rep 2006;55(RR-11):1–100.

2. Centers for Disease Control and Prevention. Update to CDC's sexually transmitted diseases treatment guidelines 2006: fluoroquinolones no longer recommended for treatment of gonococcal infections. MMWR Morb Mortal Wkly Rep 2007;56:332–336.

3. Burstein GR, Murray PJ. Diagnosis and management of sexually transmitted disease pathogens among adolescents. Pediatr Rev 2003;24:75–82.

4. Burstein GR, Murray PJ. Diagnosis and management of sexually transmitted diseases among adolescents. Pediatr Rev 2003;24:119–127.

5. Geisler WM. Management of uncomplicated *Chlamydia trachomatis* infections in adolescents and adults: evidence reviewed for the 2006 Centers for Disease Control and Prevention. Sexually transmitted diseases treatment guidelines. Clin Infect Dis 2007;44:S77–S83.

6. Walker CK, Wiesenfeld HC. Antibiotic therapy for acute pelvic inflammatory disease: the 2006 Centers for Disease Control and Prevention. Sexually transmitted diseases treatment guidelines. Clin Infect Dis 2007;44:S111–S122.

7. Holland-Hall C. Sexually transmitted infections: screening, syndromes, and symptoms. Prim Care Clin Office Pract 2006:33:433–454.

8. Wendel KA, Workowski KA. Trichomoniasis: challenges to appropriate management. Clin Infect Dis 2007;44:S123–129.

9. Centers for Disease Control and Prevention. Quadrivalent human papillomavirus vaccine: recommendations of the Advisory Committee on Immunization Practices. MMWR Morb Mortal Wkly Rep 2007;56(RR-02):1–32.

126

SYPHILIS

The Great Impostor. . . . . .Level I

Marc H. Scheetz, PharmD, MSc

LEARNING OBJECTIVES

After completing this case study, the reader should be able to:

- Discuss the diagnosis of syphilis and differentiate among the temporal stages of the disease.

- Develop a pharmacotherapeutic treatment plan individualized for the patient's stage of syphilis.

- Recommend alternate treatment regimens when the primary therapeutic option is contraindicated.

- Describe appropriate monitoring, follow-up, and counseling of patients with a syphilitic infection to ensure success of treatment.

PATIENT PRESENTATION

▓ Chief Complaint

"I've had trouble walking for the past 10 years. Lately, it has been getting worse."

▓ HPI

Bill Baker is a 79-year-old man who has been seen by a neurologist for benign tremors in his hands, difficulty walking, and extremity numbness. As part of his work-up, he was found to have both a positive RPR and FTA-ABS. The patient is not aware of any previous syphilis tests or diagnoses. The patient is a professor at a small university and states that he has no perceptible mental changes.

The patient describes hand shakes for greater than 50 years. He has had difficulty standing on one foot and walking for the last 10 years. In addition, the patient suffers from numbness in the bottom of the feet that also began about 10 years before today's presentation.

▓ PMH

Hypertension
Left ankle surgery (including placement of hardware) 2 years ago
Back surgery for leg/foot weakness 12 years ago
Back surgery for leg/foot weakness 22 years ago
Eye surgery 25 years ago

▓ FH

Wife died of breast CA in 1983
Brother alive and well (age 76)
Son died in MVA in 1973
Mother died of pneumonia (age 81)
Father died of heart attack (age 66)

▓ SH

Smokes a pipe (50-year history, approximately once per day)
Social alcohol usage (average four drinks per week)
Previous MSM Hx although currently no sexual contacts (no Hx of STDs)

▓ Meds

Amoxicillin/clavulanic acid 875 mg po BID (prescription written for 10 days; today is day 7/10)
Toprol XL 100 mg po daily
ASA 81 mg po daily
Ibuprofen 200 mg po Q 6 h PRN

▓ All

NKDA

▓ ROS

General: No fever or chills; no change in weight; no change in appetite

Skin: No generalized rash or eruptions

HEENT: No headache; no visual changes; no sore throat; no dizziness or syncope; no head trauma; no auditory changes

Respiratory: No shortness of breath, cough, or wheezing

Cardiac: No CP or palpitations

Gastrointestinal: No NV; no abdominal pain; no diarrhea or constipation

Urinary: No dysuria or increased urinary frequency; no hematuria; no urinary incontinence

Musculoskeletal: Chronic lower back pain; no extremity swelling

Neurologic: Numbness on bottom of feet bilaterally; no Hx of seizures or loss of consciousness

Hematologic: No history of bleeding or easy bruising

Psychiatric: No depression or anxiety

▓ Physical Examination

Gen

Well-nourished man in NAD

VS

BP 131/73, P 77, RR 18, T 98.5°F (36.9°C); Wt 97.5 kg

Skin

Warm, dry, non-jaundiced; without bruising or lesions; hair quantity, distribution, and texture unremarkable

HEENT

Normocephalic/atraumatic; TMs pearly gray, revealing good cone of light bilaterally, no evidence of auditory dysfunction; PERRLA, no Argyll-Robertson pupils, EOMI, optic disk margins appropriately sharp; nasal mucous membranes moist; no oropharyngeal lesions, dentures in place

Neck/Lymph Nodes

Supple; no lymphadenopathy, bruits, JVD, or thyromegaly

Chest

CTA bilaterally

CV

RRR; no MRG

Abd

(+) BS; nontender; no masses or organomegaly

GU

No penile lesions or inguinal lymphadenopathy

Rectal

No lesions or hemorrhoids

MS/Ext

Unna's boot on left foot; no rashes observed

Neuro

A & O × 3; CN II–XII intact; no nystagmus; no Babinski sign; locomotor ataxia due to left side weakness/favoring; no reflexes elicited in the knees or ankles; resting tremor in hands bilaterally

▓ Labs

Na 140 mEq/L	Hgb 14.5 g/dL
K 3.7 mEq/L	Hct 41.3%
Cl 103 mEq/L	WBC $6.9 \times 10^3/mm^3$
CO_2 23 mEq/L	Plt $211 \times 10^3/mm^3$
BUN 13 mg/dL	ESR 30 mm/h
SCr 1.0 mg/dL	
Glu 84 mg/dL	

▓ Other

Lumbar puncture: deferred by patient
RPR: Titers positive at 1:16
FTA-ABS: positive

▓ Assessment

1. The patient is a 79-year-old man with newly-diagnosed syphilis. It is unclear if this represents neurosyphilis or tertiary syphilis without CNS involvement.

2. High-risk individual based on sexual history and recent STD finding.

QUESTIONS

Problem Identification

1.a. Which populations are most at risk for syphilis?

1.b. What information (signs, symptoms, laboratory values) indicates the presence or stage of syphilis?

1.c. What laboratory tests are used in the diagnosis of syphilis, and how should they be interpreted?

Desired Outcome

2. What are the goals of pharmacotherapy in this case?

Therapeutic Alternatives

3.a. What pharmacotherapeutic alternatives are available for this patient?

3.b. What nondrug measures should be implemented in this case?

Optimal Plan

4. What is the recommended treatment (drug, dose, and duration) for this patient?

Outcome Evaluation

5. What clinical and laboratory parameters are necessary to evaluate the therapy for achievement of the desired therapeutic outcome and to detect or prevent adverse effects?

Patient Education

6.a. What information should be provided to the patient to enhance compliance, ensure successful therapy, and minimize adverse effects?

6.b. What information should be provided to the patient to prevent a future sexually transmitted disease?

▓ SELF-STUDY ASSIGNMENTS

1. Describe the differences in syphilis presentation in relation to disease progression.

2. Discuss the tests or procedures that should be used to diagnose and monitor the progression/regression of syphilis over time.

3. Describe a methodology to desensitize a patient to penicillin.

CLINICAL PEARL

Patients with neurosyphilis and a history of anaphylactic reaction to penicillin require allergy testing and possible desensitization prior to penicillin or ceftriaxone use.

CHAPTER 127

REFERENCES

1. Centers for Disease Control and Prevention. Sexually transmitted disease surveillance, 2005. Atlanta, U.S. Department of Health and Human Services, November 2006. Available at *www.cdc.gov*. Accessed January 3, 2007.
2. Centers for Disease Control and Prevention. Sexually transmitted diseases treatment guidelines. MMWR Morb Mortal Wkly Rep 2006;55(RR-11):22–35. Available at *www.cdc.gov*. Accessed January 3, 2007.
3. Tramont EC. *Treponema pallidum* (syphilis). In: Mandell GL, Bennett JE, Dolin R, eds. Principles and Practice of Infectious Diseases, 6th ed. Philadelphia, Churchill Livingstone, 2005:2768–2783.
4. Centers for Disease Control and Prevention. Inadvertent use of Bicillin C-R to treat syphilis infection—Los Angeles, California, 1999–2004. MMWR Morb Mortal Wkly Rep 2005;54:217–219.
5. Wendel GO Jr, Stark BJ, Jamison RB, et al. Penicillin allergy and desensitization in serious infections during pregnancy. N Engl J Med 1985;312:1229–1232.
6. United States Pharmacopoeia Drug Information: advice for the patient, Vol. 2, 20th ed. Englewood, Colo., Micromedex. 2000:1173-1177.

127

GENITAL HERPES, GONOCOCCAL, AND CHLAMYDIAL INFECTIONS

Triple Challenge . . . . Level II

Suellyn J. Sorensen, PharmD, BCPS

LEARNING OBJECTIVES

After completing this case study, the reader should be able to:

- Identify subjective and objective data consistent with genital herpes, gonorrhea, and chlamydia.

- Recommend appropriate therapies for the treatment of genital herpes, gonorrhea, and chlamydia.

- Provide effective and comprehensive counseling for patients with genital herpes, gonorrhea, and chlamydia.

- Identify drug interactions of clinical significance and provide recommendations for managing them.

PATIENT PRESENTATION

▓ Chief Complaint

"I have painful blisters in my genital area, and I have terrible headaches and muscle aches."

▓ HPI

Sally Simpson is a 22-year-old nulligravida woman who presents to the county health STD clinic for evaluation of genital lesions that have been present for 3 days. She has also noticed a white non-odorous vaginal discharge that has lasted 14 days. She admits to anal and vaginal intercourse with two regular partners in the last 60 days. It has been 5 days since her last sexual encounter.

▓ PMH

Recurrent UTIs; most recent 3 months ago
Vaginal candidiasis; most recent 6 months ago
Gonorrhea 5 years ago
Trichomonas vaginalis 2 years ago

▓ FH

Mother with Type 2 DM; father died at age 50 of an acute MI

▓ SH

Lives with her boyfriend and works at a local bar as a waitress. She admits to occasional use of alcohol and marijuana.

▓ Meds

Junel 21 1/20 1 tablet po daily
Multivitamin with iron 1 tablet po daily
Ibuprofen 200 mg po PRN
Ciprofloxacin 250 mg po once daily

▓ All

Penicillin (hives and tongue swelling)

▓ ROS

(−) cough, night sweats, weight loss, dysuria, or urinary frequency; (+) diarrhea and anorectal pain; LMP 6 weeks ago

▓ Physical Examination

Gen

Thin, young woman in NAD

VS

BP 136/71, P 78, RR 17, T 37.8°C; Wt 51 kg, Ht 5'5"

Skin

Dry, no lesions, normal color and temperature

HEENT

PERRLA, EOMI without nystagmus

Neck

Supple; no adenopathy, JVD, or thyromegaly

Chest

Air entry equal; no crepitations or wheezing

CV

RRR, normal S_1 and S_2; no S_3 or S_4; no murmurs or rubs

Abd

Soft, mild tenderness to palpation in RLQ, (+) bowel sounds, no HSM

Genit/Rect

Tender inguinal adenopathy. External exam clear for nits and lice, several extensive shallow small painful vesicular lesions over vulva and labia, swollen and red. Vagina red, rugated, moderate amounts of creamy white discharge. Cervix pink, covered with above discharge, nontender, ~3 cm. Corpus nontender, no palpable masses. Adnexa with no palpable masses or tenderness. Rectum with no external lesions; (+) diffuse inflammation and friability internally, no masses.

Ext

Peripheral pulses 2+ bilaterally, DTRs 2+, no joint swelling or tenderness

Neuro

Alert and oriented, CN II–XII intact

▦ Labs

Na 135 mEq/L	Hgb 12.9 g/dL	WBC $6.3 \times 10^3/mm^3$	RPR nonreactive
K 4.0 mEq/L	Hct 37.3%	PMNs 64%	Preg test: hCG pending
Cl 102 mEq/L	Plt $255 \times 10^3/mm^3$	Bands 2%	HIV serology: ELISA
CO_2 27 mEq/L		Eos 1%	pending
BUN 11 mg/dL		Lymphs 24%	
SCr 0.9 mg/dL		Monos 9%	
Glu 72 mg/dL			

▦ Other

Vaginal discharge-"whiff" test (–); pH <4.5; wet mount *Trichomonas* (–), clue cells (–), yeast (+)

▦ Clinical Course

The following results were reported 2 days later:

Vulval swab DFA monoclonal stain: HSV-2 isolated

Vaginal and rectal swab gonorrhea NAAT (PCR): *Neisseria gonorrhoeae* (+)

Vaginal and rectal swab chlamydia NAAT (PCR): *Chlamydia trachomatis* (+)

The following results were reported 5 days later:

Viral culture at base of genital vesicular fluid: HSV-2 isolated

Rectal and cervical bacterial cultures: *N. gonorrhoeae* (+)

Rectal and cervical cultures: *C. trachomatis* (+)

▦ Assessment

22-year-old woman who may be pregnant and has primary genital HSV-2 infection, vaginal candidiasis, and gonococcal and chlamydial infections of the vagina, cervix, and rectum.

QUESTIONS

Problem Identification

1.a. Create a list of the patient's drug therapy problems.

1.b. What subjective and objective clinical data are consistent with a primary genital herpes infection?

1.c. Could any of the patient's problems have been caused by drug therapy?

Desired Outcome

2. What are the goals of pharmacotherapy in this case?

Therapeutic Alternatives

3.a. What nondrug therapies might be useful for this patient?

3.b. What feasible pharmacotherapeutic alternatives are available for treatment of genital herpes, chlamydia, and gonorrhea?

Optimal Plan

4.a. What drug, dosage form, dose, schedule, and duration of therapy are best for treating this patient's genital herpes, chlamydial, and gonococcal infections?

4.b. If a nucleic acid amplification test (NAAT) (PCR) was not performed in this case and the culture result was negative for chlamydia but positive for gonorrhea, would treatment for chlamydia still be warranted?

Outcome Evaluation

5. What clinical and laboratory parameters are necessary to evaluate the therapy for achievement of the desired therapeutic outcome and to detect or prevent adverse effects?

Patient Education

6. What information should be provided to the patient to enhance compliance, ensure successful therapy, and minimize adverse effects?

■ FOLLOW-UP QUESTIONS

1. Five months later, Sally calls the STD clinic complaining of genital lesions that look and feel the same as the lesions she had 5 months earlier when seen and treated in the clinic. Should this episode of recurrent genital herpes be treated? If so, what therapies would be appropriate?

2. Is daily suppressive therapy indicated because she had a recurrent episode?

3. When is herpes treatment indicated for sexual partners?

4. When are chlamydia and gonorrhea treatment indicated for sexual partners?

5. What additional pharmacotherapeutic interventions should be made to address the drug therapy problems that were identified in question 1.a.?

■ SELF-STUDY ASSIGNMENTS

1. Determine whether there is a role for vaccines in the future management of herpes simplex disease.

2. Recommend alternative agents for the treatment of acyclovir-resistant herpes.

3. Explain the relationship between herpes simplex and HIV infections. Is there a role for herpes simplex virus suppressive therapy in preventing HIV transmission?

4. Describe herpes simplex complications that may require hospitalization, and recommend an appropriate treatment regimen.

CLINICAL PEARL

Most genital herpes infections are transmitted by persons who have asymptomatic viral shedding and are unaware that they have the infection. Systemic antiviral drugs control the signs and symptoms of genital herpes infection, but they do not eradicate latent virus.

REFERENCES

1. Centers for Disease Control and Prevention. Sexually transmitted diseases treatment guidelines 2006. MMWR Morb Mortal Wkly Rep 2006;55(RR-11):1–94. Available on the Internet at *www.cdc.gov/std/treatment.*

2. Valtrex caplets package insert. Research Triangle Park, NC, GlaxoSmithKline, July 2006.

3. Anonymous. Treatment guidelines from The Medical Letter—Drugs for sexually transmitted diseases. September 2007;61:81–90.

4. Famvir tablets package insert. East Hanover, NJ, Novartis Pharmaceuticals Corporation, December 2006.

5. Workowski KA, Berman SM. Centers for Disease Control and Prevention sexually transmitted diseases treatment guidelines. Clin Infect Dis 2007;44(Suppl 3):S73–S174.

6. Update to CDC's sexually transmitted diseases treatment guidelines 2006: fluoroquinolones no longer recommended for treatment of gonococcal infections. MMWR Morb Mortal Wkly Rep 2007;56: 332–336. Available at *http://www.cdc.gov/mmWR/preview/mmwrhtml/ mm5614a3.htm*

7. CDC Updated recommended treatment regimens for gonococcal infections and associated conditions—United States, April 2007. Available on the Internet at www.cdc.gov/std/treatment.

8. Corey L, Wald A, Patel R, et al. Once daily valacyclovir to reduce the risk of transmission of genital herpes. N Engl J Med 2004;350:11–20.

128

OSTEOMYELITIS AND SEPTIC ARTHRITIS

My Brother's Kicker . . . . .Level I

Edward P. Armstrong, PharmD, FASHP

Allan D. Friedman, MD, MPH

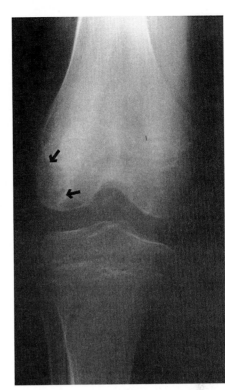

FIGURE 128-1. Lytic lesion of the distal right femur indicating osteomyelitis *(arrows)*.

LEARNING OBJECTIVES

After completing this case study, the reader should be able to:

- Recognize the most common presenting signs and symptoms of acute osteomyelitis and septic arthritis.

- Outline a treatment plan for empiric therapy of acute osteomyelitis and septic arthritis in a pediatric patient.

- Recommend alternative treatment approaches for acute osteomyelitis and septic arthritis in a pediatric patient if the initial treatment regimen fails.

- Outline monitoring parameters for antibacterial treatment of osteomyelitis and septic arthritis, including efficacy and toxicity of therapy.

PATIENT PRESENTATION

▦ Chief Complaint

"My knee still hurts."

▦ HPI

Jake Wilson is a 5-year-old boy referred to the Infectious Disease Clinic because of persistent right knee pain 1 month after being kicked in the right knee by his brother. The day after the incident, he was seen in urgent care because of right knee pain and was sent home with symptomatic therapy. He returned to urgent care 1 week later (3 weeks ago) because of persistent tenderness in that knee.

He was again sent home only to be seen 1 week later (2 weeks ago), at which time physical examination suggested and x-rays confirmed the diagnosis of osteomyelitis of the distal right femur (Fig. 128-1). He had a WBC count of $8.0 \times 10^3/mm^3$, an ESR of 21 mm/h, and tenderness over the right lateral femoral condyle. He underwent aspiration of the lesion, which revealed no pus. He was started on home IV therapy with cefuroxime 500 mg IV Q 6 h. He had continued to play soccer during the first 2 weeks after his injury.

He was seen 1 week ago because of increasing knee pain after 1 week of antibiotic therapy. He denied any systemic symptoms and was afebrile. His ESR had risen to 48 mm/h; x-rays showed an increased size of the femoral lytic lesion. Aspiration of the knee joint revealed purulent fluid. The bone culture and the knee aspirate revealed no growth. Arthroscopic surgery of the knee was performed and cefuroxime was continued.

Three days ago at an office visit with the orthopedic surgeon, his mother reported mild improvement of the pain. She related that his pain had diminished during the preceding 3 days; he could now sleep through the night. He was still unable to bear weight on his right leg and was only able to ambulate with crutches. His ESR was 56 mm/h.

▦ PMH

No prior history of serious diseases or infections
Immunizations are up-to-date

▦ FH

No family history of early childhood deaths secondary to severe infection

▦ SH

Mother and father live in the household and are well, as are three siblings. There are three dogs in the home.

▦ Meds

Cefuroxime 500 mg IV Q 6 h

▦ All

NKA

▦ ROS

No positive findings with regard to head, eyes, ears, nose, throat, cardiorespiratory systems, skin lesions, or recent illness. No recent travel. No other significant trauma.

■ **Physical Examination**

Gen

His general appearance is that of a thin, apprehensive boy in no distress unless his right knee is flexed, extended, or palpated.

VS

BP 93/50, P 104, RR 22, T 36.0°C; Wt 26.6 kg, Ht 4'4"

Skin

No lesions

HEENT

Eyes without corneal lesions, normal fundi; throat and pharynx without exudate; nose without discharge or congestion

Neck/Lymph Nodes

No lymphadenopathy or thyromegaly

Lungs/Thorax

Chest is clear to percussion and auscultation

CV

Normal S_1 and S_2; no murmurs present

Abd

Soft without hepatosplenomegaly

Genit/Rect

Genitalia are normal; circumcised male

MS/Ext

Swollen, slightly tender right knee held in flexion with marked decreased ROM. He has developed some tightness around the joint and is unable to bear weight on standing and preferred use of a posterior splint.

Neuro

Reflexes 2+; plantar reflexes downgoing; no cerebellar or sensorial abnormalities; normal strength and tone except where not measurable at the right knee

■ **Assessment**

Continued distal femoral osteomyelitis and adjacent septic arthritis of the right knee, secondary to delayed and partial treatment of a presumed staphylococcal infection. The persistently elevated ESR and slow resolution of knee symptoms are of concern.

QUESTIONS

Problem Identification

1.a. Create a list of the patient's drug therapy problems.

1.b. What information (signs, symptoms, laboratory values) indicates the presence or severity of acute osteomyelitis?

1.c. What information (signs, symptoms, laboratory values) indicates the presence of septic arthritis?

Desired Outcome

2. What are the goals of pharmacotherapy in this case?

Therapeutic Alternatives

3.a. What nondrug therapies might be useful for this patient?

3.b. What feasible pharmacotherapeutic alternatives are available for the empiric treatment of acute osteomyelitis?

Optimal Plan

4. What drug, dosage form, dose, schedule, and duration of therapy are best for this patient?

■ CLINICAL COURSE

An x-ray taken after low-dose antibiotic treatment showed a persistent lesion (Fig. 128-2). The I.D. consultant changed the therapy to cefazolin 100 mg/kg/24 h given in 3 divided doses. She recommended clinical reevaluation with repeat WBC and ESR in 1 week. If his ESR is the same, or (preferably) lower, cefazolin is to be discontinued and oral cephalexin 100 mg/kg/day in 4 divided doses is to be initiated. Reevaluation of the patient after 1 week of oral therapy was planned.

Ten days later, the patient was again seen in the Pediatric Infectious Disease Clinic where clinical evaluation revealed no additional findings. The patient continued to be afebrile and his ESR was 12 mm/h. He was still on crutches, but he had recently removed the right posterior leg splint. His mother had been helping him perform some passive range-of-motion exercises. His right leg was still maintained in a flexed position at the knee. He had full range of motion at the right hip but decreased flexion and extension at the right knee. The gastrocnemius circumference was slightly diminished on the right side, but strength on both plantar flexion and dorsiflexion of the right foot was normal. He had been tolerating the oral antibiotic regimen without apparent abdominal discomfort, diarrhea, or rash. Oral cephalexin was to be continued for at least three additional weeks at the same dose of 100 mg/kg/day.

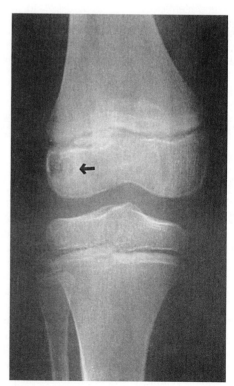

FIGURE 128-2. Persistent lesion of the distal right femur *(arrow)* after low-dose antibiotic treatment.

Outcome Evaluation

5. What clinical and laboratory parameters are necessary to evaluate the therapy for achievement of the desired therapeutic outcome and to detect or prevent adverse effects?

Patient Education

6. What information should be provided to the patient's caregiver to enhance compliance, ensure successful therapy, and minimize adverse effects?

■ SELF-STUDY ASSIGNMENTS

1. Plan alternative IV and oral treatment regimens in the event that the patient could not tolerate the antibiotic initially used.

2. Compare optimal oral treatment strategies for osteomyelitis in adults with those in children.

CLINICAL PEARL

The ultimate prognosis of acute osteomyelitis and septic arthritis is based on the speed of diagnosis, prompt initiation of appropriate antimicrobial therapy, and surgical drainage, if needed.

REFERENCES

1. Martinez-Aguilar G, Hammerman WA, Mason EO, et al. Clindamycin treatment of invasive infections caused by community-acquired, methicillin-resistant and methicillin-susceptible *Staphylococcus aureus* in children. Pediatr Infect Dis J 2003;22:593–598.

2. Karwowska A, Davies HD, Jadavji T. Epidemiology and outcome of osteomyelitis in the era of sequential intravenous-oral therapy. Pediatr Infect Dis J 1998;17:1021–1026.

3. Burnett MW, Bass JW, Cook BA. Etiology of osteomyelitis complicating sickle cell disease. Pediatrics 1998;101:296–297.

4. Nelson JD. Skeletal infections in children. Adv Pediatr Infect Dis 1991;6:59–78.

5. Unkila-Kallio L, Kallio MJ, Eskola J, et al. Serum C-reactive protein, erythrocyte sedimentation rate, and white blood cell count in acute hematogenous osteomyelitis of children. Pediatrics 1994;93:59–62.

6. Dagan R. Management of acute hematogenous osteomyelitis and septic arthritis in the pediatric patient. Pediatr Infect Dis J 1993;12:88–92.

7. Lew DP, Waldvogel FA. Osteomyelitis. N Engl J Med 1997;336:999–1007.

8. Kaplan SL, Deville JG, Yogev R, et al. Linezolid Pediatric Study Group. Linezolid versus vancomycin for treatment of resistant Gram-positive infections in children. Pediatr Infect Dis J 2003;22:677–686.

129

SEPSIS

Question the Source . . . . Level III

Christopher M. Scott, PharmD, BCPS

Tate N. Trujillo, PharmD, BCPS, FCCM

LEARNING OBJECTIVES

After completing the case study, the reader should be able to:

- Differentiate between SIRS, sepsis, septic shock, and severe sepsis with an understanding of the continuum that exists between them.

- List the variables (general, inflammatory, hemodynamic, organ dysfunction and tissue) used by health care professionals to diagnose sepsis.

- List the hemodynamic parameters that should be met during the first 6 hours of the diagnosis or identification of sepsis.

- Discuss the different components of the Surviving Sepsis Campaign as they relate to pharmacotherapy.

PATIENT PRESENTATION

■ Chief Complaint

The patient's primary caregiver reports that the patient has been vomiting a lot in the last few days.

■ HPI

Laura McChessney is a 74-year-old woman with a PMH significant for asthma and HTN who was sent from subacute care facility with hypokalemia, reports of nonbloody, nonbilious emesis (three to four episodes per day for 2–3 weeks), loose stools, decreased appetite, and chills. Patient denies dysuria/hematuria, chest pain, or dyspnea.

■ PMH

Asthma
HTN
OA
Morbid obesity
Depression

■ PSH

Partial SBO/ventral hernia 3 months ago
Cholecystectomy (unknown time frame)

■ FH

No HTN, DM, CA, or vascular disease

■ SH

One to two cigarettes every other day; stopped in the 1980s. Also stopped drinking alcohol in the 1980s.

■ Meds PTA

Albuterol MDI 2 puffs Q 6 h PRN
Ipratropium MDI 2 puffs Q 6 h
Theophylline ER 400 mg Q AM
Fluticasone inhaler 2 puffs BID
Lisinopril 10 mg po daily
Propoxyphene/acetaminophen 100 mg po Q 6 h PRN pain
Mirtazapine 15 mg po at bedtime
Promethazine 25 mg po Q 6 h PRN nausea/vomiting

■ All

NKDA

■ Physical Examination

Gen

Morbidly obese, white female in moderate distress

VS

BP 87/43, P 120–153, RR 14–33, T 37.8°C, SpO$_2$: 94% on 4L NC, Ins/Outs (24 hours): 8,489 mL/25 mL; Wt 145.5 kg, Ht 5'2"

HEENT

NCAT, PERRLA, no JVD, cap refill >3 seconds

Chest

Positive for expiratory wheezes throughout; tachypnea

CV

Tachycardia, regular rhythm; NL S_1/S_2, no MRG

Abd

+ pannus, unable to palpate organs, tenderness to deep palpation

Ext

No cyanosis/edema, 2+ pedal pulses

Neuro

A & O × 2 (not oriented to place)

▉ Labs

Na 133 mEq/L	Mg 2.5 mg/dL	Hgb 13.6 g/dL	pH 7.14
K 2.9 mEq/L	Phos 2.5 mg/dL	Hct 42%	pCO_2 26 mm Hg
Cl 98 mEq/L	Alb 2.1 g/dL	Plt 261 × 10³/mm³	pO_2 189 mm Hg
CO_2 12 mEq/L	Alk phos 127 IU/L	WBC 25.5 × 10³/mm³	HCO_3 8.9 mmol/L
BUN 13 mg/dL	T. bili 0.2 mg/dL	PMNs 58%	Base deficit −18.6
SCr 1.1 mg/dL	AST 11 IU/L	Bands 15%	mmol/L
Glu 100 mg/dL	ALT 7 IU/L	Lymphs 22%	Lactate 9.8 mmol/L
Ca 6.9 mg/dL		Monos 5%	
		Theophylline 39 mcg/mL	

EKG: sinus tach (113), but with artifacts, QRS 98/QT-QT_c 358/425

▉ Clinical Course

After spending several hours waiting in the ED for a ward bed, Ms. McChessney developed hypotension (systolic in the low 50–60s) refractory to fluids, altered mental status, and decreased urine output. Ms. McChessney also required intubation and was placed on the mechanical ventilator at that time secondary to respiratory failure and the inability to protect her airway. The primary team is concerned about septic shock. Over the next 30 minutes to 1 hour, she was started on the following medications:

> Norepinephrine 20 mcg/min
> Vasopressin 0.04 units/min
> Propofol 25 mcg/kg/min
> Fentanyl 50 mcg/h
> Levofloxacin 500 mg IV daily

▉ Assessment

74-year-old female in septic shock with acute respiratory and renal failure; probable intra-abdominal infection.

QUESTIONS

Problem Identification

1.a. Create a list of this patient's drug therapy and disease state problems.

1.b. What information (signs, symptoms, laboratory values) indicates the presence or severity of the problem or disease?

Desired Outcome

2. What are the goals of patient care in this case?

Therapeutic Alternatives

3.a. What interventions and/or therapies should be accomplished within the first 6 hours of all septic shock or severe sepsis patients?

3.b. What type of fluid should be recommended to appropriately resuscitate patients with septic shock and/or severe sepsis?

3.c. When should vasopressor agents be considered in the treatment of hypotension related to sepsis, and which agents are appropriate?

3.d. When should you consider inotropic agents in this patient's therapy, and which agents are appropriate?

3.e. When are corticosteroids used to treat septic shock?

3.f. When would you recommend recombinant human activated protein C (rhAPC) or drotrecogin alfa (activated) (Xigris) for this patient?

3.g. What other supportive care issues should be implemented for all severe sepsis patients?

3.h. What economic and ethical considerations are applicable to this patient?

Optimal Plan

4. The surgical critical care team has determined that Ms. McChessney has severe sepsis with a possible intra-abdominal source. Design an optimal sepsis treatment regimen for Ms. McChessney.

Outcome Evaluation

5. What clinical and laboratory parameters are necessary to evaluate the therapy for achievement of the desired therapeutic outcome and to detect or prevent an adverse effect?

▉ SELF-STUDY ASSIGNMENTS

1. Design evidence-based usage criteria for drotrecogin alfa (activated) taking into account the contraindications, precautions, and the patient population in whom this agent may be most beneficial.

2. Compare and contrast the available literature supporting the use of corticosteroids in severe sepsis focusing on the dosing and diagnosis of relative adrenal insufficiency.

CLINICAL PEARL

Propofol often precipitates hypotension in patients who do not have adequate intravascular volumes. Alternative sedative agents should be sought when hypotension is encountered with propofol. Propofol may cause other problems in severe sepsis patients because it is formulated in a lipid emulsion that may contribute to the inflammatory process as well as provide unnecessary fat calories (1.1 kcal/mL).

REFERENCES

1. Levy MM, Fink MP, Marshall JC, et al. 2001 SCCM/ESICM/ACCP/ATS/SIS International Sepsis Definitions Conference. Crit Care Med 2003;31:1250–1256.

2. Rivers E, Nguyen B, Havstad S, et al. Early goal-directed therapy in the treatment of severe sepsis and septic shock. N Engl J Med 2001;345:1368–1377.

3. Dellinger RP, Carlet JM, Masur H, et al. Surviving Sepsis Campaign guidelines for management of severe sepsis and septic shock. Crit Care Med 2004;32:858–873.

4. Annane D, Sebille V, Charpentier C, et al. Effect of treatment with low doses of hydrocortisone and fludrocortisone on mortality in patients with septic shock. JAMA 2002;288:862–871.

5. Marik PE, Kiminyo K, Zaloga GP. Adrenal insufficiency in critically ill patients with human immunodeficiency virus. Crit Care Med 2002;30: 1267–1273.

6. Eli Lilly and Company. Xigris package insert. Indianapolis, Indiana; April 2007. Available at: *www.xigris.com*. Accessed July 21, 2007.

7. Bernard GR, Vincent JL, Laterre PF, et al. Efficacy and safety of recombinant human activated protein C for severe sepsis. N Engl J Med 2001;344:699–709.

8. van den Berghe G, Wouters P, Weekers F, et al. Intensive insulin therapy in the critically ill patients. N Engl J Med 2001;345:1359–1367.

9. ASHP therapeutic guidelines on stress ulcer prophylaxis. ASHP Commission on Therapeutics and approved by the ASHP board of directors on November 14, 1998. Am J Health Syst Pharm 1999;56:347–379.

10. Solomkin JS, Mazuski JE, Baron EJ, et al. Guidelines for the selection of anti-infective agents for complicated intra-abdominal infections. Clin Infect Dis 2003;37:997–1005.

130

DERMATOPHYTOSIS

Toeing the Line . . . . .Level I

Scott J. Bergman, PharmD

Douglas Slain, PharmD, BCPS

LEARNING OBJECTIVES

After completing this case study, the reader should be able to:

- Recognize the signs and symptoms of a dermatophyte infection.
- Discuss the risk factors for developing a dermatophyte infection.
- Recommend an appropriate treatment plan for a dermatophyte infection.
- Explain the best way for the patient to use a selected antifungal product.

PATIENT PRESENTATION

Chief Complaint

"My socks and underwear itch."

HPI

Dave Harvester is a 21-year-old man who presents to the local pharmacy because of recent itching in the area of his undergarments. He is a college football player who plays offensive line for the local college football team. Two-a-day practices started several weeks ago in preparation for the upcoming football season, and the temperature has been extremely hot outside. He sweats profusely during practice but always showers in the locker room before going home. He has not changed laundry detergent recently, nor does he think that the equipment manager has changed detergents. He admits that he doesn't wash his uniform between practices. He also admits that his feet have always smelled bad, but he first started to notice the burning and itching about 4 weeks ago. He started applying some moisturizing cream to his feet a few days ago, but it

has only made a very slight improvement thus far. Now his groin is beginning to itch as well.

PMH

Appendectomy 4 years ago
GERD diagnosed 2 years ago

SH

Denies recent sexual activity (within past year)
Denies tobacco use
Drinks beer on weekends after games and practice

Meds

Pantoprazole 20 mg daily
Multivitamin daily
Whey protein shakes every morning
Grapefruit juice (8 ounces) every morning

All

Penicillin (rash as a baby)

ROS

Denies fever and chills. Fatigued from football practice. Reports frequent trauma to feet while playing football. Complains of itching between his toes and in his groin area.

Physical Examination (limited)

Gen

An obese, but athletic-looking young man wearing sandals, shorts, and a T-shirt.

VS

BP 118/78, P 60, RR 18; Wt 105 kg, Ht 5'11"

Skin

Visible regions are moist and soft

Abd

Fat rolls can be seen around his belly

Genit/Rect

Not directly examined, but patient reports pruritus and burning of skin around groin, not on penis or scrotum. Redness can be seen on the medial aspects of the upper thighs.

MS/Ext

Foul-smelling, dry, scaling feet with white flaking between toes
Toenails on both feet appear to have yellow-brown discoloration
The toenails of the some of the toes appear to be thicker than the rest, particularly on the right foot

Labs

None available

Assessment

1. Athlete's foot (tinea pedis)
2. Possible onychomycosis
3. Jock itch (tinea cruris)
4. Unsanitary foot and body hygiene

QUESTIONS

Problem Identification

1.a. What are this patient's drug therapy problems?

1.b. What information leads you to this conclusion?

1.c. What risk factors does the patient have for these conditions?

1.d. What pathogen is most likely to cause these infections?

1.e. What tests could be done at a doctor's office to confirm diagnosis of these conditions?

Desired Outcome

2. What are the goals of treatment in this case?

Therapeutic Alternatives

3.a. What nonpharmacologic measures should be recommended to this patient?

3.b. What pharmacologic treatments can be sold to this patient without a prescription?

3.c. What additional pharmacologic treatments could be used if a prescription is obtained from the patient's physician?

Optimal Plan

4.a. What treatment option would you recommend for this patient and why? Include drug, dosage form, strength, frequency, and duration of therapy.

4.b. If this treatment fails to work, what would you suggest and why?

Outcome Evaluation

5.a. How would you determine whether your treatment succeeded?

5.b. What side effects would you monitor for?

Patient Education

6. What would you say to the patient (in layman's terms) when counseling on how to treat his condition with the selected antifungal product? Include how to take the medication and what to expect from it in terms of efficacy and possible side effects.

■ CLINICAL COURSE

You see the patient in your pharmacy 2 months later and find out that his tinea infections have been successfully treated. He has not had any more difficulty with itching at practice or in games. He tells you that his doctor started him on itraconazole capsules for the toenail infection, based on the laboratory evaluation of his nail specimens. Despite 2 months' worth of treatment, his nails have not improved at all. This is frustrating to him because the medication is very expensive and he was told to limit his beer drinking while taking the drug.

■ FOLLOW-UP QUESTIONS

1. What were this patient's risk factors for developing onychomycosis?

2. What are the differences between appropriate treatment of onychomycosis and tinea pedis?

3. What are some possible reasons for the lack of efficacy of itraconazole after 2 months of treatment?

■ SELF-STUDY ASSIGNMENTS

1. Explain the situations where it is necessary to refer a patient to a physician for the treatment of dermatophytes and when oral therapy is preferred over topicals.

2. Read about the mechanisms of action of the azole and allylamine antifungals.

3. Review the association of oral terbinafine and oral itraconazole-associated hepatotoxicity.

CLINICAL PEARL

Over 70% of the population will experience a mycotic infection of the skin, hair, or nail at some point in their lifetime.

REFERENCES

1. Goldstein AO, Smith KM, Ives TJ, et al. Mycotic infections. Effective management of conditions involving the skin, hair, and nails. Geriatrics 2000;55:40–42, 51–52.

2. Nadalo D, Montoya C, Hunter-Smith D. What is the best way to treat tinea cruris? J Fam Pract 2006;55:256–258.

3. Gupta AK, Ryder, Chow M, et al. Dermatophytosis: the management of fungal infections. Skinmed 2005;4:305–310.

4. Singal A, Pandhi D, Agrawal S, et al. Comparative efficacy of topical 1% butenafine and 1% clotrimazole in tinea cruris and tinea corporis: a randomized, double-blind trial. J Dermatolog Treat 2005;16:331–335.

5. Patel A, Brookman SD, Bullen MU, et al. Topical treatment of interdigital tinea pedis: terbinafine compared with clotrimazole. Australas J Dermatol 1999;40:197–200.

6. Gupta AK, Tu LQ. Therapies for onychomycosis. Dermatol Clin 2006;24:375–379.

7. Penzak SR, Gubbins PO, Gurley BJ, et al. Grapefruit decreases the systemic availability of itraconazole capsules in healthy volunteers. Ther Drug Monit 1999;21:304–309.

8. Crawford F, Young P, Godfrey C, et al. Oral treatments for toenail onychomycosis: a systematic review. Arch Dermatol 2002;138:811–816.

131

BACTERIAL VAGINOSIS

Competition among Bacteria . . . . Level I

Charles D. Ponte, BS, PharmD, BC-ADM, BCPS, CDE, FAPhA, FASHP, FCCP

LEARNING OBJECTIVES

After completing this case study, the reader should be able to:

• Identify predisposing factors associated with bacterial vaginosis.

• List the common clinical and diagnostic findings associated with bacterial vaginosis.

• Develop a therapeutic plan for the management of bacterial vaginosis.

• Describe the role of the pharmacist in the overall management of infectious vaginitis.

PATIENT PRESENTATION

Chief Complaint

"I'm here for a follow-up visit."

HPI

Charlotte Webber is a 25-year-old female graduate student who comes to the Family Practice Center for a rescheduled follow-up visit for acute urethral syndrome. She missed her initial follow-up appointment 2 weeks ago. She was diagnosed 1 month ago and started on doxycycline 100 mg po BID × 7 days. At that time, a test for chlamydia was subsequently reactive. She states that she has completed her course of doxycycline despite some mild diarrhea attributed to the drug. Her sexual partners had been informed and were scheduled for treatment. She has resumed sexual activity since finishing the doxycycline and mentions that her period is 7 days late. She also complains of some mild vaginal discomfort (worse with intercourse) and a "fishy" vaginal odor. Her last period was approximately 5 weeks ago. She admits to inconsistent use of a diaphragm for contraception.

PMH

Noncontributory

FH

Noncontributory

SH

Is a graduate student in the School of Social Work. Has multiple sexual partners (including women); male partners rarely use condoms. Has smoked one pack of cigarettes per day since age 18. Alcohol use consists of a glass of wine nightly and occasional beer. Smokes an occasional marijuana joint.

Meds

Doxycycline 100 mg po BID × 7 days (completed with no problems except some mild diarrhea)
Multivitamin 1 po daily
Calcium supplement with vitamin D 1 po daily

All

Cats→itchy eyes and sneezing; house dust→watery eyes, sneezing; penicillin→hives-like pruritic rash

ROS

Noncontributory except that she has noticed a small amount of thin, white mucus on her underclothing.

Physical Examination

Limited because of follow-up for specific gynecologic complaint

Gen

Patient is a healthy appearing 25-year-old woman in NAD

VS

BP 110/70, P 90, RR 16, T 37°C; Wt 61.5 kg, Ht 5'5"

Genit/Rect

External genitalia WNL; no discharge expressed from the urethra, vagina with a small amount of thin white mucus; positive "whiff" test; pH 5.0. Cervix—not completely visualized; appears clear with a small amount of mucoid discharge from the os. Uterus is slightly enlarged, nontender, retroflexed, no cervical motion tenderness. Adnexa without tenderness or masses.

Labs

Microscopic examination of vaginal secretions: 20–25 WBC/hpf; 10–15 clue cells/hpf; 0 Lactobacilli/hpf; 15–20 squamous epithelial cells/hpf
Serum pregnancy test—positive

Assessment

Acute urethral syndrome—resolved
Bacterial vaginosis
Early pregnancy

QUESTIONS

Problem Identification

1.a. Create a list of the patient's drug therapy problems.

1.b. What clinical or laboratory information indicates the presence of bacterial vaginosis (Table 131-1)?

1.c. What is the pathophysiologic basis for the development of bacterial vaginosis?

1.d. Could the patient's problem have been caused by drug therapy?

Desired Outcome

2. What are the goals of pharmacotherapy in this case?

Therapeutic Alternatives

3.a. What feasible pharmacotherapeutic alternatives are available for the treatment of bacterial vaginosis?

TABLE 131-1	Characteristics of Different Types of Vaginitis			
Characteristic	**Candida**	**Bacterial**	**Trichomonas**	**Chemical**
Pruritus	++	+/-	+/-	++
Erythema	+	+/-	+/-	+
Abnormal discharge	+	+	+/-	–
Viscosity	Thick	Thin	Thick/thin	–
Color	White	Gray	White, yellow, green-gray	–
Odor	None	Foul, "fishy"	Malodorous	–
Description	Curd-like	Homogeneous	Frothy	–
pH	3.8–5.0	>4.5	5.0–7.5	–
Diagnostic tests	Potassium hydroxide prep. shows long, thread-like fibers of mycelia microscopically	+ "whiff test," "clue cells"	Pear-shaped protozoa, cervical "strawberry" spots	–

3.b. What economic, psychosocial, and ethical considerations are applicable to this patient?

Optimal Plan

4.a. What drug, dosage form, dose, schedule, and duration of therapy are best for this patient?

4.b. What alternatives would be appropriate if the initial therapy fails or cannot be used?

Outcome Evaluation

5. What clinical and laboratory parameters are necessary to evaluate the therapy for achievement of the desired therapeutic outcome and to detect or prevent adverse effects?

Patient Education

6. What information should be provided to the patient to enhance adherence, ensure successful therapy, and minimize adverse effects?

■ CLINICAL COURSE

After completion of the treatment you recommended, the patient returns to the clinic for follow-up. She voices no complaints except that she has been experiencing some vaginal itching and continued painful intercourse. Physical examination reveals a thick, whitish material adherent to the vaginal mucosa. Several white plaques are seen on the cervix. The vulva appears erythematous with excoriations on the labia majora. Microscopic analysis of vaginal secretions revealed hyphae and budding yeast. No white cells are noted. Vaginal pH is normal. The patient is diagnosed with vaginal candidiasis.

■ FOLLOW-UP QUESTIONS

1. What is the most likely cause of this patient's vaginal candidiasis?

2. What other issues should be addressed with the patient during this follow-up visit?

3. What is the role of the pharmacist in the management of patients with infectious vaginitis?

■ SELF-STUDY ASSIGNMENTS

1. Discuss the management of a patient who fails a specific course of treatment for bacterial vaginosis.

2. Discuss the pros and cons of screening asymptomatic pregnant women for the presence of bacterial vaginosis.

3. Describe the best therapeutic approach for a woman diagnosed with bacterial vaginosis who is breast-feeding her infant.

4. Discuss the role of sexual transmission in the pathogenesis of bacterial vaginosis.

CLINICAL PEARL

Patients should be counseled that oral metronidazole may cause a brownish discoloration of the urine resulting from the excretion of metabolites of the parent drug. This change in urine color does not reflect underlying urinary tract pathology.

REFERENCES

1. Yudin MH. Bacterial vaginosis in pregnancy: diagnosis, screening, and management. Clin Perinatol 2005;32:617–627.
2. Tam MT, Yungbluth M, Myles T. Gram stain method shows better sensitivity than clinical criteria for detection of bacterial vaginosis in surveillance of pregnant, low-income women in a clinical setting. Infect Dis Obstet Gynecol 1998;6:204–208.
3. Burstein GR, Murray PJ. Diagnosis and management of sexually transmitted disease pathogens among adolescents. Pediatr Rev 2003;24:75–82.
4. Nasraty S. Infections of the female genital tract. Prim Care 2003; 30:193–203.
5. Centers for Disease Control and Prevention. Diseases characterized by vaginal discharge. 2006 guidelines for treatment of sexually transmitted diseases. MMWR Morb Mortal Wkly Rep 2006;55(RR-11):1–94. Available at: www.cdc.gov.
6. Sobel JD. What's new in bacterial vaginosis and trichomoniasis? Infect Dis Clin North Am 2005;19:387–406.
7. Monif GRG. Bacterial vaginosis: a new perspective. Infect Med 2001;18:25–26.
8. Okun N, Gronau KA, Hannah ME. Antibiotics for bacterial vaginosis or *Trichomonas vaginalis* in pregnancy: a systematic review. Obstet Gynecol 2005;105:857–862.

132

CANDIDA VAGINITIS

When OTC Beats Rx. . . . . Level I

Rebecca M. T. Law, BS Pharm, PharmD

LEARNING OBJECTIVES

After completing this case study, the reader should be able to:

• Distinguish *Candida* vaginitis from other types of vaginitis.

• Know when to refer a patient with symptoms of vaginitis to a physician for further evaluation and treatment.

• Choose an appropriate product for the patient with *Candida* vaginitis.

• Educate patients with vaginitis about proper use of pharmacotherapeutic treatments and nonpharmacologic management strategies.

PATIENT PRESENTATION

■ Chief Complaint

"I'm having the same problem I had 2 weeks ago, and my doctor is away until next Monday. Can you give me some more of these suppositories?"

■ HPI

Sophie Kim is a 32-year-old woman who presents to your pharmacy with the above complaint. Upon further questioning, you find that she was diagnosed 3 weeks ago by her physician as having another vaginal *Candida* infection. She was prescribed nystatin suppositories 100,000 units intravaginally for 14 nights, which was the same as what she had been prescribed for her previous episode of vaginal candidiasis 2 months earlier. She stated that she had finished the prescription 1 week ago and had felt better then. However, 3 days ago she began to notice mild vaginal itching again. She thought it was her new control-top panty hose and stopped wearing them, but the itching got worse and became fairly severe with a burning sensation. There was also a white, dry, curd-like vaginal discharge that was nonodorous. This seemed to be identical to what she had experienced 3 weeks ago. Her physician is away until next week, and she wondered if the pharmacy can give her some more suppositories.

PMH

Diabetes type 1 since age 11. Her blood glucose is well controlled, and her physician is keeping a close eye due to her pregnancy.

Recurrent leg ulcers and foot infections for which she has been prescribed antibiotics on a frequent basis. Currently, there are no ulcers or infections, and she is not on antibiotics.

Last month, she began using tights (with an adjustable waist) to help prevent varicose veins.

SH

Nonsmoker; drinks alcohol in moderate amounts (one to two drinks maximum) at social functions. She is married and is $7^1/_2$ months pregnant.

Meds

Insulin glargine 15 units SC Q AM for past year
Insulin lispro 6 units SC 15 minutes prior to breakfast, 8 units 15 minutes prior to lunch, and 10 units 15 minutes prior to dinner, for past 4 months
Materna 1 po Q AM

All

NKDA

ROS

Not performed

Physical Examination

VS

BP 120/78; Wt 70 kg, Ht 5'5"

Note: No further assessments performed

Labs

Not available

QUESTIONS

Problem Identification

1.a. What signs and symptoms indicate the presence and severity of *Candida* vaginitis (Table 132-1)?

1.b. What predisposing factors for *Candida* vaginitis might exist in this patient?

Desired Outcome

2. What are the goals of therapy for this patient?

Therapeutic Alternatives

3. What pharmacotherapeutic alternatives are available for the treatment of *Candida* vaginitis?

Optimal Plan

4. Design a pharmacotherapeutic plan for this patient.

Outcome Evaluation

5. What parameters should be monitored to assess the efficacy of the treatment and to detect adverse effects?

Patient Education

6. What information should the patient receive about her treatment?

CLINICAL COURSE

The recommended treatment was successful. Two months later, Sophie had another episode of vaginal candidiasis, which was again successfully treated. She delivered a healthy 7-lb baby boy born at term. A month after that, she had another episode of *Candida* vaginitis, and she is now nursing.

FOLLOW-UP QUESTION

1. What is the most appropriate course of action for management of this patient's recurrent vaginitis?

SELF-STUDY ASSIGNMENTS

1. Obtain information on tests used to diagnose different types of vaginitis.

2. Compare the retail cost of nonprescription vaginitis treatments in your area.

TABLE 132-1 Characteristics of Different Types of Vaginitis

Characteristic	Candida	Bacterial	Trichomonas	Chemical
Pruritus	++	+/–	+/–	++
Erythema	+	+/–	+/–	+
Abnormal discharge	+	+	+/–	–
Viscosity	Thick	Thin	Thick/thin	–
Color	White	Gray	White, yellow, green-gray	–
Odor	None	Foul, "fishy"	Malodorous	–
Description	Curd-like	Homogeneous	Frothy	–
pH	3.8–5.0	>4.5	5.0–7.5	–
Diagnostic tests	Potassium hydroxide prep. shows long, thread-like fibers of mycelia microscopically	+ "whiff" test, "clue cells"	Pear-shaped protozoa, cervical "strawberry" spots	–

For some discussion of above conditions and diagnostic considerations see: Diseases characterized by vaginal discharge. CDC sexually transmitted diseases treatment guidelines, 2006. MMWR 2006;55(No. RR-11):49–56; and: Management and treatment of specific syndromes: vaginal discharge (bacterial vaginosis, vulvovaginal candidiasis, trichomoniasis). Canadian guidelines on sexually transmitted infections, 2006 edition. Public Health Agency of Canada. Available at: http://www.phac-aspc.gc.ca/std-mts/sti_2006/sti_intro2006_e.html.

3. Outline your plans for communicating your treatment recom mendations to the patient's physician.

CLINICAL PEARL

Patients with symptoms suggestive of bacterial vaginitis or sexually transmitted disease (fever, abdominal or back pain, foul-smelling discharge) should be referred to a physician for further evaluation and treatment.

REFERENCES

1. Diseases characterized by vaginal discharge. CDC sexually transmitted diseases treatment guidelines, 2006. MMWR 2006;55(No. RR-11):49–56.

2. Management and treatment of specific syndromes: vaginal discharge (bacterial vaginosis, vulvovaginal candidiasis, trichomoniasis). Canadian guidelines on sexually transmitted infections, 2006 edition. Public Health Agency of Canada. Available at: *http://www.phac-aspc.gc.ca/std-mts/sti_2006/sti_intro2006_e.html*. Accessed August 3, 2007.

3. Young GL, Jewell D. Topical treatment for vaginal candidiasis (thrush) in pregnancy (review). In: The Cochrane Library, Issue 3, 2007. Chichester, UK: John Wiley & Sons, Ltd. Abstract available at: *http://www.cochrane.org/reviews/en/ab000225.html*. Accessed on August 3, 2007.

4. Pappas PG, Rex JH, Sobel JD, et al. Guidelines for treatment of candidiasis. Clin Infect Dis 2004;38:161–189. Also available at National Guidelines Clearinghouse: *http://www.guideline.gov/summary/summary.aspx?ss=15&doc_id=4545&nbr=3359*. Accessed on July 30, 2007.

5. Sobel JD, Chaim W, Nagappan V, et al. Treatment of vaginitis caused by *Candida glabrata*: use of topical boric acid and flucytosine. Am J Obstet Gynecol 2003;189:1297–1300.

6. Briggs, GG, Freeman RK, Yaffe SJ. Drugs in Pregnancy and Lactation, 7th ed. Baltimore, MD, Williams and Wilkins, 2005.

7. U.S. FDA Center for Drug Evaluation and Research, CDER Drug Information. Miconazole vaginal cream and suppositories safety information. March 8, 2001. Available at: *http://www.fda.gov/cder/drug/infopage/miconazole/default.htm*. Accessed on August 6, 2007.

8. Sanchez JM, Moya G. Fluconazole teratogenicity. Prenat Diagn 1998;18:862–863.

9. Jick SS. Pregnancy outcomes after maternal exposure to fluconazole. Pharmacotherapy 1999;19:221–222.

10. Falagas ME, Betsi GI, Athanasiou S. Probiotics for prevention of recurrent vulvovaginal candidiasis: a review. J Antimicrob Chemother 2006;58:266–272.

11. Hilton E, Isenberg HD, Alperstein P, et al. Ingestion of yogurt containing Lactobacillus acidophilus as prophylaxis for Candidal vaginitis. Ann Intern Med 1992;116:353–357.

12. Ray D, Goswami D, Goswami R, et al. Prevalence of *Candida glabrata* and its response to boric acid vaginal suppositories in comparison with oral fluconazole in patients with diabetes and vulvovaginal candidiasis. Diabetes Care 2007;30:312–317.

Additional Resource: Clinical resources, CCHS Digital Library, University of Alabama. Available at: *http://cchs-dl.slis.ua.edu/clinical/std/vaginaldischarge/candidiasis.htm*. Accessed on July 30, 2007.

133

INVASIVE FUNGAL INFECTIONS

Fungus among Us. . . . . Level II

Douglas Slain, PharmD, BCPS

LEARNING OBJECTIVES

After completing this case study, the reader should be able to:

- Construct a prudent, empiric, antifungal regimen for a patient with invasive candidiasis or candidemia.

- Identify situations in which systemic antifungal therapy is warranted in patients with candiduria.

- Determine appropriate situations to use echinocandins for invasive *Candida* infections.

PATIENT PRESENTATION

HPI

Mary Yeasted is a 60-year-old woman who underwent an antrectomy via Billroth II procedure 7 days ago at a smaller outside hospital for intractable peptic ulcer disease. Postoperatively, the patient initially did well and diet was restarted on postoperative day 3. On postoperative day 5, the patient started complaining of increased intra-abdominal distention and increased pain. The patient had free air on her x-ray and was taken to the operating room for exploratory laparotomy, where she was found to have a pancreatic head necrosis and abscess and peritonitis. Peritoneal fluid (several PMNs) grew moderate Gram-negative rods and very rare budding yeast. The patient remained intubated postoperatively on propofol and was started on piperacillin-tazobactam, gentamicin, metronidazole, and phenylephrine for a septic appearance (Tmax = 38.2°C [100.8°F]). *Escherichia coli* was isolated from the peritoneal fluid. The organism was sensitive to piperacillin-tazobactam and gentamicin. The patient was started on IV fluconazole 200 mg × 1, then 100 mg daily 2 days ago for yeast that grew in the urine. The patient was transferred to our hospital last night. She was admitted to our MICU upon arrival. Work-up included CT abdomen/pelvis, an MRCP, and culture of blood, urine and abdominal drain fluid. The patient was transferred on TPN, hydromorphone 1–2 mg IV Q 4 h PRN, IV forms of home medications, piperacillin-tazobactam (3.375 mg Q 8 h), gentamicin (6 mg/kg/day), and metronidazole (500 mg Q 8 h). Lisinopril was held. It was determined that she had a duodenal stump leak, which was controlled via the right upper abdominal percutaneous drain. There was some drainage from her midline incision. Her skin was open and a wound vac was in place. The drain output was approximately 300 cc/day.

PMH

PUD
GERD
Seizure disorder
HTN

PSH

S/P vagotomy and pyloroplasty 1 year ago
S/P partial hysterectomy and bladder repair 10 years ago

FH

Mother died of colon cancer, aunt died of breast cancer

SH

Homemaker. Married, has three adult children. Denies smoking or ethanol use.

Home Meds

Pantoprazole 40 mg po once daily
Lisinopril 20 mg po once daily

Phenytoin 200 mg po BID
Acetaminophen 650 mg PRN aches and pains
Prevpac (lansoprazole, amoxicillin, and clarithromycin)—course completed 3 weeks ago

■ All

NKDA

■ Physical Examination

Gen

Patient is 60-year-old Caucasian woman who is intubated and ventilated (PC mode)

VS

BP 100/55, P 90, RR 20/14 (vent), T 38.2°C, O$_2$ sat 100%; Wt 120 lb, Ht 5'7"

Skin

Mildly clammy

HEENT

PERRLA, EOMI, nares patent

Neck/Lymph Nodes

Neck supple; no lymphadenopathy

Lungs/Thorax

CTA

Breasts

No rashes or palpable masses

Heart

Tachycardic. On dopamine to maintain MAP >60.

Abd

Tender, mildly distended
Midline supraumbilical incision, skin open with abscess drain and retention sutures, margins clean

GU

Grossly normal, Foley catheter in place (day 6)
ARF (SCr was 1.5 mg/dL yesterday)

MS/Ext

No deformity, +2 edema
Venodynes for DVT prophylaxis

Neuro

GCS: 3/intub/6

■ Labs

Na 135 mEq/L	Hgb 14.0 g/dL	WBC 16.8 × 10³/mm³	AST 35 IU/L
K 4.4 mEq/L	Hct 42%	PMNs 67%	ALT 30 IU/L
Cl 101 mEq/L	Plt 152 × 10³/mm³	Bands 13%	Alk phos 140 IU/L
CO$_2$ 21 mEq/L	Unbound serum	Lymphs 14%	LDH 240 IU/L
BUN 28 mg/dL	phenytoin:	Monos 5%	T. bili 2.1 mg/dL
SCr 1.4 mg/dL	2.2 mcg/mL	Eos 1%	PT 13 Sec
Glu 90 mg/dL	Gentamicin (trough):	Lipase 102 U/L	INR 1.2
Mg 1.9 mg/dL	1.2 mcg/mL	Amylase 412 U/L	Albumin 2.8 g/dL
			Pre-albumin 12 mg/dL

■ UA

Cloudy yellow, trace protein, glucose (–), ketones (–), pH 7.1, RBC 1/hpf, WBC 8/hpf, bacteria none, rare yeast (germ-tube-negative), nitrite (–)

■ Chest X-ray

No infiltrates

■ Assessment

1. Sepsis (peritonitis, UTI, or other source?)
2. Probable pancreatitis
3. Post-surgical duodenal stump leak
4. Elevated liver enzymes
5. Elevated phenytoin concentration
6. Malnutrition

■ Plan

Continue antibiotics and pressor support. Increase fluconazole to 400 mg IV daily. Change Foley catheter. Culture, blood, urine, and wound drainage. Monitor hemodynamics and end-organ function and hydrate with IV fluids.

For pancreatitis: Supportive care, IV fluids, PRN hydromorphone for pain and GI rest.

Drainage and consider surgical re-exploration when stable.

Monitor and avoid non-essential hepatic metabolized medications.

Hold phenytoin.

TPN.

QUESTIONS

Problem Identification

1.a. Create a list of the patient's drug therapy problems.

1.b. What information (signs, symptoms, laboratory values) indicates the presence or severity of each of the drug therapy problems?

Desired Outcome

2. What are the goals of pharmacotherapy for this patient's drug therapy problems?

Therapeutic Alternatives

3.a. What nondrug therapies might be useful for this patient?

3.b. What feasible pharmacotherapeutic alternatives are available for treating this infection?

Optimal Plan

4. What drug, dosage form, dose, schedule, and duration are best for this patient?

Outcome Evaluation

5. What clinical and laboratory parameters are necessary to evaluate the therapy for achievement of the desired therapeutic outcome and to detect or prevent adverse effects?

Patient Education

6. What information should be provided to the patient and/or the patient's caregiver to enhance compliance, ensure successful therapy, and minimize adverse effects?

■ CLINICAL COURSE

Despite 3 more days of continued broad spectrum antibiotic therapy the patient continues to be septic, but slightly improved. Her requirement for phenylephrine to maintain her blood pressure (around 110/60) has been titrated down. Notable abnormal labs include: SCr: 1.2 mg/dL, AST 40 IU/L, ALT 41 IU/L, Alk phos 140 IU/L, T. bili 2.0 mg/dL, amylase 386 U/L, and lipase 95 U/L.

Culture and sensitivity data are now available:

- *Abdominal Drainage Fluid* (drawn on admission to our MICU):
  - ✓ Many PMNs
  - ✓ Moderate *Candida glabrata*
  - ✓ Sensitivities:

Amphotericin B	1 mcg/mL	S
Fluconazole	32 mcg/mL	S-DD
Caspofungin	0.5 mcg/mL	No interpretation available
Voriconazole	0.5 mcg/mL	No interpretation available

- *Urine Culture* (drawn on admission to our MICU):
  - ✓ (+) for *C. glabrata* 1,000 cfu/hpf
- *Blood Cultures* (drawn 2 days ago):
  - ✓ Central catheter: Rare budding yeast
  - ✓ Right peripheral: No growth

The team decided to change fluconazole to IV caspofungin 70 mg × 1, then 50 mg Q day. The central line was changed. They also ordered an ophthalmology consult to check her for *Candida* endophthalmitis. After three more days, the patient continued to improve and was weaned off mechanical ventilation and transferred out of the MICU. A subsequent CT scan of the abdomen showed no evidence of any abnormalities that should be managed surgically. She will require surgical re-exploration when more stable and when her nutritional status is improved.

■ FOLLOW-UP QUESTIONS

1. What risk factors does Mrs. Yeasted have for invasive candidiasis?
2. Does the switch from fluconazole to caspofungin make good clinical sense in this patient after seeing the susceptibility report? Why or why not?

■ SELF-STUDY ASSIGNMENTS

1. Describe situations in which antifungal "prophylaxis" may be beneficial in the surgical intensive care setting.
2. Discuss treatment options for patients with candidemia and *Candida* endophthalmitis.
3. Explain how use of PNA FISH technology in the microbiology laboratory can reduce antifungal drug expenditures.

CLINICAL PEARL

Despite the general enhanced *in vitro Candida* activity of voriconazole over fluconazole, therapy with voriconazole may be affected by azole-class resistance mechanisms.

REFERENCES

1. Pappas PG, Rex JH, Sobel JD, et al. Guidelines for the treatment of candidiasis. Infectious Diseases Society of America. Clin Infect Dis 2004;38:161–189.

2. Dupont H, Pauggam-Burtz C, Muller-Serieys C, et al. Predictive factors of mortality due to polymicrobial peritonitis with *Candida* isolation in peritoneal fluid in critically ill patients. Arch Surg 2002;137:1341–1346.

3. Sobel JD, Bradshaw SK, Lipka CJ, et al. Caspofungin in the treatment of symptomatic candiduria. Clin Infect Dis 2007;44:e46–e49.

4. Mora-Duarte J, Betts R, Rotstein C, et al. Comparison of caspofungin and amphotericin B for invasive candidiasis. N Engl J Med 2002;347:2020–2029.

5. Deck DH, Guglielmo BJ. Pharmacological advances in the treatment of invasive candidiasis. Expert Rev Anti Infect Ther 2006;4:137–149.

134

INFECTIONS IN IMMUNOCOMPROMISED PATIENTS

Fever Pitch . . . . Level II

Douglas Slain, PharmD, BCPS

LEARNING OBJECTIVES

After completing this case study, the reader should be able to:

- Construct a prudent empiric antibiotic regimen for a febrile neutropenic patient.
- Determine appropriate situations to use vancomycin in empiric antimicrobial regimens for the treatment of febrile neutropenic episodes.
- Describe situations in which antibiotic monotherapy versus combination therapy would be warranted in the empiric treatment of febrile neutropenia.

PATIENT PRESENTATION

▓ Chief Complaint

"I have a fever and feel shaky."

▓ HPI

Tim P. Spiker is a 67-year-old man with stage IV prostate cancer with metastases to lymph nodes who is presenting with a 1-day history of fever (up to 39.4°C [102.9°F]) and chills. He underwent a second course of chemotherapy 5 days ago with liposomal doxorubicin and cyclophosphamide for hormone-refractory disease. He was given a dose of pegfilgrastim 2 days later. His wife reports that he had decreased energy starting 2 days ago. He initially had a temp of 38.3°C (100.9°F). He took some acetaminophen but still mounted a fever of 39.4°C (102.9°F) 3 hours later. He now has a cough with whitish sputum. He denies sinus or chest pain, but he has some mild body aches. He has been constipated for 2 days. His white blood count was $4.5 \times 10^3/mm^3$ in the ER, with 94% polys and 4% bands. He received a dose of ceftazidime 2 g, tobramycin 440 mg, and a ketorolac 30-mg injection in the ER.

▓ PMH

Stage IV prostate cancer with metastases
S/P external radiation
GERD

HTN
Hyperlipidemia
Diastolic heart failure (EF—60%)
Type 2 DM

Surgical History

Orchiectomy—5 years ago
Prostatectomy—radical 8 years ago
Hickman (tunneled central) catheter placed for chemo

FH

Mother died of pancreatic cancer, father died of MI at age 65

SH

Retired major league baseball umpire. Denies smoking or ethanol use.

Home Meds

Glipizide 20 mg po in AM, 10 mg po in PM
Atorvastatin 40 mg po once daily
Hydrochlorothiazide 12.5 mg po once daily
Furosemide 40 mg po once daily
Ferrous sulfate 300 mg po once daily
Promethazine suppositories pr PRN
Docusate sodium 100 mg po once daily
Omeprazole 20 mg po once daily
Diltiazem ER 180 mg po once daily
Aspirin 81 mg po once daily
Hydrocodone/acetaminophen 10 mg/500 mg po Q 6 h PRN

All

Codeine

ROS

(+) Diarrhea, (+) nausea; denies vomiting, cough, fever, or chills

Physical Examination

Gen

Patient is 67-year-old Caucasian man who appears to be very somnolent

VS

BP 98/50, P 110, RR 20, T 38.2°C, O_2 sat 98%; Wt 170 lb, Ht 5'9"

Skin

Warm and dry. No erythema or induration around port on left chest.

HEENT

PERRLA, EOMI, nares patent, moist mucous membranes; (+) mucositis

Neck/Lymph Nodes

Neck supple; no lymphadenopathy

Lungs/Thorax

Slightly decreased breath sounds at the bases

Heart

RRR, no murmurs, rubs, or gallops

Abd

Soft, NT, (+) bowel sounds, no masses palpable

Genit/Rect

Deferred

MS/Ext

No deformity, mild weakness, no peripheral edema

Neuro

A & O × 3; CN II–XII grossly intact, mild dysphagia, agnosia (per family)

Mental Status

Oriented to person and place

Lymphatic

No cervical lymphadenopathy

Labs

Na 135 mEq/L	Hgb 8.0 g/dL	WBC $4.5 \times 10^3/mm^3$	AST 53 IU/L
K 3.6 mEq/L	Hct 24.2%	PMNs 82%	ALT 51 IU/L
Cl 98 mEq/L	RBC $3.2 \times 10^6/mm^3$	Bands 4%	Alk phos 121 IU/L
CO_2 22 mEq/L	Plt $220 \times 10^3/mm^3$	Lymphs 14%	LDH 220 IU/L
BUN 38 mg/dL			T. bili 0.9 mg/dL
SCr 1.9 mg/dL			
Glu 100 mg/dL			
Ca 8.5 mg/dL			

UA

Pending

Blood Cultures

Left peripheral catheter: Pending
Right peripheral catheter: Pending
Hickman port: Pending

Chest X-Ray

Unremarkable

Assessment

1. Stage IV prostate cancer with metastases to lymph nodes
2. Febrile episode
3. Possible sepsis/hypotension
4. Elevated SCr; decreased renal function
5. Anemia (chronic)

Plan

1. Continue next chemotherapy cycle after resolution of neutropenia.
2. Draw another set of blood cultures and begin empiric antimicrobials:

    Ceftazidime 2 g IV Q 8 h (infused over 30 minutes)

    Ciprofloxacin 400 mg IV Q 8 h (infused over 30 minutes)
3. Hold BP medications while hypotensive.
4. Monitor renal function and hydrate with IV fluids.
5. Transfuse PRBCs and recheck in AM. Continue iron. Consider iron studies when stable.
6. Continue home medications except where noted, and add a laxative.

QUESTIONS

Problem Identification

1.a. Create a list of the patient's drug therapy problems.

1.b. What information (signs, symptoms, laboratory values) indicates the presence or severity of each of the drug therapy problems?

Desired Outcome

2. What are the goals of pharmacotherapy in this patient's case?

Therapeutic Alternatives

3.a. What nondrug therapies might be useful for this patient?

3.b. What feasible pharmacotherapeutic alternatives are available for treating this febrile episode?

Optimal Plan

4. What drug(s), dosage form(s), dose(s), schedule, and duration of therapy are best for the empiric treatment of this febrile episode in this patient?

Outcome Evaluation

5. What clinical and laboratory parameters are necessary to evaluate the therapy for achievement of the desired therapeutic outcome and to detect or prevent adverse effects?

Patient Education

6. What information should be provided to the patient to enhance compliance, ensure successful therapy, and minimize adverse effects?

■ CLINICAL COURSE

On day 2 of admission, the patient is still febrile and the following laboratory results are reported: SCr 1.6 mg/dL, Hgb 9.1g/dL, Hct 26.7%, platelets $205 \times 10^3/mm^3$. The WBC was $4.6 \times 10^3/mm^3$ with 46% PMNs and 4% bands (ANC $2.3 \times 10^3/mm^3$).

BP 130/70, P 110, RR 20, T 38.2°C, O$_2$ sat 98% RA

Blood cultures

- Left peripheral catheter: No growth at 24 hours

- Right peripheral catheter: No growth at 24 hours

- Hickman port: No growth at 24 hours

The team continued to monitor the patient as planned. On day 4 (ANC = $0.620 \times 10^3/mm^3$) of the admission, one-third of the blood culture bottles (the Hickman sample) were positive for Gram-positive cocci in pairs and clusters. The team added vancomycin 1 g Q 12 h at this point, stopped ciprofloxacin, and had the central line removed. On day 5 (ANC = $0.300 \times 10^3/mm^3$), the final identification of the organism in the blood was reported as *Staphylococcus aureus*, sensitive to oxacillin and vancomycin. Later that day, the team adjusted Mr. Spiker's antibiotic doses per his renal function. His SCr was 1.4 mg/dL. On day 7 (ANC = $0.150 \times 10^3/mm^3$), the patient became afebrile. Vital signs T 36.6°C, BP 125/75, P 70, RR 18. All subsequent blood and urine cultures were negative for microbial growth. A transesophageal echocardiogram did not show any vegetations. Mr. Spiker's neutropenia resolved (ANC ≥$1.0 \times 10^3/mm^3$) 4 days after becoming afebrile. Ceftazidime was stopped 2 days after resolution of neutropenia. Therapy with vancomycin was continued for a total of 2 weeks.

■ FOLLOW-UP QUESTIONS

1. What other antibiotic therapies could have been used for the treatment of Mr. Spiker's bacteremia?

2. Was the 2-week duration of vancomycin appropriate for this patient?

■ SELF-STUDY ASSIGNMENTS

1. Review the criteria for classification of febrile neutropenic patients as either "low" or "high" risk. What types of neutropenic patients would be considered "low risk" and might benefit from oral antibiotic regimens?

2. Perform a literature search to review the available data on the use of extended-interval aminoglycoside dosing in febrile neutropenia. Is there evidence to support the use of high-peak, extended-interval aminoglycoside dosing in the empiric treatment of febrile neutropenia?

3. Review the treatment of endocarditis. If a vegetation were found on Mr. Spiker's echocardiogram, would his bacteremia treatment have changed?

CLINICAL PEARL

Use of fluoroquinolones has been identified as an independent risk factor for both MRSA and *Clostridium difficile* infections.

REFERENCES

1. Klastersky J. Science and pragmatism in the treatment and prevention of neutropenic infection. J Antimicrob Chemother 1998;41(Suppl D):13–24.

2. Hughes WT, Armstrong D, Bodey GP, et al. 2002 guidelines for the use of antimicrobial agents in neutropenic patients with cancer. Clin Infect Dis 2002;34:730–751.

3. Mermel LA, Farr BM, Sherertz RJ, et al. Guidelines for the management of intravascular catheter-related infections. Clin Infect Dis 2001;32:1249–1272.

4. Paul M, Soares-Weiser K, Leibovici L. Beta lactam monotherapy versus beta lactam-aminoglycoside combination therapy for fever with neutropenia: systematic review and meta-analysis. BMJ 2003;326:1111–1119.

5. Donowitz GR, Maki DG, Crinch CJ, et al. Infections in the neutropenic patient: new views of an old problem. Hematology 2001;(Suppl):113–139.

135

ANTIMICROBIAL PROPHYLAXIS FOR SURGERY

In Life, Preparation Is Everything. . . . . .Level II

Curtis L. Smith, PharmD, BCPS

LEARNING OBJECTIVES

After completing this case study, the reader should be able to:

- Recommend appropriate antimicrobial prophylaxis for a given surgical procedure.

- Discuss the timing of antimicrobial prophylaxis for surgery, including doses prior to surgery and dosing after surgery.

- Describe the controversy regarding mechanical bowel preparation prior to colorectal surgery.

- Identify the pros and cons to using oral antimicrobial decontamination prior to colorectal surgery.

PATIENT PRESENTATION

Chief Complaint

"I have colon cancer."

HPI

Edward Adler is a 72-year-old man who was recently diagnosed with anemia and generalized weakness. The work-up for anemia included a colonoscopy, which showed a malignant neoplasm of the proximal ascending colon. The neoplasm was identified and the biopsy revealed moderately differentiated adenocarcinoma. The patient denies any current abdominal pain or change in bowel habits, but reports a 20-pound weight loss over the past several months. He is eating but has less of an appetite than normal.

PMH

Positive for hypertension, TIA, and chronic rhinitis; also mild osteoarthritis, for which he has required no regularly scheduled medications in the past. History of gastritis and anemia.

PSH

Tonsillectomy, left inguinal hernia repair, colonoscopy with biopsy

SH

Positive for smoking history of one-half of a pack daily; quit 20 years ago

Meds

Atenolol 100 mg po daily
Hydrochlorothiazide 12.5 mg po daily
Omeprazole 20 mg po daily
Aspirin 81 mg po daily
Nasacort nasal spray, two sprays in the morning
Ferrous sulfate 325 mg po TID
Multivitamin one po once daily

All

None

ROS

Cardiopulmonary: Denies chest pain, shortness of breath, or wheezing.
Gastrointestinal: Denies history of hepatitis, ulcers, or jaundice.
Genitourinary: He has no history of hematuria or renal calculi.
Musculoskeletal: Positive for arthritis of both wrists and hands.
Psychiatric: Positive for some depression.

Physical Examination

Gen

He has the appearance of a normally developed white male who appears his stated age. He is alert, awake, and in no obvious distress.

VS

BP 132/86, P 68, RR 11, T 37.1°C; Wt 69 kg, Ht 5'8"

Skin

Warm and dry. Multiple seborrheic dermatomes over the abdomen and chest.

HEENT

Face reveals no asymmetry. Pupils are equal. Eyes have no icterus or exophthalmus, extraocular muscles intact. He is wearing corrective lenses.

Neck/Lymph Nodes

No adenopathy or thyromegaly. There is no jugular venous distention.

Lungs/Thorax

Clear to auscultation

CV

Regular rate and rhythm without murmurs

Abd

The patient does have a faint, left inguinal scar from prior left inguinal hernia repair. The abdomen is without palpable masses, splenomegaly, or hepatomegaly. No tenderness noted.

Genit/Rect

Not examined

MS/Ext

No scoliosis. He has normal lordotic, kyphotic components to the vertebral curvature. No paravertebral tenderness or spasm. Leg lengths and shoulder heights are grossly equal. He was examined in the sitting and supine position. Extremities: no gross deformities, rashes, or ecchymoses. 2+ pulses in all four extremities.

Neuro

No gross motor or sensory deficits or hyperreflexia. Good grip strength bilaterally.

Labs

Na 132 mEq/L	Hgb 9.9 g/dL	WBC $6.0 \times 10^3/mm^3$
K 4.1 mEq/L	Hct 30.2%	PMNs 70%
Cl 97 mEq/L	RBC $4.06 \times 10^6/mm^3$	Bands 0%
CO_2 26 mEq/L	Plt $324 \times 10^3/mm^3$	Eos 5%
BUN 14 mg/dL	MCV 74 μm^3	Lymphs 13%
SCr 0.9 mg/dL	MCHC 32.8 g/dL	Monos 12%
Glu 93 mg/dL		
Alb 3.9 g/dL		

Assessment

1. Adenocarcinoma of the proximal ascending colon
2. Right hemicolectomy planned

QUESTIONS

Problem Identification

1.a. Based on the planned surgical procedure, what is the risk for a surgical wound infection in this patient postoperatively?

1.b. List all of the patient's drug-related problems, including potential postoperative problems.

Desired Outcome

2. What are the goals of antimicrobial pharmacotherapy for prevention of a surgical wound infection?

Therapeutic Alternatives

3.a. Discuss the pharmacologic options available for this patient to prevent a surgical wound infection. When would you dose antimicrobials related to the surgical procedure, and how long would you continue antibiotics after the procedure?

3.b. Will a mechanical bowel preparation prior to surgery benefit this patient?

3.c. What are the potential advantages and disadvantages associated with giving oral antibiotics prior to a colorectal surgical procedure?

Optimal Plan

4. What would you recommend for antimicrobial prophylaxis prior to this surgical procedure? Will this patient require additional antimicrobial dosing during the procedure? How long would you continue antibiotics following the procedure?

Outcome Evaluation

5. What clinical parameters should be monitored to assess the development of a surgical wound infection?

Patient Education

6. What information should be provided to this patient regarding the risk of surgical wound infections and the use of antibiotics to prevent this risk?

■ SELF-STUDY ASSIGNMENTS

1. Construct a chart listing surgical procedures requiring preoperative antimicrobial prophylaxis and the recommended agent(s) to use.

2. Perform a literature search and assess the current information regarding the use of oral antibiotics prior to colorectal surgery.

3. Perform a literature search and assess the current information regarding using postoperative antibiotics (for both less than and more than 24 hours).

CLINICAL PEARL

Patients who receive antibiotics for surgical prophylaxis within 3 hours after the surgical incision have a three-times higher risk of surgical wound infection compared to patients who receive antibiotics within 2 hours before the incision.

REFERENCES

1. National Nosocomial Infections Surveillance (NNIS) system report, data summary from January 1992 to June 2004, issued October 2004. Am J Infect Control 2004;31:470–485.
2. Burger W, Chemnitius JM, Kneissl GD, et al. Low-dose aspirin for secondary cardiovascular prevention—cardiovascular risks after its perioperative withdrawal versus bleeding risks with its continuation—review and meta-analysis. J Intern Med 2005;257:399–414.
3. Fleisher LA, Beckman JA, Brown KA, et al. ACC/AHA 2006 Guideline Update on Perioperative Cardiovascular Evaluation for Noncardiac Surgery: Focused Update on Perioperative Beta-Blocker Therapy. A Report of the American College of Cardiology/American Heart Association Task Force on Practice Guidelines (Writing Committee to Update the 2002 Guidelines on Perioperative Cardiovascular Evaluation for Noncardiac Surgery). J Am Coll Cardiol 2006; 47:2343–2355.
4. Geerts WH, Pineo GF, Heit JA, et al. Prevention of venous thromboembolism. Chest 2004;126:338S–400S.
5. Bratzler DW, Houck PM. Surgical Infection Prevention Guidelines Writers Workgroup. Antimicrobial prophylaxis for surgery: an advisory statement from the National Surgical Infection Prevention Project. Clin Infect Dis 2004;38:1706–1715.
6. Scher KS. Studies on the duration of antibiotic administration for surgical prophylaxis. Am Surg 1997:63:59–62.
7. Antimicrobial Prophylaxis for Surgery. Treatment Guidelines from the Medical Letter. 2006;4:83–88.
8. Lewis RT. Oral versus systemic antibiotic prophylaxis in elective colon surgery: a randomized study and meta-analysis send a message from the 1990s. Can J Surg 2002;45:173–180.
9. Classen DC, Evans RS, Pestotnik SL, et al. The timing of prophylactic administration of antibiotics and the risk of surgical-wound infection. N Engl J Med 1992;326:281–286.
10. Fonseca SNS, Kunzle SRM, Junqueira MJ, et al. Implementing 1-dose antibiotic prophylaxis for prevention of surgical site infection. Arch Surg 2006;141:1109–1113.
11. Guenaga KF, Matos D, Castro AA, et al. Mechanical bowel preparation for elective colorectal surgery. Cochrane Database Syst Rev 2005: CD001544.

136

PEDIATRIC IMMUNIZATION

Shots for Tots . . . . .Level II

Jean-Venable "Kelly" R. Goode, PharmD, BCPS, FAPhA, FCCP

LEARNING OBJECTIVES

After completing this case study, the reader should be able to:

• Develop a plan for administering any needed vaccines, when given a patient's age, immunization history, and medical history.

• Describe appropriate use of pediatric vaccines.

• Educate a child's parents on the risks associated with pediatric vaccines and ways to minimize adverse effects.

• Recognize *inappropriate* reasons for deferring immunization.

PATIENT PRESENTATION

■ Chief Complaint

"My son is here for the 'Shots for Tots' program."

■ HPI

Tim Madison is a 12-month-old boy who is generally healthy. He presents today (August 30, 2008) to the pharmacy with his mother for evaluation and to receive any needed immunizations.

■ PMH

Some prenatal care, delivered at 42 weeks' gestation via uncomplicated vaginal delivery; birth weight 7 lb, 4 oz. Mother states that her child has had several ear infections and three or four "colds," no other illnesses.

■ FH

Nonsignificant

SH

Mother age 26, father age 28. No siblings. Mother works part-time. Father works as an electrician.

Meds

Amoxicillin suspension 300 mg po TID
No recent OTC medication use

All

NKDA

ROS

Negative

Physical Examination

Gen

Alert, happy, appropriately developed 12-month-old infant in NAD. Wt 11.4 kg (77th percentile), length 31 in (80th percentile)

VS

BP 102/53, P 115, RR 28, T 36.7°C (axillary)

HEENT

AF open, flat; PERRL; funduscopic exam not performed; ears slightly red; normal looking TMs, landmarks visualized, no effusion present; nose clear; throat normal

Lungs

Clear bilaterally

Cor

RRR, no murmurs

Abd

Soft, nontender, no masses or organomegaly; normal bowel sounds

Genit/Rect

Normal external genitalia; rectal exam deferred, no fissures noted

Ext

Normal

Neuro

Alert; normal DTRs bilaterally

Labs

No other labs obtained

Assessment

Normal-appearing infant, in need of immunizations

Immunization Record Card

Name: Tim Madison

Vaccine	Dose/Route/Site	Date	Health Professional	VIS
Hepatitis B	0.5 mL IM thigh	8/15/2007	Colter, RN	Hep B
Pediarix (DTaP, Hep B, IPV)	0.5 mL IM thigh	10/20/2007	Edwards, RN	Hep B, IPV, DTaP
PCV	0.5 mL IM thigh	10/20/2007	Edwards, RN	PCV
Hib (HibTITER)	0.5 mL IM thigh	10/20/2007	Edwards, RN	Hib
Pediarix	0.5 mL IM thigh	12/29/2007	Edwards, RN	DTaP, Hep B, IPV
PCV	0.5 mL IM thigh	12/29/2007	Edwards, RN	PCV
Hib (HibTITER)	0.5 mL IM thigh	12/29/2007	Edwards, RN	Hib

QUESTIONS

Problem Identification

1. Create a list of the patient's immunization-related problems including any contraindications or precautions for vaccination.

Desired Outcome

2.a. What immediate goals are reasonable in this case?

2.b. What long-term goals are appropriate for comprehensive management of this patient?

Therapeutic Alternatives

3.a. How do health care providers determine which vaccines an infant or child needs?

3.b. What is the proper immunization administration technique for infants and toddlers, including location and needle size?

3.c. What vaccines should be administered to this child today, including dose, route, and any alternatives?

Optimal Plan

4.a. What immunization schedule should be followed for this patient today?

4.b. In addition to immunizations received today, what should be the plan for providing additional immunizations and when should they be administered?

Outcome Evaluation

5. How should the response to the immunization plan be assessed?

Patient Education

6. What important information about vaccination needs to be explained to this infant's mother?

■ FOLLOW-UP QUESTION

1. The next year, the mother brings the child to a pediatric influenza immunization clinic. The child's immunization record reveals influenza vaccine 0.25 mL × 1 dose last fall. What is your recommendation for influenza vaccine for this child?

■ SELF-STUDY ASSIGNMENTS

1. Review the most current immunization recommendations for persons aged 0–6 years, and provide a summary of how your recommendations for this case would be different if a 6-month-old patient in need of immunizations came into your clinic today.

2. Surf the Internet for immunization-related websites about vaccine associated adverse effects; compare and contrast these sites and evaluate them against reliable websites for vaccine information.

CLINICAL PEARL

Even though childhood immunization rates surpassed the Healthy People 2010 goal for 19–35 months of age, it is estimated that only 2–26% of children receive vaccinations as recommended. Pharmacists should advocate for parents and caregivers to have their children immunized on time to protect them against vaccine-preventable diseases.

REFERENCES

1. American Academy of Pediatrics. Active and passive immunization. In: Red Book—Report of the Committee on Infectious Diseases, 27th ed. Elk Grove Village, IL, American Academy of Pediatrics, 2006:1–103.
2. CDC. Advisory Committee on Immunization Practices. Recommended immunization schedules for persons aged 0–18 years—United States, 2008. MMWR 2008;57;Q1–Q4 (updated annually at *http://www.cdc.gov/vaccines/recs/schedules/child-schedule.htm#printable*).
3. CDC. General Recommendations on Immunization. Recommendations of the Advisory Committee on Immunization Practices (ACIP). MMWR 2006;55(No. RR-15):1–37.

137

ADULT IMMUNIZATION

Immunizations: Not Just Kid Stuff . . . . Level II

Jean-Venable "Kelly" R. Goode, PharmD, BCPS, FAPhA, FCCP

LEARNING OBJECTIVES

After completing this case study, the reader should be able to:

- Develop a plan for administering any needed vaccines when given a patient's age, immunization history, and medical history.
- Recognize appropriate precautions and contraindications for vaccination, including inappropriate reasons for deferring vaccination.
- Explain appropriate administration of vaccines, including timing and spacing of both inactive and live attenuated vaccines.
- Recognize the differences in vaccines for young adults currently in use in the United States.

PATIENT PRESENTATION

Chief Complaint

"I'm here to get my new prescription filled."

HPI

Sandra Williams is a 23-year-old woman who presents to your pharmacy with a new prescription for prednisone 40 mg BID for 10 days in January. She has had a moderate asthma exacerbation. She just started her new job as an elementary school teacher. She is a new patient to your pharmacy. She inquires about your "One less" signs about a new vaccine available.

PMH

Moderate persistent asthma
Chickenpox at age 5 per patient

FH

One sister—healthy
Mother—healthy
Father with Type 2 diabetes

SH

Does not smoke
Drinks alcohol socially

Meds

Albuterol MDI 2 inhalations PRN
Pulmicort DPI 2 inhalations once daily

All

NKDA

Immunization Record

No vaccines since kindergarten except:

Meningococcal vaccine before she started her freshman year in college
One dose of hepatitis B vaccine before she started her freshman year in college
MMR vaccine before she started her freshman year in college
Td 10 years ago at her adolescent well-check-up

ROS

WDWN Caucasian woman in NAD

VS

BP 120/72 (left arm, large cuff, seated) P 76; Wt 60 kg, Ht 5'5"

Physical Examination

Deferred

Assessment

23-year-old woman recently treated for a moderate asthma exacerbation. She is in need of immunizations today.

QUESTIONS

Problem Identification

1.a. Create a list of the patient's immunization-related problems, including any contraindications or precautions for vaccination.

1.b. Create a list of this patient's drug-related problems.

Desired Outcome

2.a. What immediate immunization goals are reasonable in this case?

2.b. Provide the rationale for administering each of the recommended vaccines to this patient.

2.c. What long-term goals are appropriate for comprehensive management of this patient?

Therapeutic Alternatives

3. Identify the therapeutic alternatives for addressing this patient's immunization needs.

Optimal Plan

4. What immunization schedule should be followed for this patient today, including dose and route of administration and the plan for providing additional immunizations?

Outcome Evaluation

5. How should the response to the immunization plan be assessed?

Patient Education

6. What important information about vaccination needs to be explained to this patient?

■ FOLLOW-UP QUESTIONS

1. What screening questions should a patient be asked prior to administering any vaccinations?

2. What must be documented after a health care practitioner administers a vaccination?

■ SELF-STUDY ASSIGNMENTS

1. Review the most current immunization recommendations for adults, and provide a summary of how your recommendations for this case would be different if this person were 62 years of age with diabetes.

2. Develop a list of diseases and medications indicating that a patient may be a candidate for immunization.

3. Research the laws in your state to verify which vaccines pharmacists may administer. Also, explore how to implement an immunization service in your practice.

4. Review the guidelines for vaccination of pregnant women.

5. Surf the Internet for immunization-related websites about vaccine-associated adverse effects; compare and contrast these sites; and evaluate them against reliable websites for vaccine information.

CLINICAL PEARL

Delays in vaccination put patients at risk of vaccine-preventable diseases. However, there is no need to restart an immunization series if the interval between doses is longer than that recommended in the routine schedule. Instead of starting over, merely count the doses administered (provided that they were given at an acceptable minimum interval) and complete the series.

REFERENCES

1. Centers for Disease Control and Prevention. General Recommendations on Immunization. Recommendations of the Advisory Committee on Immunization Practices (ACIP). MMWR 2006;55(No. RR-15):1–37.

2. Centers for Disease Control and Prevention. Prevention of Varicella. Recommendations of the Advisory Committee on Immunization Practices (ACIP). MMWR 2007;56(No. RR04):1–40.

3. Centers for Disease Control and Prevention. Prevention and Control of Influenza. Recommendations of the Advisory Committee on Immunization Practices (ACIP). MMWR 2007;56(No. RR06):1–54.

4. Centers for Disease Control and Prevention. Quadrivalent Human Papillomavirus Vaccine. Recommendations of the Advisory Committee on Immunization Practices (ACIP). MMWR 2007;56(No. RR-2):1–23.

5. Centers for Disease Control and Prevention. Preventing tetanus, diphtheria, and pertussis among adolescents: use of tetanus toxoid, reduced diphtheria toxoid and acellular pertussis vaccine. Recommendations of the Advisory Committee on Immunization Practices ACIP). MMWR 2006;55(No. RR-3):1–34.

6. Centers for Disease Control and Prevention. A Comprehensive Immunization Strategy to Eliminate Transmission of Hepatitis B Virus Infection in the United States. Recommendations of the Advisory Committee on Immunization Practices ACIP. MMWR 2006;55(No. RR-16):1–33.

7. Centers for Disease Control and Prevention. Prevention of Hepatitis A through Active or Passive Immunization. Recommendations of the Advisory Committee on Immunization Practices ACIP. MMWR 2006;55(No. RR-07):1–23.

138

HIV INFECTION

The Antiretroviral-Naive Patient . . . . .Level II

Mariela Díaz-Linares, PharmD

Keith A. Rodvold, PharmD, FCCP

LEARNING OBJECTIVES

After completing this case study, the reader should be able to:

• Describe situations in which antiretroviral therapy should be initiated in patients with HIV infection, and determine the desired outcome of such therapy.

• Recommend appropriate first-line antiretroviral therapies for the antiretroviral-naive person.

• Provide patient education on the proper dose, administration, and adverse effects of antiretroviral agents.

PATIENT PRESENTATION

■ Chief Complaint

"I am here for routine care."

■ HPI

Sally Smith is a 27-year-old woman diagnosed with HIV infection 2 years ago during routine exam. At the time of diagnosis, the patient was asymptomatic. During the 2 years since her diagnosis, her disease has been stable with regular clinic and laboratory follow-up every 4 months.

Today she returns for a routine follow-up visit.

■ PMH

HIV infection diagnosed 2 years ago; risk factor heterosexual contact
Appendectomy age 15

■ FH

Noncontributory

■ SH

History of crack cocaine use, last use 3 years ago.
Tobacco 1 PPD, ETOH 1–2 drinks on weekends.
Full-time employed at candy factory—stable shift.
Sexually active with stable partner; 100% condom use. He is HIV (–) and is aware of her HIV status.

■ Medications

Multivitamin one daily
Pepcid AC 20 mg PRN

■ All

NKDA

■ ROS

No active problems

Physical Examination

Gen

Thin, well-developed black female in NAD, alert and oriented × 3

VS

BP 107/54, P 68, RR 18, T 36.4°C; Wt 55 kg, Ht 5'2"

Skin

Anicteric, has large tattoo on back of neck. No other skin lesions noted.

HEENT

No oral lesions, sinuses nontender, PERRLA, ears and nose clear

Neck

Supple, no thyromegaly, L neck lymph node 0.5 cm in diameter

Chest

Lungs clear

CV

S_1, S_2 without S_3, S_4 or murmur

Abd

(+) BS, soft, nontender, without HSM

GU

The pelvic exam reveals normal external genitalia. The vaginal vault is within normal limits. Perineum and perianal regions are free of grossly visible lesions. Guaiac (−) stools.

Ext

No wasting, no CCE

Neuro

No focal deficits

Labs

See Table 138-1

Assessment

27-year-old woman with HIV infection and no other comorbidities, shows steady decline in CD4 cell count and rising levels of HIV viremia since her initial diagnosis 2 years ago

TABLE 138-1	Laboratory Values for the Previous Visit and for Subsequent Visits			
Parameter (units)	**2 Years Ago**	**This Visit**	**6 Weeks Later**	**12 Weeks Later**
General				
Weight (kg)	60	55	56	58
Hematology				
Hgb (g/dL)	13.6	12.9	12.7	13.1
Hct (%)	39.9	37.0	38.5	38.6
Plt (× 10³/mm³)	220	114	145	161
WBC (× 10³/mm³)	3.9	3.3	3.3	3.4
Lymphs (%)	34.6	28.4	34.3	40.1
Monos (%)	5.0	4.7	5.8	5.5
Eos (%)	1.0	1.9	1.5	1.0
Basos (%)	0.7	0.5	0.7	0.8
Neutros (%)	55.0	60.2	53.6	58.4
ANC (× 10³/mm³)	2.1	1.9	1.7	1.9
Chemistry				
BUN (mg/dL)	12	11	14	13
SCr (mg/dL)	0.4	0.5	0.6	0.5
T. bili (mg/dL)	–	0.6	–	0.6
Alb (g/dL)	–	4.4	–	4.4
AST (IU/L)	21	22	–	25
ALT (IU/L)	19	18	–	20
Fasting glucose	78	88		80
Fasting lipid profile				
T. chol	–	153	–	163
Triglycerides	–	81	–	98
LDL	–	125	–	128
Surrogate Markers				
CD4 (%)	33	18	–	15
CD4 (cells/mm³)	568	269	–	450
CD8 (%)	40	54	–	51
HIV RNA (RT-PCR)[a] (copies/mL)	25,000	350,000	1,000	<50
Antiviral resistance test (genotypic resistance test)	No antiviral resistant mutations detected	–	–	–
Hepatitis virus serologies				
HBV Ab	Negative			
HBV Core Ab total	Negative			
HBV Ag	Negative			
HCV Ab	Negative			
HAV Ab	Negative			

[a]Reverse transcriptase polymerase chain reaction assay.

QUESTIONS

Problem Identification

1.a. What information (signs, symptoms, laboratory values) indicates the severity of HIV disease?

1.b. Is prophylactic therapy for any associated opportunistic pathogen indicated in this patient? Why or why not?

1.c. What is your recommendation regarding antiretroviral therapy for this patient?

Desired Outcome

2. What are the goals of pharmacotherapy in this case?

Therapeutic Alternatives

3.a. What therapeutic options are available for treating this antiretroviral-naive patient?

3.b. What economic, psychosocial, racial, and ethical considerations are applicable to this patient?

3.c. How would you evaluate patient readiness for antiretroviral treatment initiation?

Optimal Plan

4.a. Propose an antiretroviral regimen for this woman. Indicate the drug name, dosage form, dose, schedule, and duration of therapy for the regimen you choose.

4.b. Design an antiretroviral regimen that would be appropriate if the patient informs you that she would like to consider becoming pregnant once her HIV infection is under control.

4.c. Recommend an antiretroviral regimen that would be appropriate if this patient has a history of chronic kidney disease, not requiring hemodialysis.

4.d. Discuss the role of HIV resistance testing in designing a regimen for the antiretroviral treatment-naive patient.

CHAPTER 139

Outcome Evaluation

5. What clinical and laboratory parameters are necessary to evaluate the clinical efficacy and toxicity of the antiretroviral regimen selected? Specify frequency with which you will monitor these parameters. Indicate therapeutic goal.

Patient Education

6.a. What important information would you provide to this patient about her therapy?

6.b. Explain in non-technical terms the surrogate markers and their use in monitoring HIV disease.

6.c. Identify potential barriers to medication adherence, and discuss potential strategies to overcome these barriers and maximize treatment adherence.

■ CLINICAL COURSE

The provider and patient accepted your treatment recommendations. The patient returns to the clinic for follow-up 6 weeks and 12 weeks after treatment initiation. Her treatment flow sheet is as follows:

Parameter	6 Weeks Later	12 Weeks Later
HIV RNA (RT-PCR)	1,000 copies/mL	<50 copies/mL
CD4 lymphocyte count	NA	450 cells/mm^3
Symptoms of HIV infection	Asymptomatic	Asymptomatic
Adverse events reported	Mild nausea, no vomiting	None
Concomitant medications	Oral contraceptives	Oral contraceptives
	MVI	MVI

■ FOLLOW-UP QUESTIONS

1. Provide an assessment of the antiretroviral regimen efficacy at each follow-up visit.

2. Identify potential problems with her concomitant medications and discuss alternatives.

■ SELF-STUDY ASSIGNMENTS

1. Review the current literature regarding recommended therapy for the antiretroviral-naive and treatment-experienced individuals. What is the recommended first-line therapy, and what are the indications to change to alternative therapy? What is known about therapy of HIV and survival?

2. Review the current literature regarding the development of HIV resistance to antiretroviral agents and strategies for the prevention and management of resistance.

CLINICAL PEARL

Despite the increasing body of clinical data to guide initial antiretroviral therapy in treatment-naive patients, the choice of the optimal regimen remains a complex issue. The ideal time to start treatment for asymptomatic patients is constantly revised based on expert opinion and available cohort data. In addition to potency and efficacy factors, clinicians must take into account a wide range of individual factors, including comorbid conditions, transmitted resistant virus, adherence, potential adverse events, drug–drug or drug–food interactions, and consequences of virologic failure for the particular regimen selected. Clinicians should always individualize therapeutic choices based on available data and unique patient factors.

REFERENCES

1. Centers for Disease Control. 1993, AIDS surveillance case definition for adolescents and adults. MMWR Morb Mortal Wkly Rep 1992;41(RR-17):1–9.

2. Centers for Disease Control. Appendix: revised surveillance case definition of HIV infection. MMWR Morb Mortal Wkly Rep 1999;48(RR-13):29–31.

3. US Public Health Service (USPHS) and Infectious Diseases Society of America (IDSA). Guidelines for the prevention of opportunistic infections in persons infected with human immunodeficiency virus—2002. Accessed at: www.aidsinfo.nih.gov.

4. Guidelines for the use of antiretroviral agents in HIV-infected adults and adolescents. Department of Health and Human Services (DHHS) Panel on Antiretroviral Guidelines for Adults and Adolescents. October 10, 2006. Accessed at: www.aidsinfo.nih.gov.

5. Hammer SM, Saag MS, Schecter M, et al. Treatment for adult HIV infection. 2006 Recommendations of the International AIDS Society-USA Panel. JAMA 2006;296:827–843.

6. Hammer SM. Management of newly diagnosed HIV infection. N Engl J Med 2005;353:1702–1710.

7. Aberg JA, Gallant JE, Anderson J, et al. Primary care guidelines for the management of persons infected with human immunodeficiency virus: recommendations of the HIV Medicine Association of the Infectious Diseases Society of America. Clin Infect Dis 2004;39:609–629.

8. Patterson DL, Swindells S, Mohr J, et al. Adherence to protease inhibitor therapy and outcomes in patients with HIV infection. Ann Intern Med 2000;133:21–30.

9. Novak RM, Chen L, MacArthur RD, et al. Prevalence of antiretroviral drug resistance mutations in chronically HIV-infected, treatment-naive patients: implications for routine resistance screening before initiation of antiretroviral therapy. Clin Infect Dis 2005;40:468–474.

10. Little SJ, Holte S, Routy JP, et al. Antiretroviral-drug resistance among patients recently infected with HIV. N Engl J Med 2002;347:385–394.

139

HIV AND HEPATITIS C CO-INFECTION

Viral Invasion. . . . . Level III

Jennifer J. Kiser, PharmD

Peter L. Anderson, PharmD

Courtney V. Fletcher, PharmD

LEARNING OBJECTIVES

After completing this case study, the reader should be able to:

- Identify when changes in antiretroviral therapy are warranted.

- Identify important considerations for choosing alternative antiretroviral therapies.

- Understand the concept of HIV genotyping.

- Identify pharmacologic interactions between antiretroviral drugs and medications used to treat hepatitis C.

- Utilize the primary and secondary literature to provide pharmacotherapy recommendations for conditions without definitive treatment guidelines.

PATIENT PRESENTATION

Chief Complaint

"I am here to find out if I need to switch my HIV meds, and I feel very weak and tired."

HPI

Erica Edwards is a 54-year-old woman with HIV and hepatitis C virus (genotype 1b) co-infection. She has been taking zidovudine, lamivudine, and efavirenz to treat HIV for approximately 5 years. Nine weeks ago, she began treatment with peginterferon alfa-2a and ribavirin for hepatitis C. Although her HIV viral load was undetectable when she began treatment for hepatitis C (HIV RNA <20 copies/mL, CD4 283 cells/mm^3), it has been elevated at her last two clinic visits. Complete hematology profile, fasting lipids, CMP, and HIV genotype were obtained 1 week ago and the results have returned.

PMH

Pneumocystis carinii pneumonia 5 years ago
HIV infection diagnosed 10 years ago—precise duration of infection unknown
Hepatitis C infection diagnosed 5 years ago—precise duration of infection unknown
Tubal ligation 15 years ago
Type 2 diabetes
Hypertension

FH

Noncontributory

SH

Single, lives with her three teenage children and her elderly mother. Works full-time as a waitress. IV drug use approximately 15 years ago. Smokes one pack of cigarettes per day. Recovering alcoholic, last drink 1 year ago.

Meds

Bactrim DS 1 po daily
Zidovudine 300 mg po BID (as Combivir)
Lamivudine 150 mg po BID (as Combivir)
Efavirenz 600 mg po at bedtime
Peginterferon alfa-2a 180 mcg SC every Friday
Ribavirin 600 mg po BID
Metformin 1000 mg po BID
HCTZ 25 mg po daily

All

NKDA

Immunizations

Influenza annually
Pneumococcal vaccine 5 years ago

ROS

Persistent fatigue/weakness, occasional flu-like symptoms from interferon injections, longstanding mild numbness and tingling in lower extremities bilaterally

Physical Examination

Gen

Somnolent, African-American woman in NAD, 10 lb (intentional) weight loss over the past 3 months

VS

BP 127/73, P 68, RR 18, T 36.8°C; Wt 72 kg, Ht 5'6"

Skin

No visible lesions

HEENT

PERRLA; no papilledema; fundi normal; ears and nose clear; oral cavity without inflammation, exudate, or lesions

Neck/Lymph Nodes

Supple; good range of motion; no fat accumulation on upper back/neck

Lungs/Thorax

CTA

CV

NSR, normal S$_1$ and S$_2$; no rubs, murmurs, or gallops

Abd

No pain or tenderness, no hepatosplenomegaly, BS (+), some accumulation of fat in abdominal area

Genit/Rect

Guaiac (–) stool; no visible genital or anal lesions; pap smear/vaginal exam not performed

MS/Ext

Pedal pulses 2+, no edema, nails normal, normal ROM, no cyanosis, no clubbing

Neuro

A & O × 3; Babinski (–); CN II–XII intact; normal strength, coordination, and gait, depressed ankle reflexes, decreased sensation and response to painful stimuli in lower extremities bilaterally, prior nerve conduction studies reveal slightly slowed nerve conduction velocity in lower extremities bilaterally

Labs

See Table 139-1

Liver Biopsy Findings Approximately 1 Year Ago

Grade 2 inflammation and stage 3–4 fibrous portal extension

HIV Genotype

K103N, no other significant mutations

Assessment

Failure to suppress plasma HIV RNA levels to "below detection" (i.e., persistent HIV viremia)
Hepatitis C responding to peginterferon alfa-2a and ribavirin treatment
Anemia
Peripheral neuropathy

QUESTIONS

Problem Identification

1.a. Create a list of the patient's drug therapy problems.

TABLE 139-1 Serial Laboratory Values Beginning 1 Year Prior to the Present Visit

Parameter (units)	1 Year Ago	6 Months Ago	9 Weeks Ago (Start IFN/RBV)	5 Weeks Ago	1 Week Ago
Liver Panel					
Albumin (g/dL)	3.2	3.5	3.4	3.3	3.1
AST (IU/L)	280	47	46	51	38
ALT (IU/L)	527	75	85	64	42
Alk phos (IU/L)	85	77	72	86	121
T. bili (mg/dL)	0.6	0.6	0.8	0.7	0.6
INR (sec)		1.12			
Chemistry					
Na (mEq/L)	137	136	138	139	140
K (mEq/L)	3.7	3.5	4.3	3.9	4.2
Cl (mEq/L)	99	102	104	103	106
CO_2 (mEq/L)	26	25	24	26	25
BUN (mg/dL)	15	11	8	10	14
SCr (mg/dL)	1.2	1.1	1.3	1.0	1.0
Glu (mg/dL)	115	89	91	98	102
Ca (mg/dL)	9.5	8.9	8.2	8.9	9.7
Fasting Lipid Profile					
Cholesterol (mg/dL)	176			163	
Triglycerides (mg/dL)	184			172	
Thyroid Function					
TSH (mIU/L)	3.3		3.1		3.3
Hemoglobin A1C					
A1C (%)	8.5	8.0	6.2		6.0
Hematology					
RBC ($\times 10^6/mm^3$)	4.39	4.68	3.88	3.32	2.95
Hgb (g/dL)	14.9	15.2	14.8	12.3	11.4
Hct (%)	44.7	45.6	44.4	36.9	34.2
Plt ($\times 10^3/mm^3$)	170	162	160	152	148
MCV (μm^3)	107	111	109	106	109
WBC count ($\times 10^3/mm^3$)	9.4	7.8	6.8	4.2	4.0
Lymphs (%)	26.3	34.4	64.2	44.9	40.9
Monos (%)	7.5	10.8	10.9	10.2	10.3
Eos (%)	0.6	0.8	0.2	0.4	0.1
Basos (%)	0.0	0.2	0.2	0.0	1.3
Neutros (%)	65.6	53.8	24.6	44.5	47.3
Virology					
CD4 (cells/mm^3)	276		283		272
HIV RNA (copies/mL) by RT-PCR method	<20	143	<20	566	4,324
HCV RNA (copies/mL)	>500,000				<60

1.b. What information (signs, symptoms, laboratory values) indicates the presence or severity of the patient's drug therapy problems?

1.c. What additional information is needed to satisfactorily assess this patient?

Desired Outcome

2. What are the desired goals of pharmacotherapy in this case?

Therapeutic Alternatives

3. What nondrug and pharmacologic treatments are available for this patient's drug therapy problems?

Optimal Plan

4. What drug(s), dose(s), and schedule(s) should be used to treat the HIV infection in this patient?

Outcome Evaluation

5. What clinical and laboratory parameters are necessary to evaluate each of the patient's drug regimens for achievement of the desired therapeutic outcomes and to detect or prevent adverse effects?

Patient Education

6. What information should be provided to the patient to enhance adherence, ensure successful therapy, and minimize adverse effects?

■ CLINICAL COURSE

The patient presents to the emergency department approximately 12 weeks after her last clinic visit. At her last visit, the zidovudine, lamivudine, and efavirenz were discontinued, and she initiated an antiretroviral regimen of tenofovir disoproxil fumarate 300 mg po once daily (as Truvada), emtricitabine 200 mg po once daily (as Truvada), and atazanavir/ritonavir 300/100 mg po once daily. She has had two undetectable HIV viral loads (HIV RNA <20 copies/mL) since switching to this antiretroviral regimen. Her anemia has improved with the treatment you recommended, and she continues to receive peginterferon alfa-2a and ribavirin for the treatment of hepatitis C. However, she reports a 3-day history of muscle weakness, myalgias, fatigue, and polyuria. On physical exam, she exhibits slow motor function, poor fine-motor control, diffuse muscle tenderness, and decreased muscle strength in all four extremities. The rest of her physical exam is normal. Abnormal laboratory findings include: serum potassium 1.9 mEq/L, serum chloride 107 mEq/L, serum bicarbonate 19 mEq/L—with an anion gap of 9, demonstrating a hyperchloremic non-anion gap metabolic acidosis; serum phosphorus is 1.2 mg/dL, urine protein 30 mg/dL, urine glucose 500 mg/dL, creatinine kinase 755 IU/L, and serum creatinine 2.5 mg/dL.

■ FOLLOW-UP QUESTIONS

1. Which medications may have contributed to the development of Fanconi syndrome in this patient?

2. What pharmacotherapeutic interventions would you make at this time?

■ SELF-STUDY ASSIGNMENTS

1. Review the current literature on treatment of hepatitis C in patients co-infected with HIV.

2. Review the current literature regarding the use of combination antiretroviral therapy, with special regard to new agents, potential drug interactions, and the use of ritonavir to increase plasma exposures of other concomitant protease inhibitors.

3. Review the literature regarding resistance testing for patients with HIV disease.

4. Review the current guidelines for treating opportunistic infections, including when to initiate and withdraw primary and secondary prophylaxis.

5. Review the literature on HIV-associated renal diseases and highly active antiretroviral therapy–induced nephropathy.

CLINICAL PEARL

Approximately 25% of patients infected with HIV are also infected with hepatitis C virus. Although data regarding optimal treatment of patients co-infected with HIV and HCV are incomplete, the threat of liver disease is too great to delay treatment. Clinicians must be vigilant in identifying and managing the additive toxicities of concomitant HIV and HCV therapy.

REFERENCES

1. Guidelines for the prevention of opportunistic infections in persons infected with HIV—November 28, 2001. Available at: *www.aidsinfo.nih.gov/guidelines.*

2. Tien PC. Management and treatment of hepatitis C virus infection in HIV-infected adults: recommendations from the Veterans Affairs Hepatitis C Resource Center Program and National Hepatitis C Program Office. Am J Gastroenterol. 2005;100:2338–2354.

3. Luciano CA, Pardo CA, McArthur JC. Recent developments in the HIV neuropathies. Curr Opin Neurol 2003;16:403–409.

4. Guidelines for the use of antiretroviral agents in HIV-infected adults and adolescents—October 10, 2006. Available at: *www.aidsinfo.nih.gov/guidelines.*

5. Fried MW. Side effects of therapy of hepatitis C and their management. Hepatology 2002;36:S237–S244.

6. Torriani FJ, Rodriguez-Torres M, Rockstroh JK, et al. Peginterferon alfa-2a plus ribavirin for chronic hepatitis C virus infection in HIV-infected patients (APRICOT). N Engl J Med 2004;351:438–450.

7. Dieterich DT, Spivak JL. Hematological disorders associated with hepatitis C virus infection and their management. Clin Infect Dis 2003;37:533–541.

8. Brau N. Update on chronic hepatitis C in HIV/HCV-coinfected patients: viral interactions and therapy. AIDS 2003;17:2279–2290.

9. Lai AR, Tashima KT, Taylor LE. Antiretroviral medication considerations for individuals coinfected with HIV and hepatitis C virus. AIDS Patient Care and STDs 2006;20:678–692.

10. Röling J, Schmid H, Fischereder M, et al. HIV-associated renal diseases and highly active antiretroviral therapy-induced nephropathy. Clin Infect Dis 2006;42:1488–1495.

140

BREAST CANCER

Neoadjuvant Therapy in Locally
Advanced Disease. . . . . Level II

Chad Barnett, PharmD, BCOP

LEARNING OBJECTIVES

After completing this case study, students should be able to:

- Design a pharmacotherapeutic plan for treatment of locally advanced breast cancer.
- Develop an appropriate monitoring plan for patients receiving adjuvant hormonal therapy for treatment of breast cancer.
- Describe appropriate follow-up for patients after definitive treatment of breast cancer.
- Provide patient education on the proper dosing, administration, and adverse effects of capecitabine.

PATIENT PRESENTATION

Chief Complaint

"I have a lump in my breast."

HPI

Rosalita Garza is a 61-year-old woman presenting for evaluation of a new mass in her left breast. She first noticed a palpable breast mass on self-examination approximately 14 months ago but was unable to have this further investigated due to loss of health insurance. The patient describes the mass as intermittently painful. A mammogram was performed prior to her current visit, which was suspicious for malignancy.

PMH

Musculoskeletal injury in 2000. Fell from a chair while at work and suffered injuries to her cervical spine. She has required bone grafting from her right hip to her cervical spine. She is taking multiple medications for pain control.
Depression (diagnosed 7 years ago).

FH

Sister diagnosed with breast cancer at age 60, now 5 years post-surgery. The patient was unable to recall any further details. No other significant cancer history is noted.

SH

Lives with and acts as primary caretaker for her mother, who has dementia. Denies alcohol use and is a non-smoker. Has a 35-year-old daughter who also lives with her.

Endocrine History

Menarche age 13; menopause age 55; first child age 26; $G_1P_1A_0$. Last PAP smear at age 40. Took Premarin as HRT for 5 years after the onset of menopause.

Meds

Pepcid 20 mg po BID
Zoloft 50 mg po once daily
Ambien 10 mg po at bedtime PRN sleep
Neurontin 300 mg po TID
Darvon 65 mg 1–2 po Q 4 h PRN pain

All

NKDA

ROS

Negative except for complaints noted above

Physical Examination

Gen

WDWN 61-year-old Hispanic female. Awake, alert, in NAD.

VS

BP 127/71, P 89, RR 16, T 36.7°C; Wt 163 lb, Ht 5'5"

HEENT

NC/AT; PERRLA; EOMI; ear, nose, throat are clear

Neck/Lymph Nodes

Supple. No lymphadenopathy, thyromegaly, or masses. No supra-clavicular or infraclavicular adenopathy.

Breasts

Left: Notable for a 2.5-cm mass at the 6 o'clock position, approximately 3 cm from the nipple margin, not fixated to skin; no nipple retraction or discharge is visualized; the mass is exquisitely tender to palpation; 1.5 cm, nontender, palpable mass in the axilla noted.
Right: Without mass or lymphadenopathy.

Lungs

CTA and percussion

CV

RRR; no murmurs, rubs, or gallops

Abd

Soft, NT/ND, normoactive bowel sounds. No appreciable hepato-splenomegaly.

Spine

Slight tenderness to percussion

Ext

No CCE

Neuro

No deficits noted

▓ Labs

Na 142 mEq/L	Hgb 12.9 g/dL	WBC $8.7 \times 10^3/mm^3$	AST 36 IU/L
K 3.7 mEq/L	Hct 37.6%	Neutros 55%	ALT 17 IU/L
Cl 102 mEq/L	RBC $4.13 \times 10^6/mm^3$	Lymphs 35%	LDH 488 IU/L
CO_2 26 mEq/L	Plt $410 \times 10^3/mm^3$	Monos 8%	T. bili 0.2 mg/dL
BUN 9 mg/dL	PT 11.9 sec	Eos 2%	CA 27.29 36.2 U/mL
SCr 0.7 mg/dL	INR 1.09		CEA 1.2 ng/mL
Glu 83 mg/dL	aPTT 30.1 sec		

▓ Chest X-Ray

Lungs are clear

▓ Other

Diagnostic bilateral mammogram (Fig. 140-1):

1. American College of Radiology Category V, highly suspicious for malignancy in the left breast. There is a high density, irregular mass measuring 2.2 cm with indistinct margins seen in the left breast lower hemisphere at 6 o'clock located 3 cm from the nipple.

2. In the right breast, no dominant mass, distortion, or suspicious calcifications are identified.

Unilateral ultrasound left breast and left axilla with biopsy:

1. An ill-defined, hypoechoic mass is noted in the 5:00–6:00 region. This measures approximately $2.5 \times 2.3 \times 1.5$ cm and is located 3 cm from the nipple. A core biopsy of this mass was performed.

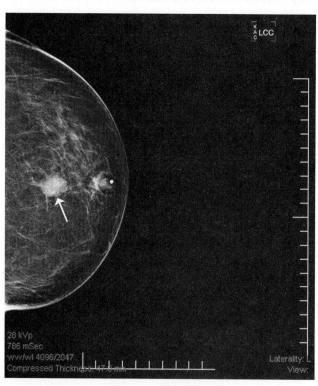

FIGURE 140-1. Mammogram of left breast. *Arrow* indicates area of abnormality highly suspicious for malignancy.

2. Suspicious lymph nodes are noted in the axilla. The largest node measures $1.8 \times 1.8 \times 1.4$ cm. A fine needle aspiration of this lymph node was performed. In the infraclavicular region, a few hypoechoic lymph nodes were also seen and were located in the lateral aspect. The largest node measured $0.8 \times 0.8 \times 0.8$ cm. A fine needle aspiration of this infraclavicular lymph node was performed. No suspicious internal mammary or supraclavicular lymph nodes were seen.

Core needle biopsy of left breast mass:

Left breast, 6 o'clock: infiltrating ductal carcinoma, modified Black's nuclear grade II (moderately differentiated), ER 95%, PR 95%, Her2 overexpression 2+, Her2 FISH negative (no amplification), ki67 30% (moderate).

Fine needle aspiration (FNA) of left axillary and infraclavicular lymph nodes:

1. Left axillary lymph node: metastatic adenocarcinoma consistent with breast primary.

2. Left infraclavicular lymph node: metastatic adenocarcinoma consistent with breast primary.

Bone scan:

1. No definite evidence of osseous metastases.

2. Abnormality in cervical spine consistent with previous history of bone grafting.

Ultrasound liver:

No lesions suggestive of metastases.

QUESTIONS

Problem Identification

1.a. Create a list of potential drug therapy problems in the patient's medication regimen.

1.b. Given this clinical information, what is this patient's clinical stage of breast cancer?

Desired Outcome

2.a. What is the primary goal for cancer treatment in this patient?

2.b. What is the prognosis for this patient based on tumor size and nodal status?

2.c. In addition to the stage of disease, what other factors are important for determining the prognosis for breast cancer?

Therapeutic Alternatives

3. List the treatment modalities available for this patient's breast cancer, and discuss their advantages and disadvantages.

Optimal Plan

4. Design an appropriate plan for treating this patient's breast cancer, focusing on pharmacologic and nonpharmacologic measures. If the plan includes chemotherapy, identify a specific regimen, and provide your rationale for selecting it.

Outcome Evaluation

5.a. What parameters should be monitored to evaluate the efficacy and adverse effects of the therapy you recommended?

Clinical Course

The patient tolerated your treatment plan well. Twelve months after its completion, the patient returns to clinic complaining of lower back pain for the past 3–4 weeks. She had been taking pro-poxyphene more regularly, "about two or three pills per day." The patient is restaged with a bone scan, chest x-ray, abdominal CT, and laboratory tests. Bone scan reveals metastases to the lumbar spine without spinal cord compression. Abdominal CT shows a solitary liver metastasis. LFT's are within normal limits. Ca 27.29 is 100.7 U/mL. The physician's assessment is that this patient's breast cancer is now metastatic to the bone and liver. The previous therapy is discontinued, and the patient is started on capecitabine.

5.b. What is this patient's current clinical stage of breast cancer, and what is the primary goal for cancer treatment for this patient now?

5.c. Using this patient's information, calculate her dose and schedule of capecitabine.

Patient Education

6. What information should be provided to the patient regarding her new therapy for breast cancer?

■ CLINICAL COURSE

Rosalita responds to 6 cycles of capecitabine. She is starting to show signs of palmar plantar erythrodysesthesias, with dry and cracked skin on her hands and feet. She states that the pain is bearable, and she would like to continue treatment with capecitabine.

CLINICAL PEARL

Even though metastatic breast cancer is usually considered to be incurable, some patients can live for a relatively long time with the use of palliative chemotherapy and (if hormone receptor-positive disease) hormonal therapy. These therapies are administered to increase the patient's quality of life and prolong disease progression, and are typically used in a sequential manner until they are no longer effective, or side effects preclude their use. Although the average life span after diagnosis of metastatic disease is a few years, some patients can live a decade or more with the disease.

■ SELF-STUDY ASSIGNMENTS

1. Perform a literature search to obtain recent information regarding adjuvant clinical trials utilizing trastuzumab in patients with Her2 overexpressing breast cancer.

2. Perform a literature search to obtain recent information regarding adjuvant clinical trials using aromatase inhibitors (anastrozole, letrozole, or exemestane) in patients with hormone receptor-positive breast cancer.

3. Develop a treatment plan for a patient presenting to the emergency center with febrile neutropenia after administration of chemotherapy.

4. Provide educational information for a patient with hormone receptor-positive metastatic breast cancer who will be starting treatment with fulvestrant.

REFERENCES

1. Singletary SE, Allred C, Ashley P, et al. Revision of the American Joint Committee on Cancer staging system for breast cancer. J Clin Oncol 2002;20:3628–3636.

2. Hanrahan EO, Hennessy BT, Valero V. Neoadjuvant systemic therapy for breast cancer: an overview and review of recent clinical trials. Expert Opin Pharmacother 2005;6:1477–1491.

3. Early Breast Cancer Trialists' Collaborative Group (EBCTCG). Effects of chemotherapy and hormonal therapy for early breast cancer on recurrence and 15-year survival: an overview of the randomised trials. Lancet 2005;365:1687–1717.

4. Dang C, Hudis C. Adjuvant taxanes in the treatment of breast cancer: no longer at the tip of the iceberg. Clin Breast Cancer 2006;7:51–58.

5. ATAC Trialists' Group. Results of the ATAC (arimidex, tamoxifen, alone or in combination) trial after completion of 5 years' adjuvant treatment for breast cancer. Lancet 2005;365:60–62.

6. Thurlimann B, Keshaviah A, Coates AS, et al. A comparison of letrozole and tamoxifen in postmenopausal women with early breast cancer. N Engl J Med 2005;353:2747–2757.

7. Khatcheressian JL, Wolff AC, Smith TJ, et al. American Society of Clinical Oncology 2006 update of the breast cancer follow-up and management guidelines in the adjuvant setting. J Clin Oncol 2006;24:5091–5097.

8. Winer EP, Hudis C, Burstein HJ, et al. American Society of Clinical Oncology technology assessment on the use of aromatase inhibitors as adjuvant therapy for postmenopausal women with hormone receptor-positive breast cancer: status report 2004. J Clin Oncol 2005;23:619–629.

141

NON–SMALL CELL LUNG CANCER

It Takes Your Breath Away . . . . .Level II

Michelle L. Rockey, PharmD, BCOP

Jane M. Pruemer, PharmD, BCOP, FASHP

LEARNING OBJECTIVES

After completing this case study, students should be able to:

- Recognize the most common symptoms of non–small cell lung cancer (NSCLC).

- Monitor carboplatin and paclitaxel therapy.

- Educate patients on the anticipated side effects of carboplatin, paclitaxel, and radiation therapy.

- Identify potential complications associated with NSCLC.

- Design a pharmacotherapeutic plan for the treatment of hypercalcemia.

- Recommend potential second-line chemotherapy agents for treating refractory NSCLC.

- Describe appropriate treatment strategies for brain metastases.

PATIENT PRESENTATION

▓ Chief Complaint

"I have been coughing up blood."

▓ HPI

This 50-year-old woman presents to her PCP with complaints of a dry, non-productive cough for 2 months, dyspnea on exertion, and hemoptysis for 1 week.

PMH

Hyperlipidemia
Anemia of unknown etiology × 1 year
DM Type 2
PPD (–)

FH

Father died of colorectal cancer at age 68

SH

Married, lives with son and daughter; 30 pack-year cigarette smoking history (approximately 1 ppd × 30 years); occasional ETOH use; no known recent exposure to TB

Meds

Folic acid 1 mg po daily
Ferrous sulfate 325 mg po TID
Simvastatin 20 mg po daily
Metformin 500 mg BID
Protonix 40 mg po daily

All

NKDA

ROS

(+) for pulmonary symptoms as in noted in HPI; no headaches, dizziness, or blurred vision

Physical Examination

Gen

Mildly overweight Caucasian woman in slight distress

VS

BP 120/65, P 90, RR 30, T 37.2°C; Wt 81 kg, Ht 5'9"

Skin

Patches of dry skin; no lesions

HEENT

PERRLA; EOMI; fundi benign; TMs intact

Neck/Lymph Nodes

No lymphadenopathy; neck supple

Lungs

Wheezing in RUL; remainder of lung fields clear

Heart

RRR; slight systolic murmur on left lateral side; normal S_1, S_2

Abd

Soft, non-tender; no splenomegaly or hepatomegaly

Genit/Rect

Normal female genitalia; guaiac (–) stool

Neuro

A & O × 3; sensory and motor intact, 5/5 upper, 4/5 lower; CN II–XII intact; (–) Babinski

Labs

Na 138 mEq/L	Hgb 11.9 g/dL	Ca 9.1 mg/dL
K 3.8 mEq/L	Hct 36.8%	Mg 2.0 mg/dL
Cl 99 mEq/L	Plt 267 × 10³/mm³	
CO_2 23 mEq/L	WBC 9.4 × 10³/mm³	
BUN 13 mg/dL		
SCr 1.1 mg/dL		
Glu 125 mg/dL		

Chest X-Ray

PA and lateral views reveal a possible mass in right upper lobe (Fig. 141-1)

Assessment

A 50-year-old woman with new-onset hemoptysis is admitted for work-up of a possible lung mass.
She has anemia and a history of hyperlipidemia and diabetes mellitus.

Clinical Course

The patient was further evaluated for lung cancer on an outpatient basis. A bronchoscopy (with biopsy) was performed that identified squamous cell carcinoma. The chest CT scan revealed a 2.5-cm × 2-cm right lung mass (Fig. 141-2). A mediastinoscopy was performed to determine the resectability of the tumor. The mediastinoscopy and biopsy revealed unresectable stage IIIB NSCLC with metastases to the contralateral mediastinal nodes. PFTs included FEV_1 1.49 L, FVC 1.9 L. An echocardiogram showed mild LVH with an LVEF of 55%.

QUESTIONS

Problem Identification

1.a. Identify the patient's drug therapy problems.

1.b. What signs, symptoms, and other information indicate the presence of NSCLC in this patient?

Desired Outcome

2. What is the goal for treatment of NSCLC in this patient? What is the likelihood of achieving this goal?

Therapeutic Alternatives

3.a. What chemotherapeutic regimens may be considered for NSCLC?

3.b. What nondrug therapies may be used for NSCLC?

Optimal Plan

4.a. Design a specific chemotherapeutic regimen to treat this patient, and explain why you chose this regimen.

4.b. What additional measures should be taken to ensure the tolerability of the regimen and to prevent adverse effects?

4.c. What additional laboratory and clinical information is needed before administration of the chemotherapy?

4.d. Calculate the patient's BSA, creatinine clearance, and the amount of each drug to be administered based on the regimen chosen.

Outcome Evaluation

5. What clinical and laboratory parameters are necessary to evaluate the therapy for achievement of the desired therapeutic outcome and the occurrence of adverse effects?

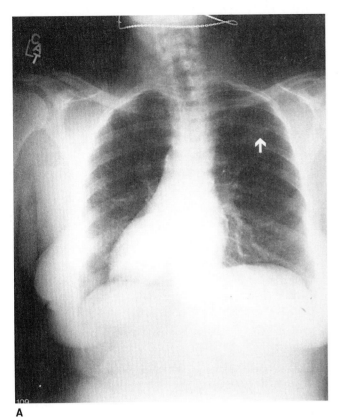

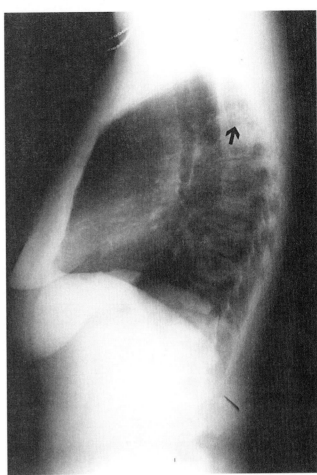

A

B

FIGURE 141-1. Chest x-ray with PA *(A)* and lateral *(B)* views showing a possible mass in the right upper lobe *(arrows)*.

Patient Education

6. What information should be provided to the patient to optimize therapy and minimize adverse effects?

■ CLINICAL COURSE

The patient's subsequent courses were further complicated by the occurrence of DVT, weight loss, neutropenic fever, anemia, nausea/vomiting, and infections. At one point, the patient presented with a serum calcium level of 12 mg/dL and an albumin of 1.9 g/dL, with symptoms of weakness, confusion, nausea, and vomiting.

Follow-Up Questions

1. Calculate the patient's corrected calcium level and provide an interpretation of that value.

2. What treatment modalities may be used to correct hypercalcemia?

■ CLINICAL COURSE

A repeat chest CT before cycle 3 of carboplatin/paclitaxel shows an increase in the size of the initial mass and several new suspicious lesions.

Follow-Up Questions

1. What treatment options are available for the patient at this time?

2. Design a specific chemotherapeutic regimen to treat this patient.

■ CLINICAL COURSE

Six weeks after beginning the new chemotherapy regimen, the patient presents to the ED with complaints of headache and mental

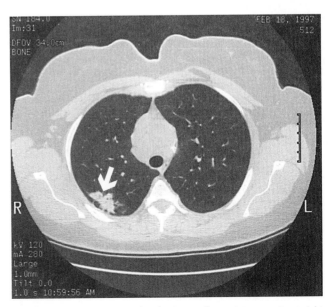

FIGURE 141-2. CT scan of the chest revealing a 2.5-cm × 2-cm right lung mass *(arrow)*.

status changes as per the patient's husband and caregiver. An MRI of the head reveals multiple lesions, most likely brain metastases.

Follow-Up Questions

1. Briefly discuss options (drug and nondrug) to treat brain metastases.

2. What is the role of anticonvulsant agents in the setting of brain metastases?

■ SELF-STUDY ASSIGNMENTS

1. Review clinically important drug interactions for cancer patients started on phenytoin. Include appropriate monitoring parameters. Extend your review beyond the medications this patient is currently receiving.

2. The oncologist has decided to place this patient on erlotinib. Design a patient education session for this new drug therapy.

CLINICAL PEARL

More than 90% of lung cancers are attributable to cigarette smoking. Smoking cessation is the only method proven to decrease the risk of lung cancer.

REFERENCES

1. Pfister DG, Johnson DH, Azzoli CG, et al. American Society of Clinical Oncology treatment of unresectable non-small-cell lung cancer guideline: update 2003. J Clin Oncol 2004;22:330–353.

2. Sause W, Kolesar P, Taylor S, et al. Final results of phase III trial in regionally advanced unresectable non-small cell lung cancer: Radiation Therapy Oncology Group, Eastern Cooperative Oncology Group, and Southwest Oncology Group. Chest 2000;117:358–364.

3. Pritchard RS, Anthony SP. Chemotherapy plus radiotherapy compared with radiotherapy alone in the treatment of locally advanced, unresectable, non-small-cell lung cancer. A meta-analysis. Ann Intern Med 1996;125:723–729.

4. Smit EF, VanMeerbeeck JP, Lianes P, et al. Three-arm randomized study of two cisplatin-based regimens and paclitaxel plus gemcitabine in advanced non-small-cell lung cancer: a phase III trial of the European Organization for Research and Treatment of Cancer Lung Cancer Group—EORTC 08975. J Clin Oncol 2003;21:3909–3917.

5. Solomon B, Ball DL, Richardson G, et al. Phase I/II study of concurrent twice-weekly paclitaxel and weekly cisplatin with radiation therapy for stage III non-small-cell lung cancer. Lung Cancer 2003;41:353–361.

6. Furuse K, Fukuoka M, Kawahara M, et al. Phase III study of concurrent versus sequential thoracic radiotherapy in combination with mitomycin, vindesine, and cisplatin in unresectable stage III non-small-cell lung cancer. J Clin Oncol 1999;17:2692–2699.

7. Curran WJ, Scott C, Langer C, et al. Phase III comparison of sequential vs. concurrent chemoradiation for patients with unresected stage III non-small cell lung cancer (NSCLC). Initial Report of Radiation Therapy Oncology Group (RTOG) 9410. Proc Am Soc Clin Oncol 2000;19:1891. Abstract.

8. Kris MG, Hesketh PJ, Somerfield MR, et al. American Society of Clinical Oncology guideline for antiemetics in oncology: update 2006. J Clin Oncol 2006;24:2932–2947.

9. Weiss GJ, Langer C, Rosell R, et al. Elderly patients benefit from second-line cytotoxic chemotherapy: a subset analysis of a randomized phase III trial of pemetrexed compared with docetaxel in patients with previously treated advanced non-small-cell lung cancer. J Clin Oncol 2006;24:4405–4411.

10. Shepherd FA, Pereira JR, Ciuleanu T, et al. Erlotinib in previously treated non-small-cell lung cancer. N Engl J Med 2005;353:123–132.

142

COLON CANCER

Intestinal Fortitude . . . . Level II

Lisa E. Davis, PharmD, FCCP, BCPS, BCOP

LEARNING OBJECTIVES

After completing this case study, students should be able to:

- Identify common symptoms associated with colon cancer at presentation and with disease progression.

- Describe the treatment goals associated with early and advanced stages of colon cancer.

- Design an appropriate chemotherapy regimen for colon cancer based on patient-specific data.

- Formulate a monitoring plan for a patient receiving a prescribed chemotherapy regimen for colon cancer based on patient-specific information.

- Recommend alterations in a drug therapy plan for a patient with colon cancer based on patient-specific information.

- Educate patients on the anticipated side effects of irinotecan, capecitabine, oxaliplatin, and epidermal growth factor receptor inhibitors.

PATIENT PRESENTATION

■ Chief Complaint

"The pain in my belly is much worse."

■ HPI

Frank Carter is a 42-year-old man who presents with increasing abdominal pain. He was diagnosed with stage IIB (T3, N0, M0) colon cancer 3 years ago after presenting with abdominal pain, cramping, and diarrhea. He underwent surgical resection and lymphadenectomy for an obstructing lesion in the transverse colon. The pathology revealed poorly differentiated adenocarcinoma with increased vascular invasion through the entire thickness of the bowel wall. None of 18 lymph nodes resected was positive for tumor. His operative recovery was uneventful, and he remained in good health until he presented with RUQ abdominal pain 5 months ago. A CT scan showed numerous metastases in both lobes of the liver, with the largest measuring 3.4 cm on the right side. A CT scan of the chest showed no evidence of lung metastases. His CEA was 6.2 ng/mL. Chemotherapy was initiated with FOLFIRI. Sixteen days later, he presented to an outside hospital with complaints of abdominal pain, nausea, vomiting, and constipation. He had not had a bowel movement for 4 days. During his 4-day hospital stay, he was managed with bowel rest, IV fluids, and morphine, and his symptoms resolved. FOLFIRI was continued, and he did not experience any dose-limiting toxicities that required dose reduction or treatment delays. After five cycles of chemotherapy, he achieved a partial response in his liver metastases. The largest metastasis in his right hepatic lobe had decreased to 2.1 cm, and his LDH level decreased to normal values. Ten days ago, he received his ninth cycle of FOLFIRI chemotherapy.

PMH

Hypercholesterolemia × 6 years

FH

The patient is the youngest of three brothers; both siblings are alive and well. He has been married for 5 years and has one daughter who is 3 years old. His mother and father are both in good health. His paternal grandfather died in his 60s from colon cancer; he is aware of no other family history of malignancy.

SH

Self-employed as an organizational consultant. He smoked cigarettes, $1^1/_2$–2 packs per day since age 20 but quit 1 year ago. He does not drink alcohol and has never tried illicit drugs.

Meds

Fentanyl transdermal patch 100 mcg/h; apply 2 patches every 3 days
Bisacodyl 10 mg suppository rectally as needed
Pantoprazole 40 mg po once daily
Simvastatin 20 mg po once daily

All

NKDA

ROS

The patient reports diffuse abdominal pain that is continuous with a "grabbing, gnawing" sensation. He rates the pain severity as 5 out of 10. He denies fever, headaches, shortness of breath, cough, nausea, vomiting, or diarrhea. He reports no lesions in his mouth or difficulty swallowing. He has been experiencing difficulty moving his bowels, but there is no pain or blood with passage of stool. He denies burning on urination. He hasn't noticed any bleeding or excessive bruising. He notes some swelling in his lower legs.

Physical Examination

Gen

Patient is a thin white man who appears fatigued

VS

BP 130/70, P 79, RR 22, T 35.6°C; Wt 65 kg, Ht 5'8"

Skin

No rash or lesions

HEENT

PERRLA; EOMI; no scleral icterus; moist mucous membranes; no lesions in oral cavity

Neck/Lymph Nodes

Supple neck; no lymphadenopathy

Lungs/Thorax

Symmetric chest expansion with respiratory effort; clear to A & P; regular breath sounds

CV

Normal heart sounds; regular rate and rhythm; no MRG

Abd

Diffuse abdominal tenderness to palpation; no rebound tenderness; decreased bowel sounds

Genit/Rect

Prostate normal size; no masses palpated; stool heme negative

MS/Ext

Full ROM in all four extremities; 2+ pedal edema bilaterally in LE

Neuro

A & O × 3

Labs

Na 137 mEq/L	Hgb 9.6 g/dL	WBC $8.1 \times 10^3/mm^3$	AST 62 IU/L
K 4.4 mEq/L	Hct 29%	Neutros 40%	ALT 20 IU/L
Cl 98 mEq/L	Plt $332 \times 10^3/mm^3$	Bands 3%	Alk phos 189 IU/L
CO_2 26 mEq/L	MCV 87 μm^3	Eos 2.6%	LDH 400 IU/L
BUN 17 mg/dL	MCHC 33 g/dL	Lymphs 44.6%	
SCr 1.0 mg/dL		Monos 9.5%	
Glu 122 mg/dL			

Abdominal CT

Multiple liver metastases, with increase in the main liver lesion by about 20% and three new liver metastases

Chest CT

No evidence of pulmonary metastases

Assessment

Colon cancer stage IV, with disease progression on FOLFIRI chemotherapy

QUESTIONS

Problem Identification

1.a. Identify all of the patient's drug therapy problems.

1.b. What clinical, laboratory, and other information is consistent with colon cancer?

Desired Outcome

2. What are the goals of pharmacotherapy for this patient?

Therapeutic Alternatives

3. What chemotherapeutic options are appropriate for this patient?

Optimal Plan

4.a. What drugs, dosage forms, treatment schedule, and duration of therapy are best for treating this patient's colon cancer?

4.b. What additional drug treatment interventions should be considered for this patient?

Outcome Evaluation

5.a. How is the response to the treatment regimen for the colon cancer assessed?

5.b. What acute adverse effects are anticipated with the chemotherapy regimen, and what parameters should be monitored?

5.c. What pharmacologic measures can be instituted to prevent or manage the acute toxicities associated with the chemotherapy regimen?

5.d. What are the potential late-onset toxicities of the chemotherapy regimen, and how can they be detected and prevented?

Patient Education

6. What information should you provide to the patient to enhance compliance, ensure successful therapy, and minimize adverse effects?

■ CLINICAL COURSE

The first two cycles of the regimen you recommended were complicated by severe nausea and vomiting, which were controlled during further cycles with aggressive antiemetic prophylaxis. After four cycles of chemotherapy, an abdominal CT scan showed a 25% decrease in size of the main liver lesion, and the current regimen was continued. He received PRBC transfusions when his hemoglobin dropped below 9 g/dL. Hydrochlorothiazide was initiated for an elevated SBP that developed after the first month of therapy, and his SBP has been maintained in the low 130s, with an average DBP of 80 mm Hg. His transdermal fentanyl dose was increased to 150 mcg/h every 72 hours, and oral immediate-release morphine sulfate, every 4 hours as needed for pain, was started. A scheduled regimen of docusate sodium, 100 mg orally plus 2 senna tablets daily, maintained a regular pattern of bowel movements. Eight months after starting chemotherapy, he presented with worsening pain, fatigue, and new-onset dyspnea. An abdominal CT scan showed the main liver lesion increased in size to 4.2 cm, and the chest CT revealed new pulmonary metastases. His ALT and AST increased to three times the upper limit of normal, and simvastatin was discontinued.

■ FOLLOW-UP QUESTION

1. What treatment options would be appropriate to consider at this time?

■ ADDITIONAL CASE QUESTION

1. How should a patient who develops a thrombotic event during bevacizumab therapy be managed?

■ CLINICAL COURSE

The patient expressed interest in receiving further treatment for his colon cancer. After considering various treatment options with his oncologist, he agreed to treatment with an epidermal growth factor receptor inhibitor. His analgesic therapy was modified, and his pain control was acceptable. His metastatic lesions remained stable (by clinical symptoms and CT scans) for 4 months.

■ SELF-STUDY ASSIGNMENTS

1. Develop an algorithm for treatment of colon cancer chemotherapy-induced diarrhea.
2. Develop patient-specific education materials regarding management of cutaneous toxicities of agents used in colon cancer treatment.

CLINICAL PEARL

A variety of active agents are available for colon cancer. The optimal combination, sequence, and treatment duration are unknown, but the ability of an individual to receive all active agents during the course of the disease is associated with the greatest likelihood of increasing overall survival.

REFERENCES

1. Gill S, Blackstock AW, Goldberg RM. Colorectal cancer. Mayo Clin Proc 2007;82:114–129.
2. Hochster HS, Hart LL, Ramanathan RK, et al. Safety and efficacy of oxaliplatin/fluoropyrimidine regimens with or without bevacizumab as first-line treatment of metastatic colorectal cancer (mCRC): final analysis of the TREE Study. In: J Clin Oncol, 2006 ASCO Annual Meeting Proceedings Part I Vol 24, No 18S (June 20 Suppl) 2006: 3510.
3. Giantonio BJ, Catalano PJ, Meropol NJ, et al. Bevacizumab in combination with oxaliplatin, fluorouracil, and leucovorin (FOLFOX4) for previously treated metastatic colorectal cancer: results from the Eastern Cooperative Oncology Group Study E3200. J Clin Oncol 2007;25:1539–1544.
4. Cunningham D, Humblet Y, Siena S, et al. Cetuximab monotherapy and cetuximab plus irinotecan in irinotecan-refractory metastatic colorectal cancer. N Engl J Med 2004;351:337–345.
5. Van Cutsem E, Peeters M, Siena S, et al. Open-label phase III trial of panitumumab plus best supportive care compared with best supportive care alone in patients with chemotherapy-refractory metastatic colorectal cancer. J Clin Oncol 2007;25:1658–1664.
6. Tournigand C, Cervantes A, Figer A, et al. OPTIMOX1: a randomized study of FOLFOX4 or FOLFOX7 with oxaliplatin in a stop-and-go fashion in advanced colorectal cancer—a GERCOR study. J Clin Oncol 2006;24:394–400.
7. Grothey A. Clinical management of oxaliplatin-associated neurotoxicity. Clin Colorectal Cancer 2005;5(Suppl 1):S38–S46.

143

PROSTATE CANCER

Missed Opportunity . . . . .Level II

Diana Hey Cauley, PharmD, BCOP

LEARNING OBJECTIVES

After completing this case study, students should be able to:

- Describe typical symptoms associated with prostate cancer at initial diagnosis and at disease progression.

- Describe the standard initial treatment options for androgen-dependent metastatic prostate cancer.

- Recommend a pharmacotherapeutic plan for patients with androgen-independent metastatic prostate cancer.

- Counsel patients regarding the toxicities associated with the pharmacologic agents used in prostate cancer treatment.

PATIENT PRESENTATION

■ Chief Complaint

"I have blood in my urine, and my shoulder is really hurting."

■ HPI

Don Walton is a 73-year-old man who usually has yearly physicals and PSA checks by his local physician. The levels have always been in the range of 4–6 ng/mL. He did not go in for his yearly physical last year, and he now presents with painless gross hematuria, shoulder pain, and a PSA level of 35.7 ng/mL.

■ PMH

Hypercholesterolemia
Congestive heart failure

Diabetes mellitus
Kidney stones
Cataracts
Diverticulitis
Severe GERD

■ SH

Retired highway maintenance employee. Christian by faith, Protestant by denomination. He has an associate degree. He denies alcohol use. He smoked 10 cigarettes a day for 21 years; stopped smoking at age 42. He is married with two children. He is an only child. Family history of cancer: father, lung: diagnosed age 71, died age 73; mother, breast: died at age 93. He has a paternal aunt and paternal grandmother who both were diagnosed with unspecified malignancies.

■ ROS

He reports significant fatigue and severe pain in right shoulder. No fever, chills, or sweats. No epistaxis or dysphagia. Reports no chest pain, shortness of breath, dyspnea, or cough. No nausea, vomiting, diarrhea, or constipation. He denies dysuria but has recurring hematuria. He reports dribbling and nocturia two to three times per night. He denies memory loss, diplopia, or neuropathy; he has had no falls recently. He reports a 15- to 20-year history of tinnitus.

■ Meds

Diovan 160 mg po daily
Lasix 40 mg po daily
Klor-Con 10 mEq po daily
Allopurinol 300 mg po daily
Flomax 0.4 mg, 2 capsules po daily
Prozac 20 mg po daily
Gemfibrozil 600 mg po daily
Metformin 500 mg po QID
Tylenol 500 mg po 6 times daily PRN
Motrin 400 mg po 6 times daily PRN
Nexium 40 mg po BID

■ All

None

■ Physical Examination

Gen

This is a pleasant, elderly gentleman who appears to be in moderate discomfort. Pain is 7 over 10 multifocally. ECOG performance status 1+.

VS

BP 136/61, P 80, RR 20, T 36.9°C; Wt 91.5 kg, Ht 5'6"

Skin

Warm and dry; no lesions or rashes

HEENT

Sclerae are anicteric. PERRLA; EOMI. Tympanic membranes are within normal limits bilaterally.

Neck/Lymph Nodes

No cervical or supraclavicular adenopathy

Lungs/Thorax

Lungs are clear in all fields. Respirations are even and unlabored.

CV

Normal rate and rhythm; S_1, S_2 normal; no murmurs, gallops, or rubs

Abd

There is a large midline abdominal hernia that does not appear incarcerated. No hepatosplenomegaly.

Genit/Rect

Patient is circumcised with a normal phallus. There are bilaterally descended testicles. No inguinal hernia on examination. Prostate is markedly enlarged and is asymmetric on the right. Texture is firm, but no discrete nodule palpated. Normal rectal tone.

MS/Ext

He has significant pain to touch on the superior aspect of the right shoulder; there is also pain on range of motion. There is tenderness in lumbar area. 1+ ankle and pedal edema is present. Pedal pulses are 2+ bilaterally.

Neuro

CN II–XII grossly normal. Cerebellar function remains intact.

■ Labs

Na 139 mEq/L	Hgb 9.5 g/dL	WBC $7.2 \times 10^3/mm^3$	Total bilirubin 0.2
K 4.0 mEq/L	Hct 27.1%	Neutros 70.3%	mg/dL
Cl 107 mEq/L	RBC $3.6 \times 10^6/mm^3$	Baso 0.2%	ALT <12 IU/L
CO_2 24 mEq/L	Plt $215 \times 10^3/mm^3$	Eos 2.3%	AST 20 IU/L
BUN 21 mg/dL	MCV 75 μm^3	Lymphs 16.6%	LDH 742 IU/L
SCr 0.9 mg/dL	MCHC 35.1 g/dL	Monos 10.6%	Alk phos 912 IU/L
Glu 188 mg/dL		PSA 35.7 ng/mL	Albumin 4 g/dL
		Testosterone 276 ng/dL	Calcium 8.7 mg/dL

■ Bone Scan

Skeletal metastases involving the skull and right shoulder

■ Cystoscopy and Bladder Neck Biopsy

High-grade carcinoma consistent with prostatic adenocarcinoma, Gleason score 8 (4 + 4), extensively involving the bladder neck biopsy tissue

■ Perineal Prostate Biopsy

Prostatic adenocarcinoma, Gleason score 9 (4 + 5), positive perineural invasion

■ CT Abdomen

No significant retroperitoneal adenopathy. Multiple small, external iliac lymph nodes are present, predominantly on the left. Small, deep inguinal lymph nodes are also present.

■ Urinalysis

Clear; negative for glucose, ketones, leukocyte esterase, nitrites, and protein; trace hemoglobin; rare bacteria

■ Assessment

73-year-old male with newly diagnosed T4N2M1b (D2) prostate cancer presenting with painless gross hematuria and elevated PSA of 35.7 ng/mL. Patient has metastatic androgen-dependent hormone-sensitive disease and is here for consideration of initial treatment options.

QUESTIONS

Problem Identification

1. What signs, symptoms, and other information are consistent with metastatic prostate cancer in this case?

Desired Outcome

2. Considering this patient's disease stage and history, what are reasonable therapeutic goals?

Therapeutic Alternatives

3. Create a list of the feasible options for initial therapy of this patient's androgen-dependent prostate cancer, including the advantages, potential side effects, and complications associated with each option.

Optimal Plan

4. Design an optimal pharmacotherapeutic plan for the treatment of this patient's metastatic prostate cancer.

Outcome Evaluation

5. How should the therapy you recommended be monitored for efficacy and adverse effects?

Patient Education

6. What information should be provided to the patient about his new therapy?

■ CLINICAL COURSE

Mr. Walton has been compliant with his treatment plan. His testosterone has been castrate since therapy was begun 20 months ago. His PSA 3 months ago was mildly elevated at 0.6 ng/mL, whereas it had been undetectable previously. His PSA has now increased to 38.5 ng/mL and his testosterone level is 22 ng/mL. He is complaining of increased pain in his pelvis and more bone pain in his ribs and back over the last 2 months, although he is still able to participate in church social activities and play golf on the weekends. A CT of the pelvis shows a soft tissue mass on the posterolateral aspect of the urinary bladder on the right side and multiple blastic lesions in the pelvis and spine. His bone scan shows numerous intense foci in the skull, scapulae, spine, and femurs.

Follow-Up Questions

1. What pharmacotherapeutic options are available to the patient for his progressive androgen-independent metastatic prostate cancer?

2. What therapeutic options are available for managing this patient's pain?

Self-Study Assignments

1. Locate information resources that are available to prostate cancer patients and their families.

2. Provide the rationale for intermittent LHRH hormone ablation for locally advanced and metastatic prostate cancer patients.

3. Define the role of secondary hormonal agents (e.g., ketoconazole, estrogens) for metastatic disease relapse.

4. Describe the clinical rationale for starting an antiandrogen 1–4 weeks before giving the first dose of an LHRH agonist.

5. Define the role of bisphosphonates in men with prostate cancer.

CLINICAL PEARL

An LHRH agonist is not discontinued when a metastatic prostate cancer patient progresses to an androgen-independent state.

REFERENCES

1. NCCN Clinical Practice Guidelines in Oncology, V1. 2007. Prostate Cancer. Available at: *www.nccn.org*. Accessed Feb. 10, 2007.
2. Sooriakumaran P, Khaksar SJ, Shah J. Management of prostate cancer. Part 2: localized and locally advanced disease. Expert Rev Anticancer Ther 2006;6:595–603.
3. Shah J, Khaksar SJ, Sooriakumaran P. Management of prostate cancer. Part 3: metastatic disease. Expert Rev Anticancer Ther 2006;6:813–821.
4. Tannock IF, de Wit R, Berry WR, et al. Docetaxel plus prednisone or mitoxantrone plus prednisone for advanced prostate cancer. N Engl J Med 2004;351:1502–1512.
5. Petrylak DP, Tangen CM, Hussain MH, et al. Docetaxel and estramustine compared with mitoxantrone and prednisone for refractory prostate cancer. N Engl J Med 2004;351:1513–1520.
6. Tannock IF, Osoba D, Stockler MR, et al. Chemotherapy with mitoxantrone plus prednisone or prednisone alone for symptomatic hormone-resistant prostate cancer: a Canadian randomized trial with palliative end points. J Clin Oncol 1996;14:1756–1764.
7. NCCN Clinical Practice Guidelines in Oncology, V1. 2006. Adult Cancer Pain. Available at: *www.nccn.org*. Accessed Feb. 10, 2007.

144

NON-HODGKIN'S LYMPHOMA

Music Soothes the Savage Tumor. . . . . Level II

Keith A. Hecht, PharmD, BCOP

LEARNING OBJECTIVES

After completing this case study, students should be able to:

- Identify and describe the components of the staging work-up and the corresponding staging and classification systems for non-Hodgkin's lymphoma (NHL).

- Describe the pharmacotherapeutic treatment of choice and the alternatives available for treating NHL.

- Identify acute and chronic toxicities associated with the drugs used to treat NHL and the measures used to prevent or treat these toxicities.

- Identify monitoring parameters for response and toxicity in patients with NHL.

- Provide detailed patient education for the chemotherapeutic regimen.

PATIENT PRESENTATION

■ Chief Complaint

"What's the next step for my lymphoma?"

■ HPI

Nathan Nightingale is a 58-year-old man who presents to his oncologist's office for recommendations about treatment of a newly diagnosed diffuse, large B-cell lymphoma. He had been in relatively good health since being diagnosed with COPD 10 years ago. He initially presented to the ED 2 weeks ago with new onset of worsening cough with hemoptysis and fevers up to 100.8°F (38.2°C). He was then hospitalized for further evaluation and treatment. At that time, he stated that he had lost weight over the past few months. Physical examination findings were significant for decreased breath sounds (worse on the left side than the right) and enlarged, painless supraclavicular lymph nodes on the left side. The largest palpable lymph node measured approximately 2 cm in diameter. Splenomegaly was also noted. Chest x-ray revealed a large heterogeneous mass at the apex of the left lung also involving the mediastinum. Given the patient's lengthy smoking history, he was presumed to have lung cancer. CT-guided biopsy of the mass was performed. Pathology revealed cells consistent with lymphoma, but definitive diagnosis could not be made. An excisional biopsy of the enlarged supraclavicular lymph node was performed. Pathology showed diffuse large non-Hodgkin's B-cell lymphoma. The oncologist on call was consulted, and it was recommended for him to follow up as an outpatient for further evaluation and treatment recommendations.

▨ PMH

HTN × 15 years
Hypercholesterolemia × 5 years
COPD × 10 years

▨ FH

The patient is the oldest of seven children (four brothers and two sisters), all alive and well. He has two children, both in good health. Family history of terminal prostate cancer in his father (died at age 63). No other history of malignancy that he is aware of.

▨ SH

The patient is employed as a piano player in the lounge of a Las Vegas casino. He previously smoked 1–2 ppd for 32 years. He quit when he was diagnosed with COPD, and he complains about the tourists who smoke in the lounge where he works. He drinks one to two martinis nightly when working. Diet is mostly buffet food. He states that he does not eat many vegetables, as he must save room for "the good stuff" on the buffet. He has been married for 34 years. His wife is with him today in the clinic.

▨ ROS

The patient reports continuing fever, typically ranging from 100.2°F to 101°F (37.9° to 38.3°C) and cough with occasional hemoptysis. In addition, he describes an unexplained weight loss of approximately 25 pounds over the last 3 months. He denies headaches, changes in vision, or fainting episodes. He reports no lesions in his mouth, difficulty swallowing, or nosebleeds. He states that he occasionally has some dyspnea on exertion, but he is able to carry out activities of daily living without limitations. He denies tachycardia or swelling in the extremities. He also denies burning on urination, frequency, dribbling, or blood in the urine. He has not noticed any additional bleeding or bruising. He has not received any prior transfusions.

▨ Meds

Lisinopril 10 mg po once daily
HCTZ 25 mg po once daily
Albuterol/ipratropium MDI 2 inhalations po QID
Simvastatin 20 mg po at bedtime
Famotidine 20 mg po BID
Hydrocodone/acetaminophen 5/500 1–2 tablets Q 4–6 h PRN pain

▨ All

Penicillin: rash

▨ Physical Examination

Gen

Patient is a thin white man in no apparent distress

VS

BP 140/95, P 95, RR 14, T 37.9°C; Wt 72 kg, Ht 5'9"

Skin

No rashes or moles noted

HEENT

PERRLA; TMs clear; no masses in the tonsils, palate, or floor of the mouth; no stomatitis. Several missing teeth, but no gingival inflammation is noted.

Neck

Supple; no masses; small scar from excisional biopsy of supraclavicular lymph node noted

Chest

Decreased breath sounds bilaterally, more on the left than the right

CV

RRR; no MRG

Abd

Soft and non-tender, non-distended. The spleen is palpable just below the costal margin. No hepatomegaly. Bowel sounds are normoactive.

Genit/Rect

Normal male genitalia

Ext

Without edema, warm to the touch; pulses palpable bilaterally

Neuro

Symmetric cranial nerve function. Symmetric facial muscle movement, and the tongue is midline. The palate is symmetric. Balance and coordination of the upper extremities are intact, with no evidence of tremor. There is symmetric coordination of rapidly alternating movements. Motor strength in the upper and lower extremities is normal and symmetric.

Lymph Node Survey

The lymph node survey is negative for any palpable peripheral nodes in the preauricular, postauricular, cervical, supraclavicular, infraclavicular, or axillary areas. No palpable inguinal nodes present. Small scar noted from excisional biopsy of left supraclavicular node.

▨ Labs

Na 138 mEq/L	Hgb 10 g/dL	AST 29 IU/L	Phos 4.0 mg/dL
K 4.2 mEq/L	Hct 30%	ALT 27 IU/L	Uric acid 3.6 mg/dL
Cl 98 mEq/L	Plt 438 × 10³/mm³	Alk phos 75 IU/L	PT 12.2 sec
CO₂ 28 mEq/L	WBC 9.9 × 10³/mm³	LDH 123 IU/L	aPTT 21.7 sec
BUN 17 mg/dL	Neutros 70%	T. bili 0.6 mg/dL	
SCr 0.7 mg/dL	Bands 2%	T. prot 6.3 g/dL	
Glu 131 mg/dL	Lymphs 18%	Alb 3.7 g/dL	
	Monos 9%		
	Eos 1%		

▨ CT Chest

Large lobular heterogeneous mass within the left chest and mediastinum that extends from the level of the left lung and apex of the diaphragm

■ Chest X-Ray

Large heterogeneous mass at the apex of the left lung also involving the mediastinum

■ Tumor Pathology

Diffuse large cell lymphoma, B-cell type; CD20+, CD45+, CD3–

■ Initial Assessment

Diffuse large cell lymphoma. Further staging will include bilateral BM biopsies, gallium scan or PET scan, HIV test, CT of the abdomen, and a baseline cardiac assessment in light of the patient's longstanding history of HTN.

■ Clinical Course

Bone marrow biopsies are negative for lymphoma. PET scanning revealed multiple foci of increased FDG (fluorodeoxyglucose) uptake; increased uptake noted in the spleen, mediastinum, and left side supraclavicular lymph nodes. The HIV test is negative. CT of the abdomen shows large heterogeneous soft tissue mass within the left upper quadrant that may be contiguous with previously noted left chest mass. The mass extends inferiomedially to the tail of the pancreas. There is an additional 4-cm low-density mass near the head of the pancreas. The spleen is enlarged. MUGA scan reveals an LVEF of 55%.

■ Assessment

Diffuse large B-cell lymphoma, stage IIISB; International Prognostic Index (IPI) score of 1

QUESTIONS

Problem Identification

1.a. Identify all of the drug therapy problems of this patient.

1.b. What clinical and other information is consistent with the diagnosis of non-Hodgkin's lymphoma?

1.c. Explain what system of staging was used and how his stage of disease was determined.

1.d. What laboratory and clinical features does this patient have that may affect his prognosis? How is the IPI determined?

Desired Outcome

2. What are the goals of therapy in this case?

Therapeutic Alternatives

3. What alternative drug therapies are available for treatment of his non-Hodgkin's lymphoma?

Optimal Plan

4.a. What drug, dosage form, schedule, and duration of therapy are best for treating this patient's non-Hodgkin's lymphoma?

4.b. What other interventions should be made to maintain control of the patient's other concurrent diseases?

4.c. What nondrug therapies might be useful for this patient?

Outcome Evaluation

5.a. How is the response to the treatment regimen for the non-Hodgkin's lymphoma assessed?

5.b. What acute adverse effects are associated with the chemotherapy regimen, and what parameters should be monitored?

5.c. What pharmacologic measures should be instituted to treat or prevent the acute toxicities associated with the chemotherapy regimen?

5.d. What are potential late complications of the chemotherapy regimen, and how can they be detected and prevented?

Patient Education

6. What information would you provide to the patient about the agents used to treat the non-Hodgkin's lymphoma?

■ CLINICAL COURSE

The patient tolerated the first few cycles of chemotherapy well, with only some minimal nausea and vomiting. He was initiated on darbepoetin, 500 mcg every 3 weeks, and ferrous sulfate, 325 mg 3 times daily. The darbepoetin dose was subsequently reduced to 300 mcg every 3 weeks due to hemoglobin increase above 11 g/dL. His antihypertensive medication was modified, increasing the lisinopril to 20 mg daily and maintaining the HCTZ at 25 mg, achieving average systolic BPs in the 120s and average diastolic BPs in the 70s. His fasting lipid panel was checked and was found to be within his goals. Two weeks after completing the fourth cycle of chemotherapy, he presented to the ED with worsening dyspnea, fatigue, and peripheral edema. He was admitted to the hospital for evaluation. Complete work-up including MUGA scan revealed new-onset heart failure with an ejection fraction of 38%. The patient was stabilized, and appropriate modifications were made to his home medications for treatment of new-onset heart failure. Imaging studies were also performed while he was in the hospital to evaluate his lymphoma. PET and CT scans showed that he achieved a complete response.

■ FOLLOW-UP QUESTION

1. What non–anthracycline-containing regimens are available for this patient to complete his chemotherapy course?

■ CLINICAL COURSE

The patient was presented with various treatment options. He and his wife decided that they did not want to undergo any more chemotherapy because he is currently in remission after just four cycles of chemotherapy. Eighteen months later, the patient returns to the oncologist office after being diagnosed with relapsed lymphoma during a hospital admission for worsening dyspnea.

■ SELF-STUDY ASSIGNMENTS

1. What is the role of bone marrow or stem cell transplantation for aggressive non-Hodgkin's lymphoma?

2. What therapeutic options are available for the treatment of relapsed diffuse large B-cell lymphomas?

3. If the patient experienced tumor lysis syndrome, what options are there for treating the hyperuricemia?

CLINICAL PEARL

Enrollment in clinical trials is considered the treatment of choice in patients with advanced (stage IV) or relapsed/refractory diffuse large B-cell lymphomas. Numerous clinical trials are under way evaluating the role of hematopoietic stem cell transplantation, different chemotherapy combinations, and new monoclonal antibodies with different targets (e.g., the CD22 receptor).

REFERENCES

1. The International Non-Hodgkin's Lymphoma Prognostic Factors Project. A predictive model for aggressive non-Hodgkin's lymphoma. N Engl J Med 1993;329:987–994.
2. Rodriguez J, Cabanillas F, McLaughlin P, et al. A proposal for a simple staging system for intermediate grade lymphoma and immunoblastic lymphoma based on the "tumor score." Ann Oncol 1992;3:711–717.
3. Fisher RI, Gaynor ER, Dahlberg S, et al. Comparison of a standard regimen (CHOP) with three intensive chemotherapy regimens for advanced non-Hodgkin's lymphoma. N Engl J Med 1993;328:1002–1006.
4. Vose JM, Link BK, Grossbard ML, et al. Long-term update of a phase II study of rituximab in combination with CHOP chemotherapy in patients with previously untreated, aggressive non-Hodgkin's lymphoma. Leuk Lymphoma 2005;46:1569–1573.
5. Feugier P, Van Hoof A, Sebban C, et al. Long-term results of the R-CHOP study in the treatment of elderly patients with diffuse large B-cell lymphoma: a study by the Groupe d'Etude des Lymphomes de l'Adulte. J Clin Oncol 2005;23:4117–4126.
6. Basser RL, Green MD. Strategies for prevention of anthracycline cardiotoxicity. Cancer Treat Rev 1993;19:57–77.
7. Smith TJ, Khatcheressian J, Lyman GH, et al. 2006 update of recommendations for the use of white blood cell growth factors: an evidence-based clinical practice guideline. J Clin Oncol 2006;24:3187–3205.
8. Ganz WI, Sridhar KS, Ganz SS, et al. Review of tests for monitoring doxorubicin-induced cardiomyopathy. Oncology 1996;53:461–470.

145

HODGKIN'S DISEASE

The Operating Room Nurse . . . . Level I

Cindy L. O'Bryant, PharmD, BCOP

LEARNING OBJECTIVES

After completing this case study, students should be able to:

- Recognize the signs and symptoms commonly associated with Hodgkin's disease (HD).

- Discuss the pharmacotherapeutic treatment of choice and the alternatives available for treating HD.

- Identify acute and chronic toxicities associated with the medications used to treat HD and the measures used to prevent or treat these toxicities.

- Determine monitoring parameters for response and toxicity in patients with HD.

- Formulate appropriate educational information to provide to a patient receiving chemotherapy treatment for HD.

PATIENT PRESENTATION

▦ Chief Complaint

"Swollen lymph nodes in my neck that come and go and a painful, swollen right axillary node for the last 2 months."

▦ HPI

Elaine Johnson is a 28-year-old woman who presents with 2 months of swollen lymph nodes in her neck and right axilla. She states that the nodes in her neck "come and go" but are always somewhat swollen; she relates this to a sore throat. The node in the axilla has been consistently swollen and painful during this time. She also complains of new-onset fatigue and general low back pain for the last 4–5 months. She denies any shortness of breath but has experienced fever, night sweats, and weight loss for the past few months. An ultrasound of the neck and axilla showed a number of lymph nodes ranging from 1.5 to 3 cm. As a result, a lymph node biopsy was performed that demonstrated nodular sclerosing HD.

▦ PMH

GERD × 7 years

▦ FH

The patient's parents and five siblings are all in good health. There is a history of breast cancer and colon cancer in her family.

▦ SH

Works as an OR nurse in the local hospital. Drinks socially about two glasses of wine per week. She began smoking at the age of 18 and smoked socially, two cigarettes a week, until the age of 24. She has not smoked since. She does not use street drugs. The patient is recently married and wishes to have a family.

▦ Meds

Ranitidine 300 mg po once daily for GERD

▦ All

NKDA

▦ ROS

Reports fevers, night sweats, and weight loss of approximately 5 kg over the past 2 months. She denies any vision changes, headaches, shortness of breath, or chest pain. She also denies nausea, vomiting, diarrhea, constipation, or urinary symptoms. Generally feels fatigued. All other systems are negative. Her performance status is 1 on the Zubrod scale.

▦ Physical Examination

Gen

The patient is a young, healthy-appearing woman in no apparent distress.

VS

BP 132/80, P 80, RR 17, T 36.6°C; Wt 68 kg, Ht 5'6^1/$_2$"

Skin

Soft, diffusely enlarged soft tissue swelling around neck and right axilla; no erythema or warmth; no rashes or moles

HEENT

PERRL; EOMI; TMs intact

Lymph Nodes

Anterior cervical lymph nodes are enlarged on the right. Right inferior axillary node is palpable. No other lymph nodes are palpable bilaterally.

Chest

Respirations with normal rhythm; clear to auscultation

Breasts

Normal appearance; no masses on palpation

CV

RRR; no JVD, murmurs, or gallops

Abd

Soft and nontender with no masses; bowel sounds are normoactive

Genit/Rect

Normal female genitalia; stool is guaiac (–)

MS/Ext

Without edema

Neuro

A & O × 3; CN II–XII intact; remainder of exam is non-focal

▓ Labs

Na 135 mEq/L	Hgb 12.5 g/dL	AST 19 IU/L	PT 12.9 sec
K 4.1 mEq/L	Hct 37.8%	ALT 22 IU/L	aPTT 27.1 sec
Cl 103 mEq/L	Plt 390 × 10³/mm³	Alk phos 94 IU/L	Phos 3.1 mg/dL
CO₂ 24 mEq/L	WBC 10.9 × 10³/mm³	LDH 293 IU/L	Magnesium 1.7 mEq/L
BUN 14 mg/dL	Neutros 80.5%	T. bili 0.4 mg/dL	Uric acid 4.5 mg/dL
SCr 0.7 mg/dL	Lymphs 13.2%	T. prot 7.7 g/dL	
Glu 93 mg/dL	Monos 5.4%	Alb 3.2 g/dL	
	Eos 0.9%		

▓ Ultrasound

There are multiple, enlarged abnormal lymph nodes in the neck and right axilla. The largest node in the neck measures 3.4 × 1.4 × 2.4 cm and is palpable to the patient. In the right axilla the largest node is 3.0 × 2.5 × 2.9 cm. The nodes contain solid echogenic material and have increased vascular flow.

▓ Tumor Pathology

Identification of lacunar cells (a variant of Reed-Sternberg cells) classifying this as Hodgkin's disease, nodular sclerosis (NS) type

▓ PET/Helical CT Scan

Enlarged nodes demonstrating hypermetabolic activity in the bilateral jugulodigastric chains and right subclavian axillary chain. There is involvement of the superior middle mediastinum and hilar nodal chains within the chest. The bilateral lungs and myocardium are negative for disease. Normal physiologic liver, GI, and urinary activity is noted. There are multiple, enlarged para-aortic and right iliac lymph nodes in the abdomen and pelvis. Diffuse increased uptake within the bone marrow; it is unclear whether this is lymphoma or hyperplasia.

▓ Bone Marrow Biopsy

Bilateral biopsies are negative for Hodgkin's disease

▓ Assessment

Nodular sclerosis Hodgkin's disease, stage IIIB

QUESTIONS

Problem Identification

1.a. What clinical and other information is consistent with the diagnosis of Hodgkin's disease?

1.b. Explain what system of staging was used and how her stage of disease was determined.

Desired Outcome

2. What are the goals of therapy in this case?

Therapeutic Alternatives

3. What treatment options are available for managing this patient's Hodgkin's disease?

Optimal Plan

4. What drug, dosage form, schedule, and duration of chemotherapy are best for treating this patient's Hodgkin's disease?

Outcome Evaluation

5.a. What clinical and laboratory parameters are necessary to evaluate the therapy for achievement of the desired therapeutic outcome for treatment of Hodgkin's disease?

5.b. What acute adverse effects are associated with the chemotherapy regimen?

5.c. What clinical or laboratory parameters are necessary to detect and prevent acute and long-term adverse events commonly associated with treatment of Hodgkin's disease?

Patient Education

6. What information should be provided to the patient to enhance compliance, ensure successful therapy, and minimize adverse effects for treatment of Hodgkin's disease?

▓ CLINICAL COURSE

The patient's treatment was administered in the outpatient setting. She received day 1 of her first cycle of chemotherapy and experienced acute nausea and vomiting. She also experienced a low neutrophil count of 0.500 × 10³/mm³ during the first cycle. Treatment was withheld until her neutrophil count improved to >1.5 × 10³/mm³. At that time, the patient restarted her chemotherapy regimen and received pegfilgrastim 24 hours after her chemotherapy to maintain her current dose of chemotherapy without dose reduction and dose delay. As a result of pegfilgrastim, the patient experienced severe bone pain that was relieved by oxycodone/acetaminophen. She returned to the outpatient clinic for the next three cycles of chemotherapy. After her fourth cycle, she was restaged with a PET/CT to assess her response to the chemotherapy treatment. Restaging showed the patient had a complete response and on subsequent follow-up is in remission.

CLINICAL PEARL

Hodgkin's disease can be cured with chemotherapy, even if it is in advanced stages.

▓ SELF-STUDY ASSIGNMENTS

1. What are unfavorable prognostic factors for Hodgkin's disease, and how does this influence treatment?

2. What is the antiemetic regimen of choice to prevent acute nausea and vomiting for highly emetogenic chemotherapy?

3. What are the salvage therapy options for patients with relapsing Hodgkin's disease?

4. What is the role of bone marrow or stem cell transplantation for Hodgkin's disease?

REFERENCES

1. Fuchs M, Diehl V, Re D. Current strategies and new approaches in the treatment of Hodgkin's lymphoma. Pathobiology 2006;73:126–140.
2. Hasenclever D, Diehl V. A prognostic score for advanced Hodgkin's disease: International Prognostic Factors Project on Advanced Hodgkin's Disease. N Engl J Med 1998;339:1506–1514.
3. Johnson PW, Radford JA, Cullen MH, et al. Comparison of ABVD and alternating or hybrid multidrug regimens for the treatment of advanced Hodgkin's lymphoma: results of the United Kingdom Lymphoma Group LY09 Trial (ISRCTN97144519). J Clin Oncol 2005;23:9208–9218.
4. Friedman DL, Constine LS. Late effects of treatment for Hodgkin lymphoma. J Natl Compr Canc Netw 2006;4:249–257.

146

OVARIAN CANCER

Family Ties............................ Level II

William C. Zamboni, PharmD, PhD

Margaret E. Tonda, PharmD

LEARNING OBJECTIVES

After completing this case study, students should be able to:

- Recognize the signs and symptoms of ovarian cancer.
- Describe the genetic factors associated with ovarian cancer.
- Recommend a pharmacotherapeutic plan for the chemotherapeutic treatment of newly diagnosed and relapsed ovarian cancer.
- Describe the uses and potential pharmacologic advantages of intraperitoneal therapy for treatment of ovarian cancer.
- Recognize the dose-limiting and most common toxicities associated with the chemotherapeutic agents used in the treatment of ovarian cancer.

PATIENT PRESENTATION

Chief Complaint

"This is my first cycle of chemotherapy, and I am worried about getting sick."

HPI

Julia Erving is a 53-year-old woman who presented to the ED 9 weeks ago with a 3-day history of acute abdominal pain. She also reported a weight gain of approximately 9 kg over the previous 3 months. CT scans of the abdomen and pelvis showed a large, soft-tissue pelvic mass. Exploratory laparotomy revealed a 20 × 10 cm mass near the left ovary and positive microscopic disease in the omentum. A TAH and left oophorectomy were performed at that time. The CA 125 was 380 IU/mL. Tumor biopsies from the ovary were positive for epithelial ovarian cancer with serous histology.

Residual disease (1.5 cm) persists in the peritoneal cavity. She is now admitted to undergo her first cycle of consolidative chemotherapy.

PMH

Right-sided oophorectomy for ruptured ectopic pregnancy 12 years ago
S/P conjugated estrogens and progesterone × 5 years for HRT
Type 2 DM × 10 years
HTN × 5 years
Bilateral numbness in feet

FH

Divorced with no children; mother, maternal aunt, and cousin all have ovarian cancer; father is alive and well

SH

Social alcohol use; denies smoking

Meds

Nifedipine XL 60 mg po daily
Glipizide 10 mg po daily

All

Penicillin (seizures)
Aspirin (stomach cramps)

ROS

Stomach area feels heavy and painful; she sometimes feels nauseated

Physical Examination

Gen

Patient is an African-American woman appearing to be her stated age

VS

BP 130/80, P 110, RR 22, T 37.6°C; Wt 60 kg, Ht 5'4"

Skin

No erythema, rash, ecchymosis, petechiae, or breakdown

Lymph Nodes

No cervical or axillary lymphadenopathy

HEENT

PERRLA, EOMI; TMs intact; fundus benign; OP with dry mucous membranes

Breasts

Without masses, discharge, or adenopathy; no nipple or skin changes

Cor

RRR; no murmurs, rubs, or gallops

Pulm

Lungs are clear to auscultation, with a slight decrease at the left base; mainly resonant throughout all lung fields

Abd

Soft and nontender without hepatosplenomegaly

Genit/Rect

Normal female genitalia; heme (–) dark brown stool; no rectal wall tenderness or masses

Ext

No CCE

Neuro

Speech: no dysarthria, rate normal. CN II–XII intact. Motor: normal strength throughout; tone normal. Sensation decreased to light touch and pinprick below the knees bilaterally. Vibration sense diminished at the great toes bilaterally. Reflexes 2+ and symmetric throughout. Babinski negative bilaterally. Cerebellar: finger-to-nose and heel-to-shin are without dysmetria. Rapid alternate movements are normal as are gross and fine motor coordination. Good sitting and standing balance without an assistive device. Gait: able to toe and tandem walk without difficulty. Gait normal in speed and step length. Cognition: A & O × 3. Able to do serial 7s. Able to abstract. Short- and long-term memories are intact.

■ Labs

Na 137 mEq/L	Hgb 13.6 g/dL	AST 21 IU/L
K 3.1 mEq/L	Hct 38%	ALT 24 IU/L
Cl 99 mEq/L	Plt 150 × 10³/mm³	T. bili 0.8 mg/dL
CO_2 22 mEq/L	WBC 5.2 × 10³/mm³	Amylase 129 IU/L
BUN 20 mg/dL	Neutros 60%	Lipase 62 IU/L
SCr 1.5 mg/dL	Bands 3%	CA 125 380 IU/mL at presentation
Glu 180 mg/dL	Lymphs 30%	
	Monos 5%	
	Eos 1%	
	Basos 1%	

■ UA

WBC 5–10/hpf; RBC 1/hpf; 1+ ketones; 1+ protein, pH 5.0

■ Genetic Results from DNA Analysis from a Blood Sample

BRCA1 (+)

QUESTIONS

Problem Identification

1.a. What are the patient's drug therapy problems?

1.b. What information (signs, symptoms, laboratory values) indicates the presence and severity of ovarian cancer?

1.c. What stage of ovarian cancer does this patient have, and how does the stage of disease affect the choice of therapy?

1.d. What is the significance of the size of residual tumor after primary cytoreductive surgery?

Desired Outcome

2. What are the goals of therapy for this patient?

Therapeutic Alternatives

3.a. How do her genetic results influence the choice of therapy and prognosis?

3.b. What are the consolidative chemotherapy options for this patient?

3.c. What are the specific toxicities and logistical issues related to intraperitoneal (IP) therapy?

Optimal Plan

4.a. Which consolidative chemotherapy regimen and ancillary treatment measures would you recommend for this patient?

4.b. Regardless of whether you recommended IV carboplatin, use the Calvert equation to calculate the carboplatin dose required to achieve a target AUC of 5 mg/mL/min.

Outcome Evaluation

5. How would you monitor the therapy for efficacy and adverse effects?

Patient Education

6. What information would you provide to the patient about this therapy?

■ CLINICAL COURSE

Ms. Erving completed six cycles of an intense combination of IV and IP therapy. The regimen consisted of IV paclitaxel on day 1 in combination with IP cisplatin on day 2 and IP paclitaxel on day 8. Cycles were repeated every 21 days. Her serum CA 125 level slowly declined over the treatment course (110 IU/mL, 95 IU/mL, 85 IU/mL, 40 IU/mL, and 25 IU/mL after the first, second, third, fourth, and fifth cycles, respectively) and was 12 IU/mL 2 weeks after her sixth cycle. Based on her CA 125 levels and negative CT scans, Ms. Erving was defined as a clinical complete response. Treatment was discontinued, and CA 125 levels were followed monthly.

Over the next 4 months the CA 125 levels were as follows: 20 IU/mL, 30 IU/mL, 43 IU/mL, and 88 IU/mL. Five months after completing the last cycle of chemotherapy, a CT scan of the abdomen and pelvis revealed a mass (5 × 6 × 6 cm) arising from the retroperitoneum and a 2-cm mass in the head of the pancreas. Biopsies of the pancreas and abdominal/pelvic mass were positive for recurrent epithelial ovarian cancer. Laboratory data were normal except for a CA 125 level of 150 IU/mL. Ms. Erving is now admitted for her first cycle of chemotherapy for her relapsed ovarian cancer.

■ FOLLOW-UP QUESTIONS

1. What chemotherapeutic options are available for this patient's relapsed ovarian cancer?

2. Which of the chemotherapeutic regimens would you suggest for the patient's locally relapsed ovarian cancer? Why?

3. What are the potential toxicities of pegylated liposomal doxorubicin? How can they be prevented and treated?

■ CLINICAL COURSE

After four cycles of salvage chemotherapy with pegylated liposomal doxorubicin 40 mg/m² every 28 days, CA 125 levels were decreasing, and radiographic findings showed no progression of disease. However, the patient complained of having trouble putting on her shoes and her feet hurt when she walked. On physical examination, the patient's feet were red, swollen, and cracked. The fifth cycle of pegylated liposomal doxorubicin therapy was delayed for 2 weeks, and the redness on her feet resolved. The pegylated liposomal doxorubicin was restarted at 30 mg/m² every 28 days.

After three additional cycles of pegylated liposomal doxorubicin, the pain, redness, and swelling in Ms. Erving's feet returned. In addition, her CA 125 levels over this 3-month period where 92 IU/mL, 150 IU/mL, and 182 IU/mL.

Considering the poor prognosis and aggressive nature of her disease, she was enrolled in a phase I trial of gemcitabine and topotecan. Even though gemcitabine and topotecan are approved for clinical use, the combination has not been evaluated in patients. Thus, a phase I trial of the combination was developed to determine the maximum tolerated dose of gemcitabine in combination with a fixed dose of topotecan. She was treated with topotecan, 0.75 mg/m^2/day IV over 30 minutes on days 1–4; gemcitabine 1,000 mg/m^2/day IV over 1 hour on day 1, repeated every 21 days. Filgrastim, 5 mcg/kg/day, was started 24 hours after the last dose of chemotherapy and continued until the ANC was >1.0 × 10^3/mm^3 for 2 consecutive days. Her treatment is ongoing.

■ SELF-STUDY ASSIGNMENTS

1. What are the pharmacologic advantages of IP therapy versus IV therapy?

2. Why is the size of the residual tumor important with regard to IP therapy?

3. As an alternative treatment option, calculate the dose of carboplatin for IV therapy.

4. What is the probable cause of paclitaxel and docetaxel hypersensitivity?

5. What are the issues related to maintenance therapy in patients with advanced ovarian cancer after complete response to consolidative chemotherapy?

6. How does the polymorphism in cytochrome P450 3A5 potentially affect docetaxel therapy in the treatment of ovarian cancer?

CLINICAL PEARL

The primary objective of a phase I clinical trial is to determine the maximum tolerated dose and dose-limiting toxicities. In phase I trials, the dose of a chemotherapeutic agent is increased in cohorts of patients until dose-limiting toxicity is achieved.

REFERENCES

1. Boyd J, Sonoda Y, Federici MG, et al. Clinicopathologic features of BRCA-linked and sporadic ovarian cancer. JAMA 2000;283:2260–2265.

2. McGuire WP, Hoskins WJ, Brady MF, et al. Cyclophosphamide and cisplatin compared with paclitaxel and cisplatin in patients with stage III and stage IV ovarian cancer. N Engl J Med 1996;334:1–6.

3. Ozols RF, Bundy BN, Greer BE, et al. Phase III trial of carboplatin and paclitaxel compared with cisplatin and paclitaxel in patients with optimally resected stage III ovarian cancer: a Gynecological Oncology Group study. J Clin Oncol 2003;21:3194–3200.

4. du Bois A, Luck HJ, Meier W, et al. A randomized clinical trial of cisplatin/paclitaxel versus carboplatin/paclitaxel as first line treatment of ovarian cancer. J Natl Cancer Inst 2003;95:1320–1330.

5. Morgan RJ, Copeland L, Gershenson D, et al. NCCN ovarian cancer practice guidelines. The National Comprehensive Cancer Network. Oncology (Huntingt) 1996;10(11 Suppl):293–310.

6. Armstrong DK, Bundy B, Wenzel L, et al. Intraperitoneal cisplatin and paclitaxel in ovarian cancer. N Engl J Med 2006;354:34–43.

7. Calvert AH, Newell DR, Gumbrell LA, et al. Carboplatin dosage: prospective evaluation of a simple formula based on renal function. J Clin Oncol 1989;7:1748–1756.

8. Parmar MK, Ledermann J, Colombo N, et al., ICON and AGO Collaborators. Paclitaxel plus platinum-based chemotherapy versus conventional platinum-based chemotherapy in women with relapsed ovarian cancer: the ICON4/AGO-OVAR-2.2 trial. Lancet 2003;361:2099–2106.

9. Alberts DS, Liu PY, Hannigan EV, et al. Intraperitoneal cisplatin plus intravenous cyclophosphamide versus intravenous cisplatin plus intravenous cyclophosphamide for stage III ovarian cancer. N Engl J Med 1996;335:1950–1955.

10. Safra T, Muggia F, Jeffers S, et al. Pegylated liposomal doxorubicin (Doxil): reduced clinical cardiotoxicity in patients reaching or exceeding cumulative doses of 500 mg/m^2. Ann Oncol 2000;11:1029–1033.

147

ACUTE LYMPHOCYTIC LEUKEMIA

Jenny's Long Battle . . . . .Level II

Mark T. Holdsworth, PharmD, BCOP

LEARNING OBJECTIVES

After completing this case study, students should be able to:

- Identify common drug-induced diseases and disease-related complications in children with acute lymphocytic leukemia (ALL).

- Design effective prophylactic and treatment strategies for drug-induced diseases and disease-related complications in children with ALL.

- Describe a contemporary management strategy for tumor lysis syndrome.

- Interpret the laboratory values that signify the response of ALL to chemotherapy.

- Discuss key information that should be presented to a child's family when educating them about the chemotherapy agents used for ALL and the response to chemotherapy.

- Describe the ancillary medications and supportive care measures that are necessary when administering chemotherapy to children with ALL.

PATIENT PRESENTATION

■ Chief Complaint

Fatigue and low-grade fever

■ HPI

Jenny Martinez is a 3-year-old girl brought to the pediatric clinic by her parents, who report that for the past week she has been quite fatigued and has had fevers, easy bruising, and puffiness of the extremities.

■ PMH

Up-to-date on immunizations; no prior surgeries or serious medical problems

■ FH

No family history of cancer; resides near a site with a history of radioactive contamination

■ SH

Not applicable

■ ROS

Noncontributory

■ Meds

None

All

NKDA

Physical Examination

Gen

Alert, interactive, well-developed but ill-appearing child

VS

BP 130/83, P 95, RR 34, T 36.8°C; Wt 17.3 kg, Ht 38", BSA 0.6 m²

Skin

Diffuse pallor; random tan macular bruises just inferior to the hairline, face, and over the proximal upper extremity, with a petechial-appearing rash over the buttocks and lower left flank

HEENT

Head is NC/AT; PERRLA; EOMI; nares are clear bilaterally; throat shows no erythema. Question of petechial hemorrhage of mucous membranes.

Neck/Lymph Nodes

Neck supple and nontender with shotty cervical and submandibular lymphadenopathy

Lungs/Thorax

CTA bilaterally without wheezes or crackles, and there is good air movement throughout

Breasts

Undeveloped

CV

Heart has RRR without murmur

Abd

Soft and nontender, without distention. There are good bowel sounds and no masses present. Hepatosplenomegaly is noted.

Genit/Rect

No tenderness, bruising, or blood observed

MS/Ext

Shotty lymphadenopathy in the inguinal area; femoral pulses are 2+ bilaterally. Extremities display no CCE, and there is no bone pain elicited with palpation.

Neuro

Without dysmorphic features or deformities. Frequent rapid eye blinking (R > L); eyes seemed briefly disconjugate when asked to focus. Fixes and follows well with conjugate eye movements. Hearing appears intact. Motor examination shows normal muscle tone and bulk. Gait is essentially normal. DTRs are normal. General muscle strength is symmetric and normal. Facial strength appears symmetric and normal.

Labs

Hgb 5.7 g/dL	AST 93 IU/L	SCr 0.6 mg/dL
Hct 17.2%	ALT 60 IU/L	PT 12 sec
WBC 17.5 × 10³/mm³	LDH 1,875 IU/L	aPTT 24 sec
Segs 2%	T. bili 0.7 mg/dL	Varicella titer (+)
Bands 0%	T. prot 6.9 g/dL	Anti-HAV (–)
Lymphs 85%	Alb 3.5 g/dL	HBsAg (–)
Monos 4%	Ca 8.3 mg/dL	Anti-HBs (–)
Myelos 1%	Phos 3.6 mg/dL	Anti-HCV (–)
Blasts 8%	Uric acid 2.3 mg/dL	

BM Aspirate

90% blasts; 3% erythroid precursors; 2% lymphocytes; 2% metamyelocytes; 1% promyelocytes; 2% myelocytes. DNA index 1.4. Early pre-B cell ALL with L1 morphology. Real-time quantitive polymerase chain reaction (RQ-PCR) was positive for TEL-AML 1 fusion transcript and negative for E2A-PBX1.

Chest X-Ray

Normal with no mediastinal mass noted

LP

Glucose 55 mg/dL; T. protein 15 mg/dL; no blasts present

Assessment

Acute lymphocytic leukemia with pancytopenia and replacement of normal bone marrow elements

Clinical Course

The patient was admitted to the pediatric subacute care unit. Medications and treatments on admission included the following:

Day 1 (day of admission):

- 1 unit of irradiated/filtered platelets
- 1 unit PRBCs
- 5% dextrose in 0.2% sodium chloride IV with 30 mEq NaHCO₃/L at 2,000 mL/m²/day
- Allopurinol 50 mg po TID

Day 2 induction chemotherapy orders:

- Vincristine 1 mg IV Q week × 4 (on days 1, 8, 15, and 22)
- Dexamethasone 2 mg po in the morning and 1.5 mg po in the evening × 28 days
- PEG asparaginase 1,500 units IM on chemotherapy day 3
- Intrathecal therapy (IT) with methotrexate 12 mg on chemotherapy days 1 and 15

Four hours after the first chemotherapy (day 2), she developed moderate nausea and vomiting, with four vomiting episodes. The patient also developed a fever of 39.5°C on day 2. Antibiotic therapy with cefipime 50 mg/kg IV Q 8 h is initiated.

Week 1 of induction therapy:

The patient remained in the hospital for the first 8 days. On day 2, serum uric acid was 4.2 mg/dL and then began to further increase throughout the week, with values of 6.8 mg/dL on day 3 and 8.5 mg/dL on day 5. On day 5, the patient received rasburicase 0.15 mg/kg IV × 1 dose. On day 6, the serum uric acid was 0.3 mg/dL and remained within or below normal limits thereafter. She became afebrile after day 4. Hematology tests obtained during the following 2 weeks of induction therapy were as follows:

Parameter (units)	Week 2 (day 7)	Week 3 (day 15)
Hgb (g/dL)	8.7	11.7
Hct (%)	25.1	35.3
Plt (× 10³/mm³)	22.0	70.0
WBC (× 10³/mm³)	0.670	2.35
Segs (%)	5	18
Bands (%)	0	0
Lymphs (%)	92	68
Monos (%)	1	12
Myelos (%)	0	2
Blasts (%)	2	0
Serum creatinine (mg/dL)	0.9	0.5

On day 15 of chemotherapy, a second BM aspirate revealed 1% blasts; 4% promyelocytes; 2% myelocytes; 4% metamyelocytes; 63% erythroblasts and other erythroid precursors; 9% lymphocytes; 4%

plasma cells; 10% bands; 1% neutrophils; 0% eosinophils; 0% basophils; 1% reticulum cells; and 1% monocytes. Day 15 LP showed CSF glucose 47 mg/dL and T. prot 14 mg/dL; no blasts present.

QUESTIONS

Problem Identification

1.a. Identify the patient's drug therapy and disease-related problems during the first week of induction therapy.

1.b. Because vincristine and the IT methotrexate are to be administered on the same day, what precautions must be observed to avoid severe drug toxicity?

Desired Outcome

2.a. What are the initial goals of pharmacotherapy in this patient, and were they achieved?

2.b. What are the long-term treatment goals in this patient?

Therapeutic Alternatives

3. List the therapeutic alternatives for the drug therapy and disease-related problems that developed during induction therapy, and discuss the risks and benefits of each.

Optimal Plan

4. Outline the optimal treatment schedule and duration for the drug therapy and disease-related problems described in the previous answer. What therapeutic alternatives should be considered if initial therapy fails?

Outcome Evaluation

5. What key laboratory parameters are indicative of an adequate response to induction therapy?

Patient Education

6.a. What information should be provided to the patient's parents about the potential beneficial and adverse effects from the chemotherapy agents used during induction therapy?

6.b. Jenny's parents believe that the term "remission" is the same as "cure" or "absence of disease." Explain to them the meaning of *remission*.

■ CLINICAL COURSE—INDUCTION WEEK 3

During week 3, Jenny develops abdominal pain and constipation. Her parents attempt to use the docusate liquid that was provided to them, but Jenny has trouble taking (and eventually refuses) this medication; after 2 additional days without bowel movements, Jenny's abdominal pain worsens. Her parents bring her to the clinic, and the PE reveals an ill-appearing child with severe abdominal pain. Vital signs are BP 100/60, P 98, RR 30, and T 37°C. The remainder of her PE is WNL. The following laboratory values are reported:

Hgb 11.7 g/dL	Glu 85 mg/dL	Ca 9.7 mg/dL
Hct 35.3%	Lactate 8 mg/dL	Phos 5.2 mg/dL
Plt 70 × 10³/mm³	AST 53 IU/L	Uric acid 2.3 mg/dL
WBC 2.35 × 10³/mm³	ALT 35 IU/L	PT 14 sec
Segs 18%	LDH 170 IU/L	aPTT 27 sec
Bands 0%	T. bili 0.5 mg/dL	
Lymphs 68%	D. bili 0.2 mg/dL	
Monos 12%	T. prot 7.3 g/dL	
Myelos 2%	Alb 4.1 g/dL	
Blasts 0%		

She is scheduled to receive day 22 of chemotherapy in 2 days, and orders are written to continue chemotherapy on the current schedule.

Follow-Up Question—Induction Week 3

1. What modifications in the therapeutic plan should be made?

■ CLINICAL COURSE—INDUCTION WEEK 4

On day 28 of chemotherapy (end of induction), her laboratory values are:

Hgb 12.8 g/dL	WBC 11.0 × 10³/mm³
Hct 38.2%	Segs 86%
Plt 326 × 10³/mm³	Bands 0%
	Lymphs 10%
	Monos 4%
	Myelos 0%
	Blasts 0%

The results of the day 28 BM aspirate showed 2% blasts; 3% promyelocytes; 5% myelocytes; 7% metamyelocytes; 8% bands; 8% neutrophils; 56% erythroblasts and other erythroid precursors; 5% lymphocytes; 1% monocytes; and 5% eosinophils and precursors.

■ CLINICAL COURSE—CONSOLIDATION PHASE

After completion of induction therapy and resolution of her acute illness, she entered an initial consolidation phase × 4 weeks that consisted of weekly vincristine, daily mercaptopurine, a dose of PEG asparaginase, and 3 weekly treatments with IT methotrexate. This phase of therapy was well tolerated, and she then proceeded to an intensified consolidation phase consisting of the following:

- Mercaptopurine 50 mg/m² po daily on days 1–14 and 29–42
- Cyclophosphamide 1 g/m² IV × 1 dose on days 1 and 29
- Cytarabine 75 mg/m² IV daily × 4 days on days 1–4, 8–11, 29–32, 36–39
- Vincristine 1.5 mg/m² IV × 1 dose on weeks 15, 22, 43, and 50
- IT with methotrexate 12 mg × 1 dose on days 1, 8, 15 and 22

At the start of this phase of therapy, her CBC is as follows:

Hgb 10.4 g/dL	WBC 5.1 × 10³/mm³
Hct 31.1%	Segs 50%
Plt 256 × 10³/mm³	Bands 0%
	Lymphs 35%
	Monos 10%
	Eos 3%
	Basos 2%

On day 14 of intensified consolidation, Jenny develops severe pancytopenia as illustrated by the following CBC:

Hgb 7.5 g/dL	WBC 0.3 × 10³/mm³
Hct 22.2%	Segs 46%
Plt 25 × 10³/mm³	Bands 0%
	Lymphs 50%
	Monos 2%
	Eos 1%
	Basos 1%

Follow-Up Questions—Intensified Consolidation (Week 10)

2. What supportive care medications should she receive with the chemotherapy that is scheduled on days 1–14?

3. What are the likely explanations for the pancytopenia?

4. Should her chemotherapy be withheld at this point on day 14 until her CBC returns to normal?

5. When would her CBC results be used to decide on whether to administer further chemotherapy?

■ CLINICAL COURSE—WEEKS 16–58

After completing the intensified consolidation phase, the plan is for Jenny to receive additional phases of therapy, including interim maintenance × 8 weeks, augmented interim maintenance × 6 weeks, standard delayed intensification × 6 weeks, augmented delayed intensification × 8 weeks, a second augmented interim maintenance × 6 weeks and a second augmented delayed intensification × 8 weeks.

Jenny proceeds through the first above three courses uneventfully and is now ready to begin standard delayed intensification. This course of chemotherapy is to begin on week 30 and is composed of the following:

- Dexamethasone 10 mg/m^2 po, divided BID on days 1–21
- Doxorubicin 25 mg/m^2 IV on days 1, 8, and 15
- PEG asparaginase 2,500 units/m^2 IM on days 4, 5, or 6 (*Note:* 1 day only)
- Vincristine 1.5 mg/m^2 IV × 1 dose on weeks 1, 8, and 15
- Methotrexate 12 mg IT on days 1 and 29
- Cyclophosphamide 1 g/m^2 IV × 1 dose on day 29
- Cytarabine 75 mg/m^2 IV daily × 4 days on days 29–32, 36–39
- Thioguanine 60 mg/m^2 po on days 29–42

Instructions are for this chemotherapy to begin on days 1 and 29 when the ANC is ≥750/mm^3 and platelets are ≥75,000/mm^3. In addition, instructions are to continue therapy on days 1–21 and 29–42 despite uncomplicated myelosuppression.

Her CBC on day 1 is as follows:

Hgb 11.5 g/dL	WBC 2.1 × 10^3/mm^3
Hct 34.5%	Segs 45%
Plt 157 × 10^3/mm^3	Bands 0%
	Lymphs 43%
	Monos 7%
	Eos 3%
	Basos 2%

Jenny's physical examination on day 1 is unremarkable.

Follow-Up Questions—Standard Delayed Intensification

6. Based upon the above CBC results, should Jenny receive chemotherapy on day 1?

7. Outline a supportive care plan for the chemotherapy that is scheduled on days 1–21.

■ CLINICAL COURSE

Once this phase of chemotherapy begins, Jenny has her CBC drawn again on day 8, which reveals the following:

Hgb 10.8 g/dL	WBC 9.1 × 10^3/mm^3
Hct 33.1%	Segs 71%
Plt 135 × 10^3/mm^3	Bands 0%
	Lymphs 21%
	Monos 3%
	Eos 3%
	Basos 2%

Jenny is clinically well on day 8.

Follow-Up Questions

8. What is the most likely reason for her increased WBC count, and what is your interpretation of the WBC differential?

■ CLINICAL COURSE

After completing all of the above chemotherapy courses through week 58, Jenny is scheduled to receive maintenance therapy for 1.5 years. The following is a summary of her maintenance chemotherapy schedule:

- Methotrexate 20 mg/m^2 po × 1 dose weekly
- Mercaptopurine 75 mg/m^2 po daily
- Vincristine 2 mg/m^2 IV every 4 weeks
- Dexamethasone 6 mg/m^2 po divided BID × 5 days every 4 weeks
- IT with methotrexate × 1 dose every 12 weeks

Follow-Up Questions

9. During the maintenance phase of her chemotherapy protocol, which laboratory test is closely monitored to gauge the adequacy of her chemotherapy doses?

10. What is the target value for this laboratory measurement, and how will the chemotherapy doses be changed if the laboratory test is above the target range?

■ CLINICAL COURSE

Jenny does well on her maintenance chemotherapy, and her parents report no significant complications from this therapy. After 15 weeks on this therapy, her CBC values are all within normal limits, and her last 4 ANC values over the past 6 weeks are as follows: 6 weeks ago 0.230 × 10^3/mm^3, 4 weeks ago 0.270 × 10^3/mm^3, 2 weeks ago 0.320 × 10^3/mm^3, today 0.240 × 10^3/mm^3.

Follow-Up Questions—Week 73

11. What is your interpretation of these ANC values? Should Jenny's maintenance therapy be changed because of these results?

■ SELF-STUDY ASSIGNMENTS

1. Provide evidence to support the value of maintaining adequate dose intensity in the maintenance phase of ALL therapy (focus on trials that report the actual received-dose intensity).

2. Discuss the value of colony-stimulating factors in the prophylaxis or treatment of therapy-related complications in children with ALL.

3. Discuss the influence of pharmacogenetics on the dynamics of pharmacotherapy during treatment of ALL.

CLINICAL PEARL

Although most chromosomal translocations in ALL confer a worse prognosis, the TEL-AML 1 fusion transcript [associated with t(12;21)] in this patient indicates a good prognosis case of B-ALL. However, relapses can still occur and tend to occur late in children with this translocation. For this reason, it is still not recommended to reduce the intensity of chemotherapy for children with this translocation.

REFERENCES

1. Holdsworth MT, Raisch DW, Winter SS, et al. Assessment of the emetogenic potential of intrathecal chemotherapy and response to prophylactic treatment with ondansetron. Support Care Cancer 1998;6:132–138.
2. Holdsworth MT, Nguyen P. Role of i.v. allopurinol and rasburicase in tumor lysis syndrome. Am J Health Syst Pharm 2003;60:2213–2224.
3. Holdsworth MT, Mathew P. Efficacy of colony-stimulating factors in acute leukemia. Ann Pharmacother 2001;35:92–108.
4. ASHP Commission on Therapeutics. ASHP therapeutic guidelines on the pharmacologic management of nausea and vomiting in adult and pediatric patients receiving chemotherapy or radiation therapy or undergoing surgery. Am J Health Syst Pharm 1999;56:729–764.

148

CHRONIC MYELOGENOUS LEUKEMIA

Philadelphia Freedom? . . . . Level II

Christine M. Walko, PharmD, BCOP

LEARNING OBJECTIVES

After completing this case study, students should be able to:

- Identify the presenting signs and symptoms of chronic myelogenous leukemia (CML).

- Identify important prognostic indicators for CML.

- Construct treatment options for newly diagnosed and refractory or relapsed CML.

- List appropriate parameters to monitor efficacy and potential adverse effects of treatment for CML.

- Educate patients on treatment complications and the most common side effects of therapy for CML.

PATIENT PRESENTATION

Chief Complaint

"I've been really tired lately."

HPI

John Pella is a 46-year-old man who complains of shortness of breath on exertion, an unintentional weight loss of 6.4 kg, and fatigue beginning 4 months ago. He also notes fullness in his left upper quadrant and early satiety.

PMH

Tonsillectomy (1968)
Appendectomy (1977) complicated with infection
Hernia repair (2000)

FH

Father died of pulmonary embolism at age 54. Mother is 73 years old with Type 2 diabetes. His 47-year-old sister and 23-year-old son are in good health. Grandparents may have had CAD. No history of cancer.

SH

Married and lives with his wife of 25 years. He works full-time in the maintenance department of a local packaging company. Smoked one-half to three-fourths a pack of cigarettes per day for more than 20 years until he quit 4 years ago. Denies alcohol consumption.

Meds

None

All

Penicillin (skin rash—31 years ago)

ROS

Increased weakness and tiredness. Occasional fever, chills, and night sweats; shortness of breath on exertion. Denies bleeding, headaches, nausea, vomiting, chest pain, or urinary symptoms.

Physical Examination

Gen

WDWN white man in NAD who appears his stated age

VS

BP 120/88, P 84, RR 18, T 37°C; actual Wt 90.9 kg, Ht 6'1"

Skin

Warm, dry, with good turgor; no evidence of rash, ecchymoses, petechiae, or cyanosis

HEENT

PERRLA; EOMI; sclerae anicteric; TMs clear; no sinus discharge or tenderness; oral mucosa moist and intact

Neck

Supple without masses; no carotid bruits auscultated; no thyromegaly appreciated

Lymph Nodes

Approximately 1-cm, nontender palpable node in right inguinal area; no other lymphadenopathy noted

Chest

CTA; no rales or rhonchi

CV

NSR; normal S_1 and S_2 without murmur

Abd

Soft, symmetric, and nontender. Spleen palpable 8 cm below costal margin. Normoactive bowel sounds. No hepatomegaly noted. Well-approximated abdominal surgical scar noted.

Rect

Deferred

MS/Ext

No joint deformities or peripheral edema; ROM and muscle strength symmetric throughout

Neuro

CN II–XII intact; DTRs 1+ throughout; gait steady. A & O × 3.

Labs

Na 143 mEq/L	Hgb 12.1 g/dL	AST 30 IU/L	Ca 8.9 mg/dL
K 4.4 mEq/L	Hct 32%	ALT 86 IU/L	Mg 3.0 mEq/L
Cl 109 mEq/L	Plt 456 × 10³/mm³	Alk phos 29 IU/L	Phos 4.8 mg/dL
CO₂ 24 mEq/L	WBC 97.0 × 10³/mm³	LDH 325 IU/L	Uric acid 0.9 mg/dL
BUN 50 mg/dL	Segs 24%	T. bili 4.9 mg/dL	LAP absent
SCr 0.7 mg/dL	Bands 8%	T. prot 2.9 g/dL	
Glu 148 mg/dL	Lymphs 64%	Alb 1.6 g/dL	
Retic 2.3%	Myelos 3%		
	Monos 1%		

Bone Marrow Biopsy

Cytogenetic studies revealed a translocation involving the long arms of chromosomes 9 and 22 [t(9q;22q)] (Philadelphia chromosome), with 95% of malignant cells analyzed found to be Ph-positive. The marrow was hypercellular and consisted of 2–3% myeloblasts, but showed no other blastic abnormalities. This information is consistent with the characteristics of CML in chronic phase (CML-CP).

QUESTIONS

Problem Identification

1.a. What information in the patient's history is consistent with a diagnosis of CML-CP (Fig. 148-1)?

1.b. Describe the natural progression of CML.

1.c. List factors that signal a poor prognosis for CML patients in chronic phase.

Desired Outcome

2. What are long-term therapy goals for this patient?

Therapeutic Alternatives

3. What nonpharmacologic and pharmacologic alternatives should be considered for this newly diagnosed patient?

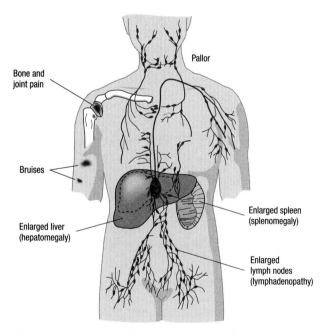

FIGURE 148-1. Common signs and symptoms of chronic myelogenous leukemia.

Optimal Plan

4. Considering all patient factors, describe the optimal initial treatment plan for this patient.

Outcome Evaluation

5. Describe parameters for monitoring disease response and toxicity for the treatment option you recommended.

Patient Education

6. What information should be given to the patient prior to treatment?

■ CLINICAL COURSE

The regimen you recommended was initiated. At the 2-week follow-up visit, the patient's WBC count was 28 × 10³/mm³. At the 4-week follow-up visit, his WBC count had decreased to 8.0 × 10³/mm³. After 6 months of treatment, his WBC count remained stable at 7.6 × 10³/mm³. He achieved a complete cytogenetic response, as evidenced by a bone marrow biopsy that revealed no positive metaphases for the Philadelphia chromosome. Molecular analysis using real-time quantitive polymerase chain reaction (RQ-PCR) reveals less than a 3-log reduction of BCR-ABL transcripts in leukocyte RNA. The patient discussed further treatment options with his physician. An allogeneic HSCT from a matched-related sibling was chosen, using IV busulfan and fludarabine as the preparative regimen.

■ FOLLOW-UP QUESTIONS

1. What is the goal of therapy for allogeneic HSCT in the management of CML-CP?

2. Is this CML patient an optimal candidate for an HSCT? Why or why not?

3. List common complications of allogeneic HSCT and this preparative regimen.

4. Identify important laboratory and clinical values to monitor during the HSCT course.

5. If relapse occurs after allogeneic HSCT, what treatment alternatives remain for this patient?

6. What are the potential mechanisms for resistance to imatinib?

■ SELF-STUDY ASSIGNMENTS

1. Describe the hematologic and cytogenetic response criteria (complete, partial, minor, and no response) for therapy in patients with CML, including WBC count, splenomegaly, and percent of Ph+ marrow cells.

2. How does the treatment of a Ph– CML patient differ from Ph+ disease?

3. Discuss the role of non–ATP-competitive BCR-ABL inhibitors in the management of CML. These include farnesyl transferase inhibitors, homoharringtonine, hypomethylating agents, histone deacetylase inhibitors, and immunologic agents such as vaccines.

CLINICAL PEARL

Fluorescence in situ hybridization (FISH) and real-time quantitative polymerase chain reaction (RQ-PCR) enable the use of peripheral blood samples, rather than bone marrow, to monitor molecular remission and minimal residual disease in patients receiving imatinib.

REFERENCES

1. Baccarani M, Saglio G, Goldman J, et al. Evolving concepts in the management of chronic myeloid leukemia: recommendations from an expert panel on behalf of the European LeukemiaNet. Blood 2006;108:1809–1820.

2. Savage DG, Antman KH. Imatinib—a new oral targeted therapy. N Engl J Med 2002;346:683–693.

3. O'Brien SG, Guilhot F, Larson RA, et al. Imatinib compared with interferon and low-dose cytarabine for newly diagnosed chronic-phase chronic myeloid leukemia. N Engl J Med 2003;348:994–1004.

4. Druker B, Guilhot F, O'Brien SG, et al. Five-year follow-up of patients receiving imatinib for chronic myeloid leukemia. N Engl J Med 2006;355:2408–2417.

5. Devergie A, Apperley JF, Labopin M, et al. European results of matched unrelated donor bone marrow transplantation for chronic myeloid leukemia. Impact of HLA class II matching. Bone Marrow Transplant 1997;20:11–19.

6. Deininger MW, O'Brien SG, Ford JM, et al. Practical management of patients with chronic myeloid leukemia receiving imatinib. J Clin Oncol 2003;21:1637–1647.

7. Talpaz M, Shah NP, Kantarjian H, et al. Dasatinib in imatinib-resistant Philadelphia chromosome-positive leukemias. N Engl J Med 2006;354:2531–2541.

8. Kantarjian H, Giles F, Wunderle L, et al. Nilotinib in imatinib-resistant CML and Philadelphia chromosome-positive ALL. N Engl J Med 2006;354:2542–2551.

149

MELANOMA

Don't Let the Sun Get You . . . . Level II

J. Michael Vozniak, PharmD, BCOP

LEARNING OBJECTIVES

After completing this case study, students should be able to:

• Identify risk factors for developing melanoma.

• Discuss appropriate pharmacotherapeutic management options for metastatic melanoma.

• List appropriate parameters to monitor for aldesleukin adverse effects.

• Educate patients with melanoma about the common toxicities associated with aldesleukin.

• Describe the two types of melanoma prevention strategies and their goals.

PATIENT PRESENTATION

■ Chief Complaint

"I'm here for round 2 of high-dose IL-2 treatment."

■ HPI

James Kelly is a 47-year-old white man who has a history of Stage IA superficial spreading melanoma diagnosed 2½ years ago. The mela-

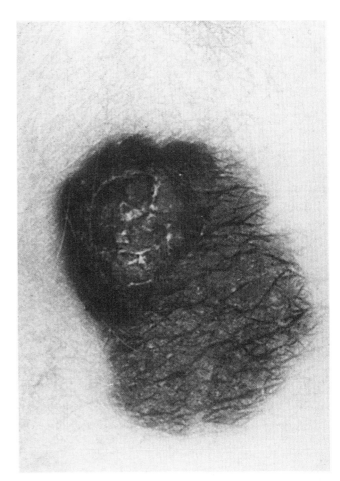

FIGURE 149-1. Superficial spreading melanoma developing in contiguity with a dysplastic nevus. *(Reprinted with permission from Lejeune FJ, Chaudhuri PK, Das Gupta TK, eds. Malignant Melanoma: Medical and Surgical Management. New York, McGraw-Hill, 1994:Plate 5b.)*

noma lesion was on his right scapula and was surgically removed with a wide excision. Since then, he has had annual dermatology appointments, and at his last visit 2 months ago, was found to have a suspicious mole on his left scapula that was asymmetric with color changes (Fig. 149-1). The mole was removed by excisional biopsy and was also found to be a superficial spreading melanoma. The patient underwent a surgical excision and sentinel lymphadenectomy. The tumor was found to be 2.18 mm thick without ulceration or satellitosis and involved one lymph node. Laboratory studies revealed an elevated LDH of 492 IU/L. CT scans of the chest, and pelvis revealed solitary lesions in both the left lung and liver consistent with metastatic disease. He was diagnosed with Stage IV (T3aN1M1c) melanoma.

Mr. Kelly presents to the hospital today for his second course of high-dose aldesleukin therapy. He was admitted 2 weeks ago for his first course, and he received 10 of 14 planned doses in the first of two 5-day treatment cycles. His initial course was discontinued prematurely secondary to hypotension, renal dysfunction, and edema. All of these complications resolved within 48 hours of aldesleukin discontinuation.

■ PMH

Hypertension
Hyperlipidemia
Melanoma (Stage IA)
S/P appendectomy (1979)

■ FH

Father age 70 alive with HTN and CAD; mother age 68 alive and well. Patient has 2 siblings, both alive and well. No family history of cancer.

SH

Patient is married with two children (ages 12 and 14). He is employed as a bank executive. He reports a history of numerous blistering sunburns as a child while at his parent's summer home at the New Jersey shore. No smoking or illicit drugs. He drinks one glass of Scotch each night before bed.

Meds

Lisinopril 20 mg po once daily
Hydrochlorothiazide 25 mg po once daily
Rosuvastatin 10 mg po once daily

All

NKDA

ROS

No fever or chills; no headaches; no nausea or vomiting

Physical Examination

Gen

WDWN white man, slightly anxious

VS

BP 119/78, P 78, RR 16, T 37.2°C; Wt 92.8 kg, Ht 6'2", BSA 2.2 m^2

Skin

Fair in complexion; left and right upper scapula wounds present; well healed with no drainage; multiple scattered dysplastic nevi, mostly on trunk

HEENT

PERRLA, EOMI; oropharynx without lesions

Neck/Lymph Nodes

Supple without adenopathy; thyroid without masses

Lung/Thorax

CTA bilaterally without rales or rhonchi

CV

RRR; normal S$_1$ and S$_2$; no MRG

Abd

Soft, NT/ND; (+) BS; appendectomy scar present

Genit/Rect

Deferred

MS/Ext

No CCE; normal ROM and sensation; distal pulses 2+ throughout

Neuro

A & O × 3; CN II–XII intact; DTRs 2+ and symmetric

Labs

Na 138 mEq/L	Hgb 15.5 g/dL	WBC 6.7 × 10^6/mm^3	T. bili 0.6 mg/dL
K 4.2 mEq/L	Hct 45%	Neutros 65%	AST 33 IU/L
Cl 101 mEq/L	RBC 5.0 × 10^6/mm^3	Bands 4%	ALT 29 IU/L
CO$_2$ 26 mEq/L	Plt 289 × 10^3/mm^3	Eos 1%	Alk phos 77 IU/L
BUN 14 mg/dL		Lymphs 26%	Alb 4.8 g/dL
SCr 1.1 mg/dL		Monos 4%	LDH 308 IU/L
Glu 82 mg/dL			Ca 8.2 mg/dL
			Mg 2.2 mg/dL
			pO$_4$ 3.4 mg/dL

Assessment

1. 47-year-old man with metastatic melanoma involving liver and lung admitted for his second course of high-dose IL-2.

2. Toxicities experienced during prior course have all resolved.

QUESTIONS

Problem Identification

1.a. Create a list of the patient's drug therapy problems.

1.b. What information (signs, symptoms, laboratory values) indicates the presence or severity of his melanoma?

1.c. What risk factor(s) does this patient have for developing melanoma?

Desired Outcome

2. What are the goals of using high-dose aldesleukin therapy for this patient?

Therapeutic Alternatives

3. What feasible chemotherapeutic alternatives to high-dose aldesleukin are available for treating this patient's metastatic melanoma?

Optimal Plan

4. Calculate the dose of aldesleukin this patient should receive.

Outcome Evaluation

5. What clinical and laboratory parameters are necessary to evaluate the therapy for achievement of the desired therapeutic outcome and to detect or prevent adverse effects?

Patient Education

6. What information would you provide to the patient about aldesleukin therapy?

■ CLINICAL COURSE

Mr. Kelly has tolerated six of seven doses of aldesleukin so far, missing dose 4 due to hypotension (BP 90/65), tachycardia (HR 124), and increased SCr (2.2 mg/dL). Eight hours later, when dose 5 was due, his BP and HR had normalized and he has subsequently tolerated doses 5, 6, and 7. He is now due for dose 8. His vitals are as follows: BP 84/54, HR 128, RR 18, Temp 38.1°C; Wt 98.3 kg (5.5 kg increase from baseline). On physical exam, he appears erythematous and diaphoretic; he has 2+ pitting edema bilaterally, and crackles are heard in his lungs bilaterally. The patient states that he is "itchy all over" but does not complain of headache, diarrhea, or abdominal pain. Pertinent lab results are as follows:

Na 141 mEq/L	BUN 28 mg/dL	Ca 8.1 mg/dL
K 3.2 mEq/L	SCr 2.6 mg/dL	Mg 1.2 mg/dL
	Alb 2.9 g/dL	pO$_4$ 2.8 mg/dL

■ FOLLOW-UP QUESTIONS

1. What is the cause of the toxicity occurring in this patient? Describe this adverse effect.

2. Create a list of the adverse effects the patient is experiencing from aldesleukin therapy. How would you manage each adverse effect?

■ ADDITIONAL CASE QUESTIONS

1. Mr. Kelly's two children ask how they can prevent getting melanoma. How would you advise them?

2. Describe the two types of melanoma prevention strategies.

■ SELF-STUDY ASSIGNMENTS

1. Design an antiemetic regimen for patients receiving high-dose aldesleukin therapy.

2. Discuss the role of sorafenib in the treatment of melanoma.

3. Perform a literature search on the treatment options for patients with metastatic melanoma who have failed aldesleukin therapy.

4. Describe how you would monitor the efficacy and toxicity of the patient's hyperlipidemia therapy.

CLINICAL PEARL

The incidence of melanoma in both men and women continues to rise each year. Fortunately, the majority (82–85%) of patients present with localized disease (Stage I or II), which is managed by surgical excision of the lesion.

REFERENCES

1. Greene FL, Page DL, Fleming ID, et al., eds. AJCC American Joint Committee on Cancer Staging Manual, 6th ed. New York, Springer-Verlag, 2002.

2. Atkins MB, Kunkel L, Sznol M, et al. High-dose recombinant interleukin-2 therapy in patients with metastatic melanoma: long-term survival update. Cancer J Sci Am 2000;6(Suppl 1):S11–S14.

3. Middleton MR, Grob JJ, Aaronson N, et al. Randomized phase III study of temozolomide versus dacarbazine in the treatment of patients with advanced metastatic malignant melanoma. J Clin Oncol 2000;18:158–166.

4. NCCN Melanoma Guidelines v.2.2006. Available at: www.nccn.org. Accessed January 4, 2007.

5. Rosenberg SA, Yang JC, Topalian SL, et al. Treatment of 283 consecutive patients with metastatic melanoma or renal cell cancer using high-dose bolus interleukin-2. JAMA 1994;271:907–913.

6. Schwartz RN, Stover L, Dutcher J. Managing toxicities of high-dose interleukin-2. Oncology (Huntingt) 2002;16(11 Suppl 13):11–20.

7. Ramirez R, Schneider J. Practical guide to sun protection. Surg Clin North Am 2003;83:97–107.

150

HEMATOPOIETIC STEM CELL TRANSPLANTATION

Complications of Allogeneic Stem
Cell Transplant . . . . Level III

Christopher A. Fausel, PharmD, BCPS, BCOP

LEARNING OBJECTIVES

After completing this case study, students should be able to:

- Understand the regimen-related toxicities of conditioning chemotherapy used for allogeneic stem cell transplant (SCT).

- Differentiate the presenting features of graft-versus-host disease (GVHD).

- Design appropriate pharmacotherapeutic regimens for patients who are critically ill during the peritransplant period.

PATIENT PRESENTATION

■ Chief Complaint

The patient developed acute onset of shortness of breath on day +15 following stem cell reinfusion, requiring intubation. The patient has Grade IV mucositis that was managed with parenteral opioids prior to intubation. The patient is also febrile.

■ HPI

Randall Taylor is a 45-year-old man who was admitted 22 days ago for an HLA-matched related donor allogeneic marrow transplant for AML. A triple-lumen central venous catheter had been placed prior to this admission. His transplant preparative regimen consisted of busulfan (0.8 mg/kg IV Q 6 h) × 4 days followed by high-dose cyclophosphamide (60 mg/kg/day) × 2 days. He was supported with aggressive antiemetics, including scheduled doses of a 5-HT$_3$ antagonist with each day of chemotherapy, and dexamethasone for the 2 days of cyclophosphamide. His GVHD prophylaxis consisted of tacrolimus (0.02 mg/kg/day) IV continuous infusion starting on day −1 and methotrexate (15 mg/m^2 IV) given on day +1 and (10 mg/m^2 IV) on day +3, day +6, and day +11. His course has been unremarkable with the exception of Grade IV mucositis for which he was initiated on a hydromorphone IV infusion and PCA for pain control, elevated liver function tests, and a fever spike on day +10 that prompted the initiation of broad-spectrum antibacterials with cefepime and vancomycin. The patient had already been receiving anti-infective prophylaxis with oral ciprofloxacin (which was discontinued after vancomycin and cefepime were started), fluconazole, and acyclovir.

The patient began to demonstrate signs of engraftment on day +13 when the WBC increased to $0.3 \times 10^3/mm^3$ from $<0.2 \times 10^3/mm^3$ the preceding day. On day +15 the patient's physical exam was notable for some rales in the lung bases, mild shortness of breath, and mild blood-tinged sputum. The WBC had further increased to $1.1 \times 10^3/mm^3$ with a differential of 59% polys, 15% bands, and 26% monocytes. As the day progressed, the patient became progressively more short of breath and slightly obtunded, despite the lowering of the hydromorphone PCA from settings the previous day of 0.8 mg/h IV and 0.5 mg IV Q 10 minutes with no lockout to 0.5 mg/h IV and 0.3 mg IV Q 10 minutes with a 4-hour lockout of 5.6 mg. A pulmonary consult was called, and after obtaining a chest X-ray showing bilateral infiltrates, the decision was made that elective bronchoscopy followed by intubation was the most appropriate course of action.

■ PMH

AML diagnosed 14 months prior to transplant that was initially treated with induction chemotherapy consisting of cytarabine and daunorubicin (the "7+3" regimen). The patient achieved remission, and it was decided that the best course of action was to offer post-remission chemotherapy with high-dose cytarabine × three cycles on the basis of his good-risk cytogenetic categorization with inversion 16 being identified as the only cytogenetic abnormality present in the leukemic clone. The patient tolerated the induction and post-remission chemotherapy with the exception of hospitalization for neutropenic fever after each cycle of

post-remission chemotherapy. Unfortunately, the patient relapsed and required re-induction chemotherapy with mitoxantrone, etoposide, and cytarabine (the "MEC" regimen) to achieve a second remission 2 months prior to transplant.
Hypercholesterolemia.
Hypertension.

■ FH

Married with three children. Both parents are deceased from cardiac disease.

■ Meds (at day +15)

Fluconazole 400 mg IV daily
Famotidine 20 mg IV Q 12 h
Hydromorphone infusion 0.5 mg/hour IV with PCA 0.3 mg IV Q 10 minutes—no lockout
Cefepime 2 g IV Q 8 h
Vancomycin (15 mg/kg) IV Q 12 h
Tacrolimus (0.01 mg/kg/day) IV continuous infusion
Chlorhexidine gluconate 0.12% 15 mL swish/spit QID
Acyclovir 500 mg IV Q 12 h
Filgrastim 480 mcg SC daily
Insulin coverage scale

■ All

Sulfa→rash

■ ROS

Unobtainable; patient is intubated

■ Physical Examination

Gen

Patient is a WDWN Caucasian male

VS

BP 106/53, P 92, T 38.1°C, currently intubated with FiO_2 of 90% and saturation 95%; Wt 102 kg (admission wt 94 kg); Ht 5'10"

HEENT

Face edematous, grade II–III oral/esophageal mucositis

Skin

Dry; no rash or evidence of GVHD

Neck/Lymph Nodes

Supple; no thyromegaly

Lungs

Bilateral decreased breath sounds, rales at the bases

Heart

RRR; no murmurs, rubs, or gallops; normal heart sounds

Abd

Slight distention, RUQ tenderness, mild hepatomegaly

Ext

Bilateral edema grade I–II in both LE

Neuro

Sedated on ventilator

■ Labs

Na 141 mEq/L	Hgb 7.3 g/dL	AST 55 IU/L
K 4.1 mEq/L	Hct 25%	ALT 61 IU/L
CL 109 mEq/L	Plt 7 × 10³/mm³	Alk phos 222 IU/L
CO₂ 20 mEq/L	WBC 1.1 × 10³/mm³	LDH 155 IU/L
BUN 22 mg/dL		T. bili 3.4 mg/dL
SCr 0.9 mg/dL		D. bili 2.8 mg/dL
Glu 133 mg/dL		Alb 2.8 g/dL

■ Blood Cultures

NGTD from day +10 (2/2 containers)

■ Other Cultures

All other culture sites (urine, sputum, central venous catheter) are negative

■ Assessment

New-onset respiratory distress in the face of neutrophil engraftment in allogeneic SCT patient

QUESTIONS

Problem Identification

1.a. What are the likely causes for the patient's new-onset respiratory failure?

1.b. What are potential causes for the patient's elevated liver function tests?

1.c. Assume that the LFT changes are not related to infection. Outline a therapeutic plan aimed at treating this new problem, should it progress.

Desired Outcome

2. What are the therapeutic goals in this patient?

Therapeutic Alternatives

3. What treatment options exist for managing the patient's respiratory failure from an infectious and noninfectious standpoint?

Optimal Plan

4.a. Outline changes that should be made to the patient's antibiotic regimen.

4.b. What pharmacotherapeutic intervention can be implemented to manage regimen-related pulmonary toxicities?

4.c. What drug therapies could be contributing to the elevated liver function tests?

Outcome Evaluation

5. What parameters should you monitor to assess the response to therapy and to detect adverse effects?

Patient Education

6. What appropriate counseling measures should be used for the patient's family and caregivers?

■ CLINICAL COURSE

The antibiotic regimen modifications were implemented as per discussion with pharmacy. The patient underwent bronchoscopy, and the washings came back with tinges of blood. The patient was subsequently initiated on high-dose corticosteroids with methylprednisolone 250 mg IV Q 6 h × 3 days. Following the fury of activity with the intubation and providing critical care level support, it was noted that he had some redness on his palms and a mild red blanching rash on his back. The dermatology resident was called to obtain a biopsy. Over the succeeding 48 hours, the patient had a decline in his FiO_2 from 90% to 40%, and the PEEP requirement dropped from 15 to 10. At this time, the patient continued to engraft with the WBC increasing to $2.2 \times 10^3/mm^3$ with an ANC of 1,020, and other labs included Hgb 9.7 g/dL and platelet count of $34 \times 10^3/mm^3$; both of which resulted from transfusion. Chemistries were remarkable for BUN 5 mg/dL, SCr 0.5 mg/dL, T. bili 3.9 mg/dL, AST 32 IU/L, ALT 16 IU/L, LDH 138 IU/L, and alk phos 144 IU/L. Bacterial blood cultures have remained negative and plasma PCR for CMV was <600 copies (negative). The skin biopsy report from dermatopathology came back as Grade II GVHD. The patient was afebrile after initiation of methylprednisolone and was ultimately extubated by day +22.

■ FOLLOW-UP QUESTIONS

1. What is the most appropriate medical therapy for the new finding of GVHD of the skin?
2. If the patient fails first-line treatment for GVHD, what further treatment options exist?

■ SELF-STUDY ASSIGNMENTS

1. What diseases are amenable to treatment with allogeneic stem cell transplantation?
2. Aside from the complications reviewed in this case, derive a list of potential problems that could occur after allogeneic marrow transplantation.

CLINICAL PEARL

Allogeneic stem cell transplantation often has multiple medical conditions requiring evaluation simultaneously that may be exacerbated by drug therapy.

REFERENCES

1. Armitage JO. Bone marrow transplantation. N Engl J Med 1994;330:827–838.
2. Copelan EA. Hematopoietic stem-cell transplantation. N Engl J Med 2006;354:1813–1826.
3. Zittoun RA, Mandelli F, Willemze R, et al. Autologous or allogeneic bone marrow transplantation compared with intensive chemotherapy in acute myelogenous leukemia in first remission. European Organization for Research and Treatment of Cancer (EORTC) and the Gruppo Italiano Malattie Ematologiche Maligne dell'Adulto (GIMEMA) Leukemia Cooperative Groups. N Engl J Med 1995;332:217–223.
4. Wah TM, Moss HA, Robertson RJ, et al. Pulmonary complications following bone marrow transplantation. Br J Radiol 2003;76:373–379.
5. CDC, the Infectious Diseases Society of America, and the American Society of Blood and Marrow Transplantation. Guidelines for preventing opportunistic infections among hematopoietic stem cell transplant recipients: recommendations of CDC, the Infectious Diseases Society of America, and the American Society of Blood and Marrow Transplantation. Biol Blood Marrow Transplant 2000;6:659–727.
6. Wadleigh M, Ho V, Momtaz P, et al. Hepatic veno-occlusive disease: pathogenesis, diagnosis and treatment. Curr Opin Hematol 2003;10:451–462.
7. Hughes WT, Armstrong D, Bodey GP, et al. 2002 guidelines for the use of antimicrobial agents in neutropenic patients with cancer. Clin Infect Dis 2002;34:730–751.
8. Raptis A, Mavroudis D, Suffredini A, et al. High-dose corticosteroid therapy for diffuse alveolar hemorrhage in allogeneic bone marrow stem cell transplant recipients. Bone Marrow Transplant 1999;24:879–883.
9. Ferrara JL, Levy R, Chao NJ. Pathophysiologic mechanisms of acute graft-vs.-host disease. Biol Blood Marrow Transplant 1999;5:347–356.
10. Przepiorka D, Smith TL, Folloder J, et al. Risk factors for acute graft-versus-host disease after allogeneic blood stem cell transplantation. Blood 1999;94:1465–1470.
11. Lazarus HM, Vogelsang GB, Rowe JM. Prevention and treatment of acute graft-versus-host disease: the old and the new—a report from The Eastern Cooperative Oncology Group (ECOG). Bone Marrow Transplant 1997;19:577–600.

SECTION 18
NUTRITION AND NUTRITIONAL DISORDERS

151

PARENTERAL NUTRITION

Not by Bread Alone . . . . .Level III

Michael D. Kraft, PharmD

LEARNING OBJECTIVES

After completing this case study, students should be able to:

- Describe how mesenteric ischemia can lead to malnutrition.

- Describe how fistulas can lead to nutritional, fluid, and electrolyte abnormalities.

- Characterize the severity of malnutrition based on subjective and objective data.

- Identify potential complications related to TPN in patients with malnutrition (e.g., refeeding syndrome) and steps to avoid or manage such complications.

- Design a patient-specific, parenteral nutrition (PN) prescription that is based on the nutritional diagnosis and other subjective and objective patient data.

- Construct and evaluate appropriate monitoring parameters for a hospitalized patient receiving PN.

PATIENT PRESENTATION

■ Chief Complaint

"I'm having foul-smelling liquid coming out of my surgery incision."

■ HPI

Larry Johnson is a 58-year-old man with a history of peripheral vascular occlusive disease (PVOD), hyperlipidemia, and Type 2 DM who was admitted to the hospital 9 days ago with abdominal pain, vomiting, and weight loss. For the past 6 months, he has had worsening abdominal pain that developed after eating a meal. The pain gradually worsened, and he developed vomiting over the 2 weeks prior to admission. Because of these symptoms, he avoided oral intake or took in only minimal amounts of food and liquids. He also reported an unintentional weight loss of approximately 40 pounds over the past 6 months. The patient underwent several diagnostic tests, including a CT scan and arteriogram. He was diagnosed with mesenteric ischemia and was taken to the operating room on the second hospital day for an exploratory laparotomy. He was found to have an occlusion of the superior mesenteric artery (SMA) and intestinal ischemia, and he underwent a vascular bypass

from the aorta to the SMA and a small bowel resection with primary anastomosis.

Postoperatively, the patient had persistent nausea and vomiting, requiring placement of an NG tube and remained NPO. The team placed a feeding tube into the duodenum on postoperative day (POD) 4 and initiated enteral nutrition (EN). On POD 6, he developed erythema around his surgical wound, which worsened over the next 2 days. On POD 8 he was noted to have a greenish, foul-smelling discharge from his surgical incision, as well as fluid that "looked like tube feeds" per the nurse. Physical examination of the wound revealed a likely enterocutaneous fistula, and a CT scan with contrast revealed an enterocutaneous fistula arising from the jejunum to the surgical incision site. A drain was placed into the fistula. Fistula output increased significantly when tube feeds were running, therefore EN was stopped, the feeding tube was removed, and the team placed a peripherally inserted central catheter (PICC) and ordered parenteral nutrition.

■ PMH

PVOD
Hyperlipidemia
Type 2 DM

■ PSH

None

■ FH

Remarkable for DM, HTN, and CAD in his mother. No family history of mesenteric ischemia.

■ SH

Married, lives with his wife; retired factory worker, now working at a local hardware store. Drinks alcohol socially; has a 70 pack-year history of smoking.

■ ROS

Subjectively reporting fevers, feels thirsty, no appetite. Complains of moderate abdominal pain and pain around the surgical incision site. Also complains his abdomen feels "crampy" and a little bloated. He denies chills, nausea, or other pain.

■ Meds

Pentoxyphylline 400 mg po BID
Simvastatin 40 mg po at bedtime
Glipizide XL 5 mg po BID
Metformin 1,000 mg po BID

■ All

NKDA

■ Physical Examination

Gen

Caucasian man, uncomfortable because of abdominal pain, appears malnourished, some evidence of wasting

VS

BP 114/68, P 86, RR 18, T 39.1°C; Wt 68 kg (wt 6 months ago ~86 kg), Ht 5'11"

Skin

Dry, flaking in some spots

HEENT

PERRLA, EOMI, anicteric sclerae, normal conjunctivae, mouth is dry, pharynx is clear, some evidence of wasting noted on temporal lobes, eyes appear sunken in, orbital ridge protruding somewhat.

Lungs/Thorax

CTA and percussion bilaterally

CV

RRR, no murmurs

Abd

Mild distention; hypoactive bowel sounds; diffuse tenderness throughout all quadrants with greater intensity in area of surgical incision; drain noted in fistula tract, draining approximately 250 mL over the past 8 hours, ~800 mL over the past 24 hours (off of tube feeds); draining greenish, foul-smelling fluid.

Genit/Rect

No lesions, no internal masses, stool is guaiac negative

MS/Ext

(−) Cyanosis, (−) edema, 2+ dorsalis pedis and posterior tibial pulses bilaterally, some evidence of wasting in large muscle groups (biceps, triceps, and quadriceps)

Neuro

A & O × 3; CN II–XII intact; motor 5/5 upper and lower extremity bilaterally; sensation intact and reflexes symmetric with downgoing toes

■ Labs on Admission

Na 136 mEq/L	Hgb 13.7 g/dL	AST 18 IU/L	Ca 7.1 mg/dL
K 3.6 mEq/L	Hct 38.2%	ALT 19 IU/L	Mg 1.8 mEq/L
Cl 94 mEq/L	Plt 287 × 10³/mm³	Alk phos 34 IU/L	Phos 2.9 mg/dL
CO₂ 27 mEq/L	WBC 9.6 × 10³/mm³	GGT 98 IU/L	PT 12.9 sec
BUN 9 mg/dL		T. bili 0.6 mg/dL	INR 0.9
SCr 0.5 mg/dL		T. prot 5.8 g/dL	
Glu 152 mg/dL		Alb 2.9 g/dL	

■ Labs on POD 8

Na 129 mEq/L	Hgb 10.1 g/dL	AST 18 IU/L	Ca 7.0 mg/dL
K 3.2 mEq/L	Hct 30.4%	ALT 19 IU/L	Mg 1.5 mEq/L
Cl 92 mEq/L	Plt 224 × 10³/mm³	Alk phos 34 IU/L	Phos 2.1 mg/dL
CO₂ 24 mEq/L	WBC 11.6 × 10³/mm³	GGT 98 IU/L	PT 13.7 sec
BUN 15 mg/dL		T. bili 1.1 mg/dL	INR 1.0
SCr 0.6 mg/dL		T. prot 5.1 g/dL	
Glu 145 mg/dL		Alb 2.4 g/dL	

■ Radiology

A CT scan with contrast demonstrates a fistula tract arising from the jejunum to the surgical incision site.

■ Assessment/Plan

EC fistula S/P exploratory laparotomy and small bowel resection: A drain was placed into the fistula tract, draining ~250 mL over the past 8 hours and ~800 mL over the past 24 hours, continue to monitor output, will start octreotide 100 mcg SC TID. If the patient continues to have high-output fistula (≥500 mL/day) and does not improve with octreotide, will discontinue octreotide.

Malnutrition with EC fistula: Given that this patient is malnourished and has a high-output EC fistula arising from the jejunum (and output appeared to increase with EN), success with enteral nutrition is unlikely. Initiate PN, obtain nutrition and pharmacy consults for recommendations. A PICC line was placed for administration of PN and fluids. Initiate IVF of 0.9% NaCl with KCl 20 mEq/L at 100 mL/h until PN is started. Once PN started, change IV fluids to administer 1 mL per 1 mL of fistula output.

Patient is now NPO, hold po pentoxyphylline, simvastatin, glipizide, and metformin for now; may require insulin for control of blood glucose.

QUESTIONS

Problem Identification

1.a. What clinical and laboratory data indicate the presence of malnutrition in this patient? Characterize the type and severity of malnutrition, and describe why he is at risk for further nutritional abnormalities.

1.b. How does mesenteric ischemia lead to malnutrition?

1.c. How can fistulas lead to malnutrition? What other disorders related to nutritional status and nutrition support (e.g., fluid, electrolytes, micronutrients) can develop in patients with fistulas?

1.d. Create a list of this patient's problems related to nutrition, fluid status, and electrolyte status (using laboratory values on postoperative day 8).

1.e. What are the limitations of albumin as an indication of nutritional status in the acute setting?

1.f. What additional nutritional assessment data should you obtain and why?

Desired Outcome

2. What are the goals of specialized nutrition support in this patient?

Therapeutic Alternatives

3. What are the therapeutic options for specialized nutrition intervention in this patient? Is PN indicated? Why or why not?

Optimal Plan

4.a. What are the ranges of estimated daily goals for calories (kcal/kg/day), protein (g/kg/day), and hydration (mL/day, mL/kg/day) for this patient?

4.b. Design a goal PN formulation for this patient that includes the total volume (mL/day) and goal rate (mL/h), amino acids (g/day), dextrose (g/day), and lipid emulsion (mL/day).

4.c. What other nutritional abnormalities (e.g., electrolytes, trace elements, vitamins) is this patient at risk for with the presence of an EC fistula? How would you address these with the PN prescription? Are there any other additives you would consider adding to the PN admixture?

4.d. How would you initiate PN in this patient? How quickly would you advance to goal infusion rate in this patient? Why?

4.e. What other monitoring parameters would you suggest ordering at the initiation of the PN?

CHAPTER 152

Outcome Evaluation

5.a. What parameters should be monitored to assess the efficacy and safety of PN in this patient? How frequently should each of these be monitored?

5.b. What specific parameter(s) should you monitor to assess this patient's nutritional status?

Patient Education

6. What information should be provided to the patient and family during his hospitalization regarding the PN?

■ CLINICAL COURSE

Fistula output decreased with initiation of PN and octreotide, but was still 300–500 mL/day. The surgical team determines that the best plan to manage Mr. Johnson's EC fistula is a conservative approach since he is malnourished, at high risk for postoperative complications, and has a fistula arising from the jejunum that had increased output with EN. On POD 13, the surgical team decides to send him home on PN and octreotide, maintain NPO status, and set up visiting nursing assistance for his PN therapy and care of his wound and fistula. If the EC fistula does not close spontaneously, he will be reassessed for surgical intervention in 6–8 weeks. Since he will be sent home on PN, they want to cycle his PN for home therapy.

■ FOLLOW-UP QUESTION

1. How should the PN be cycled for this patient? Develop a plan to initiate a PN cycle and advance to a goal cycle for home PN.

■ SELF-STUDY ASSIGNMENTS

1. This patient is at risk for a condition called refeeding syndrome. What is the refeeding syndrome? What are its potential complications? How can it be prevented?

2. What other specific postoperative complications are surgical patients with moderate to severe malnutrition at risk for developing? How can preoperative nutrition support impact a malnourished surgical patient's risk for postoperative complications?

3. Calculate how many mL/day of dextrose 70% and amino acids 10% stock solutions are needed to compound the daily PN prescription you determined for this patient.

4. Using the calculated daily goals for amino acids, dextrose, and IV lipid, determine the minimum PN volume that could be compounded for this patient. Assume it will be compounded using a 10% amino acid solution, 70% dextrose solution, 20% IV lipid emulsion, and use an estimate of 100 mL for all micronutrients and additives.

CLINICAL PEARLS

The refeeding syndrome can lead to serious complications, including death. It is one of the few true nutritional emergencies. A good rule of thumb in patients with moderate to severe malnutrition is to "start low and go slow" when initiating nutrition support (PN, enteral nutrition, or even an oral diet) to avoid complications, and aggressively correct electrolyte abnormalities (especially phosphorus, potassium, and magnesium) *before* initiating nutrition support, as well as during therapy.

Glycemic control in the range of 70–145 mg/dL is acceptable during PN infusion. Achieving tight glycemic control and avoiding hyperglycemia can reduce complications and mortality.

REFERENCES

1. Klein S, Kinney J, Jeejeebhoy K, et al. Nutrition support in clinical practice: review of published data and recommendations for future research directions. J Parenter Enteral Nutr 1997;21:133–156.
2. Kudsk KA, Tolley EA, DeWitt RC, et al. Preoperative albumin and surgical site identify surgical risk for major postoperative complications. JPEN J Parenter Enteral Nutr 2003;27:1–9.
3. Kraft MD, Btaiche IF, Sacks GS. Review of the refeeding syndrome. Nutr Clin Pract 2005;20:625–633.
4. Oldenburg WA, Lau LL, Rodenberg TJ, et al. Acute mesenteric ischemia: a clinical review. Arch Intern Med 2004;164:1054–1062.
5. Lloyd DA, Gabe SM, Windsor AC. Nutrition and management of enterocutaneous fistula. Br J Surg 2006;93:1045–1055.
6. ASPEN Board of Directors and the Clinical Guidelines Task Force. Guidelines for the use of parenteral and enteral nutrition in adult and pediatric patients. JPEN J Parenter Enteral Nutr 2002 (1 Suppl);26:1SA–138SA.
7. The American Society for Parenteral and Enteral Nutrition. Task force for the revision of safe practices for parenteral nutrition. Safe practices of parenteral nutrition. J Parenter Enteral Nutr 2004;28:S39–S70.
8. Sheldon GF, Grzyb S. Phosphate depletion and repletion: relation to parenteral nutrition and oxygen transport. Ann Surg 1975;182:683–689.
9. Clark CL, Sacks GS, Dickerson RN, et al. Treatment of hypophosphatemia in patients receiving specialized nutrition support using a graduated dosing scheme: results from a prospective clinical trial. Crit Care Med 1995;23:1504–1511.
10. Van Den Berghe G, Wouters PJ, Weekers F, et al. Intensive insulin therapy in critically ill patients. N Engl J Med 2001;345:1359–1367.
11. Finney SJ, Zekveld C, Elia A, et al. Glucose control and mortality in critically ill patients. JAMA 2003;290:2041–2047.

152

ADULT ENTERAL NUTRITION

Gut Check . . . . Level III

Carol J. Rollins, MS, RD, PharmD, BCNSP

LEARNING OBJECTIVES

After completing this case study, students should be able to:

• List contraindications to enteral nutrition therapy.

• Calculate the protein, calorie, and fluid requirements for a patient who is to receive enteral nutrition therapy.

• Recommend an appropriate enteral formula and feeding route.

• Implement an appropriate monitoring plan to achieve the desired nutritional endpoints and avoid complications.

• Design an appropriate regimen for administering medications via a feeding tube, including recommending alternate dosage forms for medications that cannot be crushed.

PATIENT PRESENTATION

Rosa Lopez is a 32-year-old Hispanic woman referred to the nutrition support team for evaluation and possible initiation of parenteral nutrition. She was admitted to the hospital 6 days ago with c/o nausea, vomiting, and RUQ pain. Her diet has not advanced beyond clear liquids, which she failed to tolerate on two attempts. Rosa continues to c/o nausea and RUQ pain.

QUESTIONS

Problem Identification

1.a. What other information is necessary or would be helpful to evaluate the patient and provide recommendations for a nutrition support plan of care?

1.b. What is the appropriate timing for nutrition intervention?

1.c. Based on risk-versus-benefit considerations, is the consult for initiation of parenteral nutrition appropriate for this patient?

■ CLINICAL COURSE

After following appropriate procedures, you obtain the following additional information about the patient.

■ HPI

Mrs. Lopez began having symptoms of nausea and RUQ pain 7 or 8 days (per patient) prior to hospital admission. She began vomiting the day prior to going to the ED and said, "It hurt so bad I didn't know what to do. My sister brought me here (to the hospital)." Her history indicates three similar episodes in the past 4 months. These episodes started after she lost about 25 lb over 6 months (her PCP recommended weight loss of 20–25 lb when Rosa indicated she did not want to start medications for hypertension and diabetes a year ago). With previous episodes, the pain was reported as less severe and lasted only a couple days; nausea occurred, but there was no vomiting. She reported these episodes to her PCP but did not go to the hospital since the pain improved on its own. Admission weight was 75 kg and height is 62 inches.

■ PMH

Hypertension (borderline)
PUD

■ FH

Mother died from a stroke nearly 2 years ago; she had DM and HTN. Father is healthy and works as an auto mechanic. Per Rosa, her father's only health complaints are "aching bones" and need for glasses to see his work. Two sisters have DM; all four brothers are "healthy" as far as the patient knows, although one brother has a "bad leg" from an accident several years ago.

■ SH

Married, 3 children between 7 and 14 years of age; works as a kitchen assistant at a local nursing home; does not smoke; occasional alcohol use, average of one drink per week. The patient has private health insurance through her husband's employer. Per the case manager, insurance coverage provides a drug benefit for oral medications but follows Medicare Parts A and B for hospitalization and home coverage.

■ ROS

From physician's note today:

Constitutional: Moderate pain, nausea.
ENT: No vision changes or eye pain. No tinnitus or ear pain. No throat pain. No problem with swallowing.

CV: No SOB, DOE, chest pain.
Resp: No cough or sputum production.
GI: Continued persistent RUQ abdominal pain; slightly improved with increased morphine dose and more frequent breakthrough pain coverage. No emesis or diarrhea; complains of intermittent nausea and mild/moderate constipation.
GU: No nocturia or hematuria; c/o frequency and burning on urination; culture positive for *Escherichia coli*.
MS: (+) Abdominal pain; no other muscle aches or bone pain.
Skin: No rashes, nodules, or itching.
Neuro: No headaches, dizziness, unsteady gait, or seizures.
Endo: Blood glucose in 120–180 mg/dL range.
Heme/Lymph Nodes: No recent blood transfusions or swollen glands.

■ Meds

Morphine sulfate, extended release 30 mg po Q 12 h
Protonix 40 mg po every morning
Docusate sodium 100 mg po at bedtime
Ciprofloxacin 500 mg po BID × 7 days (to start today)
Heparin 5,000 units SC twice daily

■ All

NKDA

■ Physical Examination

Gen

Obese Hispanic woman; alert and conversant

VS

BP 142/90, P 88, RR 16, T 37.1°C; Wt 75 kg

Skin

No nodules, masses, or rash; no ecchymoses or petechiae; redness at edges of venous access device

HEENT

PERRLA; EOMs intact. Eyes anicteric. No mouth lesions; tongue normal size.

Neck

Neck supple; no thyromegaly or masses

Lymph Nodes

No cervical, supraclavicular, axillary, or inguinal adenopathy

Heart

RRR with no gallop, rubs, or murmur

Lungs

Clear

Abd

Abdomen obese, tender to palpitation. No masses palpable.

Genit/Rect

Deferred

MS/Ext

No clubbing or cyanosis; 1+ bilateral ankle edema; no spine or CVA tenderness

TABLE 152-1 Lab Values

Na 137 mEq/L	Hgb 10.1 g/dL	WBC 11.5 × 10³/mm³	AST 33 IU/L	T. chol 273 mg/dL
K 3.8 mEq/L	Hct 36.8%	Segs 71%	ALT 24 IU/L	Trig 135 mg/dL
Cl 101 mEq/L	RBC 2.95 × 10⁶/mm³	Bands 12%	Alk phos 187 IU/L	Ca 7.7 mg/dL
CO₂ 23 mEq/L	Plt 65 × 10³/mm³	Lymphs 14%	LDH 140 IU/L	Mg 2.1 mg/dL
BUN 5 mg/dL	MCV 104 μm³	Monos 3%	T. bili 1.5 mg/dL	Phos 3.9 mg/dL
SCr 0.7 mg/dL			T. prot 7.2 g/dL	Amylase 556 mg/dL
Glu 180 mg/dL			Alb 2.7 g/dL	Lipase 636 mg/dL

Neuro

Cranial nerves intact; DTRs active and equal

▓ Endoscopy Report

From 3 days ago. ERCP, cholelithiasis; one stone removed from the common bile duct, other stones could not be removed using the endoscope.

Surgery consult for cholecystectomy states plan is to wait 4–6 weeks so that the pancreas has time to "cool down" prior to surgery.

▓ Labs

See Table 152-1

▓ Other

Peripheral blood smear: anisocytosis 2+, poikilocytosis 2+, macrocytosis 2+, hypersegmented neutrophils

▓ Assessment

Pancreatitis secondary to cholelithiasis. Continued intolerance to advancing diet; tolerates limited volume (150–200 mL/day) of clear liquids.

Problem Identification (continued)

1.d. Create a drug therapy problem list for this patient.

1.e. What information indicates the presence or severity of malnutrition?

1.f. What type and degree of malnutrition does this patient exhibit? What evidence supports your assessment?

Desired Outcome

2.a. What are the goals of nutrition support in this patient?

2.b. What outcomes should be considered for the patient's other medical problems?

Therapeutic Alternatives

3.a. What are the potential alternatives for improving nutritional status in this patient other than initiating specialized nutrition support?

3.b. What are the potential routes for specialized nutrition support and the reason(s) why each is or is not appropriate for this patient?

3.c. By postponing surgery for several weeks, the potential of continuing nutrition support outside the hospital arises. Based on the information now available to you, does this patient meet criteria for home enteral therapy? Recall that her insurance follows Medicare guidelines for home coverage.

Optimal Plan

4.a. Estimate the protein, calorie, and fluid requirements for this patient.

4.b. What type of formula (e.g., polymeric, monomeric) is most appropriate for this patient?

4.c. What administration regimen should be used for tube feedings?

4.d. Assuming that the patient is to continue her current medications during tube feedings, how should each of these be administered?

Outcome Evaluation

5. What clinical and laboratory parameters are necessary to evaluate the therapy for detection and/or prevention of adverse effects and to evaluate achievement of the desired response?

Patient Education

6. What information should be provided to the patient or her caregiver to enhance compliance, ensure successful therapy, and minimize adverse effects of enteral nutrition therapy?

■ CLINICAL COURSE

After presenting literature related to nutrition support during acute pancreatitis to the medical team, enteral nutrition therapy was discussed with the patient. The patient agreed to feeding tube placement rather than a central venous catheter for parenteral nutrition. A 1.2 cal/mL, 55.5 g protein/L, 300 mOsm/kg polymeric formula was started using an enteral infusion pump via nasojejunal tube at 35 mL/h for 8 hours then advanced to the goal rate of 55 mL/h. Basic metabolic panel results on day 2 revealed electrolyte values WNL but a decline in platelets to 58 × 10³/mm³ and WBC to 9.2 × 10³/mm³ with 80% segs, 4% bands, 14% lymphs, and 2% monos. The basic metabolic panel on day 3 showed stable values and a prealbumin of 14 mg/dL. The plan for discharge home was confirmed and arrangements for home enteral nutrition were finalized. Surgery was scheduled in 6 weeks.

■ SELF-STUDY ASSIGNMENTS

1. Select a current patient you are following, and design an appropriate regimen for administering medications via a feeding tube, including alternate dosage forms for medications that cannot be crushed and proper dosage adjustments for different forms where necessary.

2. Educate an actual patient or do a mock education with a classmate about medication administration through a feeding tube.

3. Select a current patient you are following and determine the potential cumulative sorbitol dose if all medications were changed to oral liquid dosage forms.

4. Identify the metabolic changes associated with refeeding syndrome and the characteristics that increase the risk of this complication.

CLINICAL PEARL

Medications administered through a feeding tube frequently clog the tube; evaluate the medication regimen for alternate dosage forms that do not require crushing or administration through the tube. When a tube clogs, a buffered pancreatic enzyme preparation may be used for declogging the tube.

REFERENCES

1. ASPEN Board of Directors and the Clinical Guidelines Task Force. Guidelines for the use of parenteral and enteral nutrition in adult and pediatric patients. JPEN 2002;26(1 Suppl):1SA–138SA.
2. McClave SA, Chang WK, Dhaliwal R, et al. Nutrition support in acute pancreatitis: a systematic review of the literature. J Parenter Enteral Nutr 2006;30:143–156.
3. Marik PE, Zaloga GP. Meta-analysis of parenteral nutrition versus enteral nutrition in patients with acute pancreatitis. BJM 2004;328:1407–1412.
4. American Gastroenterology Association, Clinical Practice and Practice Economics Committee. American Gastroenterology Association medical position statement: parenteral nutrition. Gastroenterology 2001;121:966–969.
5. McClave SA, DeMeo MT, DeLegge MH, et al. North American Summit on Aspiration in the Critically Ill Patient: consensus statement. JPEN 2002;26(6, Suppl):S80–S85.
6. Eatock FC, Chong P, Menezes N, et al. A randomized study of early nasogastric versus nasojejunal feeding in severe acute pancreatitis. Am J Gastroenterol 2005;100:432–439.
7. Rollins CJ. Home care issues in nutrition support. In: Pharmacotherapy Self-Assessment Program, Module 8: Gastroenterology, Nutrition. Kansas City, MO, American College of Clinical Pharmacy, 2000.
8. Mascarenhas MR, Divito D, McClave S. Pancreatic disease. In: Merritt R, ed. The A.S.P.E.N. Nutrition Support Manual, 2nd ed. Silver Spring, MD, American Society for Enteral and Parenteral Nutrition, 2005:211–230.
9. Meier R, Beglinger C, Layer P, et al. Consensus statement: ESPEN guidelines on nutrition in acute pancreatitis. Clin Nutr 2002;21:173–183.
10. Rollins CJ. Basics of enteral and parenteral nutrition. In: Wolinsky I, Williams L, eds. Nutrition in Pharmacy Practice. Washington, DC, American Pharmaceutical Association, 2002:213–306.
11. Tiengou LE, Gloro R, Pouzoulet J, et al. Semi-elemental formula or polymeric formula: is there a better choice for enteral nutrition in acute pancreatitis? Randomized comparative study. J Parenter Enteral Nutr 2006;30:1–5.
12. Makola D, Krenitsky J, Parrish C, et al. Efficacy of enteral nutrition for the treatment of pancreatitis using standard enteral formula. Am J Gastroenterol 2006;101:2347–2355.
13. Brooks MJ, Melnick G. The refeeding syndrome: an approach to understanding its complications and preventing its occurrence. Pharmacotherapy 1995;15:713–726.
14. Marcuard SP, Stegall KL, Trogdon S. Clearing obstructed feeding tubes. J Parenter Enteral Nutr 1989;13:81–83.

153

OBESITY

To Be Single and 25 Again (BMI That Is) . . . . Level II

Dannielle C. O'Donnell, PharmD, BCPS, CDM

LEARNING OBJECTIVES

After completing this case study, students should be able to:

- Identify common obesity related comorbidities.
- Calculate body mass index (BMI), and use waist circumference to determine a patient's risk of obesity-related morbidity.
- Develop a pharmacotherapeutic plan and treatment strategy for obese patients.
- Provide patient counseling on the expected benefits, possible adverse effects, and drug interactions with weight loss medications.

PATIENT PRESENTATION

Chief Complaint

"I'm eating like a gerbil and exercising, but I just can't seem to lose any weight. I'm embarrassed to go to the community pool with my children, and I can't go to my class reunion like this. I want stomach staples and liposuction."

HPI

Mimi Bonetta is a 38-year-old woman who states that she had maintained her ideal weight, which she feels is 59 kg, until after her third child at the age of 34. With her previous two pregnancies, she was able to get back to within 2 kg of her pre-pregnancy weight within 12–18 months postpartum "without any real conscious effort." She says that in her third pregnancy she retained a lot of fluid, gained much more weight than she had with the previous pregnancies (approximately 30 kg), developed gestational diabetes, and weighed more than 90 kg prior to delivery. She had a difficult recovery after her C-section, which was complicated by incisional infection and delayed hospital discharge. She complains that weight loss was slow to nonexistent in the first 2 years after her third child was born. She attributed that to hectic schedule with three young children, sleep deprivation, irregular meals, and "eating whatever was left on the kids' plates after a meal as I hate to waste anything." She states that after her youngest turned 2, she focused on her diet and portion sizes, stopped "grazing" on leftovers and became more diligent about exercise, ensuring 30–45 minutes of aerobic exercise (power walking or "spinning") at least 3–4 days a week. After doing that for almost a year, she had lost only 8 kg and was more frustrated. She attributed part of the problem to birth control pills she was taking at the time. She thought that it could be the hormones that were causing a resistance to weight loss. As she and her husband felt their family was complete, she stopped the pills, and he got a vasectomy. Thereafter and for the next 18 months, she has sequentially tried "The SlimFast plan," low-carb, no-carb, and even the grapefruit diet, with little or transient success. She requested prescription drug therapy from her OB/GYN physician whom she reports denied her request stating that "more willpower is what you need. A pill won't give you that." She is tearful as she talks about her weight struggles, attributing physical and marital problems to her weight. She states that her goal is to get back to what she weighed and the clothes she wore at age 25 before having children.

PMH

Hypertriglyceridemia × 3 years
Asthma
Sleep apnea

PSH

C-section $4^1/_2$ years ago

FH

Mother had an MI at the age of 62 years; father died in an MVA at the age of 67. Maternal grandmother died at age 62 with diabetes.

She states that her mother and grandmother were "a little heavy, but not obese." No other family members have a significant medical history, although she states that her oldest son who is 13 is a "big boy—probably sits around too much playing video games."

■ SH

She is a married housewife who cares for her three children. Her husband is in a sales job that requires a lot of travel and is away from home for days at a time. She has never smoked and denies IVDA. She states, "I'm no couch potato. I'm running around all day caring for my house and kids, and that's good exercise." She does admit that in the last 2 months, she's become so disillusioned that she stopped her power walking and spinning classes.

■ Diet

She had instruction on a low-fat, low-cholesterol diet several years ago, to which she initially said she is still adhering, although with further prompting, she states that the kids got "bored" with her food plan and she is now more frustrated because she feels she must cook two different dinners, one for her and one for her family since "they won't eat that boring healthy stuff." She typically has only a cup of coffee with no-calorie sweetener for breakfast, a salad for lunch with some yogurt for protein, and then will either heat up a Lean Cuisine for herself for dinner while she prepares a different meal for her family, or she will just have whatever she is making for them two to three times a week. She does admit to "satisfying her sweet tooth" each night for dessert and often tasting or "finishing off" what she prepares for the kids' breakfast and lunch.

■ Meds

Albuterol inhaler PRN (uses about two canisters a year)

■ All

Adhesive tape produces rash

■ ROS

She complains of general fatigue and a constant gnawing in her stomach and preoccupation with food and her weight. She denies symptoms of cold or heat intolerance; changes in skin, hair, or nails; nervousness; irritability; lethargy; muscle pain or weakness; palpitations; diarrhea or constipation; polyuria; polydipsia; chest pain; shortness of breath.

■ Physical Examination

Gen

The patient is a pleasant, but tearful, obese Hispanic woman in NAD. She is dressed neatly and appropriately for the weather.

VS

BP 138/88, P 80, RR 16, T 36.4°C; Wt 82 kg, waist 102 cm, hip 129 cm, Ht 5'4"

Skin

Warm, with normal distribution of body hair. No significant lesions or discolorations.

HEENT

NC/AT; PERRLA; EOMI; TMs intact

CV

RRR, S_1 and S_2 normal; no murmurs, rubs, or gallops

Pulm

CTA & P bilaterally

Abd

Obese with multiple striae; NT; ND; (+) BS; no palpable masses; C-section scar present and well healed

Genit/Rect

Pelvic and rectal exams deferred

Ext

LE varicosities present. Pedal pulses 2+ bilaterally

Neuro

A & O × 3; CN II–XII intact; Romberg test (−); sensory and motor levels intact; 2+ triceps tendons and DTR; Babinski (−)

■ Labs (Fasting)

Na 138 mEq/L	AST 24 IU/L
K 3.9 mEq/L	TSH 0.9 mIU/mL
Cl 96 mEq/L	*Fasting Lipid Profile:*
CO_2 26 mEq/L	T. chol 208 mg/dL
BUN 13 mg/dL	LDL-C 106 mg/dL
SCr 1.0 mg/dL	HDL-C 41 mg/dL
Glu 109 mg/dL	Trig 305 mg/dL

QUESTIONS

Problem Identification

1.a. Create a drug therapy problem list for this patient.

1.b. Calculate the patient's BMI. By using the BMI and any other markers of adiposity, categorize her obesity and stratify her risk.

1.c. What information (signs, symptoms, laboratory values) indicates the presence or severity of obesity?

1.d. Could any of the patient's problems have been caused by her drug therapy?

1.e. What other medical conditions should be considered to exclude primary causes of her obesity?

Desired Outcome

2. What are the goals of therapy for the patient's obesity?

Therapeutic Alternatives

3.a. What nondrug therapies should be recommended for this patient?

3.b. What nonprescription product(s) could you recommend for this patient's obesity? Justify your choices.

3.c. What are the primary prescription drug classes to consider when thinking about prescription drug therapy for obesity?

Optimal Plan

4.a. What drug(s), dosage form(s), dose(s), schedule(s), and duration is/are most appropriate to treat this patient's obesity and why?

4.b. What alternatives would be appropriate if initial therapy fails?

Outcome Evaluation

5. What clinical and laboratory parameters are necessary to evaluate the therapy for achievement of the desired therapeutic outcome and to detect or prevent adverse effects?

Patient Education

6. What general and medication-specific information should be provided to the patient to enhance adherence, ensure successful therapy, and minimize adverse effects?

■ CLINICAL COURSE

Mrs. Bonetta joined her local community center gym (which has child care) and attends their kick boxing class for 90 minutes three times a week. While she stated that "I still can't do everything they are doing in there or go nonstop the whole hour and a half like a lot of the ladies in there," she identified a workout buddy who holds her accountable for attending, and the new workout style is more interesting to her. She related progress at each of her 2-week weigh-ins, averaging a 1-kg weight loss at each visit through the end of week 8. Her blood pressure was stable, and she denied any adverse effects of her medication. However, at the 10-week visit she had lost only an additional 0.5 kg.

Today at her 12-week visit, she has not lost any additional weight. She weighs 77.5 kg, and her waist circumference is 98 cm. Her FBG is now 102 mg/dL and her fasting lipid profile includes total cholesterol 202 mg/dL, LDL-C 110 mg/dL, HDL-C 45 mg/dL, and triglycerides 235 mg/dL. Her blood pressure has improved to 134/82.

She states that she is as compliant with her lifestyle modifications as in previous weeks and is in much better spirits overall. She has noticed an improvement in her clothing fit, but she is starting to become frustrated again. She wants to know if she could increase her dose or add another medication. Although she is pleased with the improvement in her blood pressure and glucose, she is concerned that her LDL-C increased and her glucose is still above goal. She wonders if she should start other medications for these, particularly to prevent diabetes since she has heard that some diabetes medicines help with weight loss.

■ FOLLOW-UP QUESTIONS

1. What changes, if any, should be made in her weight loss regimen?

2. How would you educate her regarding her question about increasing her dose or adding on another drug?

3. What, if any, pharmacotherapeutic changes should be made for her lipids, glucose, and/or blood pressure at this time?

■ SELF-STUDY ASSIGNMENTS

1. List the limitations of height-weight charts or BMI determinations. What are the most accurate methods for quantifying body fat, and why are they not routinely employed?

2. Assume that you are a member of a pharmacy and therapeutics committee for a managed-care corporation. Justify whether anti-obesity drugs should be a covered benefit, and, if so, which specific agent(s) should be added to the formulary.

3. Identify the weight loss medications (Rx and OTC) withdrawn from the U.S. market in the last decade and the reasons for withdrawal.

4. Compile a compendium of common herbal and dietary supplements that claim weight loss benefits, and make a list of the evidence for their safety and efficacy.

5. Identify the control schedule for the various prescription weight loss medications. What are the legal requirements for dispensing the various scheduled weight loss agents in your state?

CLINICAL PEARL

Intermittent use of anorectic agents (i.e., for 4 weeks every few months, over the holidays, during vacations, or during periods of stress) may be effective in preventing weight regain in the later maintenance phase.

REFERENCES

1. American Gastroenterological Association. American Gastroenterological Association medical position statement on Obesity. Gastroenterology 2002;123:879–881.

2. Campbell ML, Mathys ML. Pharmacologic options for the treatment of obesity. Am J Health Syst Pharm 2001;58:1301–1308.

3. Tuomilehto J, Lindstrom J, Eriksson JG, et al. Prevention of type 2 diabetes mellitus by changes in lifestyle among subjects with impaired glucose tolerance. N Engl J Med 2001;344:1343–1350.

4. Stern L, Iqbal N, Seshadri P, et al. The effects of low-carbohydrate versus conventional weight loss diets in severely obese adults: one-year follow-up of a randomized trial. Ann Intern Med 2004;140:778–785

5. US Food and Drug Administration. FDA approves orlistat for over-the-counter use. Available at: *www.fda.gov/bbs/topics/NEWS/2007/NEW01557.html*. Accessed February 28, 2007.

6. Halpern A, Mancini MC. Treatment of obesity: an update on anti-obesity medications. Obes Rev 2003;4:25–42.

7. Cavaliere H, Floriano I, Medeiros-Neto G. Gastrointestinal side effects of orlistat may be prevented by concomitant prescription of natural fibers (psyllium mucilloid). Int J Obes Relat Metab Disord 2001;25:1095–1099.

8. American Diabetes Association and National Institute of Diabetes, Digestive and Kidney Diseases. The prevention or delay of type 2 diabetes. Diabetes Care 2002;25:742–749.

154

CYANIDE EXPOSURE

Curtain Call . . . . Level II

Colleen Terriff, PharmD

LEARNING OBJECTIVES

After completing this case study, students should be able to:

- Given a mass casualty case, identify which signs, symptoms, and laboratory data suggest possible cyanide exposure.

- Compare and contrast the two different antidote kits or treatments for cyanide exposure.

- Recommend specific dosing regimens of antidotes and supportive care for children and adults.

- List pharmaceutical supplies that may be necessary for cyanide antidotes.

- In a scenario with multiple victims where large quantities of antidotes may be necessary, explain how providers are able to obtain necessary antidotes.

PATIENT PRESENTATION

Multiple patients present to your hospital's emergency department; some are seizing, some are comatose, and others present seemingly drunk, confused, and, if ambulating, stumbling around.

■ HPI

Dozens of seriously ill patients arrive by ambulance at all area Emergency Departments. Many more turn up by car. They were attending a high school musical and many exited into a foyer for intermission. Attendees then experienced nausea, dizziness, light-headedness, and weakness. 911 was called when approximately six people passed out. The crowd estimate was 250, and most attendees ran out to the parking lot. Initial emergency medical technicians arriving on the scene recognized a mass incident. Medical Alert was activated for the town and surrounding communities. Fifty people are believed to still be in the auditorium. A decontamination area is being set up at the scene and all local hospital emergency departments.

■ PMH, PSH, FH, and SH

Most patients arriving via ambulance are unconscious. Some are seizing. History for most of these patients is unobtainable. Patients able to communicate are providing information as needed.

■ ROS

Patients are presenting with a variety of symptoms and severity. ED nurses and doctors perform brief physical exams and start using triage tags. Some patients present with triage tags from the scene. Age, height, and weight are being estimated as needed.

■ Physical Examination

Gen

Symptomatic patients appear weak and are breathing quickly. Some unconscious and seizing patients have required intubation. Most seem to have a ruddy complexion.

VS

BP: a few have mildly elevated BP, but many have hypotension; HR: most patients have bradycardia; RR: most patients are tachypneic; T: most are normal; Pain: patients are anxious but do not have notable or consistent complaints of pain; O_2 sat: most patients are normal.

Skin

Cherry red–colored skin

HEENT

Mydriasis observed in some patients. Some nurses noted "nutty" smelling breath in a few patients; on quick exam nothing else is noted.

Neck/Lymph Nodes

No lymphadenopathy

Lungs/Thorax

Rapid respiratory rate; lungs clear to auscultation

CV

Bradycardia for most patients, too noisy in ED to listen for heart sounds

Abd

Some patients complain of abdominal pain and nausea; a few experience emesis

Genital/Rect

Digital rectal exam and guaiac not performed

MS/Ext

No abnormal movements noted

Neuro

Spectrum of symptoms reported ranging from complaints of headache and dizziness to patients seeming intoxicated and confused; some are seizing and some are unresponsive or comatose

■ Labs

Complete metabolic panel, CBC, toxicology screen: Pending
Serum cholinesterase, blood cyanide levels: Pending

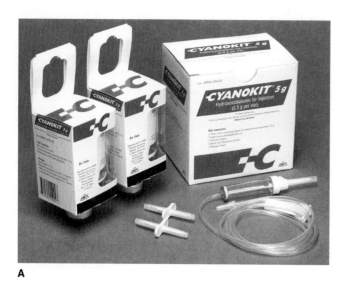
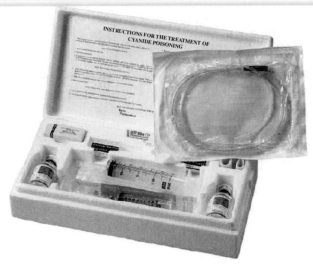

A

B

FIGURE 154-1. *A.* Cyanokit (hydroxocobalamin for injection) for the treatment of known or suspected cyanide poisoning. Dey, LP, Napa, CA, 2006. *B.* Cyanide Antidote Kit (sodium nitrite injection, sodium thiosulfate injection, amyl nitrite inhalants) for the treatment of cyanide poisoning, Taylor Pharmaceuticals, Decatur, IL, 2006.

▇ Other

Blood gases ordered on intubated patients: Pending
Multiple chest x-rays: Pending

▇ Assessment

Based on feedback from the scene and the Regional Disaster Hospital, up to 250 people may have been affected by this unknown chemical release. Paramedic services are transporting patients to all area hospitals. Medical Alert has been issued for the city. The ED staff are also alerted to obtain information from victims and save patient belongings as evidence for the FBI. Incident Command at the scene has not officially received identification of a chemical agent and asks for clinical assistance from health care providers triaging victims. First responders on the scene relayed information to Incident Command that some of the crowd complained of seeing vapor in bathrooms and in a few garbage cans, but no smoke or fire. The ED medical resident contacts the Regional Poison Control Center for guidance on identifying the agent based on patient symptoms. Cyanide exposure is suspected. The pharmacy department is also contacted for their assistance with antidote recommendations, including dosing and side-effect monitoring (Fig. 154-1).

QUESTIONS

Problem Identification

1.a. List the abnormal signs and symptoms displayed in these patients after exposure to the unknown chemical. Which of these findings are consistent with inhalation of cyanide?

1.b. List the laboratory tests that may be abnormal in patients exposed to cyanide. Explain the pathophysiology underlying these abnormalities.

1.c. What are the potential short- and long-term sequelae from this exposure?

Desired Outcome

2. What are the goals of pharmacotherapy for these patients?

Therapeutic Alternatives

3.a. What nonpharmacologic measures are available to treat cyanide poisoning?

3.b. What feasible pharmacotherapeutic alternatives are available for treating cyanide poisoning?

Optimal Plan

4.a. Outline your pharmacotherapeutic plan for treating cyanide poisoning in these patients. Include dose(s), route(s), and repeat dosing information (if any) for both adult and pediatric patients. Also describe use of administration devices or ancillary supplies required.

4.b. What supportive care measures may be necessary for optimal management?

Outcome Evaluation

5.a. Describe the clinical and laboratory parameters required to determine whether the treatment for these patients has been successful.

5.b. How often should the nursing and medical staff attempt to assess and re-assess the patients?

Patient Education

6.a. For patients who are alert and oriented, what information would you share with them about the possible immediate side effects of each of the antidotes?

6.b. How long might it take for the patients to recover from potential long-term effects of acute cyanide exposure?

■ CLINICAL COURSE

Over the next 24 hours, your ED treated 50 victims; 25 were treated and released, 20 were treated and admitted (10 to intensive care units), and 5 expired. Clinicians suspect that cyanide gas was released. This was later confirmed by HAZMAT units and federal response teams. During the next day, the FBI and local law enforcement discover that disgruntled former high school students obtained cyanide salt and a strong acid, quickly mixing and releasing a gas in bathrooms and garbage cans around the auditorium.

■ FOLLOW-UP QUESTIONS

1. If your pharmacy department runs out of antidotes and more are needed emergently, where can you obtain additional antidote supplies: locally? regionally? nationally?

2. Suppose there are 100 patients in your hospital's emergency department needing a cyanide antidote and you only have enough antidote to treat 25 patients. Who may be involved in making these ethical treatment decisions, and how would these decisions be made?

CLINICAL PEARLS

Local communities usually only have very small quantities of cyanide antidotes on hand due to their expense, short expiration dating, and rarity of use. However, some cities are stockpiling kits.

The exhaled breath of cyanide exposure victims may smell like bitter almonds. Not everyone (only 40–60% of people) can detect this odor.

■ SELF-STUDY ASSIGNMENTS

1. Research information on the Strategic National Stockpile Program. Look into various issues such as the response time and types of antidotes and treatments available with each program.

2. Describe the limitations of the antidotes for special populations, such as children.

REFERENCES

1. Leybell I, Hoffman RS, Baud FJ, et al. Emedicine [Internet]. New York: Web MD, Inc.; c1996–2006 [updated 2006 May 18, cited 2007 Apr 14]. Toxicity, cyanide. Available at: *www.emedicine.com/emerg/topic118.htm*.

2. Emergency Preparedness and Response [Internet]. Atlanta (GA): Centers for Disease Control and Prevention; [updated 2004 Jan 27; cited 2007 Apr 20]. Facts about cyanide. Available at: *www.bt.cdc.gov/agent/cyanide/basics/facts.asp*.

3. Mutlu GM, Leikin JB, Oh K. An unresponsive biochemistry professor in the bathtub. Chest 2002;122:1073–1076.

4. Cyanokit [package insert]. Napa, CA: Dey/L.P.; December 2006.

5. Baud FJ. Cyanide: critical issues in diagnosis and treatment. Hum Exp Toxicol 2007;26:191–201.

6. Gracia R, Shepherd G. Cyanide poisoning and its treatment. Pharmacotherapy 2004;24:1358–1365.

7. Ciottone G, Darling RG, Anderson PD et al., eds. Disaster Medicine, 3rd ed. Philadelphia, Elsevier Mosby, 2006, Chapter 94, Cyanide attack; 576–581.

8. Cyanide Antidote Kit [package insert]. Decatur, IL: Taylor Pharmaceuticals; February 2006.

9. Colley J, Baker DE. Hydroxocobalamin. In: Cada DJ, Baker DE, Levien TL, eds. Formulary Monograph Service. St. Louis, Wolters Kluwer Health, Inc., Jan. 2007.

155

CHEMICAL EXPOSURE

Terrorism or Freak Accident? . . . . .Level II

Colleen Terriff, PharmD

LEARNING OBJECTIVES

After completing this case study, students should be able to:

- Identify potential toxins or chemical agents that could be used in a terrorist attack.

- Determine the proper antidote or treatments and the dosing regimens for a potential chemical weapon, based on patient signs and symptoms.

- Manage seizures that may occur during severe exposure to certain chemical agents.

- Learn how to access pharmaceutical supplies for one victim as well as many victims in their health-system and communities.

PATIENT PRESENTATION

▓ Patient Scenario

Many patients present to your hospital's Emergency Department visibly teary, coughing, and having trouble breathing.

▓ HPI

Patients arrive at the ED via car, taxi, and ambulance. They were attending an all-day seminar at the downtown convention center when, after a loud explosion down the hall, they were exposed to smoke and "fumes." Paramedics also reported that patients complained of difficulty breathing and blurred vision. Patients were covering their eyes, coughing, crying, and even drooling.

Dozens of patients outside the ED are awaiting decontamination, and patients appear to be anxious and extremely concerned. Medical Alert has been activated for city and county, and the Regional Disaster Hospital has been notified of Alert. All local EDs are securing their perimeters and setting up decontamination units. Scene decontamination of patients is occurring before some are arriving via ambulance. Patients arriving by car or cab or by foot have not been decontaminated.

▓ PMH, PSH, FH, and SH

Not obtained

▓ ROS

Most patients can only nod to some questions, making individual interviews difficult. The ED lead physician instructs nurses to get patient vital signs and approximate age and weight. Medical residents are told to do brief triage physical exams on an estimated 25 patients each.

▓ Physical Examination

Gen

Patients appear anxious, breathing quickly. Some have required intubation.

VS

BP: A few patients have mildly elevated BP; P: Most have tachycardia, but a few have bradycardia; RR: Most patients are tachypneic; T: most are normal; Pain: Most patients indicate that they do not have significant pain.

Skin

Some patients are profusely sweaty; no cyanosis, clubbing, or edema present

HEENT

Bilateral pinpoint pupils, nonreactive to light, profuse rhinorrhea, and hypersalivation

Neck/Lymph Nodes

Exam not performed

Lungs/Thorax

Rapid respiratory rate, rhonchi present throughout; a few patients exhibit bronchoconstriction and excessive respiratory secretions

CV

Tachycardia for most patients; too noisy to listen for heart sounds for most patients

Abd

Some patients complain of nausea; a few experience emesis

Genital/Rect

DRE and stool guaiac not performed

MS/Ext

Facial muscle twitching noticed in a few patients who also had substantial rhinorrhea and complaints of severe vision changes

Neuro

Initially, five have flaccid paralysis and respiratory arrest requiring intubation; three of these five patients are seizing

■ Labs

Complete metabolic panel, CBC, toxicology screen: Pending
Serum cholinesterase, blood cyanide levels: Pending

■ Other

O_2 sat ordered for patients in more severe respiratory distress. Blood gases ordered on intubated patients. Multiple chest x-rays: Pending.

■ Lead Physician's Assessment

Based on feedback from the scene and the Regional Disaster Hospital, 1,000 people may have been affected by this chemical release, going to four area hospitals. The ED staff is also alerted to get information from victims and save patient belongings as evidence for FBI. Scene fire chief acting as Incident Commander asks for assistance (request relayed from combined communications center to hospitals) from health care providers triaging victims area hospitals to attempt to identify chemical agent based on symptomatology. An ED medical resident contacts the Regional Poison Control Center for guidance identifying the possible agent. The pharmacy department is also contacted for their assistance with antidote recommendations, including dosing and side effect monitoring.

QUESTIONS

Problem Identification

1.a. Create a list of potential chemical agents that the patients may have been exposed to based on presenting signs and symptoms.

1.b. How serious is this exposure, and what could be some potential sequelae?

Desired Outcome

2.a. What are the goals of pharmacotherapy in this case?

2.b. How do your goals change if there were 15 patients presenting with these symptoms and differing degrees of severity and exposure?

Therapeutic Alternatives

3.a. What nonpharmacologic measures are available to treat these patients?

3.b. What feasible pharmacotherapeutic alternatives are available for treating these patients?

3.c. Suppose there are 100 patients in your hospital's Emergency Department needing an antidote, and you only have enough antidote to treat 25 patients. How do you decide who gets life-saving treatment?

Optimal Plan

4.a. What antidotes are required for this chemical exposure? Provide the adult doses, routes, and repeat dosing information for each antidote.

4.b. There are special dosing kits and administration devices available for these antidotes (see Figs. 155-1 and 155-2). Describe how these kits should be administered.

4.c. If a patient's condition worsens and seizure activity occurs, what class of medications should be used for this chemical-induced seizure?

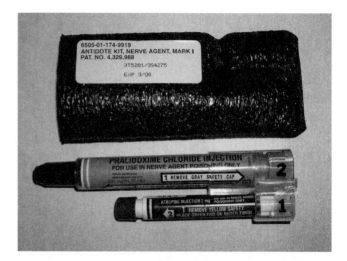

FIGURE 155-1. The Mark-I autoinjector, consisting of two antidotes to be used after exposures to a nerve or organophosphate agent in a disaster situation. The kit contains an atropine autoinjector (2 mg/0.7 mL) and a pralidoxime chloride (2-PAM) autoinjector (600 mg/2 mL).

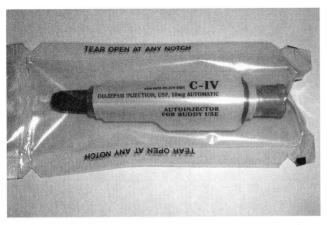

FIGURE 155-2. Diazepam provided as a 10-mg dose in a military-designed autoinjector.

Outcome Evaluation

5. Outline a monitoring plan to assess if the pharmacotherapy treatment for these patients is successful.

Patient Education

6.a. What information would you share with the patients about immediate side effects of each of the antidotes?

6.b. How long might it take for patients to recover from the ocular effects of the chemical exposure? Incorporate this information into your educational efforts.

■ CLINICAL COURSE

Students: Your instructor can provide you with the outcome of this incident.

■ FOLLOW-UP QUESTION

1. If your pharmacy department runs out of antidotes and more are needed emergently, where can you obtain additional antidote supplies: locally, regionally, nationally?

CLINICAL PEARL

Most chemical agents that could be used for a terrorist attack would likely be exploded or released as a gas in order to increase respiratory exposure and allow for rapid systemic entry into victims. Therefore, clinicians need to quickly triage patients, classify symptoms for identification, and administer appropriate treatment if available.

■ SELF-STUDY ASSIGNMENTS

1. Research information on the Strategic National Stockpile Program and the CHEMPACK program. Look into issues such as response time, types of antidotes, and treatment available with each program.

2. Review and describe the limitations of a Mark-I auto-injector for administration of nerve agent antidotes to children, especially infants.

REFERENCES

1. North Carolina Statewide Program for Infection Control and Epidemiology (SPICE). Chemical terrorism agents and syndromes. Available at: *www.unc.edu/depts/spice/chemical-generic.pdf*. Accessed August 8, 2004.

2. Field Management of Chemical Casualties Handbook, 2nd ed. US Army Medical Research Institute of Chemical Defense (USAMRICD). July 2000. Available at: *https://www.rke.vaems.org/wvems/Libraryfiles/Dis/E_04.pdf*. Accessed May 14, 2008.

3. Centers for Disease Control and Prevention. Emergency preparedness and response: chemical agents. Available at: *www.bt.cdc.gov/agent/agentlistchem.asp*. Accessed August 8, 2004.

4. Bozeman WP, Dilbero D, Schauben JL. Biologic and chemical weapons of mass destruction. Emerg Med Clin N Amer 2002;20:975–993.

5. Arnold JL. CBRNE—Chemical warfare agents. Available at: *www.emedicine.com/emerg/topic852.htm*. Accessed August 8, 2004.

6. Bartlett JG, Sifton DW, Gwynned LK. PDR Guide to Biological and Chemical Warfare Response, 1st ed. Montvale, NJ, Thomson Healthcare, 2002:79–86;94;101–102;126–127.

7. Pediatric Preparedness for Disasters and Terrorism: A National Consensus Conference. National Center for Disaster Preparedness, Columbia University Mailman School of Public Health; 2003. Available at: *http://www.bt.cdc.gov/children/pdf/working/execsumm03.pdf*. Accessed May 14, 2008.

COMPLEMENTARY AND ALTERNATIVE THERAPIES (LEVEL III)

Charles W. Fetrow, PharmD

TO THE READER

With the recent surge in the promotion and use of complementary and alternative medicine (CAM), patients have increased their desire for knowledge on the potential benefits of these therapies. The purpose of this section is to provide additional questions related to currently used dietary supplements. Ten case examples are included in this section.

Each of the 10 fictitious patient vignettes below is directly related to a patient case that was presented earlier in this book. Each scenario involves one or more questions asked by a patient about a specific remedy. Additional follow-up questions are then asked to help students provide a scientifically based answer to the patient's question(s). Students will need to refer to additional references other than the *Pharmacotherapy* textbook in order to answer these questions satisfactorily. Be sure that they rely on reputable sources to support their answers. You may wish to have them cite the literature references that they used to answer the questions. Medical literature references are provided at the end of each of these vignettes.

Here is the first general question to get you started:

1. What general questions might be asked of patients before you provide a recommendation for or against the use of any herbal or dietary supplement?

CASE 20

■ Secondary Prevention–Garlic and Omega-3 Fatty Acids

Clinical Course

While attending a wellness fair, Mr. Gonzalez engages in a discussion with a pharmacist about the safety and efficacy of natural products. The pharmacist comments that natural products are often tried for hyperlipidemia, but few possess reproducible efficacy data.

Mr. Gonzalez states that he is interested in making significant lifestyle changes after reading several nutrition guides. He is concerned about getting control of his health and preventing complications related to high cholesterol. He doesn't know where to start and how to put all of the information together. His daughter-in-law, a registered dietitian, notes that his lipid panel is not within National Cholesterol Education Program guidelines and suggests "natural approaches" to aggressively lower his lipids. She recommends a regimen consisting of garlic, guggul, and omega-3 fatty acids along with exercise.

■ FOLLOW-UP QUESTIONS

Garlic

1. Based on available data, what are the postulated antihyperlipidemic mechanisms of garlic?

2. Briefly review and critique one major clinical trial that compared the efficacy of garlic on human serum lipoprotein profiles.

3. Given this patient's medical and personal situation, would you recommend self-treatment with garlic? Why or why not?

4. What education should be provided to patients who choose to use this alternative therapy?

Omega-3 Fatty Acids

5. Based on available data, what are the postulated antihyperlipidemic mechanisms of omega-3 fatty acids?

6. Briefly review and critique one major clinical trial that compared the efficacy of omega-3 fatty acids on human serum lipoprotein profiles.

7. Given this patient's medical and personal situation, would you recommend self-treatment with fish oil? Why or why not?

8. What education should be provided to patients who choose to use this alternative therapy?

9. Are there any other dietary supplements that are claimed to be useful for hyperlipidemia?

CASE 63

■ Parkinson's Disease and Coenzyme Q10 (Co-Q10)

Clinical Course

After her initial diagnosis, Ms. Miller read some disturbing technical information from the Internet regarding levodopa and its apparent neurotoxic effects with long-term use. She appears at your pharmacy counter at 9:00 AM with pages of information she printed out regarding all types of therapies for PD. Although she is anxiously waiting to ask you a myriad of questions, you request that she return later that day when the store is less busy. She politely agrees, but not before she requests your opinion of Co-Q10 to be used instead of the medicine she has been prescribed. You kindly reply that you will be happy to discuss everything upon her return. She turns to leave as you jot yourself a note to perform a literature search on that topic before 7:00 PM tonight.

■ FOLLOW-UP QUESTIONS

1. Based on the available data, what is the postulated mechanism of action for Co-Q10?

2. Briefly review and critique one major clinical trial that compared efficacy of Co-Q10 with conventional therapies for PD.

3. Given this patient's medical and personal situation, would you recommend self-treatment with Co-Q10? Why or why not?

4. What education should be provided to patients who choose to use this alternative therapy?

5. Are there any other claims of use for Co-Q10?

CASE 69

▨ Alzheimer's Disease and Ginkgo Biloba Extract
Clinical Course

One month later, Mrs. Dale's daughter phones the clinic with a question about her mother's therapy. After attending an Alzheimer's support group, the daughter reveals that she was given literature on the medicinal use of Ginkgo biloba extract (GbE) for improving memory and mental function. Now convinced that botanical medicine offers distinct advantages over conventional therapies for dementia, the daughter asks if her mother could be titrated off the current medication and started on Ginkgo biloba with the same expected therapeutic effect. She also asks whether combination therapy with her current medication and ginkgo would be better than a single product for improving cognition, mood, memory, and behavior.

■ FOLLOW-UP QUESTIONS

1. Based on available data, what is the postulated mechanism of action for GbE?
2. Briefly review and critique one major clinical trial that compared the efficacy of GbE with conventional therapies for memory loss and impaired cognition associated with Alzheimer's disease.
3. Given this patient's medical and personal situation, would you recommend self-treatment with GbE? Why or why not?
4. What education should be provided to patients who choose to use this alternative therapy?
5. Are there any other dietary supplements that are claimed to be useful for improving memory and cognition?

CASE 73

▨ Major Depression and St. John's Wort
Clinical Course

Approximately 2 months after starting treatment, the patient returns to your pharmacy for a refill of her antidepressant medication. She also continues to take St. John's wort because she's afraid the antidepressant alone won't work well enough. She states that some of her friends have tried it and believe it helps. She believes that it is safer than her current medication because it's "natural."

■ FOLLOW-UP QUESTIONS

1. Based on the available data, what is the postulated mechanism of action for St. John's wort (SJW)?
2. Briefly review and critique one major clinical trial that compared efficacy of SJW with conventional therapies for depression.
3. Given this patient's medical and personal situation, would you recommend self-treatment with SJW? Why or why not?
4. What education should be provided to patients who choose to use this alternative therapy?
5. Are there any other dietary supplements that are claimed to be useful for depression?

CASE 75

▨ Generalized Anxiety Disorder and Kava Kava
Clinical Course

Ms. Long begins the prescribed course of therapy for anxiety. After 2 weeks, she calls her family practitioner and reveals that her restless-

ness is somewhat greater and she is not sleeping. Subsequently, her physician increases the dose and prescribes alprazolam 0.25 mg po at bedtime. One week later, she discontinues the initial anti-anxiety agent due to continued nausea and worsening of her insomnia but continues the alprazolam. A friend recommends that she try an herbal tea whose main ingredient is kava as a natural remedy to calm her nerves and allow her to sleep. Feeling that the tea made her less jittery, Ms. Long calls her local pharmacy to explore the possibility of taking kava on a regular basis in an attempt to ease her restlessness and help her sleep, thereby allowing her to be more productive during the day and attentive in class. She would like to continue the alprazolam at night and try kava for daytime anxiety. She is also concerned about the addictive and daytime sedation potential of kava. If effective, she would like to discontinue the evening alprazolam.

■ FOLLOW-UP QUESTIONS

1. Based on available data, what is the postulated mechanism of action for kava?
2. Briefly review and critique one major clinical trial that compared the efficacy of kava with conventional therapies for anxiety symptoms.
3. Given this patient's medical and personal situation, would you recommend self-treatment with kava? Why or why not?
4. What education should be provided to patients who choose to use this alternative therapy?
5. Are there any other dietary supplements that are claimed to be beneficial in patients with generalized anxiety of nonpsychotic origin?

CASE 77

▨ Insomnia and Valerian (*Valeriana officinalis*)
Clinical Course

Ms. Smith's daughter, a nurse, associates with a local herbalist and has accumulated literature on natural products as a psychotherapeutic alternative for her mother. She requests that the clinician consider valerian to help her mother sleep. Having investigated the natural products section of her pharmacy, she came across a combination of herbals touted as nature's sleep aid (kava/valerian combination). The daughter requests information about the safety of this combination product and its addiction potential.

■ FOLLOW-UP QUESTIONS

1. Based on available data, what is the postulated mechanism of action for valerian root?
2. Briefly review and critique one major clinical trial that compared the efficacy of valerian root with conventional therapies on sleep structure in patients with psychophysiological insomnia.
3. Given this patient's medical and personal situation, would you recommend self-treatment with valerian root? Why or why not?
4. What education should be provided to patients who choose to use this alternative therapy?
5. Are there any other dietary supplements that are claimed to have positive effects on sleep structure and that can be recommended for mild psychophysiological insomnia?

CASE 88

▨ Managing Menopausal Symptoms and Black Cohosh
Clinical Course

Having heard some "bad press" on hormone replacement therapy on her local television news station, the patient asks about the use of dietary supplements "that might not be as harmful for me." Specifically, she is interested in "something called black cohosh."

■ FOLLOW-UP QUESTIONS

1. Based on the available data, what is the postulated mechanism of action for black cohosh?
2. Briefly review and critique one pivotal trial that evaluated efficacy of black cohosh for postmenopausal vasomotor complaints.
3. Given this patient's medical and personal situation, would you recommend self-treatment with black cohosh? Why or why not?
4. What education should be provided to patients who choose to use this alternative therapy?
5. Are there any other dietary supplements that are claimed to be useful for postmenopausal vasomotor symptoms?

CASE 90

■ Benign Prostatic Hyperplasia and Saw Palmetto

Clinical Course

After several months on the recommended treatment with good but not total symptom relief, Mr. McLaren read an article in a magazine about the potential benefits of saw palmetto for relief of BPH symptoms. He comes to you now to ask your professional opinion about this supplement.

■ FOLLOW-UP QUESTIONS

1. Based on available data, what is the postulated mechanism of action for saw palmetto (SP)?
2. Briefly review and critique one major clinical trial that compared efficacy of SP with conventional therapies for benign prostatic hyperplasia (BPH).
3. Given this patient's medical and personal situation, would you recommend self-treatment with SP? Why or why not?
4. What education should be provided to patients who choose to use this alternative therapy?
5. Are there any other dietary supplements that are claimed to be useful for BPH?

CASE 97

■ Osteoarthritis and Glucosamine

Clinical Course

After 2 weeks on a scheduled dose of his new medication, Mr. Abernathy decides that he has waited long enough for resolution of his symptoms. Inadequate pain relief has driven him to call the doctor's office and request something else. The physician assistant who answers the phone recommends that he go to her local pharmacy and "pick up a bottle of glucosamine."

■ FOLLOW-UP QUESTIONS

1. Based on the available data, what is the postulated mechanism of action for glucosamine?
2. Briefly review and critique one major clinical trial that compared the efficacy of glucosamine with conventional therapies for osteoarthritis (OA).
3. Given this patient's medical and personal situation, would you recommend self-treatment with glucosamine? Why or why not?
4. What education should be provided to patients who choose to use this alternative therapy?
5. Are there any other dietary supplements that are claimed to be useful for OA?

CASE 115

■ Rhinosinusitis and Echinacea

Clinical Course

After experiencing bothersome diarrhea and abdominal cramps from the treatment regimen, Mr. Simmons questions you about the use of echinacea. He states that "it has to be safer than the antibiotics" he had used previously, and that he is "sick of taking antibiotics anyway because they obviously won't work for me in this case."

■ FOLLOW-UP QUESTIONS

1. Based on the available data, what is the postulated mechanism of action for echinacea?
2. Briefly review and critique one major clinical trial that compared efficacy of echinacea with conventional therapies for upper respiratory tract infections.
3. Given this patient's medical and personal situation, would you recommend self-treatment with echinacea? Why or why not?
4. What education should be provided to patients who choose to use this alternative therapy?
5. Are there any other dietary supplements that are claimed to be useful for upper respiratory tract infections?

CONVERSION FACTORS AND ANTHROPOMETRICS*

CONVERSION FACTORS

■ SI Units

SI (*le Système International d'Unités*) units are used in many countries to express clinical laboratory and serum drug concentration data. Instead of employing units of mass (such as micrograms), the SI system uses moles (mol) to represent the amount of a substance. A molar solution contains 1 mol (the molecular weight of the substance in grams) of the solute in 1 L of solution. The following formula is used to convert units of mass to moles (mcg/mL to μmol/L or, by substitution of terms, mg/mL to mmol/L or ng/mL to nmol/L).

Micromoles per Liter (μmol/L)

$$\mu mol/L = \frac{\text{drug concentration (mcg/mL)} \times 1,000}{\text{molecular weight of drug (g/mol)}}$$

Milliequivalents

An equivalent weight of a substance is that weight which will combine with or replace 1 g of hydrogen; a milliequivalent is 1/1,000 of an equivalent weight.

Milliequivalents per Liter (mEq/L)

$$mEq/L = \frac{\text{weight of salt (g)} \times \text{valence of ion} \times 1,000}{\text{molecular weight of salt}}$$

$$\text{weight of salt (g)} = \frac{mEq/L \times \text{molecular weight of salt}}{\text{valence of ion} \times 1,000}$$

Approximate Milliequivalents

Weights of Selected Ions

Salt	mEq/g Salt	mg Salt/mEq
Calcium carbonate ($CaCO_3$)	20.0	50.0
Calcium chloride ($CaCl_2 \cdot 2H_2O$)	13.6	73.5
Calcium gluceptate ($Ca[C_7H_{13}O_8]_2$)	4.1	245.2
Calcium gluconate ($Ca[C_6H_{11}O_7]_2 \cdot H_2O$)	4.5	224.1
Calcium lactate ($Ca[C_3H_5O_3]_2 \cdot 5H_2O$)	6.5	154.1
Magnesium gluconate ($Mg[C_6H_{11}O_7]_2 \cdot H_2O$)	4.6	216.3
Magnesium oxide (MgO)	49.6	20.2
Magnesium sulfate ($MgSO_4$)	16.6	60.2
Magnesium sulfate ($MgSO_4 \cdot 7H_2O$)	8.1	123.2
Potassium acetate ($K[C_2H_3O_2]$)	10.2	98.1
Potassium chloride (KCl)	13.4	74.6
Potassium citrate ($K_3[C_6H_5O_7] \cdot H_2O$)	9.2	108.1
Potassium iodide (KI)	6.0	166.0
Sodium acetate ($Na[C_2H_3O_2]$)	12.2	82.0
Sodium acetate ($Na[C_2H_3O_2] \cdot 3H_2O$)	7.3	136.1
Sodium bicarbonate ($NaHCO_3$)	11.9	84.0
Sodium chloride ($NaCl$)	17.1	58.4
Sodium citrate ($Na_3[C_6H_5O_7] \cdot 2H_2O$)	10.2	98.0
Sodium iodide (NaI)	6.7	149.9
Sodium lactate ($Na[C_3H_5O_3]$)	8.9	112.1
Zinc sulfate ($ZnSO_4 \cdot 7H_2O$)	7.0	143.8

■ Valences and Atomic Weights of Selected Ions

Substance	Electrolyte	Valence	Molecular Weight
Calcium	Ca^{2+}	2	40.1
Chloride	Cl^-	1	35.5
Magnesium	Mg^{2+}	2	24.3
Phosphate (pH = 7.4)	HPO_4^- (80%) $H2PO_4^-$ (20%)	1.8	96.0^a
Potassium	K^+	1	39.1
Sodium	Na^+	1	23.0
Sulfate	SO_4^-	2	96.0^a

^{a}The molecular weight of phosphorus only is 31; that of sulfur only is 32.1.

*This appendix contains information from Appendices 1 and 2 of Anderson PO, Knoben JE, Troutman WG, et al (eds). *Handbook of Clinical Drug Data,* 10th ed. New York: McGraw-Hill, 2002:1053–1058, with permission.

Anion Gap

The anion gap is the concentration of plasma anions not routinely measured by laboratory screening. It is useful in the evaluation of acid-base disorders. The anion gap is greater with increased plasma concentrations of endogenous species (e.g., phosphate, sulfate, lactate, and ketoacids) or exogenous species (e.g., salicylate, penicillin, ethylene glycol, ethanol, and methanol). The formulas for calculating the anion gap are as follows:

$$\text{Anion gap} = (Na^+ + K^+) - (Cl^- + HCO_3^-)$$

or

$$\text{Anion gap} = Na^+ - (Cl^- + HCO_3)$$

where the expected normal value for the first equation is 11 to 20 mmol/L, and the expected normal value for the second equation is 7 to 16 mmol/L. Note that there is a variation in the upper and lower limits of the normal range.

Temperature

Fahrenheit to Centigrade: $(°F - 32) \times 5/9 = °C$
Centigrade to Fahrenheit: $(°C \times 9/5) + 32 = °F$
Centigrade to Kelvin: $°C + 273 = °K$

Calories

1 calorie = 1 kilocalorie = 1,000 calories = 4.184 kilojoules (kJ)
1 kilojoule = 0.239 calories = 0.239 kilocalories = 239 calories

Weights and Measures

Metric Weight Equivalents

1 kilogram (kg) = 1,000 grams
1 gram (g) = 1,000 milligrams
1 milligram (mg) = 0.001 gram
1 microgram (mcg, μg) = 0.001 milligram
1 nanogram (ng) = 0.001 microgram
1 picogram (pg) = 0.001 nanogram
1 femtogram (fg) = 0.001 picogram

Metric Volume Equivalents

1 liter (L) = 1,000 milliliters
1 deciliter (dL) = 100 milliliters
1 milliliter (mL) = 0.001 liter
1 microliter (μL) = 0.001 milliliter
1 nanoliter (nL) = 0.001 microliter
1 picoliter (pL) = 0.001 nanoliter
1 femtoliter (fL) = 0.001 picoliter

Apothecary Weight Equivalents

1 scruple (Э) = 20 grains (gr)
60 grains (gr) = 1 dram (ℨ)
8 drams (ℨ) = 1 ounce (flℨ)
1 ounce (ℨ) = 480 grains
12 ounces (ℨ) = 1 pound (lb)

Apothecary Volume Equivalents

60 minims (m) = 1 fluidram (flℨ)
8 fluidrams (flℨ) = 1 fluid ounce (flℨ)
1 fluid ounce (ftℨ) = 480 minims
16 fluid ounces (flℨ) = 1 pint (pt)

Avoirdupois Equivalents

1 ounce (oz) = 437.5 grains
16 ounces (oz) = 1 pound (lb)

Weight/Volume Equivalents

1 mg/dL = 10 mcg/mL
1 mg/dL = 1 mg%
1 ppm = 1 mg/L

Conversion Equivalents

1 gram (g) = 15.43 grains
1 grain (gr) = 64.8 milligrams
1 ounce (ℨ) = 31.1 grams
1 ounce (oz) = 28.35 grams
1 pound (lb) = 453.6 grams
1 kilogram (kg) = 2.2 pounds
1 milliliter (mL) = 16.23 minims
1 minim (m) = 0.06 milliliter
1 fluid ounce (fl oz) = 29.57 milliliter
1 pint (pt) = 473.2 milliliter
0.1 milligram = 1/600 grain
0.12 milligram = 1/500 grain
0.15 milligram = 1/400 grain
0.2 milligram = 1/300 grain
0.3 milligram = 1/200 grain
0.4 milligram = 1/150 grain
0.5 milligram = 1/120 grain
0.6 milligram = 1/100 grain
0.8 milligram = 1/80 grain
1 milligram = 1/65 grain

Metric Length Equivalents

2.54 cm = 1 inch
30.48 cm = 1 foot
1.6 km = 1 mile

ANTHROPOMETRICS

Creatinine Clearance Formulas

Formulas for Estimating Creatinine Clearance in Patients with Stable Renal Function

Cockroft-Gault Formula

Adults (age 18 years and older)[1]:

$$CLcr \text{ (males)} = \frac{(140 - age) \times weight}{Cr_s \times 72}$$

$$CLcr \text{ (females)} = 0.85 \times \text{above value*}$$

where CLcr is creatinine clearance (in mL/minute), Cr_s is serum creatinine (in mg/dL), age is in years, and weight is in kilograms.

*Some studies suggest that the predictive accuracy of this formula for women is better *without* the correction factor of 0.85.

Children (age 1 to 18 years)[2]:

$$CLcr = \frac{0.48 \times height \times BSA}{Cr_s \times 1.73}$$

where BSA is body surface area (in m²), CLcr is creatinine clearance (in mL/minute), Cr_s is serum creatinine (in mg/dL), and height is in centimeters.

Formula for Estimating Creatinine Clearance from a Measured Urine Collection

$$\text{CLcr (mL/minute)} = \frac{U \times V^*}{P \times T}$$

where U is the concentration of creatinine in a urine specimen (in same units as P), V is the volume of urine (in mL), P is the concentration of creatinine in serum at the midpoint of the urine collection period (in same units as U), and T is the time of the urine collection period in minutes (e.g., 6 hours = 360 minutes; 24 hours = 1,440 minutes).

*The product of $U \times V$ equals the production of creatinine during the collection period and, at steady state, should equal 20 to 25 mg/kg per day for ideal body weight (IBW) in males and 15 to 20 mg/kg per day for IBW in females. If it is less than this, inadequate urine collection may have occurred, and CLcr will be underestimated.

MDRD Formula for Estimating Glomerular Filtration Rate (from the Modification of Diet in Renal Disease Study)[3]

Conventional calibration MDRD equation (used only with those creatinine methods that have not been recalibrated to be traceable to isotope dilution mass spectrometry [IDMS]).

For creatinine in mg/dL:

$$X = 186 \text{ creatinine}^{-1.154} \times \text{age}^{-0.203} \times \text{constant}$$

For creatinine in μmol/L:

$$X = 32,788 \times \text{creatinine}^{-1.154} \times \text{age}^{-0.203} \times \text{constant}$$

where X is the glomerular filtration rate (GFR), constant for white males is 1 and for females is 0.742, and constant for African Americans is 1.21. Creatinine levels in μmol/L can be converted to mg/dL by dividing by 88.4.

IDMS-Traceable MDRD Equation (Used Only with Creatinine Methods That Have Been Recalibrated to Be Traceable to IDMS)

For creatinine in mg/dL:

$$X = 175 \times \text{creatinine}^{-1.154} \times \text{age}^{-0.203} \times \text{constant}$$

For creatinine in μmol/L:

$$X = 175 \times (\text{creatinine}/88.4)^{-1.154} \times \text{age}^{-0.203} \times \text{constant}$$

where X is the glomerular filtration rate (GFR), constant for white males is 1 and for females is 0.742, and constant for African Americans is 1.21.

Ideal Body Weight (IBW)

IBW is the weight expected for a nonobese person of a given height. The IBW formulas below and various life insurance tables can be used to estimate IBW. Dosing methods described in the literature may use IBW as a method in dosing obese patients.

Adults (age 18 years and older)[4]:

IBW (males) = 50 + (2.3 × height in inches over 5 ft)

IBW (females) = 45.5 + (2.3 × height in inches over 5 ft)

where IBW is in kilograms.

Children (age 1 to 18 years)[2]:

Under 5 feet tall:

$$\text{IBW} = \frac{\text{height}^2 \times 1.65}{1,000}$$

where IBW is in kilograms and height is in centimeters.

Five feet or taller:

IBW (males) = 39 + (2.27 × height in inches over 5 ft)

IBW (females) = 42.2 + (2.27 × height in inches over 5 ft)

where IBW is in kilograms.

REFERENCES

1. Cockcroft DW, Gault MH. Prediction of creatinine clearance from serum creatinine. Nephron 1976;16:31–41.
2. Traub SI, Johnson CE. Comparison of methods of estimating creatinine clearance in children. Am J Hosp Pharm 1980;37:195–201.
3. Levey AS, Bosch JP, Lewis JB, et al. A more accurate method to estimate glomerular filtration rate from serum creatinine: A new prediction equation. Modification of Diet in Renal Disease Study Group. Ann Intern Med 1999;130:461–470.
4. Devine BJ. Gentamicin therapy. Drug Intell Clin Pharm 1974;8:650–655.

APPENDIX B
COMMON LABORATORY TESTS

The following table is an alphabetical listing of some common laboratory tests and their reference ranges for adults as measured in plasma or serum (unless otherwise indicated). Reference values differ among laboratories, so readers should refer to the published reference ranges used in each institution. For some tests, both SI units and conventional units are reported.

Laboratory	Conventional Units	Conversion Factor	SI Units
Acid phosphatase			
Male	2–12 units/L	16.7	33–200 nkat/L
Female	0.3–9.2 units/L	16.7	5–154 nkat/L
Activated partial thromboplastin time (aPTT)	25–40 s		
Adrenocorticotropic hormone (ACTH)	15–80 pg/mL or ng/L	0.2202	3.3–17.6 pmol/L
Alanine aminotransferase (ALT, SGPT)	7–53 IU/L	0.01667	0.12–0.88 μkat/L
Albumin	3.5–5.0 g/dL	10	35–50 g/L
Albumin:creatinine ratio (urine)			
Normal	Less than 30 mg/g creatinine		
Microalbuminuria	30–300 mg/g creatinine		
Proteinuria	Greater than 300 mg/g creatinine		
or	or		
Normal			
Male	Less than 2.0 mg/mmol creatinine		
Female	Less than 2.8 mg/mmol creatinine		
Microalbuminuria			
Male	2.0–20 mg/mmol creatinine		
Female	2.8–28 mg/mmol creatinine		
Proteinuria			
Male	Greater than 20 mg/mmol creatinine		
Female	Greater than 28 mg/mmol creatinine		
Aldosterone			
Supine	Less than 16 ng/dL	27.7	Less than 444 pmol/L
Upright	Less than 31 ng/dL	27.7	Less than 860 pmol/L
Alkaline phosphatase			
10–15 years	130–550 IU/L	0.01667	2.17–9.17 μkat/L
16–20 years	70–260 IU/L	0.01667	1.17–4.33 μkat/L
Greater than 20 years	38–126 IU/L	0.01667	0.13–2.10 μkat/L
Alpha-fetoprotein (AFP)	Less than 15 ng/mL	1	Less than 15 mcg/L
Alpha$_1$-antitrypsin	80–200 mg/dL	0.01	0.8–2.0 g/L
Amikacin, therapeutic	15–30 mg/L peak	1.71	25.6–51.3 μmol/L peak
	Less than or equal to 8 mg/L trough		Less than or equal to 13.7 μmol/L trough
Amitriptyline	80–200 ng/mL or mcg/L	3.4	272–680 nmol/L
Ammonia (plasma)	15.33–56.20 mcg NH$_3$/dL	0.5872	9–33 μmol NH$_3$/L
Amylase	25–115 IU/L	0.01667	0.42–1.92 μkat/L
Androstenedione	50–250 ng/dL	0.0349	1.7–8.7 nmol/L
Angiotensin-converting enzyme	15–70 units/L	16.67	250–1,167 nkat/L
Anion gap	7–16 mEq/L	1	7–16 mmol/L
Anti–double-stranded DNA (anti-ds DNA)	Negative		
Anti-HAV	Negative		
Anti-HBc	Negative		
Anti-HBs	Negative		
Anti-HCV	Negative		
Anti–Sm antibody	Negative		
Antinuclear antibody (ANA)	Negative		
Apolipoprotein A-1			
Male	95–175 mg/dL	0.01	0.95–1.75 g/L
Female	100–200 mg/dL	0.01	1.0–2.0 g/L

(continued)

Laboratory	Conventional Units	Conversion Factor	SI Units
Apolipoprotein B			
Male	50–110 mg/dL	0.01	0.5–1.10 g/L
Female	50–105 mg/dL	0.01	0.5–1.05 g/L
Aspartate aminotransferase (AST, SGOT)	11–47 IU/L	0.01667	0.18–0.78 μkat/L
Beta$_2$-microglobulin	Less than 0.2 mg/dL	10	2 mg/L
Bicarbonate	22–26 mEq/L	1	22–26 mmol/L
Bilirubin			
Total	0.3–1.1 mg/dL	17.1	5.13–18.80 μmol/L
Direct	0–0.3 mg/dL	17.1	0–5.1 μmol/L
Indirect	0.1–1.0 mg/dL	17.1	1.71–17.1 μmol/L
Bleeding time	3–7 min		
Blood gases (arterial)			
pH	7.35–7.45	1	7.35–7.45
Po_2	80–105 mm Hg	0.133	10.6–14.0 kPa
Pco_2	35–45 mm Hg	0.133	4.7–6.0 kPa
HCO_3	22–26 mEq/L	1	22–26 mmol/L
O_2 saturation	Greater than or equal to 95%	0.01	0.95
Blood urea nitrogen	8–25 mg/dL	0.357	2.9–8.9 mmol/L
B-type natriuretic peptide (BNP)	0–99 pg/mL	1	0–99 ng/L
BUN-to-creatinine ratio	10:1 to 20:1		
C-peptide	0.51–2.70 ng/mL	330	170–900 pmol/L or
		0.33	0.172–0.900 nmol/L
C-reactive protein	Less than 0.8 mg/dL	10	Less than 8 mg/L
CA-125	Less than 35 units/mL	1	Less than 35 kilounits/L
CA 15-3	Less than 30 units/mL	1	Less than 30 kilounits/L
CA 19-9	Less than 37 units/mL	1	Less than 37 kilounits/L
CA 27-29	Less than 38 units/mL	1	Less than 38 kilounits/L
Calcium			
Total	8.6–10.3 mg/dL	0.25	2.15–2.58 mmol/L
	4.3–5.16 mEq/L	0.50	2.15–2.58 mmol/L
Ionized	4.5–5.1 mg/dL	0.25	1.13–1.28 mmol/L
	2.26–2.56 mEq/L	0.50	1.13–1.28 mmol/L
Carbamazepine, therapeutic	4–12 mg/L	4.23	17–51 μmol/L
Carboxyhemoglobin (nonsmoker)	Less than 2%	0.01	Less than 0.02
Carcinoembryonic antigen (CEA)			
Nonsmoker	Less than 2.5 ng/mL	1	Less than 2.5 mcg/L
Smoker	Less than 5 ng/mL		Less than 5 mcg/L
Cardiac troponin I (see troponin I)	Variable ng/mL	1	Variable mcg/L
CD4 lymphocyte count	31–61% of total lymphocytes		
CD8 lymphocyte count	18–39% of total lymphocytes		
Cerebrospinal fluid (CSF)			
Pressure	75–175 mm H_2O		
Glucose	40–70 mg/dL	0.0555	2.2–3.9 mmol/L
Protein	15–45 mg/dL	0.01	0.15–0.45 g/L
WBC	Less than 10/mm^3		
Ceruloplasmin	18–45 mg/dL	10	180–450 mg/L
		0.063	1.1–2.8 μmol/L
Chloride	97–110 mEq/L	1	97–110 mmol/L
Cholesterol			
Desirable	Less than 200 mg/dL	0.0259	Less than 5.18 mmol/L
Borderline high	200–239 mg/dL	0.0259	5.18–6.19 mmol/L
High	Greater than or equal to 240 mg/dL	0.0259	Greater than or equal to 6.2 mmol/L
Chorionic gonadotropin (β-hCG)	Less than 5 milliunits/mL	1	Less than 5 units/L
Clozapine	Minimum trough 300–350 ng/mL or mcg/L	3.06	918–1,071 nmol/L
CO_2 content	22–30 mEq/L	1	22–30 mmol/L
Complement component 3 (C3)	70–160 mg/dL	0.01	0.7–1.6 g/L
Complement component 4 (C4)	20–40 mg/dL	0.01	0.2–0.4 g/L
Copper	70–150 mcg/dL	0.157	11–24 μmol/L
Cortisol (fasting, morning)	5–25 mcg/dL	27.6	138–690 nmol/L
Cortisol (free, urinary)	10–100 mcg/day	2.76	28–276 nmol/day
Creatine kinase			
Male	30–200 IU/L	0.01667	0.50–3.33 μkat/L
Female	20–170 IU/L	0.01667	0.33–2.83 μkat/L
MB fraction	0–7 IU/L	0.01667	0.0–0.12 μkat/L
Creatinine clearance (CLcr) (urine)	85–135 mL/min/1.73 m^2	0.00963	0.82–1.3 mL/s/m^2

(continued)

Laboratory	Conventional Units	Conversion Factor	SI Units
Creatinine			
Male 4–20 years	0.2–1.0 mg/dL	88.4	18–88 μmol/L
Female 4–20 years	0.2–1.0 mg/dL	88.4	18–88 μmol/L
Male (adults)	0.7–1.3 mg/dL	88.4	62–115 μmol/L
Female (adults)	0.6–1.1 mg/dL	88.4	53–97 μmol/L
Cyclosporine			
Renal transplant	100–300 ng/mL or mcg/L	0.832	83–250 nmol/L
Cardiac, liver, or pancreatic transplant	200–350 ng/mL or mcg/L	0.832	166–291 nmol/L
Cryptococcal antigen	Negative		
D-dimers	Less than 250 ng/mL	1	Less than 250 mcg/L
Desipramine	75–300 ng/mL or mcg/L	3.75	281–1,125 mmol/L
Dexamethasone suppression test (DST) (overnight)	8:00 AM cortisol less than 5 mcg/dL	0.0276	Less than 0.14 μmol/L
DHEAS			
Male	170–670 mcg/dL	0.0271	4.6–18.2 μmol/L
Female			
Premenopausal	50–540 mcg/dL	0.0271	1.4–14.7 μmol/L
Postmenopausal	30–260 mcg/dL	0.0271	0.8–7.1 μmol/L
Digoxin, therapeutic	0.5–1.0 ng/mL or mcg/L	1.28	0.6–1.3 nmol/L
Erythrocyte count (blood) See under red blood cell count			
Erythrocyte sedimentation rate (ESR)			
Westergren			
Male	0–20 mm/hour		
Female	0–30 mm/hour		
Wintrobe			
Male	0–9 mm/hour		
Female	0–15 mm/hour		
Erythropoietin	2–25 mIU/mL	1	2–25 IU/L
Estradiol			
Male	10–36 pg/mL	3.67	37–132 pmol/L
Female	34–170 pg/mL	3.67	125–624 pmol/L
Ethanol, legal intoxication	Greater than or equal to 50–100 mg/dL	0.217	10.9–21.7 mmol/L
	Greater than or equal to 0.05–0.1%	217	
Ethosuccimide, therapeutic	40–100 mg/L or mcg/mL	7.08	283–708 μmol/L
Factor VIII or factor IX			
Severe hemophilia	Less than 1 IU/dL	0.01	Less than 0.01 units/mL
Moderate hemophilia	1–5 IU/dL	0.01	0.01–0.05 units/mL
Mild hemophilia	Greater than 5 IU/dL	0.01	Greater than 0.05 units/mL
Usual adult levels	60–140 IU/dL	0.01	0.60–1.40 units/mL
Ferritin			
Male	20–250 ng/mL	1	20–250 mcg/L
Female	10–150 ng/mL	1	10–150 mcg/L
Fibrin degradation products (FDP)	2–10 mg/L		
Fibrinogen	200–400 mg/dL	0.01	2.0–4.0 g/L
Folate (plasma)	3.1–12.4 ng/mL	2.266	7.0–28.1 nmol/L
Folic acid (RBC)	125–600 ng/mL	2.266	283–1,360 nmol/L
Follicle-stimulating hormone (FSH)			
Male	1–7 mIU/mL	1	1–7 IU/L
Female			
Follicular phase	1–9 mIU/mL	1	1–9 IU/L
Midcycle	6–26 mIU/mL	1	6–26 IU/L
Luteal phase	1–9 mIU/mL	1	1–9 IU/L
Postmenopausal	30–118 mIU/mL	1	30–118 IU/L
Free thyroxine index (FT_4I)	6.5–12.5		
Gamma glutamyl transferase (GGT)	0–30 IU/L	0.01667	0–0.5 μkat/L
Gastrin (fasting)	0–130 pg/mL	1	0–130 ng/L
Gentamicin, therapeutic	4–10 mg/L peak	2.09	8.4–21.0 μmol/L peak
	Less than or equal to 2 mg/L trough		Less than or equal to 4.2 μmol/L trough
Globulin	2.3–3.5 g/dL	10	23–35 g/L
Glucose (fasting, plasma)	65–109 mg/dL	0.0555	3.6–6.0 mmol/L
Glucose, two hour postprandial blood (PPBG)	Less than 140 mg/dL	0.0555	Less than 7.8 mmol/L
Granulocyte count	$1.8–6.6 \times 10^3/\mu L$	10^6	$1.8–6.6 \times 10^9/L$
Growth hormone (fasting)			
Male	Less than 5 ng/mL	1	Less than 5 mcg/L
Female	Less than 10 ng/mL	1	Less than 10 mcg/L
Haptoglobin	60–270 mg/dL	0.01	0.6–2.7 g/L
HBeAg	Negative		

(continued)

Laboratory	Conventional Units	Conversion Factor	SI Units
HbsAg	Negative		
HBV DNA	Negative		
Hematocrit			
Male	40.7–50.3%	0.01	0.407–0.503
Female	36.1–44.3%	0.01	0.361–0.443
Hemoglobin (blood)			
Male	13.8–17.2 g/dL	10	138–172 g/L
		Alternate SI: 0.62	8.56–10.67 mmol/L
Female	12.1–15.1 g/dL	10	121–151 g/L
		Alternate SI: 0.62	7.5–9.36 mmol/L
Hemoglobin A1C	4.0–6.0%	0.01	0.04–0.06
Heparin			
Via protamine titration method	0.2–0.4 mcg/mL		
Via anti-factor Xa assay	0.3–0.7 mcg/mL		
High-density lipoprotein (HDL) cholesterol	Greater than 35 mg/dL	0.0259	Greater than 0.91 mmol/L
Homocysteine	3.3–10.4 μmol/L		
Ibuprofen			
Therapeutic	10–50 mcg/mL	4.85	49–243 μmol/L
Toxic	100–700 mcg/mL or more	4.85	485–3,395 μmol/L or more
Imipramine, therapeutic	100–300 ng/mL or mcg/L	3.57	357–1071 nmol/L
Immunoglobulin A (IgA)	85–385 mg/dL	0.01	0.85–3.85 g/L
Immunoglobulin G (IgG)	565–1,765 mg/dL	0.01	5.65–17.65 g/L
Immunoglobulin M (IgM)	53–375 mg/dL	0.01	0.53–3.75 g/L
Insulin (fasting)	2–20 microunits/mL or milliunits/L	7.175	14.35–143.5 pmol/L
International normalized ratio (INR), therapeutic	2.0–3.0 (2.5–3.5 for some indications)		
Iron			
Male	45–160 mcg/dL	0.179	8.1–31.3 μmol/L
Female	30–160 mcg/dL	0.179	5.4–31.3 μmol/L
Iron binding capacity (total)	220–420 mcg/dL	0.179	39.4–75.2 μmol/L
Iron saturation	15–50%	0.01	0.15–0.50
Lactate (plasma)	0.7–2.1 mEq/L	1	0.7–2.1 mmol/L
	6.3–18.9 mg/dL	0.111	
Lactate dehydrogenase	100–250 IU/L	0.01667	1.67–4.17 μkat/L
Lead	Less than 25 mcg/dL	0.0483	Less than 1.21 μmol/L
Leukocyte count	3.8–9.8 $\times 10^3/\mu$L	10^6	3.8–9.8 $\times 10^9$/L
Lidocaine, therapeutic	1.5–6.0 mcg/mL or mg/L	4.27	6.4–25.6 μmol/L
Lipase	Less than 100 IU/L	0.01667	1.7 μkat/L
Lithium, therapeutic	0.5–1.25 mEq/L	1	0.5–1.25 mmol/L
Low-density lipoprotein (LDL) cholesterol			
Desirable	Less than 130 mg/dL	0.0259	Less than 3.36 mmol/L
Borderline high risk	130–159 mg/dL	0.0259	3.36–4.11 mmol/L
High risk	Greater than or equal to 160 mg/dL	0.0259	Greater than or equal to 4.13 mmol/L
Luteinizing hormone (LH)			
Male	1–8 milliunits/mL	1	1–8 units/L
Female			
Follicular phase	1–12 milliunits/mL	1	1–12 units/L
Midcycle	16–104 milliunits/mL	1	16–104 units/L
Luteal phase	1–12 milliunits/mL	1	1–12 units/L
Postmenopausal	16–66 milliunits/mL	1	16–66 units/L
Lymphocyte count	1.2–3.3 $\times 10^3/\mu$L	106	1.2–3.3 $\times 10^9$/L
Magnesium	1.3–2.2 mEq/L	0.5	0.65–1.10 mmol/L
	1.58–2.68 mg/dL	0.411	0.65–1.10 mmol/L
Mean corpuscular volume	80.0–97.6 μm^3	1	80.0–97.6 fL
Mononuclear cell count	0.2–0.7 $\times 10^3/\mu$L	106	0.2–0.7 $\times 10^9$/L
Nortriptyline, therapeutic	50–150 ng/mL or mcg/L	3.8	190–570 nmol/L
NT-ProBNP (see Pro-BNP)			
Osmolality (serum)	275–300 mOsm/kg	1	275–300 mmol/kg
Osmolality (urine)	250–900 mOsm/kg	1	250–900 mmol/kg
Parathyroid hormone (PTH), intact	10–60 pg/mL or ng/L	0.107	1.1–6.4 pmol/L
Parathyroid hormone (PTH), N-terminal	8–24 pg/mL or ng/L		
Parathyroid hormone (PTH), C-terminal	50–330 pg/mL or ng/L		
Phenobarbital, therapeutic	15–40 mcg/mL or mg/L	4.31	65–172 μmol/L
Phenytoin, therapeutic	10–20 mcg/mL or mg/L	3.96	40–79 μmol/L
Phosphate	2.5–4.5 mg/dL	0.323	0.81–1.45 mmol/L
Platelet count	140–440 $\times 10^3/\mu$L	10^6	140–440 $\times 10^9$/L
Potassium (plasma)	3.3–4.9 mEq/L	1	3.3–4.9 μmol/L
Prealbumin (adult)	19.5–35.8 mg/dL	10	195–358 mg/L
Primidone, therapeutic	5–12 mcg/mL or mg/L	4.58	23–55 μmol/L

(continued)

Laboratory	Conventional Units	Conversion Factor	SI Units
ProBNP	Less than 125 pg/mL or ng/L	0.118	Less than 14.75 pmol/L
Procainamide, therapeutic	4–10 mcg/mL or mg/L	4.23	17–42 μmol/L
Progesterone			
Male	13–97 ng/dL	0.0318	0.4–3.1 nmol/L
Female			
Follicular phase	15–70 ng/dL		0.5–2.2 nmol/L
Luteal phase	200–2,500 ng/dL		6.4–79.5 nmol/L
Prolactin	Less than 20 ng/mL	1	Less than 20 mcg/L
Prostate-specific antigen (PSA)	Less than 4 ng/mL	1	Less than 4 mcg/L
Protein, total	6.0–8.0 g/dL	10	60–80 g/L
Prothrombin time (PT)	10–12 sec		
Quinidine, therapeutic	2–5 mcg/mL or mg/L	3.08	6.2–15.4 μmol/L
Radioactive iodine uptake (RAIU)	Less than 6% in 2 hours		
Red blood cell (RBC) count (blood)			
Male	$4–6.2 \times 10^6/\mu L$	10^6	$4–6.2 \times 10^{12}/L$
Female	$4–6.2 \times 10^6/\mu L$	10^6	$4–6.2 \times 10^{12}/L$
Pregnant			
Trimester 1	$4–5 \times 10^6/\mu L$	10^6	$4–5 \times 10^{12}/L$
Trimester 2	$3.2–4.5 \times 10^6/\mu L$	10^6	$3.2–4.5 \times 10^{12}/L$
Trimester 3	$3.0–4.9 \times 10^6/\mu L$	10^6	$3.0–4.9 \times 10^{12}/L$
Postpartum	$3.2–5 \times 10^6/\mu L$	10^6	$3.2–5.0 \times 10^6/L$
Red blood cell distribution width (RDW)	11.5–14.5%	0.01	0.115–0.145
Reticulocyte count			
Male	0.5–1.5% of total RBC count	0.01	0.005–0.015
Female	0.5–2.5% of total RBC count	0.01	0.005–0.025
Retinol-binding protein (RBP)	2.7–7.6 mg/dL	10	27–76 mg/L
Rheumatoid factor (RF) titer	Negative		
Salicylate, therapeutic	150–300 mcg/mL or mg/L	0.00724	1.09–2.17 mmol/L
	15–30 mg/dL	0.0724	
Sodium	135–145 mEq/L	1	135–145 mmol/L
Tacrolimus			
Renal transplant	6–12 ng/mL or mcg/L		
Liver transplant	4–10 ng/mL or mcg/L		
Pancreatic transplant	10–18 ng/mL or mcg/L		
Bone marrow transplant	10–20 ng/mL or mcg/L		
Testosterone (total)			
Men	300–950 ng/dL	0.0347	10.4–33.0 nmol/L
Women	20–80 ng/dL		0.7–2.8 nmol/L
Testosterone (free)			
Men	9–30 ng/dL	0.0347	0.31–1.04 nmol/L
Women	0.3–1.9 ng/dL		0.01–0.07 nmol/L
Theophylline			
Therapeutic	5–15 mcg/mL or mg/L	5.55	28–83 μmol/L
Toxic	20 or more mcg/mL or mg/L	5.55	111 or more μmol/L
Thrombin time	20–24 sec		
Thyroglobulin	Less than 42 ng/mL	1	Less than 42 mcg/L
Thyroglobulin antibodies	Negative		
Thyroxine-binding globulin (TBG)	1.2–2.5 mg/dL	10	12–25 mcg/L
Thyroid-stimulating hormone (TSH)	0.35–6.20 microunits/mL	1	0.35–6.20 milliunits/L
TSH receptor antibodies (TSH Rab)	0–1 unit/mL		
Thyroxine (T_4)			
Total	4.5–12.0 mcg/dL	12.87	58–155 nmol/L
Free	0.7–1.9 ng/dL	12.87	9.0–24.5 pmol/L
Thyroxine index, free (FT_4I)	6.5–12.5		
TIBC See Iron-binding capacity (total)			
Tobramycin, therapeutic	4–10 mcg/mL or mg/L peak	2.14	8.6–21.4 μmol/L
	Less than or equal to 2 mcg/mL mg/L trough	2.14	Less than or equal to 4.28 μmol/L
Transferrin	200–430 mg/dL	0.01	2.0–4.3 g/L
Transferrin saturation	30–50%	0.01	0.30–0.50
Triglycerides (fasting)	Less than 160 mg/dL	0.0113	Less than 1.8 mmol/L
Triiodothyronine (T_3)	45–132 ng/dL	0.0154	0.91–2.70 nmol/L
Triiodothyronine (T_3) resin uptake	25–35%		
Troponin I	Less than 0.6 ng/mL	1	Less than 0.6 μg/L
Uric acid	3–8 mg/dL	59.48	179–476 μmol/L
Urinalysis (urine)			
pH	4.8–8.0		
Specific gravity	1.005–1.030		

(continued)

Laboratory	Conventional Units	Conversion Factor	SI Units
Protein	Negative		
Glucose	Negative		
Ketones	Negative		
RBC	1–2 per low-power field		
WBC	3–4 per low-power field		
Valproic acid, therapeutic	50–100 mcg/mL or mg/L	6.93	346–693 μmol/L
Vancomycin, therapeutic trough for CNS infections	20–40 mcg/mL or mg/L peak	0.690	14–28 μmol/L peak
	5–20 mcg/mL or mg/L trough	0.690	3–14 μmol/L trough
	15–20 mcg/mL or mg/L trough	0.690	10–14 μmol/L trough
Vitamin A (retinol)	30–95 mcg/dL	0.0349	1.05–3.32 μmol/L
Vitamin B$_{12}$	180–1,000 pg/mL	0.738	133–738 pmol/L
Vitamin D$_3$, 1, 25-dihydroxy	20–76 pg/m	2.4	48–182 pmol/L
Vitamin D$_3$, 25-hydroxy	10–50 ng/mL	2.496	25–125 nmol/L
Vitamin E (alpha tocopherol)	0.5–2.0 mg/dL	23.22	12–46 μmol/L
WBC count	4–$10 \times 10^3/\mu$L or 4–$10 \times 10^3/mm^3$	10^6	4–10×10^9/L
WBC differential (peripheral blood)			
Polymorphonuclear neutrophils (PMNs)	50–65%		
Bands	0–5%		
Eosinophils	0–3%		
Basophils	1–3%		
Lymphocytes	25–35%		
Monocytes	2–6%		
WBC differential (bone marrow)			
Polymorphonuclear neutrophils (PMNs)	3–11%		
Bands	9–15%		
Metamyelocytes	9–25%		
Myelocytes	8–16%		
Promyelocytes	1–8%		
Myeloblasts	0–5%		
Eosinophils	1–5%		
Basophils	0–1%		
Lymphocytes	11–23%		
Monocytes	0–1%		
Zinc	60–150 mcg/dL	0.153	9.2–23.0 μmol/L

This table was reprinted with permission from: Chisholm-Burns MA, Wells BG, Schwinghammer TL, et al. (eds). Pharmacotherapy Principles and Practice. New York: McGraw-Hill, 2008.

APPENDIX C
PART I: Common Medical Abbreviations

Note: Many of the medical abbreviations contained in Part I of this appendix are used in the casebook. A more extensive list of abbreviations is available on the internet at *www.pharma-lexicon.com*.

A & O	Alert and oriented
A & P	Auscultation and percussion; anterior and posterior; assessment and plan
A & W	Alive and well
A1C	Hemoglobin A1C
aa	Of each (*ana*)
AA	Aplastic anemia; Alcoholics Anonymous
AAA	Abdominal aortic aneurysm
AAL	Anterior axillary line
AAO	Awake, alert, and oriented
ABC	Absolute band count; absolute basophil count; aspiration, biopsy, and cytology; artificial beta cells
Abd	Abdomen
ABG	Aterial blood gases
ABP	Arterial blood pressure
ABW	Actual body weight
ABx	Antibiotics
AC	Before meals (*ante cibos*)
ACE	Angiotensin-converting enzyme
ACEI	Angiotensin-converting enzyme inhibitor
ACL	Anterior cruciate ligament
ACLS	Advanced cardiac life support
ACS	Acute coronary syndrome
ACT	Activated clotting time
ACTH	Adrenocorticotropic hormone
AD	Alzheimer's disease, right ear (*auris dextra*)
ADA	American Diabetes Association; adenosine deaminase
ADE	Adverse drug effect (or event)
ADH	Antidiuretic hormone
ADHD	Attention-deficit hyperactivity disorder
ADL	Activities of daily living
ADR	Adverse drug reaction
AED	Antiepileptic drug(s)
AF	Atrial fibrillation
AFB	Acid-fast bacillus; aortofemoral bypass; aspirated foreign body
Afeb	Afebrile
AFP	α-Fetoprotein
A/G	Albumin-globulin ratio
AI	Aortic insufficiency
AIDS	Acquired immunodeficiency syndrome
AKA	Above-knee amputation; alcoholic ketoacidosis; all known allergies; also known as
AKI	Acute kidney injury
ALD	Alcoholic liver disease
ALFT	Abnormal liver function test
ALL	Acute lymphocytic leukemia; acute lymphoblastic leukemia

ALP	Alkaline phosphatase
ALS	Amyotrophic lateral sclerosis
ALT	Alanine aminotransferase
AMA	Against medical advice; American Medical Association; antimitochondrial antibody
AMI	Acute myocardial infarction
AML	Acute myelogenous leukemia
Amp	Ampule
ANA	Antinuclear antibody
ANC	Absolute neutrophil count
ANLL	Acute nonlymphocytic leukemia
AODM	Adult onset diabetes mellitus
A & O × 3	Awake and oriented to person, place, and time
A & O × 4	Awake and oriented to person, place, time, and situation
AOM	Acute otitis media
AP	Anteroposterior
APACHE	Acute Physiology and Chronic Health Evaluation
APAP	Acetaminophen (*N*-acetyl-*p*-aminophenol)
aPTT	Activated partial thromboplastin time
ARC	AIDS-related complex
ARDS	Adult respiratory distress syndrome
ARF	Acute renal failure; acute respiratory failure; acute rheumatic fever
AROM	Active range of motion
AS	Left ear (*auris sinistra*)
ASA	Aspirin (acetylsalicylic acid)
ASCVD	Arteriosclerotic cardiovascular disease
ASD	Atrial septal defect
ASH	Asymmetric septal hypertrophy
ASHD	Arteriosclerotic heart disease
AST	Aspartate aminotransferase
ATG	Antithymocyte globulin
ATN	Acute tubular necrosis
AU	Each ear (*auris uterque*)
AV	Arteriovenous; atrioventricular
AVM	Arteriovenous malformation
AVR	Aortic valve replacement
AWMI	Anterior wall myocardial infarction
BAC	Blood alcohol concentration
BAL	Bronchioalveolar lavage
BBB	Bundle branch block; blood-brain barrier
BC	Blood culture
BCG	Bacillus Calmette Guerin
BCNP	Board Certified Nuclear Pharmacist
BCNSP	Board Certified Nutrition Support Pharmacist
BCNU	Carmustine
BCOP	Board Certified Oncology Pharmacist
BCP	Birth control pill

BCPP	Board Certified Psychiatric Pharmacist
BCPS	Board Certified Pharmacotherapy Specialist
BE	Barium enema
BID	Twice daily (*bis in die*)
BKA	Below-knee amputation
BM	Bone marrow; bowel movement
BMC	Bone marrow cells
BMD	Bone mineral density
BMR	Basal metabolic rate
BMT	Bone marrow transplantation
BNP	Brain natriuretic peptide
BP	Blood pressure
BPD	Bronchopulmonary dysplasia
BPH	Benign prostatic hyperplasia
bpm	Beats per minute
BPRS	Brief Psychiatric Rating Scale
BR	Bedrest
BRBPR	Bright red blood per rectum
BRM	Biological response modifier
BRP	Bathroom privileges
BS	Bowel sounds; breath sounds; blood sugar
BSA	Body surface area
BSO	Bilateral salpingo-oophorectomy
BTFS	Breast tumor frozen section
BUN	Blood urea nitrogen
Bx	Biopsy
C & S	Culture and sensitivity
CA	Cancer; calcium
CABG	Coronary artery bypass graft
CAD	Coronary artery disease
CAH	Chronic active hepatitis
CAM	Complementary and alternative medicine
CAPD	Continuous ambulatory peritoneal dialysis
CBC	Complete blood count
CBD	Common bile duct
CBG	Capillary blood gas; corticosteroid binding globulin
CBT	Cognitive-behavioral therapy
CC	Chief complaint
CCA	Calcium channel antagonist
CCB	Calcium channel blocker
CCE	Clubbing, cyanosis, edema
CCK	Cholecystokinin
CCMS	Clean catch midstream
CCNU	Lomustine
CCPD	Continuous cycling peritoneal dialysis
CCU	Coronary care unit
CDAD	*Clostridium difficile*–associated diarrhea
CEA	Carcinoembryonic antigen
CF	Cystic fibrosis
CFS	Chronic fatigue syndrome
CFU	Colony-forming unit
CHD	Coronary heart disease
CHF	Congestive heart failure
CHO	Carbohydrate
CHOP	Cyclophosphamide, hydroxydaunorubicin (doxorubicin), Oncovin (vincristine), prednisone
CI	Cardiac index
CK	Creatine kinase
CKD	Chronic kidney disease

CLcr	Creatinine clearance
CLL	Chronic lymphocytic leukemia
CM	Costal margin
CMG	Cystometrogram
CML	Chronic myelogenous leukemia
CMV	Cytomegalovirus
CN	Cranial nerve
CNS	Central nervous system
c/o	Complains of
CO	Cardiac output; carbon monoxide
COLD	Chronic obstructive lung disease
COPD	Chronic obstructive pulmonary disease
CP	Chest pain; cerebral palsy
CPA	Costophrenic angle
CPAP	Continuous positive airway pressure
CPK	Creatine phosphokinase
CPP	Cerebral perfusion pressure
CPR	Cardiopulmonary resuscitation
CR	Complete remission
CRF	Chronic renal failure; corticotropin-releasing factor
CRH	Corticotropin-releasing hormone
CRI	Chronic renal insufficiency; catheter-related infection
CRNA	Certified Registered Nurse Anesthetist
CRNP	Certified Registered Nurse Practitioner
CRP	C-reactive protein
CRTT	Certified Respiratory Therapy Technician
CS	Central Supply
CSA	Cyclosporine
CSF	Cerebrospinal fluid; colony-stimulating factor
CT	Computed tomography; chest tube
CTB	Cease to breathe
cTnI	Cardiac troponin I
CTZ	Chemoreceptor trigger zone
CV	Cardiovascular
CVA	Cerebrovascular accident
CVAT	Costovertebral angle tenderness
CVC	Central venous catheter
CVP	Central venous pressure
Cx	Culture; cervix
CXR	Chest x-ray
D & C	Dilatation and curettage
d4T	Stavudine
D_5W	5% Dextrose in water
DBP	Diastolic blood pressure
D/C	Discontinue; discharge
DCC	Direct current cardioversion
ddC	Zalcitabine
ddI	Didanosine
DES	Diethylstilbestrol
DI	Diabetes insipidus
DIC	Disseminated intravascular coagulation
Diff	Differential
DIP	Distal interphalangeal
DJD	Degenerative joint disease
DKA	Diabetic ketoacidosis
dL	Deciliter
DM	Diabetes mellitus
DMARD	Disease-modifying antirheumatic drug
DNA	Deoxyribonucleic acid

DNR	Do not resuscitate
DO	Doctor of Osteopathy
DOA	Dead on arrival; date of admission; duration of action
DOB	Date of birth
DOE	Dyspnea on exertion
DOT	Directly observed therapy
DPGN	Diffuse proliferative glomerulonephritis
DRE	Digital rectal examination
DRG	Diagnosis-related group
DS	Double strength
DSHEA	Dietary Supplement Health and Education Act (1994)
DST	Dexamethasone suppression test
DTIC	Dacarbazine
DTP	Diphtheria-tetanus-pertussis
DTR	Deep-tendon reflex
DVT	Deep-vein thrombosis
Dx	Diagnosis
EBV	Epstein-Barr virus
EC	Enteric-coated
ECF	Extended care facility
ECG	Electrocardiogram
ECMO	Extracorporeal membrane oxygenator
ECOG	Eastern Cooperative Oncology Group
ECT	Electroconvulsive therapy
ED	Emergency Department
EEG	Electroencephalogram
EENT	Eyes, ears, nose, throat
EF	Ejection fraction
EGD	Esophagogastroduodenoscopy
EIA	Enzyme immunoassay
EKG	Electrocardiogram
EMG	Electromyogram
EMT	Emergency medical technician
Endo	Endotracheal; endoscopy
EOMI	Extraocular movements (or muscles) intact
EPO	Erythropoietin
EPS	Extrapyramidal symptoms
ER	Estrogen receptor; emergency room
ERCP	Endoscopic retrograde cholangiopancreatography
ERT	Estrogen replacement therapy
ESLD	End-stage liver disease
ESR	Erythrocyte sedimentation rate
ESRD	End-stage renal disease
ESWL	Extracorporeal shockwave lithotripsy
ET	Endotracheal
ETOH	Ethanol
FB	Finger-breadth; foreign body
FBS	Fasting blood sugar
FDA	Food and Drug Administration
FDP	Fibrin degradation products
FEF	Forced expiratory flow (rate)
FEM-POP	Femoral-popliteal
FEV_1	Forced expiratory volume in 1 second
FFP	Fresh frozen plasma
FH	Family history
FiO_2	Fraction of inspired oxygen
fL	Femtoliter
FM	Face mask
FOBT	Fecal occult blood test

FOC	Fronto-occipital circumference
FPG	Fasting plasma glucose
FPIA	Fluorescence polarization immunoassay
FSH	Follicle-stimulating hormone
FTA	Fluorescent treponemal antibody
f/u	Follow-up
FUDR	Floxuridine
FUO	Fever of unknown origin
Fx	Fracture
G6PD	Glucose-6-phosphate dehydrogenase
GAD	Generalized anxiety disorder
GB	Gallbladder
GBS	Group B *Streptococcus*; Guillain-Barré syndrome
GC	Gonococcus
G-CSF	Granulocyte colony-stimulating factor
GDM	Gestational diabetes mellitus
GE	Gastroesophageal; gastroenterology
GERD	Gastroesophageal reflux disease
GFR	Glomerular filtration rate
GGT	γ-Glutamyltransferase
GGTP	γ-Glutamyl transpeptidase
GI	Gastrointestinal
GM-CSF	Granulocyte-macrophage colony-stimulating factor
GN	Glomerulonephritis; graduate nurse
gr	Grain
GT	Gastrostomy tube
gtt	Drops (*guttae*)
GTT	Glucose tolerance test
GU	Genitourinary
GVHD	Graft-versus-host disease
GVL	Graft-versus-leukemia
Gyn	Gynecology
H & H	Hemoglobin and hematocrit
H & P	History and physical examination
H/A	Headache
HAART	Highly active antiretroviral therapy
HAM-D	Hamilton Rating Scale for Depression
HAV	Hepatitis A virus
Hb, hgb	Hemoglobin
HbA_{1C}	Hemoglobin A1C
HBIG	Hepatitis B immune globulin
HBP	High blood pressure
HBsAg	Hepatitis B surface antigen
HBV	Hepatitis B virus
HC	Hydrocortisone; home care
HCG	Human chorionic gonadotropin
HCO_3	Bicarbonate
Hct	Hematocrit
HCTZ	Hydrochlorothiazide
HCV	Hepatitis C virus
Hcy	Homocysteine
HD	Hodgkin's disease; hemodialysis
HDL	High-density lipoprotein
HEENT	Head, eyes, ears, nose, and throat
HEPA	High-efficiency particulate air
HF	Heart failure
H flu	*Haemophilus influenzae*
HGH	Human growth hormone
HH	Hiatal hernia

Hib	*Haemophilus influenzae* type b	IVF	Intravenous fluids
HIV	Human immunodeficiency virus	IVIG	Intravenous immunoglobulin
HJR	Hepatojugular reflux	IVP	Intravenous pyelogram; intravenous push
HLA	Human leukocyte antigen; human lymphocyte antigen	IVSS	Intravenous Soluset
HMG-CoA	Hydroxy-methylglutaryl coenzyme A	IWMI	Inferior wall myocardial infarction
H/O	History of	JODM	Juvenile-onset diabetes mellitus
HOB	Head of bed	JRA	Juvenile rheumatoid arthritis
HPA	Hypothalamic-pituitary axis	JVD	Jugular venous distention
hpf	High-power field	JVP	Jugular venous pressure
HPI	History of present illness	K	Potassium
HR	Heart rate	kcal	Kilocalorie
HRT	Hormone replacement therapy	KCL	Potassium chloride
HS	At bedtime (*hora somni*)	KOH	Potassium hydroxide
HSCT	Hematopoietic stem cell transplantation	KUB	Kidney, ureters, bladder
HSM	Hepatosplenomegaly	KVO	Keep vein open
HSV	Herpes simplex virus	L	Liter
HTN	Hypertension	LAD	Left anterior descending; left axis deviation
Hx	History	LAO	Left anterior oblique
I & D	Incision and drainage	LAP	Leukocyte alkaline phosphatase
I & O	Intake and output	LBBB	Left bundle branch block
IABP	Intra-arterial balloon pump	LBP	Low back pain
IBD	Inflammatory bowel disease	LCM	Left costal margin
IBW	Ideal body weight	LDH	Lactate dehydrogenase
ICD	Implantable cardioverter defibrillator	LDL	Low-density lipoprotein
ICP	Intracranial pressure	LE	Lower extremity
ICS	Intercostal space	LES	Lower esophageal sphincter
ICU	Intensive care unit	LFT	Liver function test
ID	Identification; infectious disease	LHRH	Luteinizing hormone-releasing hormone
IDDM	Insulin-dependent diabetes mellitus	LIMA	Left internal mammary artery
IFN	Interferon	LLE	Left lower extremity
Ig	Immunoglobulin	LLL	Left lower lobe
IgA	Immunoglobulin A	LLQ	Left lower quadrant (abdomen)
IgD	Immunoglobulin D	LLSB	Left lower sternal border
IHD	Ischemic heart disease	LMD	Local medical doctor
IJ	Internal jugular	LMP	Last menstrual period
IM	Intramuscular; infectious mononucleosis	LOC	Loss of consciousness; laxative of choice
IMV	Intermittent mandatory ventilation	LOS	Length of stay
INH	Isoniazid	LP	Lumbar puncture
INR	International normalized ratio	LPN	Licensed Practical Nurse
IOP	Intraocular pressure	LPO	Left posterior oblique
IP	Intraperitoneal	LPT	Licensed Physical Therapist
IPG	Impedance plethysmography	LR	Lactated Ringer's
IPI	International prognostic index	LS	Lumbosacral
IPN	Interstitial pneumonia	LTCF	Long-term care facility
IPPB	Intermittent positive pressure breathing	LUE	Left upper extremity
IPS	Idiopathic pneumonia syndrome	LUL	Left upper lobe
IRB	Institutional Review Board	LUQ	Left upper quadrant
ISA	Intrinsic sympathomimetic activity	LVH	Left ventricular hypertrophy
ISDN	Isosorbide dinitrate	MAP	Mean arterial pressure
ISH	Isolated systolic hypertension	MAR	Medication administration record
ISMN	Isosorbide mononitrate	mcg	Microgram
IT	Intrathecal	MCH	Mean corpuscular hemoglobin
ITP	Idiopathic thrombocytopenic purpura	MCHC	Mean corpuscular hemoglobin concentration
IU	International unit	MCL	Midclavicular line
IUD	Intrauterine device	MCP	Metacarpophalangeal
IV	Intravenous; Roman numeral IV; symbol for Class 4 controlled substances	MCV	Mean corpuscular volume
		MD	Medical Doctor
IVC	Inferior vena cava; intravenous cholangiogram	MDI	Metered-dose inhaler
IVDA	Intravenous drug abuse	MEFR	Maximum expiratory flow rate

mEq	Milliequivalent
mg	Milligram
MHC	Major histocompatibility complex
MI	Myocardial infarction; mitral insufficiency
MIC	Minimum inhibitory concentration
MICU	Medical intensive care unit
mL	Milliliter
MM	Multiple myeloma
MMA	Methylmalonic acid
MMEFR	Maximal midexpiratory flow rate
MMR	Measles-mumps-rubella
MMSE	Mini Mental State Examination
MOM	Milk of magnesia
MPV	Mean platelet volume
MRG	Murmur/rub/gallop
MRI	Magnetic resonance imaging
MRSA	Methicillin-resistant *Staphylococcus aureus*
MRSE	Methicillin-resistant *Staphylococcus epidermidis*
MS	Mental status; mitral stenosis; musculoskeletal; multiple sclerosis; morphine sulfate
MSE	Mental Status Exam
MSW	Master of Social Work
MTD	Maximum tolerated dose
MTP	Metatarsophalangeal
MTX	Methotrexate
MUD	Matched unrelated donor
MUGA	Multiple gated acquisition
MVA	Motor vehicle accident
MVI	Multivitamin
MVR	Mitral valve replacement; mitral valve regurgitation
MVS	Mitral valve stenosis; motor, vascular, and sensory
N/V	Nausea and vomiting
NAD	No acute (or apparent) distress
N/C	Non-contributory; nasal cannula
NC/AT	Normocephalic/atraumatic
NG	Nasogastric
NGT	Nasogastric tube
NGTD	No growth to date (on culture)
NHL	Non-Hodgkin's lymphoma
NIDDM	Non–insulin-dependent diabetes mellitus
NIH	National Institutes of Health
NKA	No known allergies
NKDA	No known drug allergies
NL	Normal
NNRTI	Non-nucleoside reverse transcriptase inhibitor
NOS	Not otherwise specified
NPH	Neutral protamine Hagedorn; normal pressure hydrocephalus
NPN	Non-protein nitrogen
NPO	Nothing by mouth (*nil per os*)
NRTI	Nucleoside reverse transcriptase inhibitor
NS	Neurosurgery; normal saline
NSAID	Nonsteroidal anti-inflammatory drug
NSCLC	Non-small cell lung cancer
NSR	Normal sinus rhythm
NSS	Normal saline solution
NTG	Nitroglycerin
NT/ND	Non-tender/non-distended

NVD	Nausea/vomiting/diarrhea; neck vein distention; non-valvular disease; neovascularization of the disk
NYHA	New York Heart Association
O & P	Ova and parasites
OA	Osteoarthritis
OB	Obstetrics
OBS	Organic brain syndrome
OCD	Obsessive-compulsive disorder
OCG	Oral cholecystogram
OD	Right eye (*oculus dexter*); overdose; Doctor of Optometry
OGT	Oral glucose tolerance test
OHTx	Orthotopic heart transplantation
OLTx	Orthotopic liver transplantation
OOB	Out of bed
OPD	Outpatient department
OPG	Ocular plethysmography
OPV	Oral poliovirus vaccine
OR	Operating room
OS	Left eye (*oculus sinister*)
OSA	Obstructive sleep apnea
OT	Occupational therapy
OTC	Over-the-counter
OU	Each eye (*oculus uterque*)
P	Pulse, plan, percussion, pressure
P & A	Percussion and auscultation
P & T	Peak and trough
PA	Physician Assistant; posterior-anterior; pulmonary artery
PAC	Premature atrial contraction
PaCO$_2$	Arterial carbon dioxide tension
PaO$_2$	Arterial oxygen tension
PAOP	Pulmonary artery occlusion pressure
PAT	Paroxysmal atrial tachycardia
PBI	Protein-bound iodine
PBSCT	Peripheral blood stem cell transplantation
PC	After meals (*post cibum*)
PCA	Patient-controlled analgesia
PCI	Percutaneous coronary intervention
PCKD	Polycystic kidney disease
PCN	Penicillin
PCOS	Polycystic ovarian syndrome
PCP	*Pneumocystis carinii* pneumonia; phencyclidine
PCWP	Pulmonary capillary wedge pressure
PDA	Patent ductus arteriosus
PDE	Phosphodiesterase
PE	Physical examination; pulmonary embolism
PEEP	Positive end-expiratory pressure
PEFR	Peak expiratory flow rate
PEG	Percutaneous endoscopic gastrostomy; polyethylene glycol
PERLA	Pupils equal, react to light and accommodation
PERRLA	Pupils equal, round, and reactive to light and accommodation
PET	Positron emission tomography
PFT	Pulmonary function test
pH	Hydrogen ion concentration
PharmD	Doctor of Pharmacy
PI	Principal investigator; protease inhibitor

PID	Pelvic inflammatory disease	RCA	Right coronary artery
PIP	Proximal interphalangeal	RCM	Right costal margin
PKU	Phenylketonuria	RDA	Recommended daily allowance
PMD	Private medical doctor	RDP	Random donor platelets
PMH	Past medical history	RDS	Respiratory distress syndrome
PMI	Point of maximal impulse	RDW	Red cell distribution width
PMN	Polymorphonuclear leukocyte	REM	Rapid eye movement
PMS	Premenstrual syndrome	RES	Reticuloendothelial system
PNC-E	Postnecrotic cirrhosis-ethanol	RF	Rheumatoid factor; renal failure; rheumatic fever
PND	Paroxysmal nocturnal dyspnea	Rh	Rhesus factor in blood
PNH	Paroxysmal nocturnal hemoglobinuria	RHD	Rheumatic heart disease
po	By mouth (*per os*)	RLE	Right lower extremity
pO_2	Partial pressure of oxygen	RLL	Right lower lobe
POAG	Primary open-angle glaucoma	RLQ	Right lower quadrant (abdomen)
POD	Postoperative day	RML	Right middle lobe
POS	Polycystic ovarian syndrome	RN	Registered nurse
PP	Patient profile	RNA	Ribonucleic acid
PPBG	Postprandial blood glucose	R/O	Rule out
ppd	Packs per day	ROM	Range of motion
PPD	Purified protein derivative	ROS	Review of systems
PPH	Past psychiatric history	RPGN	Rapidly progressive glomerulonephritis
PPI	Proton pump inhibitor	RPh	Registered Pharmacist
PPN	Peripheral parenteral nutrition	RPR	Rapid plasma reagin
pr	Per rectum	RR	Respiratory rate; recovery room
PR	Progesterone receptor; partial remission	RRR	Regular rate and rhythm
PRA	Panel-reactive antibody; plasma renin activity	RRT	Registered Respiratory Therapist
PRBC	Packed red blood cells	RSV	Respiratory syncytial virus
PRN	When necessary; as needed (*pro re nata*)	RT	Radiation therapy
PSA	Prostate-specific antigen	RTA	Renal tubular acidosis
PSCT	Peripheral stem cell transplant	RTC	Return to clinic
PSE	Portal systemic encephalopathy	RT-PCR	Reverse transcriptase-polymerase chain reaction
PSH	Past surgical history	RUE	Right upper extremity
PSVT	Paroxysmal supraventricular tachycardia	RUL	Right upper lobe
PT	Prothrombin time; physical therapy; patient	RUQ	Right upper quadrant (abdomen)
PTA	Prior to admission	RVH	Right ventricular hypertrophy
PTCA	Percutaneous transluminal coronary angioplasty	S_1	First heart sound
PTE	Pulmonary thromboembolism	S_2	Second heart sound
PTH	Parathyroid hormone	S_3	Third heart sound (ventricular gallop)
PTSD	Posttraumatic stress disorder	S_4	Fourth heart sound (atrial gallop)
PTT	Partial thromboplastin time	SA	Sinoatrial
PTU	Propylthiouracil	SAD	Seasonal affective disorder
PUD	Peptic ulcer disease	SAH	Subarachnoid hemorrhage
PVC	Premature ventricular contraction	SaO_2	Arterial oxygen percent saturation
PVD	Peripheral vascular disease	SBE	Subacute bacterial endocarditis
Q	Every (*quaque*)	SBFT	Small bowel follow-through
QA	Quality assurance	SBGM	Self blood glucose monitoring
QD	Every day (*quaque die*)	SBO	Small bowel obstruction
QI	Quality improvement	SBP	Systolic blood pressure; spontaneous bacterial peritonitis
QID	Four times daily (*quater in die*)	SC	Subcutaneous; subclavian
QNS	Quantity not sufficient	SCID	Severe combined immunodeficiency
QOD	Every other day	SCLC	Small cell lung cancer
QOL	Quality of life	SCr	Serum creatinine
QS	Quantity sufficient	SDP	Single donor platelets
R & M	Routine and microscopic	SEM	Systolic ejection murmur
RA	Rheumatoid arthritis; right atrium	SG	Specific gravity
RAIU	Radioactive iodine uptake	SGOT	Serum glutamic oxaloacetic transaminase
RAO	Right anterior oblique	SCT	Stem cell transplantation
RBBB	Right bundle branch block	SGPT	Serum glutamic pyruvic transaminase
RBC	Red blood cell	SH	Social history

SIADH	Syndrome of inappropriate antidiuretic hormone secretion
SIDS	Sudden infant death syndrome
SIMV	Synchronized intermittent mandatory ventilation
SJS	Stevens-Johnson syndrome
SL	Sublingual
SLE	Systemic lupus erythematosus
SMBG	Self-monitoring of blood glucose
SNF	Skilled nursing facility
SNRI	Serotonin-norepinephrine reuptake inhibitor
SNS	Sympathetic nervous system
SOS	Sinusoidal obstruction syndrome
SOB	Shortness of breath; side of bed
S/P	Status post
SPEP	Serum protein electrophoresis
SPF	Sun protection factor
SRI	Serotonin reuptake inhibitor
SSKI	Saturated solution of potassium iodide
SSRI	Selective serotonin reuptake inhibitor
STAT	Immediately; at once
STD	Sexually transmitted disease
SV	Stroke volume
SVC	Superior vena cava
SVR	Supraventricular rhythm; systemic vascular resistance
SVRI	Systemic vascular resistance index
SVT	Supraventricular tachycardia
SW	Social worker
SWI	Surgical wound infection
Sx	Symptoms
T	Temperature
T & A	Tonsillectomy and adenoidectomy
T & C	Type and crossmatch
TAH	Total abdominal hysterectomy
TB	Tuberculosis
TBG	Thyroid-binding globulin
TBI	Total body irradiation; traumatic brain injury
T. bili	Total bilirubin
T/C	To consider
TCA	Tricyclic antidepressant
TCN	Tetracycline
TED	Thromboembolic disease
TEN	Toxic epidermal necrolysis
TENS	Transcutaneous electrical nerve stimulation
TFT	Thyroid function test
TG	Triglyceride
THA	Total hip arthroplasty
THC	Tetrahydrocannabinol
TIA	Transient ischemic attack
TIBC	Total iron-binding capacity
TID	Three times daily (*ter in die*)
TIH	Tumor-induced hypercalcemia
TIPS	Transjugular intrahepatic portosystemic shunt
TLC	Therapeutic lifestyle changes
TLI	Total lymphoid irradiation
TLS	Tumor lysis syndrome

TM	Tympanic membrane
TMJ	Temporomandibular joint
TMP/SMX	Trimethoprim-sulfamethoxazole
TnI	Troponin I (cardiac)
TnT	Troponin T
TNTC	Too numerous to count
TOD	Target organ damage
TPN	Total parenteral nutrition
TPR	Temperature, pulse, respiration
T. prot	Total protein
TSH	Thyroid-stimulating hormone
TSS	Toxic shock syndrome
TTP	Thrombotic thrombocytopenic purpura
TUIP	Transurethral incision of the prostate
TURP	Transurethral resection of the prostate
Tx	Treat; treatment
UA	Urinalysis; uric acid
UC	Ulcerative colitis
UCD	Usual childhood diseases
UE	Upper extremity
UFC	Urinary free cortisol
UGI	Upper gastrointestinal
UOQ	Upper outer quadrant
UPT	Urine Pregnancy Test
URI	Upper respiratory infection
USP	United States Pharmacopeia
UTI	Urinary tract infection
UV	Ultraviolet
VA	Veterans' Affairs
VAMC	Veterans' Affairs Medical Center
VDRL	Venereal Disease Research Laboratory
VF	Ventricular fibrillation
VLDL	Very low-density lipoprotein
VNA	Visiting Nurses' Association
VO	Verbal order
VOD	Veno-occlusive disease
VP-16	Etoposide
V_A/Q	Ventilation/perfusion
VRE	Vancomycin-resistant *Enterococcus*
VS	Vital signs
VSS	Vital signs stable
VT	Ventricular tachycardia
VTE	Venous thromboembolism
WA	While awake
WBC	White blood cell
W/C	Wheelchair
WDWN	Well-developed, well-nourished
WHO	World Health Organization
WNL	Within normal limits
W/U	Work-up
Y-BOCS	Yale-Brown Obsessive-Compulsive Scale
yo	Year-old
yr	Year
ZDV	Zidovudine

PART II: Prevent Medication Errors by Avoiding These Dangerous Abbreviations or Dose Designations

Abbreviation or Dose Expression	Intended Meaning	Misinterpretation	Correction
Apothecary symbols	dram, minim	Misunderstood or misread (symbol for dram misread for "3" and minim misread "mL").	Use the metric system.
AU	aurio uterque (each ear)	Mistaken for OU (oculo uterque—each eye).	Don't use this abbreviation.
D/C	discharge, discontinue	Premature discontinuation of medications when D/C (intended to mean "discharge") has been misinterpreted as "discontinued" when followed by a list of drugs.	Use "discharge" and "discontinue."
Drug names			
ARA-A	vidarabine	cytarabine (ARA-C)	Use the complete spelling
AZT	zidovudine (RETROVIR)	azathioprine	for drug names.
CPZ	COMPAZINE (prochlorperazine)	chlorpromazine	
DPT	DEMEROL-PHENERGAN-THORAZINE	diphtheria-pertussis-tetanus (vaccine)	
HCl	hydrochloric acid	potassium chloride (the "H" is misinterpreted as "K")	
HCT	hydrocortisone	hydrochlorothiazide	
HCTZ	hydrochlorothiazide	hydrocortisone (seen as HCT250 mg)	
$MgSO_4$	magnesium sulfate	morphine sulfate	
MSO_4	morphine sulfate	magnesium sulfate	
MTX	methotrexate	mitoxantrone	
TAC	triamcinolone	tetracaine, ADRENALIN, cocaine	
$ZnSO_4$	zinc sulfate	morphine sulfate	
Stemmed names			
"Nitro" drip	nitroglycerin infusion	sodium nitroprusside infusion	
"Norflox"	norfloxacin	NORFLEX (orphenadrine)	
µg	microgram	Mistaken for "mg" when *handwritten*.	Use mcg.
o.d. or OD	once daily	Misinterpreted as "right eye" (OD–oculus dexter) and administration of oral medications in the eye.	Use "daily."
TIW or tiw	three times a week	Mistaken as "three times a day."	Don't use this abbreviation.
per os	orally	The "os" can be mistaken for "left eye."	Use "PO," "by mouth," or "orally."
q.d. or QD	every day	Mistaken as q.i.d., especially if the period after the "q" or the tail of the "q" is misunderstood as an "i."	Use "daily" or "every day."
qn	nightly or at bedtime	Misinterpreted as "qh" (every hour).	Use "nightly."
qhs	nightly at bedtime	Misread as every hour.	Use "nightly."
q6PM, etc.	every evening at 6 PM	Misread as every 6 hours.	Use 6 PM "nightly."
q.o.d. or QOD	every other day	Misinterpreted as "q.d." (daily) or "q.i.d." (four times daily) if the "o" is poorly written.	Use "every other day."
sub q	subcutaneous	The "q" has been mistaken for "every" (e.g., one heparin dose ordered "sub q 2 hours before surgery" misunderstood as every 2 hours before surgery).	Use "subcut." or write "subcutaneous."
SC	subcutaneous	Mistaken for SL (sublingual).	Use "subcut." or write "subcutaneous."
U or u	unit	Read as a zero (0) or a four (4), causing a 10-fold overdose or greater (4U seen as "40" or 4u seen as 44").	"Unit" has no acceptable abbreviation. Use "unit."
IU	international unit	Misread as IV (intravenous).	Use "units."
cc	cubic centimeters	Misread as "U" (units).	Use "mL."
x3d	for 3 days	Mistaken for "three doses."	Use "for 3 days."
BT	bedtime	Mistaken as "BID" (twice daily).	Use "hs."
ss	sliding scale (insulin) or 1/2 (apothecary)	Mistaken for "55."	
> and <	greater than and less than	Mistakenly used opposite of intended.	Use "greater than" or "less than."
/ (slash mark)	separates two doses or indicates "per"	Misunderstood as the number 1 ("25 unit/10 units" read as "110" units.	Do not use a slash mark to separate doses. Use "per."
Name letters and dose numbers run together (e.g., Inderal40 mg)	Inderal 40 mg	Misread as Inderal 140 mg.	Always use space between drug name, dose, and unit of measure.
Zero after decimal point (1.0)	1 mg	Misread as 10 mg if the decimal point is not seen.	Do not use terminal zeros for doses expressed in whole numbers.
No zero before decimal dose (.5 mg)	0.5 mg	Misread as 5 mg.	Always use zero before a decimal when the dose is less than a whole unit.

Reprinted with permission from the Institute of Safe Medication Practices (*www.ismp.org*). Originally printed in: Cohen MR. Medication Errors. Washington, DC, The American Pharmaceutical Association, 1999. To report real or potential medication errors, contact the ISMP by telephone (215-947-7797), fax (215-914-1492), or e-mail (*ismpinfo@ismp.org*).

37

PEDIATRIC GASTROENTERITIS

One Thing You *Can* Try at Home . . . . Level II

William McGhee, PharmD

Christina M. Lehane, MD, FAAP

CASE SUMMARY

A 3-day history of vomiting, diarrhea, and other symptoms causes a young mother to seek medical attention at the emergency department for her 9-month-old daughter. The patient has signs of moderate dehydration on physical and laboratory examination. The presumed diagnosis is viral gastroenteritis probably caused by rotavirus. Students should understand that replacement of fluid and electrolyte losses is critical to the effective treatment of acute diarrhea. Oral rehydration therapy (ORT) with carbohydrate-based solutions is the primary treatment for diarrhea in children with mild to moderate dehydration. When caregivers are properly instructed, therapy can begin at home. IV fluids may be needed for cases of severe dehydration. Early feeding of patients with an age-appropriate diet helps to reduce stool volume after completion of rehydration therapy. Although antidiarrheal and antiemetic products are available, they have limited effectiveness, can cause adverse effects, and most important, may divert attention from appropriate fluid and electrolyte replacement. Families should have a commercially available oral rehydration solution (ORS) at home to start treatment as soon as diarrhea begins. The availability of a new rotavirus vaccine is expected to dramatically reduce the morbidity and mortality of rotavirus-induced diarrhea worldwide.

QUESTIONS

Problem Identification

1.a. Create a list of the patient's drug therapy problems.

- This patient has typical viral gastroenteritis and diarrhea, a common pediatric problem in the United States, where it is estimated that 16.5 million children younger than 5 years of age experience 21–37 million episodes of diarrhea annually. Peak incidence is in the 6- to 24-month age group. Every year, it accounts for approximately 220,000 hospital admissions, 1.5 million outpatient visits, and 300 deaths in children younger than age 5 in the United States.[1] Viral gastroenteritis is usually caused by rotavirus infection, which is characterized by the acute onset of emesis, progressing to watery diarrhea with diminishing emesis. Rotavirus is the most common cause of pediatric gastroenteritis in the United States, accounting for

25% of cases, with the majority of cases occurring in otherwise healthy children. Other common viruses include Norwalk-like viruses and adenovirus.[2] Rotavirus is transmitted by the fecal-oral route, and spread of the virus is common in hospitals and similar settings such as daycare. Infection occurs when ingested virus infects enterocytes in the small intestine, leading to cell damage or death and loss of brush border digestive enzymes. Approximately 48 hours after exposure, infected children develop fever, vomiting, and watery diarrhea. Fever and vomiting usually subside in 1–2 days, but diarrhea can continue for several days, leading to significant dehydration. Dehydration, along with the corresponding electrolyte losses, is the primary causes of morbidity in gastroenteritis. Children with poor nutrition also are at risk for complications.[1] Approximately 65% of hospitalizations and 85% of diarrhea-related deaths occur in the first year of life.

- The patient has moderate dehydration (acute weight loss of 9%, from 9.0 kg [19.8 lb] to 8.2 kg [18.0 lb]) as well as clinical and laboratory evidence of dehydration with metabolic acidosis.

1.b. What information (signs, symptoms, laboratory values) indicates the presence or severity of gastroenteritis?

- The most accurate indicator of the degree of dehydration is actual weight loss. Fortunately for the patient, she had a physician's office visit 5 days earlier, during which she was weighed and an actual weight loss of 0.8 kg (1.8 lb, or 9%) was documented.

- By history, the patient had a 3-day history of fever, vomiting, and diarrhea of acute onset; she had a reported decrease in the number of wet diapers; and her lips and tongue appeared to be dry.

- She has a social history of daycare attendance, where several of her daycare mates had similar illnesses recently. Attendance at daycare is part of a typical history in pediatric gastroenteritis. Children can be infected but asymptomatic and transmit the infection unknowingly. In addition, on the day she presented to the emergency room (ER), her mother developed abdominal discomfort and loose stools.

- On physical examination, she was sleepy but arousable, and her mental status was normal. Her skin turgor had mild "tenting," and the capillary refill was increased, at 2–3 seconds. Her tongue and lips were dry, and there were scant tears. Her eyes were moderately sunken and the anterior fontanelle was sunken. She was tachypneic and tachycardic.

- Her labs indicated metabolic acidosis (total carbon dioxide [CO_2] 14 mEq/L and Cl 113 mEq/L), and her urinalysis showed a specific gravity of 1.029 (indicating moderate dehydration). Ketones were 2+ in the urine, indicating fat breakdown in a hypocaloric diet. Her serum sodium was 137 mEq/L, indicating isotonic dehydration (defined as serum sodium between 130 and 150 mEq/L), and her BUN was slightly high, at 23 mg/dL.

TABLE 37-1	Clinical Assessment Guidelines for Dehydration In Children of All Ages		
Parameter	**Mild**	**Moderate**	**Severe**
Weight loss	3–5%	6–9%	≥10%
Body fluid loss	30–50 mL/kg	50–100 mL/kg	>100 mL/kg
Stage of shock	Impending	Compensated	Uncompensated
Heart rate	Normal	Increased	Increased
Blood pressure	Normal	Normal	Normal to reduced
Respiratory rate	Normal	Normal	Increased
Skin turgor	Normal	Decreased	"Tenting"
Anterior fontanelle	Normal	Sunken	Sunken
Capillary refill	<2 sec	2–3 sec	>3 sec
Mucous membranes	Slightly dry	Dry	Dry
Tearing	Normal/absent	Absent	Absent
Eye appearance	Normal	Sunken orbits	Deeply sunken orbits
Mental status	Normal	Normal to listless	Normal to lethargic to comatose
Urine volume	Slightly decreased	<1 mL/kg/h	<1 mL/kg/h
Urine specific gravity	1.020	1.025	>1.035
BUN	Upper normal	Elevated	High
Blood pH	7.40–7.22	7.30–6.92	7.10–6.8
Thirst	Slightly increased	Moderately increased	Very thirsty or too lethargic to indicate

- Table 37-1 is a dehydration assessment tool to help categorize the degree of dehydration. Dehydration is categorized clinically into mild, moderate, and severe, but rarely does a child fall entirely into one category or another. When a child does not fit into one category, the category with the most signs should be used. In assessing the degree of dehydration, changes in mental status, skin turgor, mucous membranes, and eyes are important assessment tools because they correlate with the degree of dehydration better than other signs and symptoms.

Desired Outcome

2. What are the goals of pharmacotherapy in this case?

- The goals of appropriate pharmacotherapy of dehydration include reversing dehydration, restoring normal urine output, and maintaining adequate nutrition.

- Replacement of fluid and electrolyte losses is the critical element of effective treatment. This is necessary to prevent excessive water, electrolyte, and acid–base disturbances.

- Reinstitution of an age-appropriate diet is essential to ensure adequate nutrition and to reduce stool volume. Further morbidity and unnecessary hospitalization may be prevented.

- Other secondary goals may include providing symptomatic relief and treating any curable causes of diarrhea.

Therapeutic Alternatives

3.a. What nondrug therapies might be useful for this patient?

- *ORT* with carbohydrate-based solutions is the mainstay of treatment of fluid and electrolyte losses caused by diarrhea in children with mild to moderate dehydration. ORT can be used regardless of the patient's age, causative pathogen, or initial serum sodium concentration. The basis for the effectiveness of ORT is the phenomenon of glucose-sodium co-transport, where sodium ions given orally are absorbed along with

glucose (and other organic molecules) from the lumen of the intestine into the bloodstream.[2] Once these molecules are absorbed, free water naturally follows. Any of the commercially available ORSs can be used successfully to rehydrate otherwise healthy children with mild to moderate dehydration. These products are formulated on physiologic principles and should be close to isotonic to avoid unnecessary shifts in fluid. They are to be distinguished from other nonphysiologic clear liquids that are commonly but inappropriately used to treat dehydration. Clear liquids to be avoided include colas, ginger ale, apple juice, chicken broth, and sports beverages.[3] This patient was inappropriately treated because in addition to an ORS (Pedialyte), she received a variety of clear liquids including water, cola, and diluted apple juice. These liquids have unacceptably low electrolyte concentrations, and cola beverages are hypertonic because of the high glucose concentrations, with osmolalities greater than 700 mOsm.[3]

- *Early feeding of age-appropriate foods.* Although carbohydrate-based ORT is highly effective in replacing fluid and electrolyte losses, it has no effect on stool volume or duration of diarrhea, which can be discouraging to parents. To overcome this limitation, cereal-based ORT (e.g., rice flour-based ORT) has been used investigationally and can reduce stool volume by 20–30%. However, no commercial products are available in the United States. Another ORT product based on rice-syrup solids (Infalyte) is equivalent in efficacy to carbohydrate-based ORT. Nonetheless, early feeding of patients as soon as oral rehydration is completed may provide similar reductions in stool volume.[4] Therefore, children with diarrhea requiring rehydration should be fed with age-appropriate diets immediately after completing ORT. Optimal ORT incorporates early feeding of age-appropriate foods. Unrestricted diets generally do not worsen the symptoms of mild or moderate diarrhea and decrease the stool output compared with ORT alone. For breast-fed infants, there is no need to stop breastfeeding. Supplementation with ORT between regular feedings should be considered to ensure adequate intake. In addition, most children being fed milk-based formulas tolerate them well. Children who do not tolerate them, however, can be changed to a soy-based formula for the duration of diarrhea. Older children can resume a normal diet for their age once ORT is complete.

- ORT is well established as the appropriate therapy for preventing and treating diarrhea with mild to moderate dehydration associated with pediatric gastroenteritis. The principles of ORT include early rehydration with an appropriate ORS, replacement of ongoing fluid losses from diarrhea and vomiting with an ORS, and reintroduction of age-appropriate diets as soon as rehydration is complete. As simple as this sounds, the majority of health care providers, contrary to the guidelines of the American Academy of Pediatrics (AAP) and the recommendations of the Centers for Disease Control and Prevention (CDC), overuse IV hydration, prolong rehydration, delay reintroduction of age-appropriate diets, and withhold ORT inappropriately, especially in children who are vomiting. Continuing education of health care workers and reemphasizing the value of oral rehydration versus IV rehydration is essential for the future success of ORT.

3.b. What feasible pharmacotherapeutic alternatives are available for treating this patient's diarrhea?

- Antidiarrheal compounds have been used to treat pediatric gastroenteritis. Their use is intended to shorten the course of diarrhea and to relieve discomfort by reducing stool output and electrolyte losses. However, despite a large number of antidiarrheal compounds available, none has found a place in the routine treatment of acute diarrhea associated with pediatric gastroenteritis. Their usefulness remains to be proved, and they generally should not be used. These agents have a variety of proposed mechanisms; their possible benefits and limitations are outlined below.

✓ *Antimotility agents (opioids and opioid/anticholinergic combination products)* delay GI transit and increase gut capacity and fluid retention. *Loperamide* with ORT significantly reduces the volume of stool losses, but this reduction is not clinically significant. Loperamide also may have an unacceptable rate of side effects (lethargy, respiratory depression, altered mental status, ileus, abdominal distention). *Anticholinergic agents* (e.g., atropine or mepenzolate bromide) may cause dry mouth that can alter the clinical evaluation of dehydration. Infants and children are especially susceptible to toxic effects of anticholinergics. Antimotility agents can worsen the course of diarrhea in shigellosis, antibiotic-associated pseudomembranous colitis, and *Escherichia coli* O157:H7–induced diarrhea. *Most important, reliance on antidiarrheal compounds may shift the focus of treatment away from appropriate ORT and the early feeding of the child.* They are not recommended by the AAP to treat acute diarrhea in children because of the modest clinical benefit, limited scientific evidence of efficacy, and concern for toxic effects.

✓ *Antisecretory agents (bismuth subsalicylate)* may have an adjunctive role for acute diarrhea. Bismuth subsalicylate decreases intestinal secretions secondary to cholera and *E. coli* toxins, decreases frequency of unformed stools, decreases total stool output, and reduces the need for ORT. However, the benefit is modest, and it requires dosing every 4 hours. Also, pediatric patients may absorb salicylate (but the effect on Reye's syndrome is unknown). This treatment is also not recommended by the AAP because of modest benefit and concern for toxicity.

✓ *Adsorbent drugs (polycarbophil)* may bind bacterial toxins and water, but their effectiveness remains unproved. There is no conclusive evidence of decreased duration of diarrhea, number of stools, or total stool output. Major toxicity is not a concern with these products, but they may adsorb nutrients, enzymes, and drugs. These products are not recommended by the AAP because of lack of efficacy.

✓ *Probiotics* are defined as beneficial species of bacteria that when ingested, colonize and replicate in the intestine, producing a beneficial effect in the host.[5] The rationale for using them in pediatric gastroenteritis is that they act against intestinal pathogens. Their exact mechanism is unknown, but they may act by producing antimicrobial substances, decreasing adhesion of pathogens to enterocytes, decreasing toxin production, and/or stimulating specific immune responses to pathogens.[6] Multiple meta-analyses indicate significant but modest benefit from the use of probiotics, shortening the duration of diarrhea by approximately 1 day.[7] This effect was especially seen in young children with rotavirus infections who were administered probiotics early in the course of the illness. (The most consistent effect was seen with use of *Lactobacillus* GG, a bacterial strain isolated in humans in the 1980s by Drs. Gorbach and Goldin, thus the name *Lactobacillus* GG.) Notwithstanding this evidence, probiotics are not generally recommended for the treatment of pediatric gastroenteritis. Although they generally are considered safe, there are reports of bacteremia and fungemia occurring in immunosuppressed patients. Because they are categorized as nutra-

ceuticals, the FDA has no authority to regulate or standardize the production or the purity of these products. There is great variability in product content, and some formulations have even contained no bacteria when tested. Because of these concerns, the use of probiotics is not recommended, although the availability of standardized products may make a future role possible.

✓ *Antiemetic drugs* have been used in dehydrated patients who are vomiting, but their use is discouraged. They are used with the intent of reducing the rate of dehydration and improving the efficiency of ORT. However, the possible benefits of antiemetics must be weighed against side effects that can interfere with the evaluation of the patient such as lethargy and drowsiness (e.g., *promethazine*) or dystonic reactions (*metoclopramide*).

✓ Several studies have examined the usefulness of *ondansetron* in ER settings. Although there is less emesis, an increase in the amount of diarrhea may be experienced during the first 24–48 hours after use. Currently, no study has addressed the primary question of whether ondansetron (or any antiemetic) reduces the vomiting associated with rotavirus infection, increasing the likelihood that ORT will be more successful. Thus, although ondansetron probably would decrease vomiting and might reduce the need for hospitalization, there is insufficient evidence to justify its routine use in children with mild to moderate dehydration secondary to acute gastroenteritis.[8] Perhaps ondansetron's use might be reserved for patients with intractable vomiting who cannot tolerate ORT, where avoidance of hospitalization might be possible.

✓ *Zinc supplementation* is recommended for treating acute diarrhea in children in developing countries. In those areas, zinc deficiency occurs in children not only because of increased stool losses with diarrhea, but also because of prior reduced intake of animal foods, excess dietary phytates that decrease zinc absorption, and poor food intake.[9] Oral zinc has ion absorption and antisecretory effects that result in reduced duration and severity of diarrhea as determined by stool output and frequency. Because of these benefits, in May 2004 both UNICEF and WHO jointly recommended that all children with diarrhea in developing countries be treated with zinc in addition to ORT. It has been estimated that if the UNICEF/WHO recommendations were implemented worldwide, zinc administration could save 400,000 lives annually.

Optimal Plan

4.a. What drug(s), dosage forms, schedule, and duration of therapy are best for this patient?

- Treatment of a child with dehydration is directed primarily by the degree of dehydration present.[2] This patient had diarrhea with moderate dehydration (6–9% loss of body weight). There are four potential treatment situations.[3]

  ✓ *Diarrhea without dehydration.* ORT may be given in doses of 10 mL/kg to replace ongoing stool losses. Some children may not take the ORT because of its salty taste. For these few patients, freezer pops are available in a variety of flavors. ORT may not be necessary if fluid consumption and age-appropriate feeding continues. Infants should continue to breast-feed or take regular-strength formula. Older children can usually drink full-strength milk.

  ✓ *Diarrhea with mild dehydration (3–5% weight loss).* Correct dehydration with ORT, 50 mL/kg over a 4-hour period.

Reassess the status of dehydration and volume of ORT at 2-hour intervals. Concomitantly replace continuing losses from stool or emesis at 10 mL/kg for each stool; estimate emesis loss and replace with fluid. Children with emesis can usually tolerate ORT, but it is necessary to administer ORT in small 5- to 10-mL aliquots (1–2 teaspoonfuls) every 1–2 minutes. Feeding should start immediately after rehydration is complete, using the feeding guidelines described previously.

✓ *Diarrhea with moderate dehydration (6–9% weight loss).* Although the patient presented to the emergency department, ORT is still the initial treatment of choice to reverse moderate dehydration, and it can usually be performed at home.[4] Compared with IV rehydration, oral rehydration can be initiated more quickly and is equally effective. To correct the dehydration, administer ORT, 100 mL/kg, plus replacement of ongoing losses (10 mL/kg for each stool, plus estimated losses from emesis as above) during the first 4 hours. Assess rehydration status hourly and adjust the amount of ORT accordingly. Close supervision is required, but this can be done at home. Rapid restoration of blood volume helps to correct acidosis and to increase tissue perfusion. Resume feeding of age-appropriate diet as soon as rehydration is completed.

✓ *Diarrhea with severe dehydration (≥10% weight loss).* Severe dehydration and uncompensated shock should be treated aggressively with IV isotonic fluids to restore intravascular volume. Poorly treated pediatric gastroenteritis, especially in infants, can cause life-threatening severe dehydration and should be considered a medical emergency. The patient may be in shock and should be referred to an emergency department. Administer 20 mL/kg aliquots of normal saline or Ringer's lactated solution over 15–30 minutes (even faster in uncompensated shock). Reassess the patient's status after each completed fluid bolus. Repeat boluses of up to 80 mL/kg total fluid may be used. Isotonic fluid replacement may be discontinued when blood pressure is restored, heart rate is normalized, peripheral pulses are strong, and skin perfusion is restored. Urine output is the best indicator of restored intravascular volume and should be at least 1 mL/kg/h. If the patient does not respond to rapid IV volume replacement, other underlying disorders should be considered, including septic shock, toxic shock syndrome, myocarditis, cardiomyopathy, pericarditis, and other underlying diseases. ORT may be instituted to complete rehydration when the patient's status is satisfactory. Estimate the degree of remaining dehydration and treat according to the above guidelines. IV access should be maintained until it is certain that IV therapy will not be reinstituted. After ORT is complete, resume age-appropriate feeding following the guidelines outlined previously.

4.b. What is the efficacy and safety record of the new rotavirus vaccine, and what impact is it expected to have on preventing rotavirus-induced diarrhea?

- Because rotavirus-induced disease kills approximately 500,000 children each year in developing countries and accounts for one-third of hospitalizations for diarrhea worldwide, preventing it is the most effective way to lower its impact throughout the world. A decade ago, efforts to reduce the tremendous worldwide health burden of gastroenteritis suffered a setback when the available licensed rotavirus vaccine (Rotashield) was removed from the market because of the rare side effect of intussusception. Since then, another rotavirus vaccine (Rotateq) has been approved in the United States after a safety trial in

more than 70,000 infants found no evidence of increased risk of intussusception.[10] Rotateq proved to be highly successful in preventing rotavirus-induced diarrhea caused by the common serotypes G1, G2, G3, and G4. Through the first rotavirus season after vaccination, it had 98% efficacy against severe rotavirus-induced diarrhea and 74% efficacy against any severity of diarrhea. The vaccine reduced hospitalizations and emergency department visits related to G1–G4 rotavirus-induced diarrhea by 94.5%, and clinic visits were reduced by 86%. In the United States, vaccination reduced the number of lost work days from rotavirus by 87%. Since then, the Advisory Committee on Immunization Practices (ACIP) and the CDC have recommended it for routine vaccination of U.S. infants.[11] It is an oral vaccine given in a three-dose series at 2, 4, and 6 months of age. On a worldwide basis, a future successful rotavirus immunization program would have a tremendous impact on reducing the number of rotavirus-related hospitalizations and deaths.

Outcome Evaluation

5. What clinical and laboratory parameters should be monitored to evaluate therapy for achievement of the desired therapeutic outcome?

- Vital signs should normalize with appropriate therapy, but they may be unreliable in patients with fever, agitation, pain, or respiratory illnesses. Tachycardia is usually the first sign of mild dehydration (see Table 37-1 of this instructor's guide). With increasing acidosis and fluid loss, the respiratory rate increases and breathing becomes deeper (hyperpnea). Hypotension is usually a sign of severe dehydration.

- Any existing central nervous system (CNS) alterations should be reversed. No CNS changes occur in mild dehydration; some patients may appear listless with moderate dehydration, and severely dehydrated patients appear quite ill with lethargy or irritability.

- Skin changes should be normalized. Mucous membranes should appear moist (previously dry in all degrees of dehydration). Capillary refill is normally <2 seconds and usually is not altered in mild dehydration. Capillary refill in moderately dehydrated patients is 2–3 seconds and >3 seconds in severe dehydration. Skin turgor (elasticity) should be normal. There is no change in mild dehydration; but it decreases in moderate dehydration, with "tenting" occurring in patients with severe dehydration. The anterior fontanelle should no longer be sunken, which is seen in moderate to severe dehydration.

- The eyes should appear normal. No change occurs in mild dehydration, but in moderate to severe dehydration, tearing will be absent and the eyes will appear sunken.

- Laboratory tests should be assessed appropriately. Most dehydration occurring with pediatric gastroenteritis is isotonic, and serum electrolyte determinations are unnecessary. However, some patients with moderate dehydration (those whose histories and physical examinations are inconsistent with routine gastroenteritis), those with prolonged inappropriate intake of hypotonic or hypertonic solutions, and all severely dehydrated patients should have serum electrolytes determined and corrected.

- Urine volume and specific gravity should be normalized. Progressive decreases in urine volume and increases in specific gravity are expected with increasing severity of dehydration. Urine output will be decreased to <1 mL/kg/h in both moderate and severe dehydration (see Table 37-1 of this Instructor's

Guide). Specific gravity is 1.020 in mild dehydration, 1.025 in moderate dehydration, and maximal in patients with severe dehydration. Adequate rehydration should normalize both urine output and specific gravity. During rehydration, lung sounds should be assessed periodically to determine if continued fluid administration is warranted. Lung sounds should remain clear. The development of crackles requires careful evaluation and the temporary stopping of further fluid administration until the evaluation is complete.

Patient Education

6. What information should be provided to the child's parents to enhance compliance, ensure successful therapy, and minimize adverse effects?

- Treatment of diarrhea due to gastroenteritis in your child should begin at home. It is a good idea for you to keep ORT at home at all times (especially in rural areas and poor urban neighborhoods where access to health care may be delayed), and to use it as instructed by your doctor. Sometimes doctors instruct new parents about this treatment at the first newborn visit. Be careful of information obtained from sources on the Internet. Much of the information available does not concur with the AAP guidelines for the use of ORT in pediatric gastroenteritis.
- However, infants with diarrhea should receive a medical evaluation for diarrhea. Additionally, any child with diarrhea and fever should be evaluated to rule out serious illness.[12]
- Early home management with ORT results in fewer complications such as severe dehydration and poor nutrition, as well as fewer office or ER visits.
- Any of the commercial ORSs can be used to effectively rehydrate your child. However, rehydration alone does not reduce the duration of diarrhea or the volume of stool output. Early feeding after rehydration is necessary and can reduce the duration of diarrhea by as much as one-half day.
- Effective oral rehydration always combines early feeding with an age-appropriate diet after rehydration. This corrects dehydration, improves nutritional status, and reduces the volume of stool output.
- Vomiting usually does not preclude the use of oral rehydration. Consistent administration of small amounts (1–2 teaspoonfuls) of an ORS every 1–2 minutes can provide as much as 10 ounces per hour of rehydration fluid. Parents must resist the child's desires for larger amounts of liquid. Otherwise, further vomiting may occur.
- If the child does not stop vomiting after the appropriate administration of oral rehydration (as above) and appears to be severely dehydrated, contact your doctor, who may refer you to the ER for IV rehydration therapy.
- Oral rehydration is insufficient therapy for bloody diarrhea (dysentery). Contact your doctor if this occurs.
- Additional treatments, including antidiarrheal compounds, antiemetics, probiotics, and antimicrobial therapy, are almost never necessary in the treatment of pediatric gastroenteritis. Most children can be successfully rehydrated with ORS without the use of antiemetic medication.
- Proper hand-washing technique, diaper-changing practices, and personal hygiene can help to prevent spread of the disease to other family members. The child should be kept out of daycare until the diarrhea stops.

REFERENCES

1. Elliot EJ. Acute gastroenteritis in children. BMJ 2007;334:35–40.
2. Duggan C, Santosham M, Glass RI. The management of acute diarrhea in children: oral rehydration, maintenance, and nutritional therapy. MMWR Morb Mortal Wkly Rep 1992;41(RR-16):1–20.
3. Snyder J. The continuing evolution of oral therapy for diarrhea. Semin Pediatr Infect Dis 1994;5:231–235.
4. Spandorfer PR, Alessandrini EA, Joffe MD, et al. Oral versus intravenous rehydration of moderately dehydrated children: a randomized, controlled trial. Pediatrics 2005;115:295–301.
5. Vanderhoof JA, Young RJ. Pediatric applications of probiotics. Gastroenterol Clin North Am 2005;34:451–463.
6. Szajewska H, Mrukowiz JZ. Probiotics in the treatment and prevention of acute infectious diarrhea in infants and children: a systematic review of published randomized, double-blind, placebo-controlled trials. J Pediatr Gastroenterol Nutr 2001;33:S17–S25.
7. Guandalini S. Probiotics for children: use in diarrhea. J Clin Gastroenterol 2006;40:244–248.
8. Borowitz SM. Are antiemetics helpful in young children suffering from acute viral gastroenteritis? Arch Dis Child 2005;90:646–648.
9. Bhatnagar S, Bahl R, Sharma PK, et al. Zinc with oral rehydration therapy reduces stool output and duration of diarrhea in hospitalized children: a randomized controlled trial. J Pediatr Gastroenterol Nutr 2004:38:34–40.
10. Vesikari T, Matson DO, Dennedy P, et al. Safety and efficacy of a pentavalent human-bovine (WC3) reassortant rotavirus vaccine. N Engl J Med 2006;354:23–33.
11. Anonymous. Postmarketing monitoring of intussusception after Rotateq™ vaccination—United States, February 1, 2006–February 15, 2007. MMWR Morb Mortal Wkly Rep 2007;56:218–222.
12. Centers for Disease Control and Prevention. Managing acute gastroenteritis among children: oral rehydration, maintenance, and nutritional therapy. MMWR Morb Mortal Wkly Rep 2003;52:(RR-16):1–16.

118

DIABETIC FOOT INFECTION

Watch Your Step. . . . . .Level II

A. Christie Graham, PharmD

Renee-Claude Mercier, PharmD, BCPS, PhC

CASE SUMMARY

Accidentally stepping on a piece of metal results in erythema and swelling of the right foot in a 67-year-old Native-American woman with poorly controlled Type 2 diabetes mellitus and several comorbid conditions. Laboratory evaluation reveals leukocytosis with a left shift. The patient undergoes incision and drainage of the lesion with removal of a 2-cm metallic foreign body from the foot. Empiric antimicrobial treatment must be initiated before results of wound culture and sensitivity testing are known. Because of this patient's comorbidities and the size and severity of the wound, parenteral antibiotic therapy should be initiated. Because this is an acutely infected wound, aerobic Gram-positive bacteria (especially *S. aureus*) are the most likely causative organisms. However, broad-spectrum coverage for Gram-negative and anaerobic bacteria should also be instituted due to the location of the wound (bottom of foot), its size and severity, and the patient's diabetes. This patient does have risk factors for hospital-acquired MRSA (HA-MRSA) infection (i.e., recent hospitalization, existing chronic illnesses), and empiric coverage of this organism should be considered. When tissue cultures are reported as positive for *S. aureus* (MRSA), the reader is asked to narrow to more specific therapy, which includes parenteral vancomycin or either oral or parenteral linezolid. Second-line agents include dalfopristin/quinupristin or daptomycin. This infection will require a duration of therapy of 2–4 weeks, so the patient will most likely be discharged on outpatient antibiotic therapy. Although parenteral therapy using any of a variety of agents, or oral linezolid, may be completed as an outpatient, attention must be given to the patient's social and economic situation. Better glycemic control and education on techniques for proper foot care are important components of a comprehensive treatment plan for this patient.

QUESTIONS

Problem Identification

1.a. Create a list of the patient's drug therapy problems.

- Cellulitis and infection of the right foot in a patient with diabetes, requiring treatment.

- Poorly controlled Type 2 diabetes mellitus, as evidenced by an A1C of 11.8% (goal <7%) and recent episode of hyperglycemic hyperosmolar state. Metformin is contraindicated in this patient due to her SCr 1.7 mg/dL. However, her renal function may improve with hydration, and this should be monitored.

- Nonadherence with medication administration and home glucose monitoring.

- Renal insufficiency secondary to diabetic nephropathy, appropriately treated with lisinopril.

- Coronary artery disease, post-MI w/percutaneous coronary intervention and stenting; treatment with a β-blocker should be considered.

- Hyperlipidemia, appropriately treated with simvastatin.

- History of depression, which may be inadequately treated (the patient is described as having a "dull affect").

- Fungal infection of toenails, requiring treatment.

- Language barrier requiring additional resources (i.e., translator) to optimize patient education.

1.b. What signs, symptoms, or laboratory values indicate the presence of an infection?

- Swollen, sore, and red foot.

- 2+ edema of the foot increasing in amplitude.

- White blood cell count (WBC) elevated ($16.4 \times 10^3/\text{mm}^3$) with increased polymorphonuclear neutrophil leukocytes and bands.

- X-ray showing the presence of a foreign body in the right foot.

1.c. What risk factors for infection does the patient have?

- Patient stepped on a foreign object.

- She is a patient with poorly controlled diabetes.

- Vascular calcifications in the foot per x-ray indicate a decreased blood supply.

- She has decreased sensation of bilateral lower extremities.

- Poor foot care (presence of fungus and overgrown toenails).

1.d. What organisms are most likely involved in this infection?

- Aerobic isolates: *S. aureus, Streptococcus* spp., *Enterococcus* spp., *Proteus mirabilis, Escherichia coli, Klebsiella* spp., *Pseudomonas aeruginosa*.

- Anaerobic isolates: *Peptostreptococcus, Bacteroides fragilis.*[1]

Desired Outcome

2. What are the therapeutic goals for this patient?

- Eradicate the bacteria.

- Prevent the development of osteomyelitis and the need for amputation.

- Preserve as much normal limb function as possible.

- Improve control of diabetes mellitus.

- Prevent infectious complications.

Therapeutic Alternatives

3.a. What nondrug therapies might be useful for this patient?

- Deep culture of the wound for both anaerobes and aerobes.

- Appropriate wound care by experienced podiatrists (incision and drainage, debridement of the wound, toenail clipping), nurses (wound care, dressing changes of wound, foot care teaching), and physical therapists (whirlpool treatments, wound debridement, teaching about minimal weight-bearing with a walker or crutches).

- Bedrest, minimal weight-bearing, leg elevation, and control of edema.

- Proper education about wound care and the importance of good diabetes control, glucometer use, adherence with the medication regimens, and foot care in the patient with diabetes.

3.b. What feasible pharmacotherapeutic alternatives are available for the empiric treatment of diabetic foot infection?

- Diabetic foot infections are classified into two categories:

   ✓ *Non–limb-threatening infections.* Superficial, no systemic toxicity, cellulitis extending less than 2 cm from portal of entry, ulceration not extending fully through skin, no significant ischemia.

   ✓ *Limb-threatening infections.* More extensive cellulitis, lymphangitis, and ulcers penetrating through skin into subcutaneous tissues, prominent ischemia.

- Oral antimicrobial therapy may be used in mild, uncomplicated diabetic foot infections *only*.[2] Suggested regimens include:

   ✓ *Amoxicillin/clavulanate monotherapy;* or

   ✓ Either *ciprofloxacin* or *levofloxacin in combination with clindamycin.*

   Although these regimens cover the most likely causative organisms, it is important to note that amoxicillin/clavulanate does not cover *P. aeruginosa*.

- Treatment of limb-threatening infections must include IV antibiotic therapy.[1] IV monotherapy may be used with:

   ✓ *Piperacillin/tazobactam;*

   ✓ *Ticarcillin/clavulanate;*

   ✓ *Imipenem/cilastatin;* or

   ✓ *Meropenem.*

- These agents cover all of the most likely causative organisms, including anaerobes and *P. aeruginosa*. However, imipenem/cilastatin is a potent β-lactamase inducer, so therapy with the other agents may be preferable.

   The following agents could also be used as IV therapy, but they do not cover *P. aeruginosa*:

   ✓ *Ampicillin/sulbactam;*

   ✓ *Ertapenem;*

✓ *Cefoxitin* or *cefotetan;*

✓ Third-generation cephalosporin *(ceftriaxone/cefotaxime) plus IV clindamycin combination.*

- *Clindamycin IV plus either aztreonam or an oral or IV fluoroquinolone* could be used in patients with limb-threatening infections who are allergic to penicillin.

- MRSA may be a suspected causative organism in some cases. There are two genetically distinct types of MRSA that can be of concern in diabetic foot infections: community-acquired MRSA (CA-MRSA) and HA-MRSA. While acquisition of HA-MRSA is associated with well-defined risk factors (history of prolonged hospital or nursing home stay, past antimicrobial use, indwelling catheters, pressure sores, surgery, or dialysis), risk factors for acquisition of CA-MRSA are not as well established. CA-MRSA is susceptible to more antibiotics than HA-MRSA.[3]

- *Vancomycin IV or linezolid oral or IV* may be used if HA-MRSA is a suspected causative organism. Persons who are at high risk for HA-MRSA wound infection include those who: a) have a previous history of HA-MRSA infection/colonization, b) have positive nasal cultures for HA-MRSA, c) have a recent history (within the last year) of prolonged hospitalization or intensive care unit stay, or d) receive frequent and/or prolonged courses of broad-spectrum antibiotics.[4–6] Should vancomycin or linezolid be used empirically, Gram-negative and anaerobic coverage will need to be added to provide adequate empiric coverage.

- Should CA-MRSA be more of a concern (for example, in a patient with no HA-MRSA risk factors who is admitted from an area where the CA-MRSA rate is relatively high), then the antibiotic regimen should include any of those agents active against HA-MRSA or *clindamycin, sulfamethoxazole/trimethoprim,* or *doxycycline* or *minocycline.*[3]

- Aminoglycosides should be avoided in diabetic patients as they are at increased risk for the development of diabetic nephropathy and renal failure.

- *Becaplermin 0.01% gel (Regranex)* is approved by the FDA for the treatment of diabetic ulcers on the lower limbs and feet. Becaplermin is a genetically engineered form of platelet-derived growth factor, a naturally occurring protein in the body that stimulates diabetic ulcer healing. It is to be used as adjunctive therapy, *in addition to* infection control and wound care. In one clinical trial, becaplermin applied once daily in combination with good wound care significantly increased the incidence of complete healing when compared to placebo gel (50% versus 35%, respectively). Becaplermin gel also significantly decreased the time to complete healing of diabetic ulcers by 32% (about 6 weeks faster). The incidence of adverse events, including infection and cellulitis, was similar in patients treated with becaplermin gel, placebo gel, or good diabetic wound care alone.[7] Further studies are needed to assess which patients might best benefit from becaplermin use, particularly considering its cost (average wholesale price $665 per 15 GM tube at the time of this writing).

3.c. **What economic and social considerations are applicable to this patient?**

- A simplified drug regimen (monotherapy and less-frequent dosing, whenever possible) should be selected because of her history of poor medication adherence.

- The patient receives her health care primarily at Shiprock Indian Health Services. This may become an important consideration in selecting her future therapeutic plan.

- For this patient to receive appropriate wound care and home IV therapy if judged necessary, the health care team must establish that her daughter or a home health care nurse will be able to provide assistance.

Optimal Plan

4. **Outline a drug regimen that would provide optimal initial empiric therapy for the infection.**

- This diabetic foot infection has significant involvement of the skin and skin structures with deep tissue involvement. Moreover, the area of cellulitis and induration exceeds 2 cm (4 × 5 cm). Because this is an acutely infected wound, aerobic Gram-positive bacteria (especially *S. aureus*) are the most likely causative organisms.[1] However, broad-spectrum coverage for Gram-negative and anaerobic bacteria should also be instituted due to the location of the wound (bottom of foot), its size and severity, and the patient's diabetes. This patient does have risk factors for HA-MRSA infection (i.e., recent hospitalizations, existing chronic illnesses), and empiric coverage of this organism should be considered as well. Initial empiric IV therapy is appropriate in serious, limb-threatening diabetic foot infections such as this one.

- A number of treatment options are appropriate for empiric therapy of diabetic foot infection in this patient. The antimicrobial therapy selection may be based on institutional cost and drug availability through the formulary system. It should also be adjusted for the patient's renal function. This patient's calculated creatinine clearance, based on adjusted body weight [ideal body weight + 0.4(actual − ideal body weight)] is 34 mL/min.

- The only parenteral monotherapy agent available to adequately cover all of these potential causative organisms is tigecycline 100 mg IV loading dose, followed by 50 mg IV Q 12 h. Of note is that tigecycline is not yet approved for diabetic foot infection, and does not cover *P. aeruginosa*. However, since this infection is moderate in severity and the patient does not have risk factors for pseudomonal infection (i.e., previous history of pseudomonal infection, corticosteroid use, frequent broad-spectrum antibiotic use, or nursing home residence) it is not necessary to empirically cover *Pseudomonas*. An advantage of using this drug is that it does not need to be dose adjusted for renal dysfunction and is the only monotherapy option. A drawback is that it is associated with a high rate of nausea (≥20%).

- All other antibiotic regimens appropriate for this patient include two or more antibiotics (one to cover HA-MRSA and other Gram-positive bacteria, and one or two to cover Gram-negative and anaerobic bacteria). It would be best to limit it to no more than two antibiotics to optimize nursing ease and patient adherence and to minimize drug costs and toxicity.

- To cover HA-MRSA, one of the following agents would be preferred:

✓ Vancomycin 1.5 g IV Q 48 h (or other dosing regimen to achieve vancomycin trough of 10–15 mg/L);

✓ Linezolid 600 mg po Q 12 h; or

✓ Daptomycin 380 mg IV Q 24 h is a second-line option.

- To cover Gram-negative bacteria and anaerobes, one of the following agents would be preferred (dosed for renal dysfunction when indicated):

✓ Piperacillin/tazobactam 2.25 g IV Q 6 h;

✓ Ticarcillin/clavulanate 2.0 g IV Q 6 h;

✓ Ampicillin/sulbactam 3 g IV Q 8 h;

✓ Ertapenem 1 g IV Q 24 h;

✓ Imipenem/cilastatin 250 mg IV Q 6 h; or

✓ Meropenem 1 g IV Q 12 h.

- Other acceptable IV alternatives for Gram-negative and anaerobic coverage, with dose adjustments appropriate for Ms. Littlehorse's renal function, include the combination of either clindamycin or metronidazole plus either a third-generation cephalosporin, aztreonam, or a fluoroquinolone. However, this would cause the patient to be on a three-drug empiric regimen (including the antibiotic active against HA-MRSA), which may be more costly, inconvenient, and associated with more adverse drug reactions than mono- or dual therapy options (for example, clindamycin and cephalosporins are more highly associated with *Clostridium difficile* colitis than other antibiotics).

Outcome Evaluation

5.a. What clinical and laboratory parameters are necessary to evaluate your therapy for achievement of the desired therapeutic outcomes and monitoring for adverse effects?

- Regardless of the drug chosen, improvement in the signs and symptoms of infection and healing of the wound with prevention of limb amputation are the primary endpoints.

- Observe for decreased swelling, induration, and erythema. Improvement should be observed after 72–96 hours of appropriate antimicrobial therapy and surgical debridement.

- A decrease in cloudy drainage and formation of new scar tissue are signs of positive response to therapy that may take as long as 7–14 days to be seen.

- Obtain a WBC count and differential every 48–72 hours for the first week or until normalization if less than 1 week, and weekly thereafter until the end of therapy. Continue monitoring until therapy is completed because neutropenia is associated with many antibiotics (e.g., ampicillin/sulbactam, vancomycin).

- Vancomycin is not considered nephro- or hepatotoxic, in general. Routine weekly SCr levels may be recommended to prevent vancomycin-associated ototoxicity that can develop with accumulation of the drug should the patient's renal function worsen. It would be reasonable to order a weekly vancomycin trough level also to ensure that an adequate trough level (~10 mg/L) is being achieved.

- Question the patient to detect any unusual side effects related to the drug or infusion (e.g., rash, nausea, vomiting, diarrhea) daily for the first 3–5 days and then weekly thereafter.

5.b. What therapeutic alternatives are available for treating this patient once results of cultures are known to contain methicillin-resistant *Staphylococcus aureus* (MRSA)?

- Once the culture results are available and the involved organism(s) is (are) considered pathogenic and responsible for the infectious process, therapy should be targeted at the specific organism(s).

  ✓ Vancomycin given IV is often considered the drug of choice for skin and soft tissue infections caused by MRSA, as it has established efficacy, is generally well tolerated, and is inexpensive.

  ✓ Linezolid is at least as effective as vancomycin in MRSA skin and soft tissue infections and has the advantage of oral administration, but it is expensive.[8] A weekly CBC must be obtained from patients receiving linezolid as it carries a significant risk of thrombocytopenia that may require treatment discontinuation (0.3–10.0%).

  ✓ Quinupristin/dalfopristin is another alternative, but it has the drawback of being associated with significant side effects, including severe infusion site reactions and myalgias/arthralgias.

  ✓ Daptomycin is a lipopeptide antibiotic approved for the treatment of complicated skin and soft tissue infections due to susceptible organisms including MRSA. It is expensive and its use is generally restricted to prevent the development of resistance.

  ✓ Tigecycline is also effective against MRSA, but it also has activity against Gram-negative aerobic and anaerobic bacteria, making it too broad-spectrum to be appropriate for use in this patient.

5.c. Design an optimal drug treatment plan for treating the MRSA infection while she remains hospitalized.

- The patient's therapy should be narrowed to vancomycin 1.5 g IV Q 48 h. After the third dose, a vancomycin trough level should be recommended and therapy adjusted to maintain a trough ≥10 mg/L.

- Because vancomycin only covers Gram-positive bacterial infections, it is essential to monitor for efficacy since diabetic foot infections are frequently polymicrobial. The patient's infection should be assessed daily for changes in swelling, induration, and erythema. Temperature should be assessed at least twice daily and a WBC obtained daily if it was initially increased. Improvements in these physical signs and laboratory parameters should be observed after 72–96 hours of appropriate antimicrobial therapy and surgical debridement. If the area of swelling and erythema increases, foul odor or drainage develops, or if response to therapy appears inadequate, it may be necessary to broaden therapy so that Gram-negative and anaerobic bacteria are covered as well. Response to therapy is often patient dependent, and in some cases improvement may not be seen until after 7–10 days of treatment.

- The duration of therapy is controversial and based on the patient's personal situation. Therapy should be continued until all signs and symptoms disappear and for at least 2–4 weeks total. Some patients require longer therapy, and wound healing in diabetic patients is often very slow.

- The patient should remain hospitalized until she is afebrile for 24–48 hours, has signs of improvement and positive response to therapy (decreased swelling, redness, purulent drainage; normalization of the WBC), and outpatient wound care has been established, either by proper teaching to the patient (and her daughter) or through home health care services.

5.d. Design an optimal pharmacotherapeutic plan for completion of her treatment after she is discharged from the hospital.

- The decision about completion of therapy with IV versus oral therapy is often based on clinical experience because few clinical trials have been performed on long-term treatment of diabetic foot infections.

- In this patient, continued use of IV vancomycin would probably be the best choice. The drug could be either infused at home, most likely with the daughter's assistance and frequent nursing care visits, or the patient may be required to visit her local Indian Health Services clinic to receive therapy, depending on what is economically feasible. Discharge planning should be involved in this case to ensure a smooth transition to outpatient therapy.

- The patient should be seen in clinic at least once weekly while on therapy to assess therapeutic efficacy and safety. At each visit, a CBC should be obtained to evaluate for vancomycin-associated neutropenia or thrombocytopenia. An SCr should be obtained as well, and, if any significant changes in renal function are observed, the vancomycin dose should be adjusted.

Patient Education

6. What information should be provided to the patient to enhance compliance, to ensure successful therapy, and to minimize adverse effects with IV vancomycin?

- We will need to see you in the clinic each week to make sure the antibiotic is working. At these visits, we will draw some blood so that we can check for side effects of the medication.

- Vancomycin should be infused slowly, over 1–2 hours, to prevent flushing and blood pressure decreases that are associated with rapid infusion.

- Contact your doctor or me if any unusual side effects, such as rash, shortness of breath, diminished hearing or ringing in the ears, or decreased urine production, occur while taking this medicine.

- Contact your home health care provider if pain, redness, or swelling is observed at the IV site.

- *Note:* The patient needs to be made aware that osteomyelitis and limb amputation are possible consequences of these infections in diabetic patients. She also needs to be provided with personnel resources (telephone numbers, addresses) to contact if unusual reactions occur while on therapy, if infection worsens, or if she has questions or concerns. Compliance with outpatient clinic follow-up visits is of prime importance for success in this case.

REFERENCES

1. Lipsky BA, Berendt AR, Deery G, et al. Diagnosis and treatment of diabetic foot infections. Clin Infect Dis 2004;39:885–910.
2. Levin ME. Management of the diabetic foot: preventing amputation. South Med J 2002;95:10–20.
3. Rybak JM, LaPlante KL. Community-associated methicillin-resistant *Staphylococcus aureus*: a review. Pharmacotherapy 2005;25:74–85.
4. Boyce JM. Methicillin-resistant *Staphylococcus aureus*. Detection, epidemiology, and control measures. Infect Dis Clin North Am 1989; 3:901–913.
5. Herwaldt LA. Control of methicillin-resistant *Staphylococcus aureus* in the hospital setting. Am J Med 1999;106:11S–18S; discussion 48S–52S.
6. Asensio A, Guerrero A, Quereda C, et al. Colonization and infection with methicillin-resistant *Staphylococcus aureus*: associated factors and eradication. Infect Control Hosp Epidemiol 1996;17:20–28.
7. Wieman TJ, Smiell JM, Su Y. Efficacy and safety of a topical gel formulation of recombinant human platelet-derived growth factor-BB (becaplermin) in patients with chronic neuropathic diabetic ulcers. A phase III randomized, placebo-controlled, double-blind study. Diabetes Care 1998;21:822–827.
8. Weigelt J, Itani K, Stevens D, et al. Linezolid versus vancomycin in the treatment of complicated skin and soft tissue infections. Antimicrob Agents Chemother 2005;46:2260–2266.